NATURAL HEALING WITH CHINESE HERBS

Keisetsu Otsuka
Domei Yakazu
Totoro Shimizu

Compiled and
Edited by
Hong-yen Hsu

ORIENTAL HEALING ARTS INSTITUTE
8820 SOUTH SEPULVEDA BOULEVARD, SUITE 218
LOS ANGELES, CALIFORNIA 90045 U.S.A.

**NATURAL HEALING
WITH
CHINESE HERBS**

English Copyright 1982 by the Oriental Healing Arts Institute of the United States. No part of this book may be reproduced by any mechanical, photographic, or electronic process, or in the form of a photographic recording, nor may it be stored in a retrieval system, transmitted, or otherwise copied for public or private use — other than for "fair use" — without the written permission of the publisher.

ISBN: 9-941942-05-8

Printed in Taiwan, R.O.C.

Contents

Foreword vii
Preface xi

The Characteristics of Chinese Medicine 1
   The Characteristics of Chinese Medicine 3
   The Characteristics and Constitutents of Chinese Herbal
      Formulas 22
   An Introduction to Chinese Medicine 35

**Diagnoses and Therapeutical Methods of Chinese
Medicine** 49
   The Four Kinds of Diagnoses 51
   Outlines of Therapeutical Methods 91

Diagnosis According to the Diseases 101
   Contagious Diseases 103
   Respiratory Diseases 124
   Diseases of the Circulatory System 144
   Diseases of the Alimentary System 174
   Diseases of the Kidneys 212
   Metabolic Diseases 230
   Diseases of the Joints and Nervous System 244
   Children's Diseases (Pediatric Diseases) 275
   Surgical Diseases 299
   Ophthalmic Diseases 336
   Nose and Throat Diseases 359
   Obstetric Diseases 391
   Gynecological Diseases 421
   Skin Diseases 459

Urological Diseases 510
Venereal Diseases 517
Oral Diseases 537

Explanation of Chinese Herbal Formulas 549
Explanation of Chinese Herbal Formulas 551

Herbs Used in Chinese Medicine 647
Herbs Used in Chinese Medicine 649
Herb Index 743

Glossary of Chinese Medical Terminology 751
Glossary of Chinese Herbal Formulas 785
Formula Index
English to Chinese 835
Chinese to English 875

FOREWORD

It pleases me greatly that Dr. Hong-yen Hsu, President of the Oriental Healing Arts Institute of USA, is publishing an English translation of *Manual for Medical Treatment*. He has asked me to write a few words of introduction.

In retrospect, the first edition was called *The Practice of Chinese Medical Diagnosis and Treatment*. It was published by Nanzando Press in October, 1941, during the decline and low period of Chinese medicine in Japan. The book was co-authored by Nagahisa Kimura, Keisetsu Otsuka, Domei Yakazu, and Totaro Shimuzu and arranged in monographs according to the disease categories of modern medicine. In such a way physicians educated in modern medical science could easily follow the text since diagnostic and treatment methods of traditional Chinese medical science are utterly different from modern medicine. The book built an unexpectedly good reputation and has had many reprints since its first publication.

Chinese medicine was first introduced to Japan in 1500. It is divided into three schools, namely, the Posterity School which adopts the newer medical formulations of Li and Chu's of the Chin and Yuan dynasties of China, the Ancient Prescription School which follows the rules and criteria of the classic *Shang han lun* (circa AD 200), and the Intermediate School which shuns the other two schools and bases practice on investigation and proof.

Among the authors of the book, Keisetsu Otsuka belonged to the Ancient Prescription School, Nagahisa Kimura belonged to the Intermediate School, and I to the Posterity School; hence we succeeded in carrying on the tradition of Chinese

Foreword

medical science. The fourth author, Totaro Shimizu, is an herbal pharmaceutical scholar belonging to the Ancient Prescription School. In the 1920s and '30s, the four authors taught at Takushoku University and served together as executive members of the East Asian Medical Association. They collaborated in order to have the three branches of Chinese medicine represented. After spending five years discussing and writing, the book was finally published. It was the first modern publication on Chinese herb medicine in Japan.

In October, 1945, one of the authors, Nagahisa Kimura, died in the war. The remaining three authors have since supplemented and revised the text ten times. In 1965 the book was translated into Chinese and within three years 90,000 copies were sold.

In December, 1968, the three authors again revised the book and published it under its present title *A Manual for Medical Treatment*. For the first time the type was set in horizontal lines. Ten years later, I rewrote my portion and the edition so made is the final form. To summarize, up till now the book has had 16 editions.

Today, Oriental medical science is being reassessed all over the world. Even the World Health Organization is considering implementing the use of Chinese medical science. Because of this renaissance of interest, English translations of Chinese medical literatures are strongly desired by countries the world over. Fortunately Dr. Hong-yen Hsu is doing just that, a very pleasing and welcomed act.

Dr. Hong-yen Hsu earned his doctorate of pharmacy at Kyoto University after graduating from Meiji University, School of Pharmacy, and doing graduate study on pharmacognosy at Tokyo University, School of Pharmacy. His wide work experience includes the following: former director of Taiwan Provincial Hygienic Laboratory; director of Food and Drug Control, National Health Administration of the Republic of China; director of the Brion Research Institute of Taiwan; president of the Taiwan Pharmaceutical Association for 30 years; former dean of the Department of Botany, China Culture University; and former director of Chinese Medical Research Institute, China Medical College. Dr. Hsu, an international scholar, has written twenty-four books on Chinese medicine.

He is active in research. In fact, he is a truly remarkable human being. I have been in close touch with Dr. Hsu for more than ten years and enjoy continuous academic interchanges with him.

Regretably two of the original authors, Keisetsu Otsuka and Totoro Shimizu, passed away before the advent of the publication of the English translation of their work. I, however, on behalf of the four authors, would like to express our appreciation and approval of the publication. Dr. Hsu has accomplished a worthy mission for which I have long been wishing with all my heart.

> **Domei Yakazu**, Doctor of Medicine and
> Doctor of Literature
> Director of Oriental Medicine Research
> Center of the Kitasato Institute
> Chairman of East Asian Medical Association
> July 15, 1981

PREFACE

Modern medicine began in 1858 when a German pathologist, Rudolf Virchow (1828-1902), formulated the science of cellular pathology. Since then remarkable scientific advances in all areas have often been directly applied to medicine. Another major step was the synthesis of 606 Salvarsan (a combination of arsenic developed to treat syphilis) in 1910 by Paul Ehrlich which marked the advent of antibiotic medicine. The discovery of the "miracle drugs," penicillin and sulfa, followed in the 1930s and 1940s. These developments gave the very distinct impression that modern therapeutic methods would one day solve the problem of disease. This has not happened. On the contrary, in one sense the exact opposite has occurred. A case in point is thalidomide. The West German government in 1957 approved it for use because of its excellent sedative effects. However, in 1958 a report surfaced suggesting that ingestion of the drug by pregnant women produced infants with dolphin-like hands. Following this report, medical researchers all over the world began to test thalidomide and discovered that, in addition to its teratogenous effects, it induced such symptoms as an extremely cold sensation in the limbs, disturbances in muscular equilibrium and coordination, spasms and cramps in the limbs, and purpura. Thalidomide is but one example of modern medicine's unfortunate side effects. Worse, it has been found that drug therapy can induce new diseases.

Chinese herbal medicines offer an alternative therapy to Western drugs as they are natural substances that seldom induce side effects. Further, a formula may contain 4-12 different ingredients which ameliorate each other in contrast to Western drugs which are synthetic analogues of natural substances and usually contain only one powerful ingredient. According to my research and experiments, Chinese herbs, with very few exceptions, have almost no toxicity. I selected two hundred varieties of the most frequently used Chinese herbs and extracted them with 50% ethanol. Each extract was then forcibly administered to ten selected male mice, in accordance with the Litchfield and Wilcoxon methods, in order to find the LD_{50} values and the effects on the central nervous system. Generally, the LD_{50} values were about 2-5 grams per kilogram of body weight. Thus, Chinese herbs being almost nontoxic are well suited for human consumption.

Naturally, all medical systems focus on the alleviation of human suffering, but they differ widely in theory and practice. Chinese medicine is basically preventative and as such oriented toward the maintenance of good health by revitalizing and reinforcing the body's natural resistance to disease. Dietary restraints and exercise are natural concomitants of this process. (Prevention is paramount because the Chinese are adverse to taking medicine except for acute and traumatic disorders.) The special characteristics of Chinese medicine are discussed in detail in the first chapter of this volume.

Although Chinese history extends over a period of 400,000 years, written records did not appear until the Shang period in 1766 B.C. The first known medical book is *The Yellow Emperor's Classic of Internal Medicine,* which was written during the Han dynasty in A.D. 206. The first attempt to systematize Chinese herbal medicine came with the *Shang han lun* (Treatise on Febrile Diseases). The author Chang Chung-ching, often compared with Hippocrates, is considered one of China's greatest physicians. The *Shang han lun* and *Chin kuei yao lueh* (Summaries of Household Remedies) represent the outcome of his intellectual efforts. From these medical classics a reader learns that Chinese medicine stresses treatment of conformation—the cluster of symptoms, objective and subjective, and physical traits presented by the patient. After determining the conformation, the Chinese doctor devises the appropriate therapy, usually consisting of herbal formulas. Many of the formulas still used by Chinese doctors are found in the *Shang han lun* and *Chin kuei yao lueh*, even though they were written nearly 1,800 years ago. From the very beginning Chinese medicine has combined empirical experience with philosophical theory.

Since former President Nixon's visit to China in 1972, acupuncture has enjoyed a renaissance in the United States. Yet acupuncture actually treats symptoms only and is but a small part of the Chinese medical legacy. The most important part lies in the use of medicinal herbs and diet therapy. In the West, little is known about Chinese herbal medicine due to language difficulties. Translation has been hampered particularly by the lack of a technical vocabulary to describe intertwined philosophical and medical theories. In 1976, I set up the Oriental Healing Arts Institute to introduce the theory and practice of Chinese medicine to the American public. In addition to bimonthly bulletins, we plan to publish a series of books on Chinese herbal medicine. Presently, we have already published the following:

1. *The History of Chinese Medicine*, an introduction to the major events in the history of Chinese medicine provides biographies of famous physicians

2. *Chinese Herbal Medicine and Therapy* is a comprehensive introduction to the theory and practice of Chinese medicine.

3. *Chinese Herbs and Formulas* is a practical guide on the therapeutic use of 50 commonly used Chinese herbal formulas.

4. *How to Treat Yourself with Chinese Herbs* is a manual on how the Chinese use herbs to achieve good health. It includes information on 95 herbs and 128 herb formulas, their uses and healing properties

The present volume draws extensively from a Japanese best seller entitled *Standard Practice of Chinese Herbal Medicine*, which was first published under the name *Practical Application of Chinese Herbal Therapy*. A complete revision was made in 1969 and the name changed to *Standard Practice of Chinese Herbal Medicine*. In 1980 the fourth edition of this book came out in Japan and it continues to be a best seller. Almost every Western-trained physician in Japan has a copy as it has become an indispensible reference work. In 1953 the original was translated into Chinese and in 1963 into Korean. This is the first English edition.

Additional source material for this book is as follows: (1) *The Characteristics of Chinese Medicine* (Oriental

Healing Arts Institute Bulletin, Vol. 5, No. 6, 1980); (2) *An Introduction to Chinese Medicine* (which appears in the introductory section of this book); (3) *A Description of the Four Diagnoses and the Eight Principles* (OHAI Bulletin, Vol. 3, No. 2, 1978); (4) *Theories of Diagnostic Methods* (Chih-liao ko-lun); (5) *An Explanation of Chinese Herbal Formulas* (Yao-fang chieh-shuo); (6) *Glossary of Chinese Herbal Formulas* (Chu-fang chi); (7) *Glossary of Chinese Medical Terminology* (OHAI Bulletin, Vol. 5, No. 5, 1980); (8) *An Explanation of Chinese Medicinal Herbs* (Yao-wu-pien). Items 4, 5, and 6 are adaptations of sections of *Standard Practice of Kanpo Medicine;* the remaining items are taken from my own publications.

The informed reader can use the information to great advantage because each section covers symptoms or conformation and appropriate herbal remedies. A fundamental assumption is that each person is responsible for his or her own health. By helping the reader identify symptoms that may indicate the beginning of serious illness, this book may contribute to the prevention of disease, but it is not intended as a substitute for professional medical care, especially for people with serious ailments.

I would like to thank the authors of *Standard Practice of Chinese Herbal Medicine,* Otsuka Keisetsu, Yakazu Domei, and Shimizu Totoro, and the publisher, Nanzan-do, for their permission to translate the work into English and to carry out minor alterations of the text.

I would also like to thank Mr. Wang Shih-yen for his translation of this book and Ms. Lu Yueh-ying and Wang Shu-kuei for proofreading and editing the Chinese version. I am also grateful to the staff of the Oriental Healing Arts Institute, especially Ms. Jeannine Talley Ph.D., and Mrs. Judy Haueter for editing the English translation, and Douglas Easer for translating the preface and introduction.

Hong-yen Hsu
May 1, 1981
Oriental Healing Arts Institute, U.S.A.
Los Angeles

THE CHARACTERISTICS OF CHINESE MEDICINE

THE CHARACTERISTICS OF CHINESE MEDICINE

Foreword

The basic theories of Chinese medicine are found in *Huang ti nei ching* (The Yellow Emperor's Classic of Internal Medicine), *Shang han lun* (A Treatise on Colds and Feverish Diseases) and *Chin kuei yao lueh* (Summaries of Household Remedies), the latter two of which were written by Chang Chung-ching of the Latter Han dynasty. Since then theories have gradually evolved and developed into the present day discipline. The basic rules of treatment derive from the thesis that diseases occur as a consequence of an imbalance between toxins, in the broad sense of the word, and normal vitality. Also, from the earliest times, Chinese medicine has been aware of the problem of toxicity in medicinals, hence it uses mostly natural products for the treatment of diseases. The fundamental basis of treatment is radical instead of palliative, making the various ways of diagnosing and methods regarding the treatment of disease different from those of Western medicine. Chinese medicine has characteristics not found in modern medicine: its expositions are replete with metaphysical and philosophical thoughts not readily accepted by modern medicine. It has been found to be most successful in curing chronic diseases. Modern medicine which is well advanced in therapeutics and surgery, still has not developed an effective policy toward the treatment of recalcitrant diseases; and the number of recalcitrant diseases seems to be increasing. This phenomenon is no doubt closely associated with the contamination of the environment by various pollutants, the adulteration of foods through colorings and preservatives, and the side effects of drugs.

The present article was written for the special issue of the 1978 *Exhibition of Chinese Medicines* in response to the kind request from the Chinese Medical Merchants Association in Hong Kong which was commemorating its fiftieth anniversary. It is printed here to help the reader gain a small understanding of Chinese medicine. The last section, which concerns the characteristics and constitution of Chinese medical formulas, was originally one of the sections of *Characteristics of Chinese Medicine* written by Otsuka Keisetsu, who has made an extensive study of Chinese medicine and often produces excellent and outstanding writings. In view of the persistence of many recalcitrant diseases, the author intends in the future to introduce the different views of Chinese medicine and Western medicine towards these diseases by presenting translations of sixty-one articles published in the *Modern Drug Weekly of Taiwan* during the period from May 2, 1977 to December 18, 1978.

Comparison of Chinese Medicine and Western Medicine

A study of Western medical history reveals that the art developed from the very primitive treatment of human beings and the sorcery and religious medicine of the Middle Ages. It was not until the French Revolution (1789-1799) that scientific treatment was adopted.

Modern medical science, fragmented and specialized, is based on the experimental studies of bacteriology, physiology, and pharmacology, and on clinical research in the treatment of disease. It features detailed analysis, exhaustive investigation, theoretical studies, and objective clinical examinations. The identification of a disease is desirable before treatment is conducted, and its drugs are composed mainly of synthetic and chemical substances. In addition, Western medicine excels in and uses surgery as a principal tool of treatment.

In contrast, Chinese medicine is intertwined with a philosophy of life, and is based on comprehensive, whole-body treatment. This treatment is the legacy of many thousands of years of accumulated experience. Chinese medicine pays special attention to the patient's pains or the conformation and prescribes a holistic treatment on a subjective basis before even identifying the disease by name; for example. "weakness" is supplemented, "firmness" is purged. The Chinese system designated blood, water, air, thoraco-costal distress, and food toxins as constituting another set of therapeutic theories; and when a Chinese physician diagnoses an illness, he first considers the condition of the blood, water, and air in the body.

Dr. Yakazu Domei, a leading authority in Chinese herbal medicine, lists the following differences between Chinese and Western medicine.

Chinese medicine: philosophical, synthetical, holistic, internal, conformatory, empirical, hygienic, individual, preventative, experiential, humoral, subjective, natural.

Western medicine: scientific, analytical, topical, surgical, heteropathic, theoretical, preventative, socialized medicine, bacteriological, experimental, cellular, objective, chemical.

From the above, we can see that Chinese medicine is holistic in approach. For example, if the eyes of a patient turn red, a Western doctor will use eye lotion to wash the eyes while a Chinese herb doctor will regard the disorder as "overthriving fire" and try to decrease the fire in the patient by having him take such fire-dissipating agents as coptis or gardenia. Another example is the treatment of itchy skin, a condition in Chinese medicine related to the vitality of the liver. If a person takes care of the liver, the skin takes care of itself. Thus the liver is the focal point for treatment. But Western medicine would more than likely use dermatological lotion to cure a skin ailment, focusing on the specific symptom.

Otsuka Keisetsu, a leading authority in Chinese herb medicine in Japan, points out that modern Western medicine frequently uses surgery to interrupt pregnancy or to remove cysts of the ovaries. The women afterwards often suffers from chills, headache, and paralysis of the limbs. Dr. Otsuka refers to this condition as the "hernia syndrome" and suggests that it can best be cured by *Tang-kuei-szu-ni-chia-wu-chu-yu-sheng-chiang-tang* (*Tang-kuei*, Evodia, and Ginger Combination). He says the symptoms arise because of an obstruction of the absolute-yin-liver-meridian of the feet.

The "meridian theory" of Chinese medicine is still not accepted by Western medicine because meridians, which are neither blood vessels nor part of the nervous system, have not yet been verified anatomically. However, to the Chinese doctor their functions are undeniable, and the meridians and meridian points have been used in acupuncture practice for thousands of years. The aforementioned absolute-yin-liver-meridian of the feet is just one of the meridians. It starts at the *tatun* point on the big toes, passes through the genitalia, stomach and liver and ascends to the eyes. Stimulation of this meridian by applying acupuncture to any of many points often results in healing diseases associated with the meridian. Likewise, injury of the meridian by surgery or operation will cause related diseases. Chinese herb medicinals are used then to treat all the diseases derived from injuries of the meridians.

Chinese medicine regards the universe as an organism and man as microcosm of the universe. From the every beginning Chinese medicine has regarded man as a part of the process of organismic development while Western medicine has likened the human body to a machine and developed its theories from this assumption. Unlike a machine which is constructed of component members, an organism has organs and parts that function together as a whole. The difference between these two model systems has created the differences between Chinese and Western medicine.

Diseases Caused by Passion

According to Chinese medical theory, diseases are brought about by either external or internal causes. External causes are due mainly to geography, weather, and environment and are called the "Six Excesses," namely, wind, dryness, cold, fire, moisture, and heat. Internal causes are the "Seven Emotions," namely, pleasure, anger, anxiety, pensiveness, sorrow, fearfulness, and fright. The progress of disease varies with an individual's constitution, temperament, site of the symptoms, nutrition, and circulation of his blood, water, and *"ch'i"*, (defensive energy, *wei;* physiological energy, *ch'i;* and constructive energy, *ying).* In the *Shang han lun* the various stages of diseases are the "six paths": greater yang, lesser yang, sunlight yang, lesser yin, greater yin, and absolute yin. Different herb formulas are used for different disease stages. In addition to the "six paths" theory, Chinese medicine is based on the dualism of yin and yang. It classifies the conformations of diseases into either "excessive" or "deficient" and body conditions into their "thriving" or "deteriorated" or "strong" or "weak". Accordingly there are eight key types of conformation: yin, yang, external, internal, cold, fever, weak, and firm. Once the conformation is determined, there are corresponding herbal drugs administered for treatment.

Chinese medicine pays special attention to the symptoms caused by the seven emotions. Diseases caused by seven emotions, such as excessive emotional stimulation or inhibition, are internal. Circumstances cause mental imbalances which injure the viscera, thereby inducing disease. Conformations resulting from the seven emotions are mainly disease of the *ch'i* (vitality or energy), but they may progress and affect the blood. For example, anger raises *ch'i,* pleasure calms *ch'i,* sadness subsides *ch'i,* fear suppresses *ch'i,* fright disturbs *ch'i,* thought coagulates the *ch'i,* and violent anger injures yin and agitates the blood. In addition, the seven emotions can cause visceral diseases via the heart, because all changes of the seven emotions affect the heart, it being the governing organ of the viscera.

The Japanese call diseases "bioki" literally meaning "injured *ch'i."* They believe that diseases are caused by disturbances of the body and the *ch'i. Ch'i* is invisible and omnipresent. Dr. Gonzan Goto, a Japanese authority on Chinese herbal medicine, contends that the obstruction of *ch'i* is the cause of all disease; therefore, they can be cured by chi-soothing agents such as magnolia, perilla and citrus peel.

According to Chinese medical science, the Seven Emotions are closely interrelated with the Five Elements, namely, metal, wood, water, fire, and earth. The following is a diagram showing their relationship.

Seven Emotions and Related Diseases

```
                  ┌─ yin (nerve paralysis) ................ aphasia
         toxin ───┤
                  └─ yang (nerve excitement) ....... mania ...... epilepsy
```

Anger raises *ch'i* . . . . .injures the liver leading to wildness. . . . . .epilepsy
Pleasure slows *ch'i* . . . . .injures the heart leading to mania. . . . . . .epilepsy
Sorrow subsides *ch'i* . . . . .injures the lungs leading to epilepsy . . . . . . mania
Fear suppresses *ch'i*. . . . . .injures the kidneys leading to mania . . . .wildness
Fright disturbs *ch'i* . . . . .injures the kidneys leading to mania . . . .wildness
Pensiveness coagulates *ch'i* . . . . .injures the spleen leading to epilepsy . . . . . mania

(1) Anger makes the *ch'i* soar and injures the liver; a more severe condition causes wild behavior and epilepsy. Since the liver controls moods, the principle of treatment is to inhibit, clean and nourish the liver. The herbal formulas used are *Hsiao-yao-san* (*Tang-kuei* and Bupleurum Formula), *I-kan-san* (Bupleurum Formula), *Wen-tan-tang* (Hoelen and Bamboo Combination).

(2) Pleasure slows down the *ch'i* and injures the heart. If the condition advances it becomes mania and turns into epilepsy. Since the heart equates to fire, the principle of treatment if to purge and nourish the heart. The herbal formulas used are *Huang-lien-chieh-tu-tang* (Coptis and Scute Combination), *Yang-hsin-tang* (Zizyphus and Astragalus Combination), *Kuei-pi-tang* (Ginseng and Longan Combination).

(3) Sorrow or anxiety makes *ch'i* subside and injures the lungs. If the condition advances, it becomes epilepsy and turns into mania. Sorrow equates to metal, and the principle of treatment is to nourish the lungs. The herbal formula used is *Pai-ho-ku-chin-tang* (Lily Combination).

(4) Fright is caused by external stimuli and disturbs *ch'i*, while fear originates within the individual and makes *ch'i* malfunction. Both emotions injure the kidneys. If the condition advances, it becomes mania, finally turning into wildness. Both fright and fear belong to water, and the principle of treatment is to nourish the kidneys and fortify the sperm. The herbal formulas used are *Pa-wei-ti-huang-wan* (Rehmannia Eight Formula) and *Chin-suo-ku-ching-wan* (Lotus Stamen Formula).

(5) Pensiveness coagulates *ch'i* and injures the spleen. As the

Table I

Seven Emotions	Mechanism	Manifestation
Pleasure	Excessive pleasure injures the heart by causing unease in the spirit, and it loosens the *ch'i*.	disorderly speech, abnormal behavior
Anger	Violent anger injures the liver, causing an adverse up-rush of *ch'i*. Extreme anger causes the blood to congest in the upper torso.	pallor, cyanosis or ruddy face and red eyes, even coma and sudden apoplexy; an angry or manical look in the eyes; a tendency to shout and vilify.
Anxiety	Excessive worry injures the lungs, as well as the spleen, causing obstruction of *ch'i*.	depression and agonizing, sullenness, melancholia, loss of appetite
Pensiveness	Excessive thought injures the spleen, causing coagulation of *ch'i*: psychosis.	loss of appetite, insomnia, aberated mental state
Sorrow	Excessive sorrow injures the lungs, causing subsidence of *ch'i*.	pale facial complexion, depression, sadness
Fear	Constant fears cause deficiency and weakness in renal *ch'i* and deficiency of the blood and *ch'i*.	timidity, fearfulness, irritability and uneasiness, agoraphobia, paranoia
Fright	Fright will disturb *ch'i* and agitate the heart and spirit internally.	agitation, abnormal behavior and speech

This table is drawn up according to *An Outline of Conformation in Chinese Medicine* by Dr. Hong-yen Hsu, 1977.

Natural Healing with Chinese Herbs

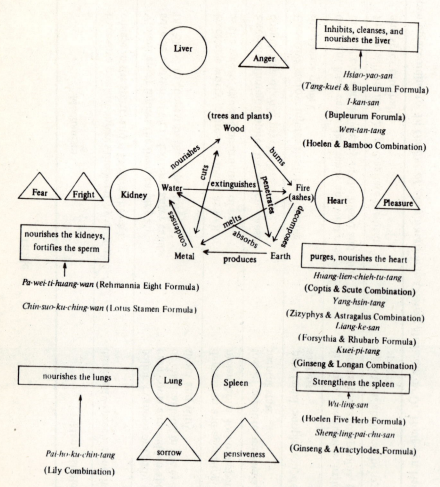

Diagram I
Relationship between the Seven Emotions and Five Elements

condition advances, it becomes epilepsy, turning into mania. Pensiveness belongs to earth, and the principle of treatment is to strengthen the spleen. The herbal formulas used are *Wu-ling-san* (Hoelen Five Herb Formula), *Sheng-ling-pai-chu-san* (Ginseng and Atractylodes Formula).

The above mentioned five elements are mutually interlinked, sometimes reciprocally producing and destroying each other. Chinese medicine also feels that weakness or firmness of the five solid viscera arouses emotional changes. This is a concept not found in Western medicine. In other words, an appraisal of the mental state can determine the disease occuring in the viscera and hence is used to prescribe the appropriate herbal therapy. Although modern Western medicine incorporates the science called "psychological medicine" which emphasizes psychological analysis and mainly uses tranquilizers for the treatment, it never approaches treating the pathological state which existed before the onset of psychoses.

The Concept of Herbal Nature

Chinese herb medicine has experimented with herbs in the human body for a long time. As long as two thousand years ago, the author of *Shen nung pen ts'ao ching* (God of Husbandry's Herbal) put forth the concept of "Four Essences and Five Flavors" to categorize various foods and medicinals. For example, diseases having fever as a symptom are treated with medicinals that have cold or cool properties. On the other hand, chill diseases, which manifest themselves in cold limbs are treated with medicinals which have hot or warm properties. Drugs with cold properties are gypsum and mirabilitum; those with cooling properties, chrysanthemum and moutan. Medicinals with hot properties are aconite, ginger, and asarum, while medicines with warm properties are *tang-kuei* and cnidium. Neutral medicinals are like licorice, to name one.

According to the concept of the Five Flavors, everything we eat is considered either sour, bitter, salty, sweet, pungent or hot (or sometimes bland). According to long term experience, each flavor has a specific function.

    Sour flavor: schizandra, terminalia; astrigent action
    Bitter flavor: coptis, rhubarb; fortifying action

Salty flavor: sargassum, mirabilitum; softening action and expectoration effect
Sweet flavor: ginseng, rehmannia; mild strengthening and supplementing actions
Pungent flavor: ginger, perilla; dispersing action
Bland flavor: hoelen, tetrapanax; diuretic action

These actions have been verified through long clinical experience.

Chinese medicine also associates the actions of herbs with the corresponding viscera. This kind of association is called the "meridian assortment". For example, according to this principle, the pungent-flavored herbs are associated with the lungs; the sour-flavored herbs, with the liver; the bitter-flavored herbs, with the heart; and the salty herbs, with the kidneys. This classification by the meridian is equivalent to what Western medical science terms invivo metabolism. Although Chinese herb medicine has learned the herbal actions through long years of observation and experiment, action still needs to be more rigorous in the application of the scientific method to verify its conclusions.

Western medicine classifies medicinals into poisons, potent drugs, and common drugs and knows the pharmacological actions of each drug. However, Western medicine overemphasizes the healing properties of drugs to the exclusion of their unfavorable side effects, such as the allergic reactions (also refer to next section of this article). Corresponding with the classification of drugs as poisons, potent drugs and common drugs by Western medicine, Chinese medicine places medicinals into upper, middle, and lower classes, according to their properties and the target of the action of the drugs. This classification can be found in the herbal classic *Shen nung pen ts'ao ching*.

Most Chinese herbs contain natural ingredients: some of the herbs actually being food, such as *tang-kuei*, dioscorea, lotus seed and coix, found in the daily diet of the Chinese people. Therefore, Chinese herbs are compatible with the functions of the human body and capable of being anabolized and absorbed easily.

Side-effects and Drug Abuse in Western Medicine

With the exception of surgery and physical therapy, most cases of human ailments call for treatment with drugs. Even though drugs are foreign substances to our bodies, small quantities can be absorbed and disposed of by the body without producing any harmful effects. On the other hand, large amounts of drugs taken continuously over long periods have harmful and cumulative effects resulting in chronic intoxication. According to the World Health Organization, a side-effect is defined as follows: "An ordinary dosage of medicine which leads to an unexpected and harmful reaction."

The Causes of Drug Side-effects Are Many

(1) Inherent toxicity

The drug itself may possess strong toxicity very harmful to the human body. For example, the once frequently-used antisyphilitic agent Salvalsan (606) contains poisonous arsenic which is effective against treponeme. For that reason since 1910, it has been known to injure the liver, causing such side-effects as jaundice. It is now no longer in use.

Another example of a drug with shocking side-effects is the tranquilizer Thalidomide. It was approved for disbursement by the government of Western Germany in October 1957 because of its excellent tranquilizing effects.

Frequently given to quiet infants so that the parents could relax and enjoy the movies, it was called "movie juice" and was very popular for some time. However, in November of 1958, a physician reported that ingestion of this drug by pregnant women produced infants with dolphin-like hands. Following this report, research on the side-effects of this drug by medical researchers all over the world continued to reveal that in addition to its teratogenous effects, it caused such symptoms as an extremely chilly sensation in the limbs, disturbances in the muscular equilibrium and coordination, spasms and cramps in the limbs, and purpura. This drug was also being sold under the name of Isomin in Japan since October of 1957. From that time up to January 1963, it was estimated that more than one thousand teratogenic children were produced in Japan, over six thousand in Germany, and perhaps over one hundred cases in Taiwan. The deleterious effects of this drug are obvious.

Another drug-induced disease found mostly in Japan was called Simon's disease. A subacute myelocular neurosis, it was caused by Chinoform, a product manufactured by a Swiss company. This drug had been on the market since 1899 and was included in various editions of *Japanese Pharmacopeia* since 1949 as a remedy for acute enteric diseases and a broad range of other diseases. Then in 1960 a physician linked the side-effects of paralytic claudication and atrophy of ocular nerve in infants to administration of this drug. This side-effect was studied until 1975 when the drug was finally abandoned. At present there are 11,033 cases of Simon's disease caused by the drug Chinoform.

Several kinds of antibiotics, such as penicillin and chloramphenicol, may cause leucocythemia (blood cancer); adrenocorticosteroid hormone cause aplastic anemia or collagen disease; and other drugs cause purpura, fulminative hepatitis, and polynecrosis. All of these diseases are related to the ingestion of drugs per se.

(2) Inappropriate use of drugs

Overdosing on drugs which are known to be harmful or addictive (intolerance due to an unsuitable body), or taking drugs which cause sleepiness such as antihistamine are included in this category.

(3) Side-effects due to anaphylactic reaction

Western medicine does not specify the nature of drugs; hence anaphylaxis is frequently encountered. For instance, phenylbutazone is used for rheumatic aches to mitigate pain but it also causes agranulocytosis or allergic reactions.

(4) Side-effects as a secondary reaction to drugs

It happens frequently that administration of Western drugs may result in an unintended side-effect. For example, the administration of the adrencorticoid hormone that presently is frequently used for the treatment of rheumatism may activate latent tubercular bacilli or cause adrenal atrophy. Antibiotics may inhibit streptomyces or staphylococcus but will also cause reproduction of *Pseudomonas aeruginosa*, molds, and the occurrence of certain other diseases.

(5) Side-effects due to drug interaction

As a rule, the fewer varieties of drugs administered the better. Statistics show that the incidence of side-effects from a combination of less than five kinds of drugs is 18.6% whereas with six kinds of drugs in combination the side effects increase to 81.4%. Drugs are first absorbed by the stomach and intestines or other digestive organs and then dissociated by the enzymes in the liver or combined with other substances (metabolism) or bound with serum; they then go to the kidneys and are excreted. If several drugs are taken simultaneously, there may well be adverse reactions. For example, administration of a certain kind of antibiotic may result in a decrease in intestinal bacteria count. This decrease in intestinal bacteria may in turn result in a disturbance in vitamin production. Then if an anticoagulant is taken, a hemorrhage may result. Another chemical, diphenylhydantoin, which is used for epiletic patients, inhibits pulmonary tubercular bacilli and in turn causes intoxication.

From the foregoing examples we have an insight into the severe side effects of some Western drugs. One may ask how many commonly used Western drugs cause side effects? According to the statistics from the United States Joint Pharmaceutical Monitoring Center in Boston, the figures are as follow:

Pharmaceuticals		Percentage of side-effects
Cardiotonic	digitalis	12.4%
Hypotensive	guanethidine	22.4%
Diuretic	hydrochlorothiazide	18.3%
Anticoagulant	heparin	17.2%
Hypoglycemic	insulin	12%
Antiphlogistic	prednisone	15%
Antibiotics	ampicillin	10.2%
	cephalothin	12.7%
Anticarcinogenic	cyclophosphamide	62.4%

Moreover with regard to the frequency of occurrence of side effects, although the data from documented sources vary, the highest percentage is as high as 35% while the lowest value is still as high as 1.5%. According to a report made by a prominent hospital in the United States, a comparison of the side effects among in-patients showed that from 6 to 15% of the total number of patients who have taken internal medicines experienced side effects, or a total of 3% of the beds in general hospitals are occupied by patients suffering from the side effects of drugs. It is estimated that in the United States the annual expenditures for the treatment of side effects reaches as high as 4.5 billion dollars, while the number of sufferers is between 30,000 and 140,000. In every country, government health organizations have attached special importance to the strict regulation of pharmaceuticals in order to reduce the occurrence of side effects and to improve drug safety.

In 1962 orders from the United States government and the Japanese government were established for rigorous evaluation of any new drug being introduced on the market. A rating system was also established for drugs which were already on the market. Thus although new drugs are subject to strict regulation, for those drugs marketed previously there is little regulation, complete evaluations and investigations being very difficult owing to budgetary limitations. For example, in 1961 an investigation was begun on 1027 patients to evaluate the antidiabetes drug tolbutamide which is taken orally. The United States has since spent 15 million dollars conducting the detailed study, the results of which are shown below.

	Total Deaths	Cardiovascular Symptoms
Control	10.2%	4.9%
Tolbutamide	14.7%	12.7%
Insulin	9.5%	6.2%

From the figures it can be readily seen that the administration of tolbutamide can result in a significant increase in cardiovascular troubles. Hence this drug is being gradually phased out. Another large scale investigation of coronary drugs divided 8300 patients into five groups for follow-up tests on side effects. The five groups were: clofibrate group, nicotinic acid group, estrogen group, dextrothyroxine group, and a control group. The results showed that in comparison with the control group, the estrogen group and the clofibrate group had extremely elevated rates of cardiac infarction and cancer.

Modern Western medicine emphasizes hypoglycemic therapy in diabetes mellitus patients and hypocholesterolemic therapy in patients with arteriosclerosis and cardiac infarction. Though hypoglycemic or hypocholesterolemic medicinals can alleviate the symptoms, the drugs administered for this purpose often adversely affect the body and even cause birth defects.

The Toxicity and Side-effects of Chinese Herbs

What can we say about the toxicity of Chinese herbs? The author chose two hundred varieties of the most frequently used Chinese herbs and extracted them with 50% ethanol. The extracts were then forceably administered to ten selected male mice in accordance with the Litchfield and Wilcoxon method in order to obtain the LD_{50} values and to observe the effects on the central nervous system. The results showed that the majority of herbs tested had an LD_{50} value of 500mg/kg which when converted to human dosages would be 250gm/50kg, i.e. 50% of a group of people having a body weight of 50kg would die only if they took a drug dosage as high as 250gm per person. The following 30 herbs have negligible effects on the central nervous system in doses of 5gm/kg: cnidium (*Cnidium officinale* Makino, or *Conioselinum univittatum* Turcz.), jujube, cinnamon. rehmannia, apricot, perilla, citrus, *tang-kuei*, morus, angelica, Japanese *tang-kuei, chih-ko*, anemarrhena, cimicifuga, *chih-shih* (unripe fruit), alisma, dioscorea, akebia, schizonepeta, ophiopogon, eriobotrya, atractylodes (chinensis), lonicera, elsholtzia, dolichos, *tang-sheng* (root), capillaris, magnolia flower, lycium bark, and polyporus. Twenty other herbs, including coix, have an effect on the central nervous system to a certain extent; for example, cinnamon and *ma-huang* function to stimulate the autonomic nerves. These specimens might have some connection with the so-called "dispersing action" in Chinese medical theory. Aconite and ginger have a behavioral inhibitive effect which might account for their efficacious action on internal chills. Herbs such as gentiana, phellodendron and lithospermum, which have the so-called heat-dissolving and detoxicating actions of the Chinese medicine, can cause diarrhea. Most of these herbs will have this effect in white mice an hour after administration. However, rhubarb causes diarrhea three hours after ingestion.

The Toxicities of the more important herbs and prescriptions are shown in Table 2.

Table 2
Toxicities with Chinese Herbs

Herb	LD_{50}	Lethal Dose in 50kg Human
Cinnamon	5000mg/kg	250gm
Paeonia	5000mg/kg	250gm
Bupleurum	5000mg/kg	250gm
Ma-huang	2500mg/kg	125gm
Ricinus	2100mg/kg	105gm
Wild Aconite slices	650mg/kg	32.5gm
Croton	180mg/kg	9.0gm
Wild Aconite	90mg/kg	4.5gm
Nux-vomica	15mg/kg	750mg
Pa-wei-ti-huang-wan (Rehmannia Eight Formula)	8000mg/kg	400gm
Pan-hsia-hou-pu-tang (Pinellia and Magnolia Combination)	8000mg/kg	400gm
Tang-kuei-shao-yao-san (*Tang-kuei* and Paeonia Formula)	7500mg/kg	375gm
Ling-kuei-chu-kan-tang (Atractylodes and Hoelen Combination)	5000mg/kg	250gm
Fang-feng-tung-sheng-san (Siler and Platycodon Formula)	5000mg/kg	250gm
Kuei-chih-fu-ling-wan (Cinnamon and Hoelen Formula)	5000mg/kg	250gm
Ma-huang-hsi-hsin-fu-tzu-tang (*Ma-huang*, Aconite, and Asarum Combination)	4000mg/kg	200gm
Ma-hsing-kan-shih-tang (*Ma-huang* and Apricot Seed Combination)	2000mg/kg	100gm
Chai-hu-kuei-chih-kan-chiang-tang (Bupleurum, Cinnamon, and Ginger Combination)	5000mg/kg	250gm

From the earliest times to the present, Chinese herb medicine has employed various processes to reduce toxicity whenever it is exhibited in a herb. This is the main reason why Chinese herb medicine continues to exist.

Chinese Herb Medicine Has Great Efficacy in Treating Recalcitrant Diseases

In recent years advancements in the medical sciences have provided human beings with long and comfortable lives. However, there are still many diseases that remain incurable. For example, cancer, Simon's disease, myasthenia gravis, collagen disease, Behcet's syndrome, sarcoidosis, aplastic anemia, purpura, multiple sclerosis, polycythemia, leukocytosis, violent hepatitis, hemolytic anemia, and progressive myatrophy. These diseases are mainly caused by the deleterious effects of medicine, food poisoning, and environmental pollution. So far modern Western medicine has found no suitable therapeutic methods for curing these diseases. Chinese herb medicine also has had difficulty in treating these diseases. However if they are treated according to the patient's constitution and conformation, these diseases are curable at times.

The therapeutic methods for the treatment of these recalcitrant diseases are presented by the author in *The Modern Drug Weekly of Taiwan* which has published seventy-two consecutive issues. These articles systematically introduced and compared the views of Chinese herb medicine to those of Western medicine.

Considerations of space prevent mentioning more than a few examples here. Below are several recalcitrant diseases and the formulas used to treat them.

(1) Progressive myatrophy. For this disease *Chen-wu-tang* (Vitality Combination) and *Shih-chuan-ta-pu-tang* (Ginseng and *Tang-kuei* Ten Combination) are recommended.

(2) Raynaud's disease. This is a disease which is characterized by a gangrenous rotting and fetid odor starting on the toes. It can be treated with *Tao-ho-cheng-chi-tang* (Persica and Rhubarb Combination).

(3) Purpura. For this disease *Kuei-chih-fu-ling-wan* (Cinnamon and Hoelen Formula) is used.

(4) Aplastic anemia. This disease can be treated with *Chiung-kuei-chiao-ai-tang* (*Tang-kuei* and Gelatin Combination), *Shih-chuan-ta-pu-tang* (Ginseng and *Tang-kuei* Ten Combination), or *Szu-wu-tang* (*Tang-kuei* Four Combination).

(5) Polycythemia. This disease can be treated with *Tao-ho-cheng-chi-tang* (Persica and Rhubarb Combination).

(6) Leucocytosis. This disease can be treated with *Chia-wei-kuei-pi-tang* (Ginseng, Bupleurum, and Longan Combination) or *Shih-chuan-ta-pu-tang*.
(7) Hemophilia. This disease can be treated with *Tang-kuei-pu-hsich-tang* (*Tang-kuei* and Astragalus Combination) or *Huang-chi-chien-chung-tang* (Astragalus Combination).
(8) Banti's disease. This disease can be treated with a modified prescription of *Kuei-pi-tang* (Ginseng and Longan Combination).
(9) Behcet's syndrome. This disease can be treated with *Wen-ching-yin* (*Tang-kuei* and Gardenia Combination).
(10) Venous thrombosis. This disease can be treated with *Tang-kuei-shao-yao-san* (*Tang-kuei* and Paeonia Formula) or prescriptions modified from it.

The foregoing prescriptions are cited for reference. Yet it should be once again noted that Chinese herb medicine treats diseases according to the patient's conformation and in so doing, it can at times easily cure diseases that are still classified as recalcitrant in Western medicine.

Why Chinese Herb Medicine Can Treat Diseases Which Western Medicine Can Not Treat

There are many diseases virtually incurable using Western medical methods which are more susceptible to cure with Chinese herbal medicine. Theoretically Chinese herbal medicine strives to achieve a holistic balance in the body by "supplementing" the "weakness" or "emptiness" and "purging" the "firmness" or "fullness". In addition, it also has the "blood", "water" and "*ch'i*" theories which Western medicine lacks. These methods which were mentioned previously are further explained below:

(1) Blood Conformation Theory

Blood conformation is also called blood stagnation and occurs most often in women, owing to the physiological consequences of menstruation and childbirth which can result in poor blood circulation and blood stagnation within the body. In some cases blood stagnation is caused by external injury. Even today, Asian women customarily visit Chinese medical doctors whenever they are sick. For this reason Chinese herb medicine has developed the "blood stagnation" theory and perfected its therapeutic methods. Blood stagnation theory is also very effective in dealing with recalcitrant diseases.

(2) **Water Conformation Theory**

Many diseases may be caused by disturbances in water metabolism, an imbalance in circulation, and or abnormal distribution of water throughout the body. Chinese herb medicine refers to the symptom of water stagnation within the stomach as *"tan yin"* (literally, sputum drink). If the stagnation occurs in the bronchi it is called *"chih yin"* (branch drink); and renal edema is called *"yi yin"* (overflow drink).

Western medicine refers to the action of increasing the excretion of urine as "diuresis", while Chinese herb medicine refers to it as "water delivery." Although there are many Western diuretics, they have pronounced side-effects. In Chinese herb medicine there are many water-delivering herbs, such as hoelen, alisma, atractylodes, and polyporus, which are very effective in treating chronic nephritis and uremia, illnesses which Western medicine regards as recalcitrant.

(3) **The *"Ch'i"* Theory in Chinese Medicine**

As mentioned before in Section III, *"ch'i"* can be divided into the "mobile *ch'i*" and the "still *ch'i*". Mobile *ch'i* refers to the up-rushing of *ch'i* causing dizziness, headache, and flushing. Cinnamon suppresses this up-rushing *ch'i*. "Still *ch'i*" means the *ch'i* is obstructed and accumulated in one place. For this condition Chinese medicine employs other *ch'i* herbs such as perilla, magnolia, and prescriptions such as *Pan-hsia-hou-pu-tang* (Pinellia and Magnolia Combination), and *Ling-kuei-chu-kan-tang* (Hoelen and Atractylodes Combination).

Another kind of disease related to *ch'i* which Dr. Fujihira Ken of Japan called the "disease of no disease" is very difficult to treat with modern Western medicine. Its symptoms are chills, stiff shoulders, habitual constipation, headache, insomnia, giddiness, hyperemesis gravidarum — all related to *ch'i* and cured more easily by Chinese herb medicine.

In conclusion, Western medicine does not possess an equivalent of the *"ch'i"* theory. Chinese herb medicine also has many other theories not found in Western medicine but due to limitations of space they are omitted here.

THE CHARACTERISTICS AND CONSTITUENTS OF CHINESE HERBAL FORMULAS

Comparison of Modern Synthetic Drugs Used in Prescriptions and the Natural Herbs Used in Chinese Formulas

Chinese medicine uses formulas instead of prescriptions. A modern medical prescription contains chemical compounds such as aminopyrine, caffeine, and phenacetine combined in a capsule and taken three or four times a day. The prescription has no particular name. The doctor writes it down according to his diagnosis. The prescriptions vary considerably from patient to patient and year to year as new drugs are discovered. By comparison, every Chinese formula has a particular name. For example, the name *Ko-ken-tang* (Pueraria Combination) refers to a specific combination of seven different herbs pueraria, *ma-huang*, cinnamon, paeonia, jujube, ginger, licorice. This formula is found in the medical classic *Shang han lun*. This book was written nearly 1800 years ago, indicating that the formula was in use long before the book was written. Moreover, this formula is still in common use today whereas it is difficult to find a Western medical prescription that has been used very long without being altered.

The formulas of the *Shang han lun* and *Chin kuei yao lueh* (Summaries of Household Remedies) are not merely used out of habit and custom but because they still work. The two books were written during the later Han dynasty, after which came the dynasties of Tang, Sung, Yuan, Ming, and Ching. In each of these succeeding dynasties, many famous doctors emerged who developed many more efficacious formulas. But none of the formulas they established could supplant those of the *Shang han lun* and the *Chin kuei yao lueh*. That is why people in earlier times referred to the two books as the works of the sages. The two were combined into one text which is called *Shang han tsa ping lun*. (Treatise on Colds and Miscellaneous Diseases).

Apart from being subtle in combination, formulas of the *Shang han tsa ping lun* use common herbs that are readily available and inexpensive. In addition, many formulas call only for three, four, five or at the most ten herbs. How simple this is in comparison with the Tang dynasty's *Chien chin yao fang* (One Thousand Precious Prescriptions) which has formulas that contain more than fifty herbs in one combination.

Generally, the formulas of *Shang han tsa ping lun* are referred to as the old formulas while those that appeared after in the Tang and Sung dynasties are considered new formulas. Old formulas are simple and plain while the new formulas are comparatively more complicated.

Preparation and Identification of Formulas

Formulas of *Shang han tsa ping lun* are named in various ways. The following is a categorization according to the methods used.

(1) According to the principal herb of the formula *Hsiao-chai-hu-tang* (Minor Bupleurum Combination), *Ko-ken-tang* (Pueraria Combination) *Jen-sheng-tang* (Ginseng and Ginger Combination).

(2) According to two principal herbs of the formula *Pan-hsia-hou-pu-tang* (Pinellia and Magnolia Combination), *Tang-kuei-shao-yao-san* (*Tang-kuei* and Paeonia Formula), *Kuei-chih-fu-ling-tang* (Cinnamon and Hoelen Combination).

(3) According to three principal herbs of the formula *Ko-ken-huang-lien-huang-chin-tang* (Pueraria, Coptis, and Scute Combination), *Chai-hu-kuei-chih-kan-chiang-tang* (Bupleurum, Cinnamon, and Ginger Combination).

(4) According to all the herbs of the formula *Kan-mai-ta-*

tsao-tang (Licorice and Jujube Combination), *Ma-huang-hsi-hsin-fu-tzu-tang* (Ma-huang, Aconite, and Asarum Combination), *Kuei-chih-kan-tsao-lung-ku-mu-li-tang* (Cinnamon, Licorice, Oyster Shell, and Dragon Bone Combination).

(5) According to the effects of the formula *Pai-nung-san* (Platycodon and Jujube Formula) *Pai-nung* means pus-discharging, *Wen-ching-tang* (*Tang-kuei* and Evodia Combination), *Tsou-ma-tang* (Croton and Apricot Seed Combination).

(6) According to designations "big," "small," and numerals *Hsiao-ching-lung-tang* (Minor Blue Dragon Combination), *Ta-chien-chung-tang* (Major Zanthoxylum Combination), *Wu-ling-san* (Hoelen Five Herb Formula).

(7) According to the names of the guardian gods *Pai-hu-tang* (Gypsum Combination, Tiger Combination), *Chen-wu-tang* (Vitality Combination).

(8) According to the deduction or addition of one or more herbs to a formula. *Kuei-chih-chia-shao-yao-tang* (Cinnamon and Paeonia Combination), *Szu-ni-chia-jen-sheng-tang* (Ginseng, Aconite, and Licorice Combination).

A Personal Experience *Kan-tsao-tang* (Licorice Combination)

Kan-tsao-tang (Licorice Combination) is a formula of the *Shang han lun.* It consists of only one herb, licorice, and is found in the chapter on "lesser yin disease." *Kan-tsao-tang* (Licorice Combination) can be used when the patient suffers from a sore throat and lack of vitality. If the use of *Kan-tsao-tang* (Licorice Combination) is ineffectual after taking for two or three days, it should be replaced by *Chieh-keng-tang* (Platycodon Combination), which is a combination of licorice and platycodon. It should be noted here that the use of *Kan-tsao-tang* (Licorice Combination) is recommended before the sore throat is seriously inflamed. When symptoms of tonsillitis appear. *Chieh-keng-tang* (Platycodon Combination) is the appropriate remedy.

The following case will serve as an example of the efficacy of *Kan-tsao-tang* (Licorice Combination). One day my daughter suddenly had a terrible pain in her throat. When I examined her throat, I could not see any particular abnormality. So I gave her *Kan-tsao-tang.* No sooner had she drunk it than she recovered.

During the war I prescribed another formula of the licorice category to a woman with unspecified, acute abdominal pain as her chief complaint. She was well in two days. She previously had been hospitalized and given medical treatment for some time for the same condition. I prescribed a formula for her which consisted of licorice, rice powder, and honey. Except for the licorice the other two ingredients of this formula are foods. An explanation of this formula, known as *Kan-tsao-fen-mi-tang* (Licorice, Oryza, and Honey Combination), can be found in *Chin kuei yao lueh*. According to this book, *Kan-tsao-fen-mi-tang* is an effective cure for abdominal pain caused by an infection of common intestinal worms if the pain has not been alleviated with drastic-acting chemical drugs. I used this formula to treat my patient because she had already been treated with drastic drugs.

An ancient Chinese medical text records that this formula is a cure for various intoxications caused by other drugs. The detoxifying functions of licorice are illustrated in the following case.

It was in 1927 that I first became interested in herbal medicine. A policeman of about fifty years of age was transferred to my village, and I had the opportunity to make friends with him. One day our conversation touched on the subject of herbal medicine. He said, "Acute abdominal pains that are not subdued by an injection can be subdued immediately by a decoction of licorice. The place where I was previously stationed was a remote border area where doctors were not readily available. So when people suffered from acute abdominal pain I would give them licorice."

That licorice is effective for abdominal pain recalcitrant to injection is definitely something worthy of our attention.

Food and drug intoxication can also be remedied by drinking concentrated decoctions of licorice in large quantities. Quoted below are the detoxifying functions of licorice which have been gleaned from various medical books.

"Licorice is the cure for thinness and can change the weak into strong." *Wai tai mi yao* (Extra Medical Secrets).

"Licorice is the master of the toxic air of the world and the mountains and rivers and the fog and dew; it eliminates the toxins of the earth and miasma." *Wai tai mi yao*.

"Licorice is the master herb of the hot and cold evil air of the viscera; it fortifies the sinews and bones and muscle growth, and doubles our strength; it cures swollen wounds due to wrenching and cutting and detoxifies. . . " *Shen nung pen tsao ching* (Shen Nung's Herbal).

"Licorice is the master of acuteness. So it cures acute abdominal pain, pressing pain, and convulsions, as well as the toxin caused by coldness and stress." *Yao cheng* (Characteristics of Drugs). It is also recorded in *Wai tai mi yao* that severe diarrhea with as many as ten discharges a day can be relieved by *Kan-tsao-tang* (Licorice Combination).

Diagnosis and Treatment

Treatment in accordance with conformation

In Chinese medicine diagnosis is linked closely to treatment, the two being virtually inseparable. In modern medicine diagnosis is done by determining the disease name according to the cause and condition. The course of treatment is decided on after the disease name has been determined. This is the basic principle of modern medicine. With regard to therapy, it is generally known that there are two methods of treatment: "treating the disease" and "treating the cause."

The method of treating the disease centers on the individual symptoms. For example, sleeping pills are used for insomnia; laxatives are used for constipation. The method of treating the cause obviously focuses on the origin of the disease. However, many diseases have an obscure cause or one that can only be inferred. Also the cause may disappear but the disease still be present.

Todo Yoshimasu, a famous scholar of Japanese herb medicine, once said, "There is really no need to find the cause. This does not mean that there is no cause. There is always a cause but during the investigation speculation tends to obscure the true origin. It is futile to establish any disease name or course of treatment with such uncertainity." Therefore, he advocated "treatment in accordance with conformation" is different from treatment in accordance with disease. The former is characteristic of Chinese medicine in which diagnosis aims at reaching a "conformation." A conformation is the objective and proof of the kind of treatment to be given. For example, when a disease is the *Ko-ken-tang* (Pueraria Combination) conformation, it means that

Ko-ken-tang (Pueraria Combination) is used for treatment. Since the determination of a conformation is very important in Chinese diagnosis, I am going to talk about it and give actual examples.

Most of the patients who visit my clinic have been to various hospitals and clinics but have not been cured. As I question them about their symptoms, they cannot give very satisfactory answers. They say, for instance, "I am suffering from severe gastroptosis," or another one suffering from chronic hepatitis will tell me about his B.S.P. test results (a laboratory test for determining hepatitis).

One particular patient was a young man who suffered from a rare disease called Wilson's disease. The disease affects the metabolism of copper in the blood. The chief symptom is tenseness and convulsions of the muscles. The patient will also have acute pain and hence insomnia. The young man was carried to me by his mother because the disease had already paralyzed him. I restored sleep to him with a formula of the paeonia and licorice category.

In Chinese medicine the conformation is the basis for treatment. In a Chinese diagnosis, the patient's complaints are of vital importance. We expect the patient to tell us the location, quality, and frequency of his pains. Subjective symptoms matter greatly in the determination of the conformation, such as cold feet, warm feet, and stiff shoulders. These mutual symptoms form the basis for the course of treatment to be given. On the other hand, modern medicine does not assign great import to the patient's subjective complaints. If nothing wrong is found objectively through the many tests administered, the patient is dismissed as all right. This, of course, is very different from the view of Chinese medicine which deems the subjective complaint a symptom of disease.

I once knew a man who was delighted when his physical examination showed nothing abnormal. However, he died five days later. His friend, on learning of the sad news, exclaimed to me, "How unreliable such physical examinations are!" I explained that although modern medicine employs a variety of methods to examine a patient, the examination is often incomplete, parts of the body outside the tests being left unexamined and hence unattended. For example, sometimes heart disease is not detected by electrocardiogram. I once told a patient of mine that he had an unhealthy heart, but he did nothing about it because he had passed an electrocardiogram examination. He died about a half year later from a massive heart failure.

The other day a woman of about fifty came to see me. Though the weather was hot, she had on woolen socks to keep her feet warm. She also had stiff shoulders and a headache, tired easily, and felt dizzy when standing up. She had been to see many doctors. Every doctor she visited considered her case to hyperesthesia and did not give her any medical treatment. Later she was examined in a hospital and found to be normal. Finally, she visited my clinic.

After I had examined her and considered her case, I said, "Your problem is a feeling of distress just as you say. Apart from this you have no disease."

The patient asked the name of her disease. I replied, "The remedy for your disease is a formula called *Tang-kuei-szu-ni-chia-wu-chu-yu-sheng-chiang-tang* (*Tang-kuei,* Evodia, and Ginger Combination). If you want a disease name, you can add the word "conformation" after the name of this formula. Thus you may call the disease the *Tang-kuei-szu-ni-chia-wu-chu-yu-sheng-chiang-tang* conformation.

My patient was unable to understand this so I went on to explain, "The so-called disease name is actually something designated by professionals for the convenience of dealing with disease. Actually the kidney is not the only place of trouble in nephritis or the liver the only place of trouble in hepatitis. The human body is a living entity, not a lifeless television set or automobile. Hence whether it is the kidney or the liver, the disease affects the whole body. Therefore, Chinese medicine gives a patient a whole-body treatment no matter what the disease may be. Chinese medicine never treats the disease alone but treats the disease-stricken patient.

One point I would like to add here is that although a disease name is not necessary in Chinese diagnosis, a doctor practicing Chinese medicine should avail himself of modern methods of examination to help him decide upon the course of treatment. Besides helping him in reaching a diagnosis, Western methods make it easier for him to convince the patient of "exactly" what he or she is suffering.

Conformation and its determination.

The data from which the conformation is determined are

symptoms like headache, dizziness, chills, buzzing in the ears, thirst, diarrhea, and so on. In approaching a patient's symptoms, the doctor should not just treat them separately.

Take for example the symptom of vomiting. If the patient reports that he has vomited, the doctor must ask for details before writing a formula. For different types of vomiting there are different formulas.

Severe vomiting often occurs in an infant after it has taken medicine for a cold or when it is suffering from acute gastroenteritis. The baby seems to have a strong desire for water yet will vomit the water after drinking it. He cannot sleep quietly but moves restlessly and noisily. The doctor must be sure to inquire about the urination in such cases because there is usually a decrease in the amount. Chinese medicine calls such a condition "reverse water vomiting" or the *Wu-ling-san* (Hoelen Five Herb Formula) conformation. One or two dosages of this formula will stop the vomiting and the thirst, increase the amount of urine discharged, calm the restlessness, and induce perspiration.

On the other hand, the vomiting of a woman during pregnancy, though belonging to the same vomiting category, is different. She will often feel nauseated, have no appetite for food and drink, become upset, and then vomit. This is the *hsiao-pan-hsia-chia-fu-ling-tang* (Minor Pinellia and Hoelen Combination) conformation and should not be confused with the *Wu-ling-san* (Hoelen Five Herb Formula) conformatin. The vormiting that sometimes accompanies migraine is the *Wu-chu-yu-tang* (Evodia Combination) conformation. Thus the Chinese doctor must find out about the kind of vomiting along with the other symptoms to which it is linked. He must investigate and evaluate other complaints such as headache, dizziness and diarrhea in like manner.

When diarrhea occurs, the doctor should find out how and when it takes place. If the diarrhea comes suddenly following a thundering sound in the stomach, the doctor should consider giving the patient *Kan-tsao-hsieh-hsin-tang* (Pinellia and Licorice Combination). Whereas if the patient has acute pains in his abdomen, has difficulty in having a bowel movement, and has to stay on the toilet for fear of sudden discharge, *Shao-yao-tang* (Paeonia Combination) or formulas in this category are suitable remedies. Diarrhea may develop in a way similar to the example above but the stool will be discharged first in small quantities and then smoothly in watery form. In this case *Chen-wu-tang* (Vitality Combination) is the remedy.

Also there are several types of coughs: cough without sputum, cough with sputum that is easily removed, cough with sputum that is difficult to remove, cough that is accompanied by stridor, cough that is acute at night, and so on. Different coughs are dealt with by different formulas.

Besides investigating and analyzing complaints, the doctor must also employ the method of palpation in determining a conformation. In addition, examination of reports of blood pressure, urine, and X-rays are very helpful. The doctor of Chinese medicine today does not reject the modern methods as he did in the past. As a matter of fact, modern physics and chemistry supplement Chinese diagnosis.

Here is an example to show the importance of using Western diagnostic methods to assist Chinese medicine. I once had a patient, a boy of ten, who was brought to my clinic because of bed-wetting at night. When I examined him, I found that he had a poor complexion and was suffering from inadequate nutrition. In addition, he suffered from thirst and abdominal convulsions. I prescribed *Hsiao-chien-chung-tang* (Minor Cinnamon and Paeonia Combination), a formula particularly effective for bed-wetting of this type. However, the patient did not improve after treatment. Therefore, I suspected that there was something wrong with my diagnosis. So I gave him a urine test and found that he had renal tuberculosis. His bladder had become ulcerated causing his control over his urination to be reduced. I changed the prescription to a combined formula of *Szu-wu-tang* (*Tang-kuei* Four Combination) and *Chu-ling-tang* (Polyporus Combination) which is often taken for this disease. The patient gradually recovered.

Some people use drugs carelessly. They take herbal medicine while they are taking modern chemical drugs and may even be taking tonics purchased over the counter at the drugstore at the same time. Using drugs in this manner may bring about changes in a conformation. For example, digitalis for heart disease will make the patient's pulse large, floating, and slow. If the doctor is unaware that the patient is taking digitalis, he may decide that the patient is of the strong type (*shih cheng*) when in fact he is not; thus the doctor may give an inappropriate formula. In order to avoid pitfalls of this kind, the patient must tell the doctor about all drugs he has taken or is taking.

Other factors that will affect a conformation and should be included as data for conformation determination are the patient's constitution, sex, age, likes and dislikes in food, living conditions, and general life style.

Arriving at a conformation and some examples of treatment in accordance with the conformation.

To conform a disease, Chinese medicine uses four methods of diagnosis: observing, listening, smelling, questioning, and palpating. Observing refers to the visual appearance of the patient; listening and smelling to the quality of his voice and body odors; questioning to the doctor's inquiry about his condition and symptoms; and palpating to the doctor's feeling the pulse and abdomen. The ancients said that diagnosing by observing is god-like, by listening is saintly, by questioning is skillful, and by palpating is clever. Present day Chinese doctors employ these same four methods along with various modern techniques. Modern medicine also employs abdomen palpation as a means of diagnosis but for different reasons than Chinese medicine. Modern medicine tries to discover certain abnormalities while palpating whereas Chinese medicine uses it as a means to determine if the patient is "substantial" or "deficient." Substantial means physically strong and deficient means physically weak. Treatments will then vary accordingly.

High blood pressure is a good example. If a patient is stout with a good complexion but a tendency to be constipated and have abdomen distention, and if he has chest distress, a stiff neck and shoulders, and a heavy feeling in the head, he is of the substantial type; formulas in the *Ta-chai-hu-tang* (Major Bupleurum Combination) category are indicated. On the other hand, if the patient is thin with a weak abdomen, has a suction-like sound under the heart, and has headaches and vertigo, he is conformed as the deficient type; formulas in the *Pan-hsia-pai-chu-tien-ma-tang* (Pinellia and Gastrodia Combination) category are indicated.

However, not all patients with high blood pressure are solely of the one type or the other. There are varying degrees of substantialness and deficiency and the doctor should prescribe accordingly.

I now would like to cite several examples of "treatment in accordance with conformation." Let's consider a patient with a fever contracted during the previous night. Modern medicine would focus on determining what the disease is and then giving treatment. Chinese medicine, however, focuses on determining the kind of therapy that would be best for the patient according to his conformation. In diagnosing a patient with fever, the symptom the Chinese doctor must look for is "harmful chills," harmful chills meaning that the body feels cold. One principle of Chinese medicine is that purgatives are not applied to feverish patients with harmful chills, whether the chills are light or severe. If the feverish patient has harmful chills, aching joints, headache, floating and strong pulse, and no natural perspiration, *Ma-huang-tang* (*Ma-huang* Combination) may be given regardless of the name of the disease. On the other hand, if harmful chills occur with a floating but weak pulse, headache, and natural perspiration, it is the *Kuei-chih-tang* (Cinnamon Combination) conformation. If the symptoms are similar to those of the *Ma-huang-tang* (*Ma-huang* Combination) conformation but accompanied by tenseness from the neck to the shoulders, it is the *Ko-ken-tang* (Pueraria Combination) conformation. *Ko-ken-tang* (Pueraria Combination) is usually used as a medication for the common cold, but its scope of application is not limited to the common cold. The formula is suitable for any diseases of the *Ko-ken-tang* (Pueraria Combination) conformation. Thus it can be taken for fifty-year shoulders, parasinusitis, conjunctivitis, and so on.

When used by an experienced physician, the same formula may be a cure for several different kinds of diseases. In the past there were physicians who treated all ailments with *Ko-ken-tang* (Pueraria Combination). People ridiculed such doctors by calling them "*Ko-ken-tang* doctors;" but, as a matter of fact, *Ko-ken-tang* (Pueraria Combination) is the basic ingredient for the cure of a wide variety of diseases. An efficacious formula can cure several diseases with the addition of one or two appropriate herbs.

If a doctor can manage to bring a formula's potential into full play and if he knows what needs to be added to the same formula in order to cure different disease, he is considered to be an excellent doctor. The fact is that as an herb doctor's experience and knowledge increase, he will find himself making use of only a few common formulas. An inexperienced doctor who has not yet reached this stage has to use many different categories tentatively.

A famous Chinese physician once said, "A formula is something that can be used freely. It would be senseless to designate one formula for one disease and another formula for another disease. A basic Chinese formula has as many uses as a basic container: It is a pot if one puts food in its; a vase if one puts dirt in it for growing flowers; a basin if one puts water in it; a pail if sand is in it; and a stepping stone if one puts it upside down on the ground." He also said. "The doctor increases in skill as the number of formulas he uses decreases." It is said that when he got old, he used only about 30 different formulas for all the various ailments.

Here is one more example of the approach that Chinese medicine takes to disease. The patient was a man of sixty-five. He had had a cold for almost a month. His body temperature was in excess of 37°C and he coughed constantly. As a result he was not able to sleep well and recently had developed constipation and a loss of appetite. He was getting weaker by the day and was very fearful of developing pneumonia.

His disease had been previously diagnosed as bronchitis. Medicine to stop the coughing, improve the appetite, and relieve the constipation had been prescribed for him. At night he took sleeping pills and an injection of glucose.

His pulse was a little large but weak. His tongue was a little dry looking with thin white fur on it. The patient coughed frequently even when being examined, but the phlegm was easily expectorated. The abdomen totally lacked elasticity. A slightly quick palpitation above the navel could be detected. The patient felt no pain. I prescribed *Chu-ju-wen-tan-tang* (Bamboo and Ginseng Combination). Two or three days later he coughed less and slept better. In addition, his constipation was gone and his appetite had returned. He was able to get out of bed and take a walk around the garden. Since that constipation and loss of appetite had probably been caused by the drugs he was taking, I advised him to discontinue taking all other drugs. Modern medicine treated his symptoms one by one with various medications: sleeping pills, laxatives, cough suppressants, and a tonic. In contrast to this, Chinese medicine determined him to be of the one conformation and treated him with one formula. The symptoms were treated as a whole, if you will, a syndrome.

Professor Hisayuki Omodaka of Osaka University in Japan

commented on the different kinds of therapy in his article "Chinese Herb Medicine and Bergsonisme." He pointed out that Chinese therapy is a whole-body treatment, the most thorough kind of treatment there is. Chinese medicine never considers symptoms separately; instead the problem is considered as a syndrome. In summary, Chinese medicine cures the patient, not the disease.

AN INTRODUCTION TO CHINESE MEDICINE

The Origins of Chinese Medicine

Chinese physicians use herbal formulas to treat disease. (The word "herbal" encompasses animals and other natural sources as well as plants.) Chinese medicine is the oldest formal medical system known to man. *The Classic of the Mountains* (Shan ching 400 B.C.) and *The Classic of the Seas* (Hai ching 120 B.C.) mention sixty-eight varieties of plants-such as apricot seed, cinnamon, and atractylodes-used as medicinals. *Shen Nung's Herbal* (Shen nung pen ts'ao ching) written around A.D. 25 contains information on 365 different herbs. This is considered to be the first systematic attempt to catalog herbs. In the years following, the number of identified species increased, and by the Ming dynasty (1368-1644), Li Shih-chen was able to identify 1,898 herbs in his monumental study *Pen ts'ao kang mu*. (For further information concerning the historical evolution of the *pen ts'ao* "herbals" tradition see table 1.) Presently, Chinese herb doctors use 522 different herbs, 235 of them commonly.

Because of China's immense landmass and long history, many questions arise concerning botanical origins, methods of preparation, formula components, effectiveness, and toxicity. Scientific research on Chinese herbal medicine has so far only added to the confusion. However, the problems are worthy of study and as

Table 1
History of Development of the Pen Ts'ao

Year	Author	Name of Writing	No. of Herbs Included
250 B.C.		*Shan ching*	68
120 B.C.		*Hai ching*	
25 A.D.	Lei Kung	*Shen nung pen tsao ching* (Shen Nung's Herbal)	365
502 A.D.	Tao Hung-ching	*Shen nung pen tsao ching* (Shen Nung's Herbal)	730
569 A.D.	Su Ching, et al.	*Shin hsiu pen tsao* (New Revised Herbal)	850
973 A.D.	Liu Han, et al.	*Kai pao pen tsao* (Kai Pao Herbal)	984
1057 A.D.	Chang Yu-hsi, et al.	*Chia yu pu chu pen tsao* (Chia Yu Herbal Supplement)	1084
1098 A.D.	Tang Shen-wei	*Ching shih chen lei pei chi pen tsao* (Classical Historical Herbal Sorted by conformations for Emergency Use)	1744
1590 A.D.	Li Shih-chen	*Pen tsao kang mu* (The General Catalogue of Herbs)	1898 *

36

Table 2
Herbs of Asia

	Chinese Mainland, Others	Taiwan	Hong Kong
蒲公英	*Taraxacum officinale* (Compositae)	*Taraxacum formosanum* *Lactuca chinensis* (Compositae)	*Elephantopus scaber* (Compositae)
萹蓄	*Polygonum aviculare* (Polygonaceae)	*Euphorbia thymifolia* *Euphorbia hirta* (Euphorbiaceae)	*Belamcanda chinensis* (Iridaceae)
王不留行	*Vaccaria pyramidata* (Caryophyllaceae)	*Melastoma candidum* var. *nobotan* (Melastomaceae)	*Ficus pumila* (Moraceae)
白頭翁	*Pulsatilla chinensis* (Ranunculaceae)	*Polycarpaea corymbosa* (Caryophyllaceae) *Gnaphalium japonicum* (Compositae)	
杜仲	*Eucommia ulmoides* (Eucommiaceae)	*Euonymus pellucidifolius* (Celastraceae) *Euonymus japonica* *Celastrus* sp.	
昆布	*Ecklonia kurome* *Undaria pinnatifida* *Laminaria japonica* (Laminariaceae)	*Ulva lactuca* (Laminariaceae)	*Ulva lactuca* (Laminariaceae)
蛇床子	*Cnidium monnieri* (Umbelliferae)	*Cnidium formosanum* (Umbelliferae)	*Cnidium formosanum* (Umbelliferae)
馬兜鈴	*Aristolochia contorta* (Aristolochiaceae)	*Lilium formosanum* *Lilium phillipensis* (Liliaceae)	*Aristolochia* sp. *A. Contoria* *A. Debilis*
仙鶴草	*Agrimonia pilosa* (Rosaceae)	*Agrimonia pilosa* (Rosaceae)	*Agrimonia eupatoria* (Rosaceae)
豨薟草	*Siegesbeckia orientalis* *S. pubescens* (Compositae)	*Anisomeles ovata* (Labiatae)	*Anisomeles indica* (Labiatae)

such need to be studied further. Chinese doctors believe that the therapeutic effectiveness of herbal formulas depends on the quality of herbs used and the quality depends on the place where the herbs are grown. Unfortunately, it is often very difficult to determine the quality of a crude drug without the assistance of an expert. To add to the confusion, different species often go by the same name. For instance, according to recent my investigations (see table 2), mainland China and Japan use the dandelion of the *Taraxacum* species of the Compositae family in formulas. On the other hand, Taiwan uses the *Lactuca* species and Hong Kong the *Elephantopus* species in the same formulas to treat the same symptoms. Knot grass, a diuretic and insecticide, is the plant *Polygonum aviculare.* In Taiwan, when a formula calls for knot grass the whole plant *Euphorbia thymifolia* of the Euphorbiaceae family is substituted, and in Hong Kong the rhizome of *Belamcanda chinensis* of the Iridaceae family. Cow herb, which is the seed of *Vaccaria pyramidata* of the Caryophyllaceae family according to the *Dictionary of Chinese Herbs,* has been replaced by the stem of *Melastoma candidum* var. *nobotan* of the Melastomaceae family in Taiwan and by the peel of *Ficus pumila* of the Moraceae family in Hong Kong. Besides this, three different plant species-*Pulsatilla chinensis* of the Ranunculaceae family, *Polycarpaea corymbosa* of the Caryophyllaceae family, and *Gnaphalium japonicum* of the Compositae family—are sold under the same name, namely, Nodding Anemone (*Pai-tou-weng*), even though the efficacy of each is different. *Tu-chung,* an herb that grows in Yunnan province bordering Vietnam, has been replaced by more than ten different species of the Eucommiaceae family. This herb is exported by Japan and Hong Kong. As can be readily seen then, nomenclature in Chinese medicine presents many problems, and the ability to differentiate between various herb species requires considerable expertise. (For further information on this subject see the *Dictionary of Chinese Medicine* and *Study of Chinese Medicinal Herbs.)*

Problem with Nomenclature

Another problem contributing to the confusion is the profusion of modern day botanical names. Normally there are three names given to Chinese herbs: the scientific name, the common name, and the Chinese name. The scientific name currently given to Chinese herbals is based upon the universal binomial system. Botanists first give a pair of Latin or Latinized words to each species. The first and second parts of the binomial, or botanical name, identify the genus and species of the plant. The genus encompasses various species that show certain common elements. The ancillary parts of the name usually denote a historical name, a physical characteristic, a usage, a geographical location, or a name of a botanist being honored. In the case of *Panax ginseng* C. A. Meyer, *Panax* is the genus name, ginseng the species name, and C. A. Meyer the name of the botanist being honored. Sometimes, as in this case, the scientific species name also becomes the common name–ginseng. Angelica is another example of confusion. The many varieties of angelica tend to confuse the reader, so the Chinese name, *tang-kuei,* with which everyone is familiar, is used. In most cases, the scientific name is used for the purpose of clarity; however, there are exceptions as noted above.

A complete exposition on major Chinese herbs can be found in *How to Treat Yourself with Chinese Herbs.* The appendix gives the Chinese name, common name, part used in formulas, Latin or scientific name, and medical use of the major herbs.

The Classification of Chinese Drugs Sold on the Market

Chinese medicine attaches much importance to the so-called "indigenous, genuine medicinals." For instance, it is doubtful whether herbs grown in different places have the same efficacy. It is thought that medicinals cultivated in their native place are the best. However, sometimes native production is not plentiful, and it then becomes necessary to use an herb grown in another area as a substitute. Moreover, high cost often necessitates the use of substitutes. Nonetheless, Chinese medical theory classifies herbs according to source and method of processing. Following is a glossary of terms used to describe herbs.

Fresh (生) unprocessed as opposed to dried or parched
Dry (乾) dehydrated, not fresh

Fresh Dried (生乾) allowed to dry naturally
Hot (熟) cooked by heating or boiling
Processed (製) cut and heated
Mountains (山) grown in the mountains, most often in Szechuan
Chuan Szechuan (川) grown in Szechuan
Not native (土) mostly substitutes
Hu (胡) native to Northeast China
Ho (和) a Japanese substitute
T'ang (唐) native to China
Kowatari (古渡) Japanese high-quality product that requires aging
Jou (肉) having a soft or fleshy quality
Shuang (霜) crystallized ash or crystalline form
Taiwanese (台) native to Taiwan or mountainous area

The Preparation of Chinese Herbal Drugs

Once again, the effectiveness of Chinese herb medicinals depends upon three conditions: (1) place of growth; (2) manner of processing; and (3) selection of ingredients. Of course, processing must be in accordance with the highest standards as judged by traditional guidelines. For instance, *The Yellow Emperor's Classic* (Nei ching) outlines the method for roasting pinellia (Pinelliae Rhizoma), and *Treatise on Febrile Diseases* (Shang han lun) describes many methods of preparation. Chinese pharmacies in Taiwan mainly follow what is called "Lei's Directions," Lei Kung being a pupil of Huang Ti, the author of the *Nei ching*. Seven chapters in *The Yellow Emperor's Classic* are attributed to him, as is a book on the art of dispensing medicinals. Drug preparation is also discussed in the following documents:

1. *Golden Precious Prescriptions* (Chien chin yao fang) Directions for preparing more than one hundred herbs are given using these methods:
    a. Manual processing–removing the outer layer, nodes, wings, and legs, peel, and core portion by hand
    b. Water processing–washing, soaking, and dipping
    c. Fire processing–roasting, broiling, burning, and frying

d. Water and fire processing—boiling and steaming
2. *Experimental Prescriptions of Physicians* (Ho chi chu fang) Discusses how to prepare 186 herbs by manual, water, and fire processes.
3. *Chinese Materia Medica* (Pen ts'ao kang mu)
   Tells how to do the following processing methods: manual, water, fire, water and fire processing; extracting; These are but a few examples of the processing methods used in the preparation of Chinese herbal drugs. Processing reduces toxicity, precludes potential side effects, and increases potency. The Brion Research Institute of Taiwan has carried out extensive research on the methods of processing herbal medicine. In addition, it has performed scientific assessments of the preparation of Chinese herbal formulas. A case of its findings is given below.

Preparation of *Ma-huang*

According to traditional Chinese materia medica, the roots and nodes are removed from Ephedrae herba (*ma-huang*) before it is processed. It is then boiled in water several times and the upper layer of foam is removed with a bamboo slip. General alkaloid tests on the treated stem, nodes, and roots determine the changes and pharmacological actions with the following conclusion:
   1. The most desirable method of preparation is to fry *ma-huang* with ginger and licorice. The frying of *ma-huang* with ginger and licorice, followed by dipping in lukewarm water or acetic acid, reduces the level of toxicity and the general alkaloid content when compared to the raw plant. Note: The *ma-huang* root alone does not contain an alkaloid.
   2. Testing of nodes, stems, and the section between the two nodes of a *ma-huang* plant on mice revealed that the nodes are the most toxic and cause convulsions, and the section between the two nodes shows no evidence of toxicity.

These tests support traditional preparation methods, in which it has been customary to prepare *ma-huang* by removing its nodes, and add evidence to the growing proof that the traditional medicinal processing reduces the level of toxicity. For further information on this subject see the article "The Scientific Problems Facing Chinese Herb Medicine," *Bulletin of the Oriental Healing Arts Institute,* vol. 5, no. 6, 1980.

Storage of Chinese Herbs

Since herbs are natural substances, they must be stored under ideal conditions; otherwise they are subject to a change in quality due to insects, excessive moisture, and so on. Excessive moisture can degrade product quality by as much as 30 percent by inhibiting enzyme activity and by creating ideal conditions for fungal growth and molds. Water content of herbs is generally 10 percent. Thus, to properly store crude herbs, refrigeration temperature of 40°C or less is needed to prevent bacterial growth. For additional information about the storage of Chinese herbs see the Chinese edition of *The Storage of Chinese Herbs* by Dr. Hsu.

Preparation and Use of Chinese Herbal Formulas

Formulas are prepared in two ways: (1) by the traditional decocting method; or (2) by the powder method. In the traditional method, raw ingredients of a given formula are purchased from a pharmacy, added to water, and decocted over a low fire. The dregs are removed, and the resulting "tea" then drunk. Pueraria Combination may serve as an example. The components of this formula are as follows:

8.0g pueraria	2.0g licorice
4.0g *ma-huang*	1.0g ginger
3.0g cinnamon	3.0g paeonia
4.0g jujube	

The pueraria and *ma-huang* are first cooked in 400cc of water over a low fire until 80cc of the water has evaporated. The white foam which forms on the surface is then removed, the other herbs added, and the formula once more simmered until the liquid is reduced to 120cc. It is decanted before being given to the patient.

In Taiwan and China people drink this combination, warm,

on an empty stomach during the day. The residue can be boiled once again during the night. In Japan people usually take a combination like this between meals—three times per day. When decocting, a porcelain, or clay vessel is used, not stainless steel or aluminum.

An example of the powder method is the formula *Tang-kuei and Paeonia Formula*. It contains the following ingredients:

3.0g *tang-kuei*	4.0g paeonia
4.0g atractylodes	3.0g cnidium
4.0g hoelen	4.0g alisma

After all the ingredients are purchased at a Chinese drug store, they are then dried, crushed, and ground into powder. It can be taken three times daily, preferably around meal times.

In the interests of clarity, formulas that have traditionally been called "soups" or "teas" are known as "combinations" in this book. The Pueraria Combination is an example of this. If the original ingredients are in powder form we call it a formula. Some formula was originally a pill. Pills are composed of powder along with 30-50% honey.

The Scientific Preparation of Chinese Herbal Formulas

Western medicine has traditionally used pharmaceuticals. Galen (about A.D. 100) first placed herbs in a solution of alcohol to extract their constituents. Since that time medicinals have been available in tinctures, syrups, injections, and gelatin capsules. Chinese herbal medicine, on the other hand, with the exception of a few powders and pills, is in most cases decocted. This method has not changed for five thousand years. However, it is not only inconvenient but also unpalatable, because decocted herbs leave a bitter taste in the mouth.

No longer does the pace of modern life allow people to use the decoction process, since the old method of preparation is time-consuming and inconvenient. Some sixty years ago, Nagakura, a pharmaceutical company of Japan, began developing ways to mass produce Chinese medicine using precision apparatus and scientific methods. At the present time there are more than twenty pharmaceutical companies producing drugs based on the

Nagakura model.

In 1963 the Sun Ten Pharmaceutical Company was established based on the Nagakura model. This was the first company of its type in Taiwan to produce Chinese herbal formulas in powder and granule form. For more than seven years the company did not sustain a profit. Time is needed for something so revolutionary to take hold. Now Sun Ten products are used throughout Taiwan, Japan, and Southeast Asia. The potency of these scientifically prepared formulations is anywhere from 6-10 times the potency of traditional decoctions and, of course, they are more convenient.

Scientifically formulated herbal medicine is produced according to the highest standards. Pharmacologists select the finest raw materials, and then vacuum condense them to reduce spoilage. The essential oils are extracted from the herbs with the latest high-speed, vacuum-baking apparatus. Modern laboratory apparatus also used the baking process to extract the essence of the herb and turn it into granule or powder from. Afterwards precision apparatus are used in quality control to examine the final product to determine whether it meets established standards.

The general daily dosage of these scientifically prepared Chinese herbal formulas is 4.5-6.0 grams divided into three equal parts. So from 1.5-2.0 grams is taken with lukewarm water three times a day, either between or just after meals.

Occasionally, the addition of other herbs to the basic formula is necessary. In this case, two-thirds of the original formula is taken while each new herb is added in the amount of one-third of the original quantity. For example, if the daily dosage of pueraria is 4.0 grams and cnidium and magnolia flower are added, these two herbs would be added in the amount of 1.0 gram each, thus maintaining the daily dosage for formulas and combinations of 4.5-6.0 grams. Presently packets can be purchased ranging from 100-1,000 grams. Chinese herbal formulas and combinations are also available in capsule form. Usually two or three capsules are taken three times daily.

In the United States, Sun Ten products are widely used. The Sun Ten product line consists of 250 herbal formulas and 400 individual herb preparations. Sun Ten products are herbal extracts.

The Side Effects of Chinese Medicine

In modern medicine, with the exception of surgery and physical therapy, drugs are used for most human ailments. And despite the fact that drugs are usually substances foreign to our bodies, small quantities can be absorbed and disposed of by the body without producing any harmful effects. On the other hand, large amounts of drugs taken continuously over long periods have cumulative and harmful effects resulting in chronic intoxication.

Western medicines are very effective for some diseases, but they do have side effects. Because of their toxicity, frequent use can be harmful to the body. By contrast, the toxicity of Chinese herb formulas is very low. For example, toxicity is expressed as LD_{50}, meaning a man weighing 60 kilograms (roughly 150 pounds) would have to ingest somewhere between 120 and 300 grams of a typical formula to endanger his life. Since Chinese dosages are never more than a few grams, this is manifestly impossible. Thus, their low toxicity is one reason Chinese herb formulas will long exist.

This is not to say that there are absolutely no side effects resulting from the ingestion of Chinese herbal formulas. Sometimes a patient who takes Chinese herbal drugs develops a hypersensitive reaction. The Cinnamon and Ginseng Combination (*Kuei-chih-jen-sheng-tang*) induces such side effects as a rash. Some patients who take large amounts of licorice develop edema. This reaction is due to the glycyrrhiza component in licorice which produces actions similar to those of cortisone. Another example is the Rehmannia Eight Formula which tends to induce indigestion and nausea in some patients, in which case they should use the Rehmannia Six Formula, a milder formula with essentially the same effects. Cinnamon and *ma-huang* overstimulate the autonomic nerves. They are known in Chinese medicine as "dispersing agents." Aconite and ginger have an inhibitive behavioral effect which might account for their effectiveness in treating internal chills. Herbs such as gentiana, phellodendron, and lithospermum, which have heat dissolving and detoxicating actions, can cause diarrhea. Most of these herbs will have this effect in white mice an hour after administration. Rhubarb on the other hand causes diarrhea three hours after ingestion.

Ming Hsuan "Hypersensitivity"

Another side effect resulting from the ingestion of Chinese herbal formulas is *ming hsuan* or hypersensitivity, but it is quite different from the side effects resulting from the use of Western drugs. The reaction is due to the detoxification effects of Chinese herbal formulas. For a short period the patient's condition will appear to be worsening. Contrary to appearance, this is an indication that the formula is working and that recovery is imminent. Dr. Yakazu Domei reports that he once had a patient with a serious asthmatic condition. He administered Minor Blue Dragon Combination and soon thereafter the patient developed uterine bleeding while at the same time her asthmatic condition disappeared. Later the uterine bleeding also stopped. Not every patient will experience these effects but people with chronic ailments will.

Where to Buy Chinese Herbs

Throughout Asia there are more than one billion people using Chinese herbal medicine, in Hong Kong, Singapore, South Korea, Japan, Taiwan, and China. Although Taiwan is only one-sixth the size of California, there are more than eight thousand Chinese herb stores in that country.

Almost all of the ingredients for the formulas mentioned in this book can be obtained in Chinese herb stores, and the formulas prepared at home. The Sun Ten Pharmaceutical Company of Taiwan produces herbal extractions in granule and powder form which can be ingested immediately. Chinese herbal medicines can be bought throughout the United States in Chinese sections of the major cities. Chinese formulas in granule and powder form can be purchased at the following companies:

Sun Ten Pharmaceutical Works Co., Ltd.
114 Chung-ching South Road, Section 3
Taipei, Taiwan   107 R. O. C.

Junkoh Medicinal Industry Co., Ltd.
2-4-8 Uehara, Shibuyaku
Tokyo 151, Japan

For further information concerning Chinese herbal medicine and the scientifically prepared Chinese herbal formulas write to:
Oriental Healing Arts Institute
8820 S. Sepulveda Blvd., Suite 218
Los Angeles, CA 90045

List of Suggested Readings

English

Chang Chung-ching. *Shang han lun* (Treatise on Febrile Diseases). Los Angeles: Oriental Healing Arts Institute, 1981. (To be Published)

Hsu Hong-yen and Peacher, William. *Chinese Herb Medicine and Therapy.* Los Angeles: Oriental Healing Arts Institute, 1976.
Chen's History of Chinese Medicine. Los Angeles: Oriental Healing Arts Institute, 1977.

Hsu Hong-yen. *Chinese Herbs and Formulas.* Los Angeles: Oriental Healing Arts Institute, 1978.
How to Treat Yourself with Chinese Herbs. Los Angeles: Oriental Healing Arts Institute, 1980.
"The Scientific Problems Facing Chinese Herb Medicine," *Bulletin of the Oriental Healing Arts Institute,* vol. 5, no. 6, 1980.
Help for Chronic Ailments via Chinese Herbal Formulas, vol. I. Los Angeles: Oriental Healing Arts Institute, 1982. (To be published)
Treating Cancer with Chinese Herbs: Help for Chronic Ailments via Chinese Herbal Formulas, vol. II. Los Angeles: Oriental Healing Arts Institute, 1982. (To be published)

Veith, Ilza. *The Yellow Emperor's Classic of Internal Medicine.* Berkeley and Los Angeles: University of California Press, 1972.

A Barefoot Doctor's Manual. Prepared by the Revolutionary Health Committee of Hunan Province. Mayne Isle and Seattle: Cloudburst Press, 1979.

Chinese

Hsieh Kuan, general editor. *Chung-kuo i-hsueh ta-tzu-tien* (The Dictionary of Chinese Medicine, 7th edition, four volumes). Taipei: Taiwan shang-wu yin-shu-kuan, 1975.

Hsu Hong-yen. *Chung-yao-tsai chih yen-chiu* (A Study of Chinese Medicinal Herbs). Taipei: Hsin i-yao chu-pan-she, 1980.

Hsu Hong-yen and Hsu Lin-run. *Chung-yao chih pao-tsun* (The Storage of Chinese Medicine). Taipei: Hsin i-yao chu-pan-she, 1980.

DIAGNOSES AND THERAPEUTICAL METHODS OF CHINESE MEDICINE

THE FOUR KINDS OF DIAGNOSES

Preface

Since ancient times, the diagnostic method of Chinese herbal medicine has been to discern conformations according to the five senses, to analyze these results, and to administer appropriate therapy. Unlike the diagnostic practice of Western medicine, this method of diagnosis uses no scientific instruments.

What does it mean "to discern conformation according to the five senses"? This refers to the four different kinds of diagnosis which are the primary steps of discerning and treating: observation, hearing, questioning, and touching. The term "observation" means that the doctor visually observes the appearance of the patient's whole body. In "hearing" the doctor listens to body sounds (through succussion and auscultation) and voice sounds. He also discerns odors of body secretions, breath, stool, pus, etc. through the sense of smell. In "questioning" the doctor asks about the patient's past symptoms and pain, while during touching" he touches the patient's body directly with his hands, feeling the pulses and palpating the abdomen.

The term "conformation" means a series of symptoms that the human body exhibits when its normal physiological functions break down. Some of these symptoms appear immediately, while others do not become apparent until later. All of the symptoms within a conformation have closely related pathological and physiological causes and effects.

Yin, yang, surface, inside, chill, fever, weakness, and firmness are the "Eight Principles" which underlie the symptoms of all diseases. Yin and yang are regarded as the main principles. Inside, chill, and weakness belong to the yin grouping, while surface, fever, and firmness belong to the yang grouping. However, during clinical practice, complicated relationships arise between yin and yang such as yin-inside-yang and yang-inside-yin, as well as surface-inside, chill-fever, weak-firm, etc. Therefore, when using the eight principles we must either analyze and discern conformations or summarize the information available and induct the diagnosis on this basis. In addition. it is necessary to consider the possibility of inversion of conformations and their validity or falsity.

Inversion. Due to variations in disease-resistance ability, the Eight Principles may invert or become interchanged with one another. If surface becomes inside, the disease condition will deteriorate; but if inside becomes surface, the disease will subside. It is a good sign if weakness inverts to firmness, but it signals danger if firmness inverts to weakness. The inversion of chill to fever is a firmness conformation, while the inversion of a fever disease to a chill disease is a weakness conformation. Therefore, it is important for physicians to pay particular attention to the inversion of diseases whenever they discern conformation.

Validity or Falsity. Generally, severe or chronic diseases will exhibit dissimilar and contradictory phenomena such as true fever-false chill or true chill-false fever, true firmness-false weakness or true weakness-false firmness. Therefore, the process of discerning should be done carefully so that the validity or falsity of the symptoms may be accurately determined.

If discernment of conformations is carried out systematically according to the Four Diagnoses and the Eight Principles, it is possible to avoid purposeless observation, unnecessary hearing, inappropriate questioning, and incorrect touching. This method will then provide a valid clinical basis for correct therapy.

The Four Kinds of Diagnosis

1. **Observation**

   In the observation diagnosis the physician notices variations in the patient's mental disposition, face and skin coloring, physical appearance, and physical state.

Mental Disposition: This refers to the attitude of the patient which may range from cheerfulness (high-spirits) to depression (low-spirits). From this observation it is possible to judge whether the case is mild or severe and whether the prognosis is favorable or unfavorable. It is said, "If the patient possesses 'spirit', he will survive; if not, he will die."

Color: This refers to the tinge and the five colors observable when looking at the skin. It indicates an abundance or weakness of *"ch'i"* (vitality) and blood in the viscera and bowels, and it reveals variations in diseases. Bright and full color is a favorable sign as opposed to dull color which is not.

Physical Appearance: This manifests the patient's growth-state and nutritional condition. It is an indication of the patient's potential resistance to toxins and the prognosis of any disease he may contract.

Physical State: This is indicative of the present status and the prognosis of a patient's disease.

Since the determination of mental disposition and color is subjective, the diagnosis is dependent upon the personal judgment of the physician. For this reason it is said, "The skillful employment resides in one's mind." On the other hand, the physical appearance and physical state of the patient are evident and can be observed objectively. Hemiplegic paralysis and stooped posture due to deterioration of cervical vertebrae are examples of evident physical appearance, while tremor, edema, and aggresive behavior show the physical state.

The determination of mental disposition, coloring, physical appearance, and physical state is based upon general observations. In addition, there are twelve guidelines of making detailed observations of the patient's whole body and appearance.

Physique: Patients with a good complexion, plump appearance, and sound muscle tone belong to the yang-firm conformation. Generally, these patients are short. Those of the yin-weak conformation have exactly the opposite qualities.

Facial and Skin Color: Patients of the yang-firm conformation have good color and supple, well-nourished skin that demonstrates proper nutrition. Their skin or mucous membranes are clear and ruddy. Patients of the yin-weak conformation have dry, shriveled skin and poor coloring. If the patient has stagnant blood, the skin is blemished or has spider nevi.

Nails: Those of the yang-firm conformation have strong, healthy-looking, pink nails; those of the yin-weak conformation have pail nails. Nails turn white when pressure is applied to them. Rapid recovery to a pink color indicates health, whereas longer recovery indicates the presence of stagnant blood.

Lips and Gums: A dark red color of the lips, gums, and oral mucous membrane indicates poor blood circulation and the presence of stagnant blood.

Fever type is also indicated by the gums. If the teeth are dry, particularly the front incisors, then *yang ming* (sunlight yang) high fever or sunstroke is present. Dry upper gums indicate severe inflammation of the stomach vein and arteries. Dry lower gums mean severe inflammation of the large intestine. Swelling of the gums indicates gastrointestinal disturbance. Turgid, painful gums and teeth indicate a stomach ailment, while chattering teeth without swollen gums indicate a kidney ailment.

Eyes: Bright, active, lively, clear eyes are a yang-firm conformation, whereas the opposite is a yin-weak conformation. Specific conditions may also be detected by examining the eyes.

a. Stagnant blood — The eyelids are reddish-violet and/or the conjunctiva are dark red.
b. Psychasthenia — The patient has difficulty reopening the eyes after closing them.
c. Mental instability — The gaze is unsteady and the patient blinks his eyes frequently.
d. Liver, heart, and lung fevers — The eyes are red.
e. Liver and stomach fevers — There is photophobia and epiphora.
f. Weakness of *"Ch'i"* (vitality) and onset of water disease — There is orbital edema.
g. Obstruction of sputum or "liver wind" (*tien tiao*) — The patient has a staring gaze which, after a while, returns to normal.
h. Eclampsia — The patient squints.
i. Fever disease and eclampsia — The patient has a fixed stare.
j. Insufficiency of "kidney water" — The pupils are dilated.

The following are remedies used for conditions indicated by

the eyes.
a. Surface conformation — A diaphoretic (50% each of *ma-huang* and cinnamon) is used.
b. Inside conformation — *Huang-lien-chieh-tu-tang* (Coptis and Scute Combination) is administered.
c. Extravasated blood — *Tao-ho-cheng-chi-tang* (Persica and Rhubarb Combination) or *Kuei-chih-fu-ling-wan* (Cinnamon and Hoelen Formula) is used. For weakness conformation, *Tang-kuei-shao-yao-san* (Tang-kuei and Paeonia Formula) is prescribed. For the weaker type, aconite is added.

Skull: A concave skull indicates inherited general weakness as well as weakness in both *ch'i* (vitality) and blood. An unfused fontanel indicates insufficient kidney *ch'i* and cerebrospinal deficiencies.

Face: Variations in facial coloring are significant.
a. Ruddy — Normal red indicates a reduction of *yang ch'i* and surface melancholy. Flushing of the cheeks in the afternoon indicates yin weakness, internal fever. A ruddy, light red and white complexion indicates *tai yang*, while a ruddy complexion similar to that of drunkenness indicates stomach fever.
b. Yellow — This is generally a sign of wet fever and weakness: Light or withered yellow is indicative of internal injury to the spleen and stomach. When the disease is protracted, the tip of the nose, the space between the eyebrows, and the face turns yellow. Bright yellow means that the patient is progressing and will be cured. Yellow with dull green indicates the presence of stagnant blood and wet fever.
c. Greenish — This is a sign of juvenile eclampsia and pain in the ribs and abdomen.
d. Black — When accompanied by dry, rough skin, this indicates the presence of stagnant blood.

Hair: Drooping hair indicates a blood deficiency and a lack of vitality. Dry, yellowish hair indicates a weakness in the blood.

Tongue: Observation of the tongue is the primary method of diagnosing acute febrile and gastrointestinal diseases. However, other symptoms should be considered also. The tongue should be evaluated with regard to three main characteristics: general

appearance, color, and the presence and color of tongue fur.
- a. Appearance of tongue.
    1) Lean and shriveled (thin, lean, small) — Light red or tender red indicates weakness of the heart and spleen or poor cardiac blood circulation. If the tongue is dry and shriveled and no saliva is present, the disease is difficult to cure.
    2) Swelling — This indicates "water disease", excessive sputum, and flushing up of wet fever.
    3) Rolling — A dry, red tongue indicates severe fever; a white, wet tongue indicates a slight chill; a short, fat tongue indicates wet sputum.
    4) Projecting — Swelling and a tendency to project the tongue is a firmness conformation and indicates sputum fever in the heart. If a child is unable to roll back his tongue after projecting it, the heart *ch'i* is weak.
    5) Stiffness — This indicates apoplexy, weak meridians, and lack of stomach *ch'i*.
    6) Protruding tongue — This indicates fever in the heart and spleen.
    7) Tongue tremor — This indicates "liver wind disease". A trembling tongue accompanied by aphonia is a symptom of weak heart and spleen *ch'i*.
- b. Color.
    1) Red — This signifies weakness of *ch'i* (vitality) in the heart and spleen. A feeling of feverishness on the outside is a sign of high fever. Weakness and internal injury is a yin weakness conformation with high fever.
    2) Deep red — This means that a dangerous fever is beginning.
    3) Purple — If the tongue is swollen, alcohol toxins (from liquor) are affecting the heart. If the tongue is dull and moist, there is an accumulation of stagnant blood. If it is bluish-purple and moist, a chill toxin is beginning to affect the liver and kidneys.
    4) Blue — This indicates an insufficiency of both *ch'i* (vitality) and blood.
- c. Tongue fur.
    1) No fur — Generally, there is no fur on a healthy person's tongue. However, during the initial stages

of febrile diseases, febrile chronic disease, and greater yang diseases, there is also no tongue fur present.

When there is no tongue fur, but the tongue is dry, it is an indication of yang disease. *Pai-hu-tang* (Gypsum Combination) is administered.

When there is no tongue fur, but the tongue is wet, it is an indication of yin disease. *Jen-sheng-tang* (Ginseng and Ginger Combination) is administered.

2) White fur — If the mouth is sticky and the throat is slightly dry, the disease has become a lesser yang disease for which *Hsiao-chai-hu-tang* (Minor Bupleurum Combination) is administered. For extensive, thin, wet fur, *Hsiao-chai-hu-tang* (Minor Bupleurum Combination) is also administered. For thick, white fur, *Pai-hu-tang* (Gypsum Combination) is prescribed.

3) Yellow fur — This means that the disease condition will deteriorate, and the patient should be given *Ta-chai-hu-tang* (Major Bupleurum Combination). If the tongue is yellow and wet, other symptoms should be considered and *Ta-chai-hu-tang* should not be used.

4) Black fur — This is caused by a febrile disease. If the tongue is hard when touched, a purgative should be used. If it is dry and soft, tonics should be given.

5) Purple fur — This signifies a gastrointestinal disease. The following are remedies used for conformations indicated by the condition of the tongue.

a. Stagnant blood conformation: This is indicated by purple spots around the edge of the tongue. Persica and moutan are prescribed.

b. Inside-firm conformation: This is indicated by a short, hard, rolling tongue. The tongue is shortened due to dryness, and it is difficult to uncurl after rolling. This signifies lack of vigor. Purgatives or tonics are used depending on the other symptoms present.

c. Yin conformation: This is indicated by a wet, thin, black tongue that looks like a hairbrush or soot. Aconite should be included in any formula used for treatment, such as *Szu-ni-tang* (Aconite, Ginger, and Licorice Combination).

d. Firmness conformation: This is indicated by a red, dry

tongue. A tongue of this appearance usually occurs in old men who are convalescing and in women after childbirth. Treatment should include rehmannia, anemarrhena, ginseng, and ophiopogon.

Abdomen and Back: There are four different syndromes of the abdomen and back.
  a. Large abdomen: A thick abdominal wall with pale coloring belongs to the *ch'i* (vitality) type. A thin wall with bright coloring belongs to the "water" type. Those with prominent green veins or red striping on the hands and feet belong to the "blood" type.
  b. Convex umbilicus: When there is edema, umbilical "wind" disease, or umbilical hernia in children, convex umbilicus is an adverse symptom.
  c. Back opposite – stretching: This is a sign of toxin disease at the *tu* pulse, and of spasms, tetanus, umbilical "wind" disease, or eclampsia.

Limbs: To diagnose whether the disease is a yin or yang type and whether or not it affects the tendons and bones, the physician observes the strength or weakness of the limbs while the patient stretches and bends.
  a. Spasmic muscular contraction – This indicates convulsive disease or eclampsia.
  b. Pain in the limbs and joints – Marked difficulty in stretching or bending indicates numbness and seasonal apoplexy.
  c. Weakness of the feet which prevents walking – This is a paralysis conformation or beriberi.
  d. Red, swollen, painful legs – This indicates erysipelas and wet, descending fever.
  e. Bending with difficulty stretching – This is indicative of a yin disease of the tendon and muscle.
  f. Difficulty bending legs that are extended – This is indicative of a bone disease.
  g. Leg tremor – This indicates insufficient flow of both *ch'i* and blood.
  h. Tense hand and feet muscles – This indicates a severe chill and tendon and muscle spasm.
  i. Limp hands – This indicates a dissipation of yang vitality.
  j. Clenched hands – This indicates apoplexy, eclampsia,

firm conformation, closeness, any yin toxin concealed inside.
k. Disease of the knee joints — This indicates "wind chill", wet fever, and extravasation of blood at the knee joints.
l. White nail color — This indicates a weakness of the blood.
m. Green nail color — This indicates pain and slow eclampsia.

Skin: The skin is observed for the following conditions:
a. Edema — This indicates obstruction of the flow of *ch'i* (vitality) and fluid accumulation.
b. Dryness and roughness — This signifies weakness in the lungs, and intestinal carbuncles. If, at the same time, the eyes are dull and black, there is dry blood inside the patient's body.
c. Spots — Red spots on the skin indicate either measles (if they do not sting when touched) or chicken pox (if they do sting when touched). Red spots are caused by either warm toxins or chill toxins entering the bloodstream. They appear in two varieties:
(1) *Tan* which are large and lumpy and (2) *Pan* which are large and flat.
d. Blisters — These appear as bright crystals in the form of fine rice. Generally, they appear on the abdomen and back, although a few may appear on the limbs. They occur mainly during the middle stage of a "wet feverish" disease and are caused when the flow of *ch'i* is blocked by the toxin of wet fever and resulting in longterm melancholy.

Human secretions or excrement is classified in four categories: sputum, blood, stool, and urine.

Sputum: Fever sputum is dense, yellow, and sticky. Chill sputum is greenish. Thin sputum (liquid) is called "chill drink". Sputum with air bubbles is called "wind sputum". Sputum with malodorous pus and blood is caused by a lung abscess. Sputum with blood only is due to injury of the lung meridian by fever. Yellow, dense sputum is due to heat and dryness. White, thin sputum is called "wet sputum". Gray sputum is called "chill sputum" and is probably due to the breathing of polluted air. A large volume of sputum that is easily expectorated is "wet sputum", while "dry sputum" has less volume and is difficult to expectorate.

Blood (from coughing or vomiting): Thin, light-colored blood indicates weakness. Dark red blood indicates fever toxin. Blood of the lung meridians is expectorated as a thin thread of blood. Blood from the liver is vomited as a blood clot. Stomach blood appears with a scrap of food, while blood from the lungs appears with sputum. Light red blood is a weakness conformation, whereas bright red blood (heat fever) is a firmness conformation. Fresh, purple, dense blood indicates abundant *ch'i* (vitality), but dark purple blood indicates weak *ch'i* (vitality). Black blood is a symptom of stagnant blood and signifies chill.

Stool: A white, thin stool signifies intestinal chill. Fever of the intestine is indicated by a thin brown or deep yellow stool. The fever is severe if the stool is hard and dry. Weakness of the large intestine and weak chill is indicated by a clear, white stool. A light yellow stool signifies weak fever.

Blood in the stool has three manifestations: 1) Fresh purple indicates that the yin veins have been injured by fever or hemorrhoids; 2) thin stool indicates a weak spleen; 3) black indicates stagnant blood.

Stool with pus is a symptom of diarrhea. If it is white in color, the disease is at *ch'i fen;* if red, the disease is at *hsieh fen.*

Indigestion is a sign of severe inside chill or insufficiency of middle yang. Green stool accompanied by indigestion indicates that liver toxins are attacking the spleen.

Diarrhea with wet fever is indicated by a fish-brain colored stool, while fever diarrhea is signified by a color resembling amaranthus juice.

A large stool means that there is insufficient spleen *ch'i.* A small stool indicated dryness of the intestine.

Urine: Turbidity of the urine indicates a wet, descending fever. If the color of the urine is light yellow, there is a weak fever of the kidney meridian. If it is red-yellow, there is a firm fever of the liver meridian. If it is yellow and turbid, there is wet fever. Deep yellow indicates jaundice. A color resembling Sappan Lignum indicates blood fever.

Clear urine may be due to weakness of the kidney yang in the chill conformation. White urine indicates weakness of *ch'i* (vitality).

Hematuria (blood in the urine) indicates fever in the bladder or kidney damage which is an indirect result of excessive sexual intercourse.

Brown urine indicates kidney disease. If edema is also present, its cause is nephrosis.

A large volume of urine indicates diabetes, while a small volume is the result of edema, excessive sweating, vomiting, or damage to the excretory system.

2. Hearing

The term "hearing" means that the physician discerns chill, fever, weak, or firm conformations by listening to a patient's body and voice sounds (whether high or low, strong or weak, etc.). This process also includes the detection of odors of the body and its secretions (whether sour, sweet, foul, or rotten smelling).

Voice: The pitch and quality of the voice is an indication of the conformation.

  a. Yang conformation – This is indicated by a loud clear voice. A loud, shrieky voice with rambling speech is the result of nightmares.
  b. Yin conformation – This is indicated by a low voice. If the patient's voice sounds like a mosquito and he has alalia, low voice during a nightmare, and repetition of his words, the prognosis is unfavorable.
  c. Weakness conformation – This is indicated by a "decadent sound", that is, a low, moaning voice. Hoarseness is usually caused by internal injury to *ch'i* (vitality).
  d. Firmness conformation – This is indicated by dysphonia which is due to "wind chills and fever". Delirium is indicated by a coarse voice and incoherent speech, and it is caused by firm fever.
  e. Strong physique – This is indicated by a loud and vigorous voice.
  f. Weak physique – This is indicated by a soft and weak voice.
  g. Neuropathy – This is indicated by slow, faltering, unclear speech and a painful chest.

Breath: The quality, quantity, and sound of respirations indicate the conformation.

  a. Firmness conformation – This is indicated by loud, rapid respirations during which the patient shrugs his shoulders.

b. Weakness conformation — This is indicated by quick, shallow respirations, a low, fearful voice, and a weak physique. There is less *ch'i* (vitality) when weakness is due to chronic disease. Yin weakness and fever is caused by shortness of breath (more exhalation than inhalation) or dyspnea due to sputum filling the chest and diaphragm.
c. Asthma — This is caused by the inner obstruction of sputum and by infection due to an externally-caused chill or overconsumption of sugar or salt.
d. Shortness of breath — This is the result of inner-firm sputum and lung weakness.

Cough: A cough which can be heard but which produces no sputum is called *ko*; a cough with sputum but which cannot be heard is called *sou*; a cough which can be heard and which produces sputum is called *ko sou*.

a. Wet cough —This indicates chest distress or "wind chill water conformation". If the sputum is wet or sticky, *Hsiao-ching-lung-tang* (Minor Blue Dragon Combination) is given. If the sputum is very sticky, *Hsiao-chai-hu-tang* (Minor Bupleurum Combination) or *Ta-chai-hu-tang* (Major Bupleurum Combination) is prescribed. If the cough sound is deep, there is infection from an exterior source and wet sputum inside the body.
b. Dry cough — Those with a dry cough should be given *Mai-men-tung-tang* (Ophiopogon Combination) with pinellia and magnolia bark.
c. Yang conformation — Those with cough who are of the yang conformation should be given *Hsiao-ching-lung-tang* (Minor Blue Dragon Combination), *Hsiao-chai-hu-tang* (Minor Bupleurum Combination), or *Yueh-pei-chia-chu-tang* (Atractylodes Combination).
d. Yin conformation — Those with cough who are of the yin conformation should be given *Chen-wu-tang* (Vitality Combination) or *Ma-huang-fu-tzu-hsi-hsin-tang* (Asarum and *Ma-huang* Combination).
e. Distressed cough — This is a continuous cough such as that of children suffering from pertussis.

Vomiting: Noisy retching or nausea is called *ou*; quiet vomiting of matter is called *tu*. Strong, noisy vomiting is a firm conformation, while weak, quiet vomiting is a weak conformation.

Hiccups: Loud, rapid hiccups are a firm-fever conformation. Soft, slow hiccups are a weakness conformation which, if intermittent, indicates weakness of a patient with chronic disease.

Sighing: If breath odor is pleasant, sighing indicates a weak stomach. If the breath odor is sour, sighing indicates indigestion.

Abdominal sounds: Borborygmus indicates mucus, chill, and fluid in the intestine. There is no sound when the large intestine contains dry stool or fever disease is present.

Body odors: These may indicate certain disease conditions.
  a. Foul body odor — This accompanies infectious diseases of a general nature and those resulting from epidemic contagion.
  b. Odor of blood — This occurs after severe hemorrhage.
  c. Malodorous sputum — This is caused by a lung abscess.
  d. Malodorous nasal discharge — This may be due to any nasal disease.
  e. Halitosis — This indicates stomach fever.
  f. Sour breath — This indicates indigestion.
  g. Fetid mouth odor — This is due to tooth decay or gum disease.
  h. Fruity breath odor — This indicates acidosis of severe diabetes.

Stool: Intestinal chill is indicated by a foul, malodorous stool. Accumulated fever in the intestine is indicated by malodorous stool also. Noxious flatus signifies indigestion.

Menses and vaginal discharge: When there is a "dirty" odor, it indicates a wet-fever conformation. If there is a rank odor, it is a sign of chill-weak conformation.

3. **Questioning**

The main purpose of questioning is to uncover the patient's subjective symptoms. Through interrogation, the physician comes to an understanding of the patient's lifestyle and habits, his subjective symptoms and various diseases, and his previous medical history. This information should be elicited in detail so that the physician may have a basis for understanding the present symptoms and for further diagnosis.

Careful questioning and observation of the patient's mental state (whether normal or abnormal) is essential for precise diagnosis. The patient should be asked about the following:

Patient history: The patient's history includes his family medical history, his prior medical history, the state of his present disease, and the treatment prescribed. From this information the physician is able to understand the patient's body condition, tendencies, and response to herb formulas and chemical drugs. When there is an acute fever disease, it is important to know both the amount of time since the onset and the nature of treatment.

Severe chill or severe wind: Severe chill means that the patient feels chilled more or less continuously. Severe wind means that the patient feels uncomfortable only when he faces the wind or is in contact with the cold air. Severe wind is the less serious of the two. Both belong to the greater yang diseases are divided into surface, yin, and yang conformations. When either of these conditions is present and there is a floating pulse with fever, it is a yang conformation. If there is a sinking pulse without fever, severe chill, and easy fatiguability, it is a yin conformation.

Sweat: The presence or lack of sweat may, in combination with consideration of other symptoms, indicate the conformation.

a. Surface-weak — This is indicated by perspiration (mostly on the head) and fever. If it is a symptom of a greater yang disease with sweat, *Kuei-chih-tang* (Cinnamon Combination) is administered. Occasionally, the patient does not sweat, in which case the conformation may be determined by feeling the pulse. For floating and weak pulse, *Kuei-chih-tang* is used.

b. Surface-strong — This is indicated when there is no perspiration but the patient has had a fever and severe chill. In this case, the patient's pulse will be floating and tight and is the surface-strong conformation of a greater yang disease.

c. Yang Disease — Lesser yang disease is indicated by perspiration on the head and night sweats. Sunlight yang disease is indicated when there is profuse diaphoresis during tide fever. In the treatment of yang disease, a diaphoretic should be given. If it does not produce sweat, the symptom has become a weakness conformation for which a diaphoretic cannot be used.

Perspiration on the head indicates stomach fever and flushing up of yang *ch'i* (vitality). Sweating of the hands and feet signifies inside-strong sunlight yang disease as well as weakness of *ch'i* (vitality). Sweating when there is no fever (cold sweat) signifies weakness of yang *ch'i*, while sweating when there is fever signifies strong yang *ch'i* (vitality).

Yin Disease — Normally there is no perspiration in yin

disease. If sweating does occur, it is called "releading sweat" and indicates a severe condition. Night sweats are a sign of yin weakness.

Certain conditions are also indicated by the circumstances and severity of the patient's sweating.
   a. Shuddering sweat — If the patient is relaxed and has a quiet pulse after sweating, his state is normal. If he is confused, irritable, and has a large pulse, his state is abnormal.
   b. Profuse diaphoresis — This condition, which looks like oil dripping from the patient's body, indicates loss of yang and weakness.
   c. Sweating over half the body — This indicates apoplexy.

Fever: The term "fever" refers not only to a rise in body temperature, but also to the patient's subjective feeling of heat within his body or a part of his body. Usually, those of yang conformation and those with a high rate of metabolism have fever. Occasionally, fever exists in diseases of yin conformation. Therefore, when considering fever it is important to discern correctly its type (yin, yang, weak, or firm) and its site in the patient's body.

Various terms are used to describe the types of fever.
   a. Dry fever — Urine volume is normal, but fever is present.
   b. Wet fever — There is oliguria with fever.
   c. Tide fever — This is a sunlight yang disease characterized only by fever. There are no chills, but the fever rises and falls regularly (like the tides). Purgatives are used.
   d. Surface fever — This is a symptom of surface disease for which *Kuei-chih-tang* (Cinnamon Combination) is used. If there is severe inside fever, *Ta-cheng-chi-tang* (Major Rhubarb Combination) is used.
   e. Alternating chills and fever — This is the primary symptoms of lesser yang disease or malaria. If symptoms occur every two days, it is tertian malaria; if they occur every three days, it is quartan malaria.
   f. Mild fever — The subjective feeling of a moderate elevation in inside body temperature is an inside conformation.
   g. Fever with anxiety — This usually occurs in patients with chest distress and is a weak fever conformation. Formulas containing rehmannia are prescribed. For fever of the

hands and feet accompanied by anxiety, *Pa-wei-ti-huang-wan* (Rehmannia Eight Formula) is prescribed.
h. Fever with severe chill — This indicates surface infections caused by external toxins.
i. Yin chill — Chilled limbs signify a large amount of yin chill. If there is a high fever, it is a true fever and not a chill conformation.
j. Accumulated fever — If fever has accumulated in the body, the patient has a burning sensation in the chest and abdomen.
k. Weakness — Patients with fever in the morning usually have *ch'i* weakness. Chills without fever indicate weakness of yang. Fever in the afternoon and bone fever indicate weakness of yin. Fever accompanied by irritability is due to weakness of yin and is a "heat strong" conformation.

Appetite: Variations in appetite and the circumstances in which they occur may indicate the conformation.
a. Firmness conformation — If patients of this type have overeaten, vomiting and diarrhea do not occur, and they are not hungry if a meal is delayed.
b. Weakness conformation — These patients have a sensation of fullness beneath the heart after overeating, and vomiting and diarrhea will also occur. If a meal is delayed, they will feel weak. They have no appetite and feel full after eating a small amount. This conformation is due to a weakness of yang.
c. Yang diseases — If the patient has a normal appetite, it is the surface conformation of greater yang disease. If the patient has a sticky feeling and a bitter taste in his mouth along with a decrease in appetite, it means that the disease has become a lesser yang conformation.
d. Yin diseases — Usually, the patient has anorexia and a dry, bitter taste in his mouth but is not thirsty. Patients of the absolute yin conformation feel hungry but do not want to eat. If they do eat, they will vomit immediately. If food is retained but fatigue occurs after eating, there is gastrointestinal weakness. *Liu-chun-tzu-tang* (Six Major Herb Combination) is suitable for use.
e. Fever disease — This is indicated by a tendency to drink

large amounts of fluids. This tendency may also be an "emaciation-thirst" symptom.
- f. Inside fever — This is indicated by a preference for hot beverages.
- g. Inside chill — This is indicated by a preference for hot beverages and is due to the presence of wet sputum inside.
- h. Overeating and continuous hunger — This indicates stomach fever.
- i. Stomach distress after eating — This indicates a stagnancy of *ch'i*, the obstruction of food, and tympanites.
- j. Pica — This indicates the presence of worms in the digestive system.
- k. Acatoposis — This is different from anorexia. If the patient finds eating difficult because of abdominal swelling, the swelling should be treated first.

Stool: The consistency and contents of the stool, the circumstances under which it is passed, and the existence of specific other symptoms are indications of the conformation.
- a. Firmness conformation — This is indicated by fecal incontinence due to high fever, and by semiconsciousness.
- b. Weakness conformation — This is indicated by constipation and/or abdominal distention with weakness. Scatacratia may also be an indication. Warm tonics are suitable for use. Constipation with shortness of breath, sweating, vertigo, and diarrhea at the Fifth Watch (3 to 5 a.m.) are signs of kidney yang weakness. Indigestion indicates spleen and kidney weakness and chill.
- c. Firmness conformation — This is indicated by constipation with a hard stool for which purgatives are used. Patients with diarrhea and pressing pain at the lower part of the heart should be given *Ta-chai-hu-tang* (Major Bupleurum Combination). Patients with diarrhea and tenesmus should be given rhubarb or paeonia. The stool of this type of patient is dry, sticky, black or dark brown in color, and malodorous. If the stool consists of pellets, moistening agents such as rehmannia and ginseng are used.
- d. Fever conformation — This is indicated by constipation,

fever, fetid breath odor, abdominal distension, reddish urine. If the patient has abdominal pain (cramping), it will be followed immediately by diarrhea with yellow-brown stool and micturition with reddish urine.

e. Chill conformation — This is indicated by constipation, pale lips, a late pulse, shivering, and a desire for warmth. If there is continuous abdominal pain, the stool will be loose.

f. Wind conformation — This is indicated by constipation, generalized itching, and a floating pulse. "Intestine wind" is the copious discharge of fresh, red blood before defecation.

g. Toxicity of the viscera — This is indicated by pain and swelling at the anus and by the excretion of dark, decomposed blood before the stool.

h. Exhaustion of the blood — This is indicated by night sweats, dry mouth with adipsia, and fever accompanied by irritability (especially at night).

i. Distant blood — This is indicated by dull red-colored blood following the excretion of stool. The patient will also become fatigued easily and have a poor complexion, both of which symptoms are due to poor blood circulation in the spleen.

Urine: Symptoms should be evaluated on the basis of frequency, volume, and color of the urine.

a. Yang conformation — The main indication is dysuria, which is divided into the categories of weak and strong. Dysuria is due to excessive sweating, diarrhea, and vomiting, all of which cause patients to lose body fluids; food and liquid intake should be increased in order to restore them. Enuresis signifies yang weakness of the kidney.

b. Yin conformation — This is indicated by excessive urinary volume.

c. Weakness conformation — Urinary incontinence and frequent micutrition with small amounts of urine are the main indication.

d. Stagnant blood — Patients with stagnant blood have a high urine volume. *Pa-wei-ti-huang-wan* (Rehmannia Eight Formula) is administered. Patients who have

stagnant blood with dysuria should be given *Ti-tang-tang* (Rhubarb and Leech Combination). Urine that is dull red or dark brown indicates a yang conformation. Light and clear urine indicates a yin conformation.
  e. Firmness conformation — This is indicated by difficulty in stool and urine excretion. After the bowels have moved, urination will usually become normal.

Thirst and Dry Mouth: The symptom of thirst is a desire to drink water and a feeling of dryness in the throat. Dryness of the mouth is due to decreased saliva secretion and is accompanied by a desire to moisten the mouth but not to drink water. Both symptoms are of the yin conformation for which mild tonic agents are administered. Patients suffering from stagnant blood may also complain of thirst.

Severe thirst is divided into yin and yang conformations:
  a. Yin conformation — This is indicated by the patient's desire for hot liquids (particularly soup). At the last stage of yin conformation, however, the preference may be for cold liquids. At this time, *Chen-wu-tang* (Vitality Combination) should be given.
  b. Yang conformation — This is indicated by the patient's desire for cold liquids, although patients of the severe yang type prefer hot liquids. *Pai-hu-tang* (Gypsum Combination) is given.

Vomiting: Vomiting with sound but no matter is called *ou*, while vomiting with matter but no sound is called *tu*. Vomiting with both sound and matter is called *"ou tu"*. The physician should ask if the patient experienced nausea, thirst, dysuria, or headache in the period during which the vomiting occurred.

When vomiting occurs immediately after eating, it may be due to indigestion, stomach heat, or dysphagia. If the patient has eaten during the morning and vomits in the afternoon, it may be due to indigestion, weakness of the stomach, and stomach chill.

Severe vomiting, called "adverse vomiting", is characterized by nausea and frequent vomiting of matter which includes thick mucus. Pinellia is prescribed. "Water flushing-up" is the condition in which the patient has a dry mouth and vomits a large amount of water. In this case, *Wu-ling-san* (Hoélen Five Herb Formula) is administered. *Wu-chu-yu-tang* (Evodia Combination) is given to patients suffering from vomiting accompanied by severe headache.

Cough: The following questions should be asked by the physician regarding cough:
- a. Does a wheezing sound accompany the cough?
- b. Is there sputum (wet cough) or not (dry cough)?
- c. Is the sputum easily expectorated?
- d. Does the face turn red with exertion when coughing?
- e. Is there any dryness of the throat? Any odor?
- f. If there is asthmatic wheezing, is it more severe at night?
- g. Is the cough more severe on arising?

Patients who are coughing and have severe chills, fever, and surface conformations should be treated first for the surface conformations. If the cough is accompanied by asthmatic wheezing and insomnia, it will be paroxysmal in nature and is due to swelling of the lungs and stagnation of the sputum. Chronic cough accompanied by sweating indicates exhaustion of lung vitality and a lack of kidney *ch'i*. Cough with chest pain indicates the presence of a lung abscess, an accumulation of sputum, and liver toxins attacking the lungs.

Palpitations: This is a throbbing sensation which is produced by the pulsation of the heart and the major arteries below the heart and abdomen. It is indicative of a weakness conformation. When palpitations are intense *Chih-kan-tsao-tang* (Baked Licorice Combination) or *Kuei-chih-chia-lung-ku-mu-li-tang* (Cinnamon and Dragon Bone Combination) is given.

Dizziness: Physicians of Western medicine believe that dizziness is caused by disorders of the nervous, digestive, or circulatory systems or by anemia eye disease, or ear disease. In the Chinese medical system, however, physicians attribute dizziness to water toxin and stagnant blood. Therefore, most prescriptions for treating dizziness contain hoelen and alisma, herbs which regulate the balance of water in the body.

Dizziness with a feeling of heaviness in the head is called *mao hsuan*. Usually, dizziness and vertigo are caused by insufficient yin, "wind fever", chills, ascites, and weakness of the blood and liver yang. Cold diseases are characterized by pallor and dizziness with a feeling of heaviness in the head.
- a. Yin conformation — This is indicated by a sunken abdomen, pallor, and weakness. *Chen-wu-tang* (Vitality Combination) and *Tang-kuei-shao-yao-san* (Tang-kuei and Paeonia Formula) are prescribed.

b. Yang conformation — When dizziness occurs in this conformation, cinnamom and hoelen are prescribed.

Headaches: This is divided into yin, yang, weak, and strong categories.
   a. Greater yang disease — This is indicated by headache at the neck and the back of the head accompanied by fever, severe chills, and a floating and tight pulse. It is a surface conformation and *Ma-huang-tang* (*Ma-huang* Combination) is prescribed.
   b. Lesser yang disease — This is indicated by headache accompanied by a sinking pulse. It is a bilious headache and *Ma-huang-hsi-hsin-fu-tzu-tang* (*Ma-huang*, Aconite, and Asarum Combination) is prescribed.
   c. Sunlight yang diseases — This is indicated by a headache located at the forehead and extending to the eyebrow edge. When the pain involves the entire head, the cause is an infection by an exterior toxin of the three yang.
   d. Lesser yin diseases — This is indicated by a severe headache with vomiting, cold limbs, and a sinking pulse. *Wu-chu-yu-tang* (Evodia Combination) is given.
   e. Weakness conformation — This is indicated by morning headache, afternoon headache, intermittent headaches with severe pain, lassitude, and fatigue.
   f. Firmness conformation — This is indicated by a continuous headache caused by a toxin.

Shoulder ache: Stiffness and aching of the shoulder may include the neck and the back of the head. Sometimes the tension may extend to the shoulder articulation as well. The pain may be unilateral or bilateral.

For shoulder stiffness in a patient with strong, tense abdominal and limb muscles, *Ko-ken-tang* (Pueraria Combination) is suitable. For shoulder stiffness in a patient with weak tendons and muscles and a weak pulse and abdomen, *Pan-hsia-pai-chu-tien-ma-tang* (Pinellia and Gastrodia Combination), *Liu-chun-tzu-tang* (Major Six Herb Combination), or *Tang-kuei-shao-yao-san* (*Tang-kuei* and Paeonia Formula) is prescribed. If the stiffness is in the left shoulder, '*Yen-nien-pan-hsia-tang* (Pinellia and Evodia Combination) is prescribed.

Lumbago: Lumbago has three causes: pathological change of the soft tissue at the waist, abnormality of articulating bone joints, and pathological change of viscera in the pelvic cavity resulting from complications of various diseases. In order to establish the direction of therapy, the physician should evaluate the pulses and results of abdominal palpation before completing his diagnosis.

    a. Lumbago with weakness and fatigue — *Pa-wei-ti-huang-wan* (Rehmannia Eight Formula) is prescribed. For sudden-onset lumbago in children, *Ko-ken-tang* (Pueraria Combination) is used.

    b. Lumbago in abdominal disease with stagnant blood — *Kuei-chih-fu-ling-wan* (Cinnamon and Hoelen Formula) or *Tao-ho-cheng-chi-tang* (Persica and Rhubarb Combination) is prescribed.

    c. Lumbago with chills — This is a recalcitrant type of lumbago in which the patient experiences pain that becomes severe and extends to the lower limbs or lower abdomen when he is chilled by cold air. In ancient times this was called "hernia". *Tang-kuei-chien-chung-tang* (*Tang-kuei*, Cinnamon, and Paeonia Combination) is prescribed.

Abdominal pain: The physician should ask clearly the following questions regarding the patient's abdominal pain:

    a. Where is the pain located?
    b. Is the pain worse when pressure is applied?
    c. Is the pain continuous or intermittent?
    d. In which direction does the pain radiate?
    e. Under what conditions is the pain more severe?
    f. If the pain is spasmodic in nature, does any other symptom follow the episodes of cramping?

The patient's answers to these questions indicate the conformation.

    a. Yang conformation — This is indicated by acute abdominal pain, constipation, abdominal distention, and a desire to become cooler. It is part of the dry firmness conformation of the sunlight yang type. Periumbilical pain is the viscera firmness conformation of sunlight yang disease. *Ta-chai-hu-tang* (Major Bupleurum Combination) and *Ta-huang-mu-tan-pi-tang* (Rhubarb and Moutan Combination) are prescribed.

    b. Yin conformation — This is indicated by chronic abdo-

minal pain, or "hernia". *Hsiao-chien-chung-tang* (Minor Cinnamon and Paeonia Combination), or *Jen-sheng-tang* (Ginseng and Ginger Combination), a mild tonic, is prescribed.
  c. Chill conformation — Periumbilical pain is an indication of a weak-chill conformation. Borborygmus and abdominal pain are signs of intestinal chill.
  d. Weakness conformation — This is indicated by a distended abdomen, an inclination to press the abdomen, a desire for warmth, and a loose stool. Generalized pain that has a tendency to shift is also characteristic of this conformation. The cause is spleen weakness.

Chest pain: When diagnosing chest pain, the physician should take into consideration the abdominal conformation and the other symptoms. Usually, bupleurum is prescribed as the main herb for chest pain or numbness.
  a. Rib pain — This is an indication of liver damage, liver heat, stagnant water in the stomach (ascites), obstruction of blood flow, and obstruction of *ch'i*.
  b. Chest distress — This is lesser yang disease and indicates liver damage and obstruction of *ch'i*.
  c. Subcardiac swelling — The patient has a feeling of blockage in the chest and has no appetite. The chest feels soft when pressure is applied. *San-huang-hsieh-hsin-tang* (Coptis and Rhubarb Combination) is prescribed.
  d. Subcardiac swelling and hardness — The patient has a feeling of distress in the heart area and has no appetite. The chest feels hard when pressed. *Ta-chai-hu-tang* (Major Bupleurum Combination) is prescribed.
  e. Cardiac swelling — The patient suffers from ascending and accumulating air in the chest. *Jen-sheng-tang* (Ginseng and Ginger Combination) is prescribed.

As the *ch'i* (vitality) of the heart becomes weak, the patient is aware of palpitations. The patient of weak-fever conformation feels depressed and becomes delirious. Delirium is also characteristic of an inside-fever conformation.

Bleeding: The physician should ask the patient where the bleeding occurs. In addition to the source of bleeding, the color of the blood, the general symptoms, the pulse, and the complexion should be taken into consideration.

Patients of fever conformation with warm hands and feet, good complexion, strong pulse, and congestion should be given *San-huang-hsieh-hsin-tang* (Coptis and Rhubarb Combination). Those with cold hands and feet, poor complexion, feeble pulse, and stagnant blood should be given *Szu-wu-tang* (*Tang-kuei* Four Combination), while those with intermediate conformations should be given *Wen-ching-yin* (*Tang-kuei* and Gardenia Combination). If profuse bleeding causes anemia, *Tu-sheng-tang* (Ginseng Combination) is prescribed. When bleeding occurs and there is stagnant blood, *Tao-ho-cheng-chi-tang* (Persica and Rhubarb Combination) is used.

Absolute Chill of the hands and feet: When both the hands and feet are chilled, *Tang-kuei-szu-ni-tang* (*Tang-kuei* and Jujube Combination) is given. If the patient feels chilled in the lower body only, *Wen-ching-yin* (*Tang-kuei* and Gardenia Combination) is recommended.

Edema: This is the retention of fluid in the tissues and is divided into "surface" and "inside" types.
    a. Surface edema — This type of edema can be either "wind swelling" or "skin swelling". The former is caused by water toxins or exterior toxins. It is characterized by the surface conformations of floating pulse, perspiration, and a feeling of being very cold. *Hsiao-ching-lung-tang* (Minor Blue Dragon Combination) is prescribed. "Skin swelling" edema is caused by water toxins and is not accompanied by fever or a feeling of being cold. *Fang-chi-fu-ling-tang* (Stephania and Hoelen Combination) is used.
    b. Inside edema — This is characterized by difficult micturition and a sinking pulse. *Yueh-pei-chia-chu-tang* (Atractylodes Combination) is prescribed.

Tinnitus: This is characterized by a continuous ringing or buzzing sound in the outer or inner ear. It is caused by water toxins, stagnant blood, or food poisoning.

Bradyecoia: There are two types of partial deafness, middle ear bradyecoia and inner ear bradyecoia. Chinese herbal physicians classify them as follows:
    a. Obstruction by heat — This is due to an ascending reaction, cerebral congestion, or hypertension. *Hsieh-hsin-tang* is given.
    b. Obstruction by toxin — This is caused by inflammation

of the middle ear. *Ko-ken-tang* (Pueraria Combination) is prescribed.
  c. Obstruction of the opening — This is caused by inflammation of the external ear.
  d. Obstruction due to weakness — This occurs during convalescence, old age, and excessive fatigue. *Pa-wei-ti-huang-wan* (Rehmannia Eight Formula) is given.
  e. Obstruction due to stagnancy of *ch'i* — *Chai-hu-tang* (Bupleurum Combination) in combination with *Hsiang-su-yin* (Cyperus and Perilla Combination) is prescribed.

Menses: The amount and color of menstrual blood as well as the regularity or irregularity of periods is indicative of particular conditions.
  a. Blood fever — This is characterized by frequent periods with excessive flow of bright red blood.
  b. Weakness of blood — This is indicated by delayed periods and a decreased flow.
  c. Stagnant blood and obstruction of *ch'i* — In this condition there is no definite period and the flow is minimal with dull, purple clots.
  d. Weakness of *ch'i* — This is indicated by a large amount of light red blood.

Leucorrhea: Determination of conformation is based on the color, odor, and amount of leucorrhea.
  a. Wet fever — Generally, the discharge is yellow in color. When it is green, there is descending wet fever of the liver meridians. Red-white color accompanied by a strong fetid odor is due to the lingering of wet fever.
  b. Wet chill — There is a malodorous discharge.
  c. Weakness of spleen and liver damage — There is a large amount of discharge.

Mental states: The following conditions are indicated by the patient's mental state:
  a. Lethargy — This condition occurs when fever attacks the spirit.
  b. Sleeping sickness — This occurs when yang is weak, yin is strong, and there is obstruction of wet sputum.
  c. Insomnia and amnesia — This is due to weakness of the heart and kidneys, anemia, exhaustion of the heart and

spleen, and yin weakness of the liver and kidneys.
d. Desire to rest and sleepiness — This is a lesser yang disease which is due to weakness of the heart and kidneys.
e. Mental aberration — This is caused by mental or emotional illness, mania, epilepsy, or dry viscera.

4. Touching

Diagnosis by "touching" means that the physician examines the patient's body directly through palpation. There are two main classifications, pulse feeling and abdominal palpation.

Pulse Feeling: The physician determines the patient's pulse rate by measuring it against the rhythm of his own normal respiration, and he discerns the state of the pulse by feeling it with his fingers. This is called "feeling the pulse.". During pulse feeling the physician should be aware of the patient's physical characteristics such as height, weight, age, and sex. Usually obese people have sinking pulses and lean people have floating pulses. A child's pulse is faster than an adult's.

The site of pulse feeling is the radial arteries. In *Huang ti nei ching* and *Su wen,* the earliest records dealing with pulse feeling, it is stated that three parts of the body, the head, hands, and feet, each have a different pulse area. However, the complete information contained in these classics has been lost for a long time. The pulse feeling method presently used is recorded in *Ling shu* and is called the *Jen Yin* pulse.

Through pulse feeling, the physician is able to diagnose various related diseases. While Western medicine emphasizes the importance of the frequency and strength of the pulse, Chinese medicine takes into consideration all of the following points:
a. Observation of the pathological site — The pathological site is determined by palpating the three points of *tsun kou, kuan shang,* and *chih chung.* On the left wrist the physician can detect symptoms relating to the heart and

small intestine by touching *tsun kou,* symptoms relating to the liver and gall bladder by touching *kuan shang,* and symptoms relating to the kidneys and bladder by touching *chih chung.* By palpating the artery in the right wrist, the physician can detect symptoms relating to the lungs and large intestine when touching *tsun kou,* symptoms relating to the spleen and stomach by touching *kuan shang,* and symptoms of *ming men* (the triple warmer) and the reproductive system and circulation of vital energy by touching *chih chung.*

b. Determination of surface, inside, weakness, and firmness conformations — Patients with a floating pulse have a surface conformation, while those with a sinking pulse have an inside conformation. Those with a floating, weak pulse belong to the surface weak type, while those with a sinking, smooth pulse are of an inisde-firm conformation.

c. Discernment of chill or fever conformation — A patient with a floating, fast pulse is of a surface fever conformation, while one with a sinking, slow pulse belongs to an inside chill conformation. Patients with a ·floating, late pulse are of the surface fever, inside chill type.

d. Simple evaluation of conformations — Patients with headache, fever, severe chill, and a floating, quick pulse are of the surface fever firmness conformation for which *Ma-huang-tang* (*Ma-huang* Combination) is prescribed. Those with a floating, weak pulse are of the surface-fever weakness conformation for which *Kuei-chih-tang* (Cinnamon Combination) is prescribed.

e. Prognosis — Patients with surface conformations and surface toxins have floating, fast pulses. If the patient's pulse is sinking and late, he may recover from his illness. If the patient's symptoms indicate a severe illness of the sunlight yang conformation, he will suffer from tide fever, delirium, and unconsciousness. If the patient has a tense pulse, he may recover; if it is obstructed, he will die within a short time.

f. Discernment of pathological physiology — By means of pulse feeling, the physician may determine what the course of the disease will be. If the patient has a smooth, fast pulse and eats excessively, he should be given purgatives. If there is edema, the pulse will be sinking and small. If there is appendicitis and suppuration has occurred, the pulse will be large and fast.

g. Discernment of the nature of the disease — Tense pulse indicates diarrhea. Fast and solid pulse indicates lung abscesses, while fast but void pulse indicates tuberculosis.

Method of pulse feeling: The method used and the physical and mental state of the physician are very important when feeling the pulse. It should be done in the early morning prior to the intake of any food, and the physician should be quiet, relaxed, and have his mind clear of other matters. He then gently places his three fingers on the patient's wrist with his index, middle, and ring fingers on the *tsun kou, kuan shang,* and *chih chung* points, respectively. Sometimes the fingers are pressed lightly, sometimes heavily. Pulse feeling is divided into the following categories:

a. Floating
1. Floating — With a light touch the physician can feel the pulse floating on the surface of skin. This is a surface yang conformation. Patients who have an acute febrile disease with a floating pulse have a surface conformation of greater yang disease. If the patient's pulse is floating and fast, it is a surface firm conformation, but if it is floating and feeble, it is a surface weak conformation.
2. Large — The breadth of the pulsation is large and wide. It is an indication of yang abundance along with strong heat diseases. Patients with a large, fast pulse often suffer from abdominal pain or intestinal parasites.
3. Stronger — The pulse is stronger than the ordinary pulse, but it does not signify great danger. This is a weakness conformation which is due to the presence of a potent toxin.
4. Hollow — This is a floating, strong pulse which feels hollow inside and like it has a hard wall similar to a scallion stalk outside. It indicates a loss of blood.
5. Soft — The pulse is very small, soft, and floating. It is caused by various weaknesses (i.e. kidney weakness or exhaustion of vitality) and the presence of wet toxin.

6. Strong — This is a large, tense pulse which feels hollow inside and hard (like a drum surface) outside. It is a symptom of accumulation and is caused by chill abundance, inside weakness, or premature delivery with excessive bleeding.
7. Tense — This pulse feels like a tight string of a drawn bow and has little up-and-down rhythm and no left-right movement. It is an indication of lesser yang disease. Patients with muscle spasm or water toxin exhibit this kind of pulse as do those suffering from liver disease, sputum accumulation, pain, or malaria.

b. Sinking Pulse
1. Sinking — This pulse becomes apparent with firmer pressure. It indicates that the disease is internal and is a yin conformation caused by a stagnancy of *ch'i* (vitality). A purgative is used for a sinking, strong pulse (an inside strong conformation). A tonic is used for a sinking, weak pulse (an inside weak conformation).
2. Hidden — This pulse is deeply concealed and can only be detected when the physician presses the artery very firmly. When disease is indicated, the site of it is very deep and the cause is an obstruction of toxin. It belongs to an absolute conformation. A sweating or vomiting agent is frequently used to expel the toxin rapidly.
3. Firm — This is a sinking, tense, solid, large, and long pulse. It is caused by inside yin chill and abdominal pain.

c. Late-Slow Pulse
1. Late — This is due to insufficient yang vitality, chilled *ch'i* (vitality) and blood, and accumulated cold. It belongs to inside chill conformation. A floating-late or sinking-late-pulse is an inside-chill-weakness conformation for which formulas containing aconite should be given. A late but strong pulse belongs to the late-strong conformation for which purgatives are used.
2. Slow — This is a normal pulse consisting of four beats per respiratory cycle, and it is a sign of alleviation. The patient with this pulse will have an early recovery

from illness.
3. Obstructed — This is a small, late pulse which feels very rough and astringent (like scraping bamboo with a knife). A patient suffering from blood loss, lack of vigor, stagnant blood, and obstruction of *ch'i* (vitality) exhibits this type of pulse.
4. Knotted — This pulse is slow with sudden interruptions. It indicates that a large amount of stagnant blood is accumulating in the body.
5. Uneven — This is an irregular pulse which is sometimes loose and weak, sometimes tense and tight, sometimes fast, sometimes late. It indicates weakness and lack of vitality in the viscera and that the disease has become very serious.

d. Fast Pulse (exceeding 90 beats per minute for adults)
1. Fast — The fast pulse has six beats per respiratory cycle and indicates fever in the body (weak-strong fever).
2. Rapid — This pulse is very fast, having seven to eight beats per respiratory cycle. It is a serious sign and indicates exhaustion of the patient's vitality.
3. Quick — This pulse is very quick with frequent interruptions and is part of the heat conformation. It indicates abundant yang, strong fever, carbuncles, and obstruction of blood, food, sputum, and *ch'i* (vitality).
4. Movable — This pulse is shaped like a pea and feels smooth, strong, and movable. Patients suffering from pain, fright, or bleeding will exhibit this pulse.
5. Tight — This is similar to the tense pulse, but it can move from left to right. A patient suffering from chill or pain will exhibit this pulse.

e. Void Pulse
1. Void — This pulse is floating, late, and slow and is very difficult to find. It is a weakness conformation.
2. Scattered — This pulse is confused and floating; the physician feels nothing when pressing the artery. It is an indication that the patient's condition is serious.
3. Feeble — This pulse is very difficult to detect; sometimes it is apparent, sometimes it is not. It indicates

loss of yang and serious blood and *ch'i* (vitality) weakness. Tonics should be given.
   4. Weak — This pulse is small, sinking, and weak. The physician will feel nothing upon deep touching. It indicates chronic disease with weak yang and insufficient *ch'i* (vitality) and blood. The patient with a floating, weak pulse should be given a sweating agent. If the pulse is too weak, however, a sweating agent should not be used.
   5. Small — This pulse is small and fine (like a tiny, soft thread). It indicates weakness of *ch'i* (vitality) and blood, exhaustion, and wet *ch'i* attacking downward.
   6. Short — This pulse arises from the middle and is small, weak, and abnormal. It indicates weak and insufficient *ch'i* (vitality) and blood.
f. Solid Pulse
   1. Solid — This pulse feels strong on either deep or light touching. It is substantial and vigorous, belonging to the firmness conformation and the heart conformation. It indicates toxin accumulation.
   2. Long — This pulse is very long and is straight from beginning to end. It indicates ascending *ch'i* and abundant heat.
   3. Smooth — This is a smooth pulse which feels warm and firm. When it occurs as part of a weakness conformation, it indicates a severe disease condition. When it occurs in a patient with an abundance of blood, it may indicate a state of good health. Patients with sputum disease, stagnant blood, or pregnancy also exhibit a smooth pulse.
f. Dying Pulse
   1. Dying — The pulse has an abnormal rhythm which is feeble and small.
   2. Boiling pot — This pulse is floating (like a pot of boiling soup). The flow is not smooth, and it indicates lung exhaustion, severe fever, and loss of Yin.
   3. Swaying fish — This pulse resembles the tail movement of a resting fish; it is a dangerous state of obstructed pulse. It indicates uneven blood circulation, heart failure, severe chill of the three yin, and

loss of yang.
4. Rebounding stone — This pulse is between the tendon and the muscles. It is quick and firm with a rebounding action and indicates kidney failure.
5. Loose rope — This pulse in on the tendon and muscles and is scattered and unconcentrated. It indicates spleen failure, depletion of kidney *ch'i,* and exhaustion of *ming men* (located between the two kidneys).
6. Rain dropping from the edge of a roof — This pulse is between the tendon and the muscles and is uneven (like rain dropping from the edge of a roof). It signifies exhaustion of the stomach.
7. Shrimp swimming — This pulse is just beneath the skin surface, and it appears irregularly. It indicates exhaustion of the large intestine.
8. Bird pecking — This pulse is between the tendon and the muscles and feels like the pecking of a bird. It indicates depletion of stomach *ch'i.*
9. Knife edge — This pulse feels like the sharp edge of a knife. It does not deviate, does not rise, does not fall. It indicates exhaustion of the liver.
10. Rotating pea — This pulse feels like a rotating pea and indicates heart failure.
11. Fast and indefinite — This pulse is small, feeble, and indefinite. A patient with this pulse will die within one day.

Complicated, abnormal pulses: During clinical pulse feeling, most patient exhibit two or more kinds of abnormal pulses such as: floating and fast; floating, late, and sinking; sinking and late; tense and small; tense and obstructed; tight and tense; sinking and tight; sinking and knotted; small and late; feeble and small; smooth and fast; large and weak.

1. Floating and fast — This floating pulse has more beats than normal. It belongs to the surface-fever conformation and indicates a surface conformation or metabolic hyperfunction of the upper body. For floating, quick, and weak pulse, *Kuei-chih-tang* (Cinnamon Combination) is given. For floating, quick, and tight pulse, *Ma-huang-tang* (*Ma-huang* Combination) is given.

2. Floating, late, and sinking — This indicates poor metabolism and chill within the body. *Jen-sheng-tang* (Ginseng and Ginger Combination) is given.
3. Sinking and late — A sinking, late, and solid pulse is an inside-firmness conformation for which *Cheng-chi-tang* (Rhubarb Combination) is prescribed. For a sinking, late, and weak pulse, *Jen-sheng-tang* (Ginseng and Ginger Combination) is administered.
4. Tense and small — *Hsiao-chai-hu-tang* (Minor Bupleurum Combination) is given.
5. Tense and obstructed — This indicates depletion of body fluids and tendon and muscle spasms. *Hsiao-chien-chung-tang* (Minor Cinnamon and Paeonia Combination) is prescribed.
6. Tight and tense — This indicates pain caused by an accumulation of water toxin in one part of the body. Warm *Ta-huang-fu-tzu-tang* (Rhubarb and Aconite Combination) is used to effect elimination of the water toxin.
7. Sinking and tight — This is an indication of shortness of breath, palpitations, decreased urine volume, and edema induced by water toxin. *Mu-fang-chi-tang* (Stephania and Ginseng Combination) is given.
8. Sinking and knotted — This is an indication of the presence of stagnant blood. *Tao-ho-cheng-chi-tang* (Persica and Rhubarb Combination) is prescribed.
9. Small and late or feeble and small — This indicates chilled hands and feet. *Tang-kuei-szu-ni-tang* (*Tang-kuei* and Jujube Combination) is administered.
10. Smooth and fast — This indicates that rapid metabolism is forming a fever disease. *Pai-hu-tang* (Gypsum Combination) is used.
11. Large and weak — This indicates physical weakness and lack of vigor. *Shih-chuan-ta-pu-tang* (Ginseng and *Tang-kuei* Ten Combination) is given.

Abdominal Touching: The purpose of abdominal touching is to determine the weakness or firmness so that therapeutic direction may be established. Using his fingers, the physician touches the patient's head, face, skin, limbs, chest, abdomen, waist, and back to determine body temperature, degree of moisture on the skin, accumulation, and the presence of tumors or swelling.

When determining skin temperature, the physician should take into consideration the temperature in the room. During chest or abdominal touching, he should try to keep the patient calm.

During abdominal touching, the patient should be down in a comfortable position with his limbs outstretched and his abdomen relaxed. If the physician detects a succussion sound beneath the heart, he should ask the patient to bend his knees and relax the abdominal muscles before continuing the examination.

The physician's hands should be warm during this part of the examination. He begins by gently touching the patient with his palms, starting with the chest and moving downwards to the abdomen. First he notes the thickness of the abdominal wall, the amount of moisture on the skin, and the presence or absence and characteristics of any palpitations. Then he proceeds with palpation of the abdomen.

1. Thickness of the abdominal wall — If the abdominal wall is thick, the patient's entire body is flexible and has a large amount of subcutaneous fat. This is part of a firmness conformation. If there is concomitant chest distress, *Ta-chai-hu-tang* (Major Bupleurum Combination) is administered. A patient with a thin abdominal wall and lack of flexibility is of a weakness conformation. *Chen-wu-tang* (Vitality Combination) is then given.
2. Abdominal distention — Usually this is part of a firmness conformation. A patient with a resistent, distended abdomen and a strong pulse is of a firmness conformation and should be given *Ta-chai-hu-tang* (Major Bupleurum Combination). A patient with a distended abdomen and a feeble pulse is of a weakness conformation and should be given tonics such as *Szu-ni-tang* (Aconite and G. L. Combination).

The Four Kinds of Diagnoses

Diagram 1. Sites of Abdominal Touching

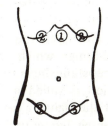 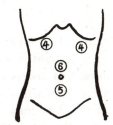

(1) Under the heart
(2) Ribs
(3) Lower abdomen

(4) Under the ribs
(5) Under the umbilicus
(6) Above the umbilicus

Diagram 2. Area of Abdominal Distention

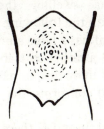

Diagram 3. Area and Types of Chest Distress

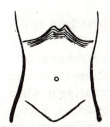 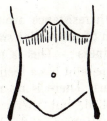 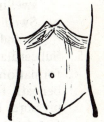

3. Chest distress — This patient has a feeling of outward pressure between the lower part of the heart and the ribs. Objective symptoms are abdominal distention with resistance on touching and pain at the affected site (substernal area). This is part of a firmness conformation. If a patient has a distended abdomen which is soft on touching and is not painful or resistant, he is of a weakness conformatin. This condition is called a "swelling chest" and may occur on either the right or the left side near the ribs. Formulas containing bupleurum are prescribed.
4. Subcardiac swelling — This patient has a feeling of distress in the area near the heart. *Pan-hsia-hsieh-hsin-tang* (Pinellia Combination) is prescribed for this condition. If the patient has asthmatic wheezing, gasping respirations, palpitations, and edema, *Mu-fang-chi-tang* (Stephania and Ginseng Combination) is prescribed. When diagnosing subcardiac swelling, the physician should take into consideration the following points:
   a. If the patient has a large amount of subcutaneous fat, he will have a rather soft abdominal surface without resistance. If upon deeper palpation, however, there is resistance, it conforms the diagnosis of subcardiac swelling.
   b. In the initial diagnosis there may seem to be subcardiac swelling when the physician presses on the abdominal wall. However, abdominal muscles that feel rigid like a board do not indicate subcardiac swelling.
   c. Swelling with resistance around the umbilicus is not an indication of subcardiac swelling.
5. Subcardiac hardness — This is part of a weakness conformation. The pateint has a feeling of distress in the area beneath the heart. There is no resistance or pain when pressure is applied, but there is a succussion sound. *Jen-sheng-tang* (Ginseng and Ginger Combination) or *Szu-chun-tzu-tang* (Four Major Herb Combination) is prescribed.
6. Subcardiac swelling and hardness — The area beneath the

patient's heart is distended and he feels distress over the heart. *Yin-chen-hao-tang* (Capillaria Combination) or *Wu-ling-san* (Hoelen Five Herb Formula) is prescribed.

7. Lower abdominal tension and lower abdominal stress — Tenseness of the abdominal muscles below the umbilicus is called "lower abdominal tension". Chinese physicians regard it as a weakness of the lower abdomen or a symptom of kidney weakness. *Pa-wei-ti-huang-wan* (Rehmannia Eight Formula) is given. Lower abdominal stress is similar to lower abdominal tension. The difference is shown in the figures below:

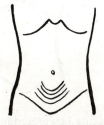 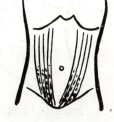

Lower Abdominal Tension   Lower Abdominal Stress

8. Abdominal seizure — The contraction or twitching of the abdominal muscles causes bar-like rigidity, and it is part of a weakness conformation. Both the right and the left sides may be rigid, or one side may be contracted while the other is not. *Hsiao-chien-chung-tang* (Minor Cinnamon and Paeonia Combination) is prescribed. If there is tenseness in the upper abdomen, *Szu-ni-san* (Bupleurum and *Chih-shih* Formula) is used.

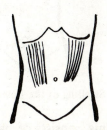 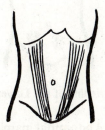

Abdominal Seizures

9. Feeling of emptiness beneath the umbilicus — The lower abdomen is loose and weak, the abdominal symptom of kidney weakness. *Pa-wei-wan* (Rehmannia Eight Formula) is given.
10. Acute lower abdominal pain — There is acute pain at the lower left side of the abdomen when it is pressed with the fingers. This is the abdominal symptom of stagnant blood. *Tao-ho-cheng-chi-tang* (Persica and Rhubarb Combination) is prescribed.

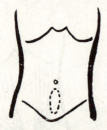
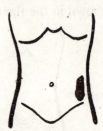

Feeling of Emptiness   Acute Lower Abdominal Pain
Beneath the Umbilicus

11. Hard swelling of the lower abdomen — On touching there are two or more places of resistance, but no swelling. This is the abdominal symptom of stagnant blood or sputum disease. *Ta-huang-mu-tan-pi-tang* (Rhubarb and Moutan Combination) is prescribed.

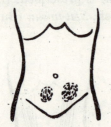
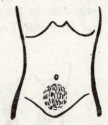

Hard Swelling of the Lower Abdomen   Swelling of the Lower Abdomen

12. Abdominal palpitation — This consists of palpitation of the abdominal arteries. A rapid pulse rate is due to poor blood circulation in the stomach and intestines due to disease or congestion. Palpitations at the heart, lower

heart, and lower umbilical area are part of a weakness conformation. Diaphoretics, purgatives, or emetics cannot be used. Either *Chih-kan-tsao-tang* (Baked Licorice Combination) or *Wu-ling-san* (Hoelen Five Herb Formula) is prescribed. *Shui-fen* is palpitation above the umbilicus, while that below the umbilicus is palpitation between the kidneys.

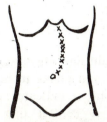
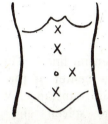

Lower Heart Palpitation

Lower Heart Palpitation
Lower Umbilical Palpitation

13. Liquid sound — This is a sound heard when the area over the lower heart is tapped with the fingers. It is a weakness conformation and indicates atony of the stomach muscles, gastroptosis, or gastrectasis. *Jen-sheng-tang* (Ginseng and Ginger Combination) or *Wu-ling-san* (Hoelen Five Herb Formula) is prescribed.
14. Inside acute — This is a type of abdominal contraction in which the patient feels as if the skin on the lower abdomen is being pulled. Purgatives cannot be used even if the patient is constipated.
15. Erratic peristalsis — The patient's abdominal walls are atonic and the movement in his intestines is irregular. This movement is clearly audible through the abdominal wall and is sometimes accompanied by abdominal pain. Usually it is a weakness conformation and purgatives cannot be used even if the patient is constipated. *Ta-chien-chung-tang* (Major Zanthoxylum Combination) is prescribed.

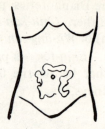

Erratic Peristalsis.

16. Central line — This is a straight line which passes through the center of the umbilicus and seems to be made of a hard substance. When present, it indicates weakness of the spleen and kidneys. A central line above the umbilicus indicates weakness of the spleen, while one below indicates weakness of the kidneys. For the former *Chen-wu-tang* (Vitality Combination) is prescribed; for the latter *Pa-wei-wan* (Rehmannia Eight Formula) is prescribed.

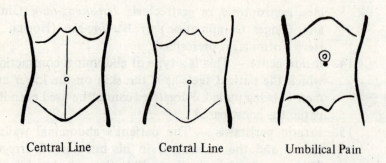

Central Line   Central Line   Umbilical Pain

17. Umbilical pain — This pain is located above the umbilicus and occurs on gentle touching. The patient also has a tight pulse and tense, strong abdominal muscles. *Ko-ken-tang* (Pueraria Combination) is prescribed.

OUTLINES OF THERAPEUTICAL METHODS

Recognition of Therapeutical Directions

In Chinese herbal medicine, the selection of an appropriate therapeutical method is based upon evaluation of the individual patient according to what is termed his or her "conformation." A patient's conformation is the constellation of an individual's symptoms, constitution, somatic state, psychological state, and history. For example, when a person is said to have a *Ko-ken-tang* conformation, his constellation calls for the formula named *Ko-ken-tang*. Hence Chinese medical diagnosis aims at determining the patient's conformation, and therapy follows the rule: "Treatment according to conformation."

Gaoku Kyoyasu said: "Conformation means to conform, to verify, to serve as evidence. What a medical practitioner uses to determine a conformation is the patient's response." The physician evaluates the responses (symptoms) of the patient to determine the conformation. Once the conformation is established the doctor can then prescribe the proper therapeutic method.

During actual clinical diagnosis, however, the practitioner often encounters problems and ambiguities. What does he do then? One rule he follows is: Treat the new disease first, then treat the old disease. In other words, if a new ailment arises in a patient with chronic disease, the rule of thumb is to treat the new disease first, then the chronic disease. As is stated in *Chin kuei yao lueh:* "When someone is suffering from a chronic and an acute disease at the same time, the acute disease should be treated first followed by treatment of the chronic one." If a new disease or complication develops during the course of treatment of a chronic disease, the new disease takes priority. For example, if acute gastroenteritis occurs during the course of treatment with the regimen of *Hsiao-ching-lung-tang* in a patient with bronchial asthma, the gastroenteritis should be treated immediately. A common cold in a hypertensive patient who has been under the therapy of *Ta-chai-hu-tang* will alter the patient's conformation; then the administration of *Ta-chai-hu-tang* should be interrupted and *Ko-ken-tang* taken. Likewise if a patient who has had thoraco-costal distress catches a common cold *Ko-ken-tang* should be administered to combat the cold symptoms, and the originally existing thoraco-costal distress may be disregarded temporarily.

Another rule of therapy is: If weakness and firmness appear simultaneously, first supplement the weakness then attack the firmness. (The concepts of weakness and firmness have been discussed in the part entitled "Explanation of Terms.") For example, a fever accompanied by stomach distention, constipation, and thirst is an internal-firmness conformation which calls for *Cheng-chi-tang*. However, if the above condition is accompanied by anemophobia (fear of chills), it is an external-weakness conformation requiring *Kuei-chih-tang* to be administered first to supplement the surface weakness. After the anemophobia disappears, *Cheng-chi-tang* is given. This conformation is termed external-weakness with internal firmness.

For simultaneous surface and internal-weakness, treatment can be either (1) simultaneous treatment of the surface and the interior or (2) surface treatment first and interior second. An illustration of this principle is a person with fever on the surface, chillphobia or anemophobia, and sweating who simultaneously has diarrhea. This condition is called "surface fever and internal chill." If the condition is not serious, *Kuei-chih-jen-sheng-tang* may be prescribed to treat the surface and the interior simultaneously. However, if the internal symptom is very serious—in this case, violent diarrhea of undigested foods, a condition considered fatal if not treated in the early stages—the interior is first cured with *Szu-ni-tang* followed by treatment of the surface condition with *Kuei-chih-tang*.

If weakness or firmness cannot be ascertained, the disease is treated as a weak condition. Without this knowledge it is difficult to establish a therapeutical method. This situation is especially true in the diagnosis and treatment of an acute feverish disease which is easily mistaken as a *Hsiao-chai-hu-tang* or a *Pai-hu-tang* conformation for a *Chen-wu-tang* conformation. The author has encountered many cases in which a weak conformation was misdiagnosed as a firm one. For example, there was one acute pneumonia case in which the patient had a temperature increase to nearly 40°C and experienced delirium and constipation for many days. The author diagnosed the illness as a *yang ming* (sunlight yang) disease, which has the typical character of internal firmness, and therefore prescribed *Tiao-wei-cheng-chi-tang*. However, a few hours after the first administration of this combination, the patient began to have frequent diarrhea, his eyes turned upward, his pulse became disorderly, and his general condition became very serious. These problems resulted from an erroneous diagnosis whereby the weak conformation was mistaken for a firm one, and an internal rebellion, as such, was fomented. After a shift to *Chen-wu-tang*, the diarrhea ceased, his pulse stabilized, and the seriousness of his condition eased. Therefore, whenever one is not confident in diagnosing the firmness or weakness of symptoms, it is safer to treat the condition as a weak conformation. If a firm condition is mistaken for a weak one and treated accordingly, the patient has less chance of lapsing into a near fatal state. On the contrary, in the event of an acute disease, if a weak conformation is erroneously attacked as a firm conformation, the result often is irreversible.

Yumoto Kyushin, the teacher of Otsuka Keisetsu, said: "The ancient school killed people quickly while the modern school kills people slowly." In other words, medical practitioners of the ancient school such as Yoshimasu Todo often misdiagnosed a weak conformation for a firm one and prescribed the wrong medication. Such a mistake killed people immediately; more recently, doctors often diagnose a firm conformation as a weak one and prescribe warm supplementary drugs as treatment (e.g. prescriptions which contain ginseng, astragalus, aconite, etc.) which allows people to live longer, often for many years. Yumoto Kyushin, who was an ancient school practitioner, remarked later: "The ancient school was less guilty than supposed while recent practitioners are extremely guilty." Nevertheless, diagnostic mistakes must be guarded against.

Precautions for Treatments

Since Chinese herbal medicine employs the principle of "treatment according to conformation," diseases are always cured successfully if the prescription complies with the conformation. However, in reality accurate determination of the disorder can be difficult. This point is especially evident when the physician thinks the prescription complies with the conformation but often, unexpectedly, it does not. A complicating factor is the patient's specific physique, which often causes an unexpected reaction to the prescription. Various conditions which practitioners of Chinese herbal medicine must understand are described below.

Drug Characters

It often happens that the patient's appetite is effected by a prescription making it necessary to change the prescription. Prescriptions effecting the appetite often contain rehmannia or *ma-huang*. This situation especially happens with such prescriptions as *Pa-wei-ti-huang-wan-liao,* or *Ma-hsing-kan-shih-tang* or *Ko-ken-tang,* all of which may induce anorexia or nausea in a patient who has a weak stomach and intestines. Therefore, a cystitis patient with a *Pa-wei-wan-liao* indication who has a weak stomach and intestines, is given *Chu-ling-tang, Ching-hsin-lien-tzu-yin* or *Wu-lin-san* instead. For patients who are suffering from a common cold but have a weak stomach and intestines, prescriptions containing no *ma-huang* are preferred. Thus a knowledge of drug characteristics is necessary to the practitioner.

What if the patient gets nauseated at the odor of the drug and can hardly drink the medication? If the prescription complies with the conformation, it can be drunk easily even though it is commonly regarded as barely drinkable. On the other hand, if the prescription does not comply with the conformation, it will hardly be drinkable even though it is commonly regarded as easily drinkable. Hence, if the patient gets sick from the drug odor the moment he smells it, the physician should suspect the possibility of a discrepancy between the prescription and the conformation. The practitioner must also question what is happening when a prescription which worked very well at the beginning and which the patient was fond of suddenly makes him sick. For example, a patient takes *Chai-hu-chia-lung-ku-mu-li-tang* or *Ta-chai-hu-tang* with good results; suddenly he becomes sick and can hardly drink it. The formula is replaced with an extract form of the same formulation, but he still cannot swallow it. Then as an alternative, *Szu-ni-san* along with *San-huang-hsieh-hsin-tang* is prescribed and drunk quite easily. The patient's condition improves. Another example is that of a *Ta-chai-hu-tang* patient who had very severe thoraco-costal distress which did not improve with the prescribed medication. Later, he was given *Hsiao-chai-hu-tang* plus rhubarb. The second prescription was easy to drink compared to the first one, and was successful in curing him.

Cases such as the above are numerous; hence it is not always advisable to stick to the established rule. It is important that one be flexible and responsive to conditions and developments.

Conditions for Purgative Agents

When a patient has constipation, one often thinks of using purgatives. However, before prescribing purgative agents, the doctor has to interrogate the patient to see if the patient has ever used them. If not, despite severe constipation, it is better not to hazard prescribing them. The author had a case of an old woman who had intolerable constipation. *Tiao-wei-cheng-chi-tang* which contained 1.0g each of rhubarb and mirabilitum was prescribed and administered. During the night after taking only one-third of the dosage, she had more than ten successive diarrhea attacks. She also experienced severe anemophobia, cold limbs, and a general condition threatening to her life. Although this is rare, there are cases in which rhubarb with as low a daily dosage as 0.5g causes severe diarrhea and other complications.

For patients in whom purgatives are contraindicated, it is necessary to administer such drugs as *Liu-chun-tzu-tang*, *Chai-shao-liu-chun-tzu-tang*, *Chia-wei-hsiao-yao-san* or *Ta-chien-chung-tang* together with *Hsiao-chien-chung-tang*, *Hsiao-chai-hu-tang*, etc. Patients who use purgatives for their constipation often request an increased dosage. However, no bowel movement, even with an increased dosage of purgatives, can be encouraged without increasing water intake. Also, rhubarb and other herbs can augment the purgative effect.

Illusion

In Chinese medicine "illusion" indicates a reaction to medication in which the patient's condition appears to be worsening. Yoshimasu Todo regards as axiomatic the words from the classics: "If a drug does not produce an illusive effect, it does not have a curative effect." This statement means that if the drug hits the bull's eye of its target, the disease can definitely be cured; but if there is no illusion exhibited, the drug has not hit the bull's eye. Hence, an illusive reaction in a patient is regarded as a sign that the disease is being cured by the drug. Todo cited a case in his *Medical Questions* about a patient who had suffered from chronic gastrointestinal disease since childhood. Todo administered *Sheng-chiang-hsieh-hsin-tang* to the patient which induced severe vomiting and diarrhea causing the patient to become comatose. After the patient came to, his chronic disease was gone as though it had been mopped away.

The author also had an experience with a patient suffering from chronic G I disease. After he administered *Sheng-chiang-hsieh-hsin-tang,* the patient vomited a large quantity of water and was cured. Of course, the illusion reaction is produced not only by *Sheng-chiang-hsieh-hsin-tang.* For instance, an old woman who had suffered from chronic bronchitis suddenly discharged a large quantity of leukorrhea after taking *Hsiao-ching-lung-tang,* thus curing her bronchitis. Another case concerns a bronchial asthmatic patient who was given *Hsiao-ching-lung-tang* which brought on violent metrorrhagia resulting in her cure. Still another case was that of a woman with eczema. After taking *Hsiao-feng-san,* her condition worsened for three days but was ameliorated from the seventh day on.

Among cases which show the illusive effect, many unexpected reactions are also observed which aggravate the disease and are thus considered reactions due to noncompliance between drug and conformation. The side effects derived from noncompliance between drug and conformation are not regarded as an illusion. The author has had the following experience concerning this circumstance. A debilitated patient suffering from chronic G I disturbance was given *Jen-sheng-tang*. Three or four days later he developed dropsy. However, this was a good sign (an illusion), because no sooner had the dropsy disappeared than the disease was cured. Nevertheless, the same condition did not yield the same result in a similar case. An old man with the anemia, debility, anorexia, and chills of adynia took *Jen-sheng-tang*. Two to three days later dropsy appeared which was taken as a good sign and the *Jen-sheng-tang* was continued. Unexpectedly, the dropsy became more and more serious. The patient was examined and found to have proteinuria, a condition indicative of chronic nephritis. Medication was shifted to *Wu-ling-san* and the dropsy disappeared. Thus the dropsy was not an illusion in this case.

Auxiliary Formulas, Modified Formulas, and Combined Formulas

During treatment it is better to avoid as much as possible the use of auxiliary, modified, or combined formulas; especially, the neophyte doctor who develops the habit of using auxiliary, modified, or combined formulas from the very beginning may become indecisive and have difficulty determining the conformation.

An auxiliary formula means that other drugs in the form of pills, powder, or potion are employed in addition to a decoction which is prescribed as the chief drug. For example, *Ta-chai-hu-tang* may be prescribed as the chief drug and *Pa-wei-wan* as the auxiliary one. Some doctors adopt the regimen of today prescribing *Hsiao-chai-hu-tang*, tomorrow *Tang-kuei-shao-yao-san*, in the morning *Ko-ken-tang* and in the evening *Shih-wei-pai-tu-tang*. This procedure is followed because the prescriber is incapable of making a clear-cut diagnosis and does not know the indicative prescription.

A modified formula denotes a formula made by adding or subtracting one, two, or more component herbs from an established formula. For example, *Kuei-chih-chia-shao-yao-ta-huang-tang*, *Chia-wei-hsiao-yao-san*, *Chia-wei-kuei-pi-tang* or *Kuei-chih-chu-shao-yao-chia-shu-chi-lung-ku-mu-li-tang* are such compounds. Modification of a prescription that has been used for a very long period of time for a corresponding conformation that is very evident is out of the question. If a formula is fabricated out of one's own head without clinical conformation, one may encounter unexpected failure. This point must be well noted. The author offers an empirical case. A young man's face was covered with *acne vulgaris*. *Ching-shang-fang-feng-tang* was administered and his condition improved by 80 percent. Because there were furuncles on the patient's head, an attempt was made to cure them, too. Peach kernels were added to *Ching-shang-fang-feng-tang*. After taking this combination the acne became unexpectedly serious and pustulent. The author was very astonished and had the sorrowful feeling that one should never make innovations.

A combined formula is two formulas made into one. The larger doses of the herbs common to the two formulas are adapted in the combined formula. (This formulation method was Yumoto Kyushin's idea.) For a combined formula, the indicated conformation is not necessarily limited to the conformations of the two or three component formulas, or all the conformations together. Because of the combined effects, the indicated conformation may be completely different from those of the component formulas. Therefore, the application of a combined formula should be guided by the ancestral sages' experience and used only when the indicated conformation is clearly discriminated. One should not attempt to combine formulas out of one's head. Neophytes especially must be cautioned against using combined formulas because such a practice will prevent them from obtaining a clear understanding of formula indications and from progressing in their acquisition of knowledge.

Shift of Formulas

The so-called shift of formulas means the change from one formula to another. As the conformation changes, the formula changes accordingly. A change of conformation in an acute disease is conspicuous but in a chronic disease indistinct. If after consideration the formula and conformation are believed to comply with each other but the result is contrary to expectation and no effect is observed, it indicates in most cases that the formula is not suitable for the conformation. One should then consider shifting the formula. For example, a young woman suffering from *alopecia areata* had not even a single strand of hair on her head. The author applied *Chai-hu-chia-lung-ku-mu-li-tang* to her head. For three months there was no change. However, the patient seemed indifferent to the alopecia and appeared very optimistic. The author then realized that if the patient's conformation was suitable for *Chai-hu-chia-lung-ku-mu-li-tang* she ought to have a nervous temperament, but she did not. Hence the author shifted medication to *Wen-ching-yin,* which is indicated for a facial complexion characterized by flushing up, ruddiness, and dry skin. One month later, pitch black hair completely covered her head. It was really astonishing. According to the author's experience, administration of *Hsiao-chai-hu-tang-chia-mu-li* or *Chai-hu-chia-lung-ku-mu-li-tang* for *alopecia areata* had often been effective within one to two months. From the above case, however, it seems that *Wen-ching-yin* may also be effective.

DIAGNOSIS ACCORDING TO THE DISEASES

CONTAGIOUS DISEASES

Typhoid Fever

The so-called *shang han* or contagious febrile diseases of ancient times included typhoid fever. The famous Chinese classic *Shang han lun* describes and analyzes the attacks, symptoms, and therapies for *shang han* and similar feverish diseases.

Typhoid fever usually begins with chills and fever, a condition which the *Shang han lun* designates a greater yang or a lesser yin disease. If the symptoms are chills and fever with a buoyant pulse, the illness is diagnosed as greater yang disease. In this stage, the patient is treated with *Ma-huang-tang* (*Ma-huang* Combination) or *Ko-ken-tang* (Pueraria Combination). If there are chills and fever but the pulse is submerged and small and the limbs are cold, the condition is diagnosed as lesser yin disease and *Ma-huang-fu-tzu-hsi-hsin-tang* (*Ma-huang,* Aconite, and Asarum Combination) or *Ma-huang-fu-tzu-kan-tsao-tang* (*Ma-huang,* Aconite, and Licorice Combination) is the proper treatment.

Patients contracting typhoid fever may begin the illness either as a greater yang or a lesser yin disease depending on the physical condition of the patient, the environment in which the patient contracted the disease, and the nature of the prevailing epidemic. It was once thought that disease in obese and stalwart people takes on greater yang characteristics and in senile or feeble people, lesser yin manifestations. Such a conclusion is erroneous, however, because there are cases in which obese and stalwart people begin with lesser yin disease and weak people begin with greater yang disease.

Within a few days the chills and fever cease. The patient may then have a headache, low back pains, lassitude, and anorexia; plus his tongue becomes white with dry fur. In one and a half weeks the patient will have a swollen spleen that is palpable and pain at the left hypochondrium. At this stage the disease has gone from a greater yang conformation to a lesser yang conformation, and the formulas of *Chai-hu-kuei-chih-tang* (Bupleurum and Cinnamon Combination) or *Hsiao-chai-hu-tang* (Minor Bupleurum Combination) are now appropriate. The pulse has become submerged and tense or chordal and thin, and the mouth has become sticky. The patient wants fresh fruits or water. As the spleen swells, thoraco-costal distress appears; the condition is now one of lesser yang disease. If this condition continues for more than ten days, the patient becomes debilitated and develops head sweating, night sweats, and thirst. At this stage suitable treatment is *Chai-hu-kuei-chih-kan-chiang-tang* (Bupleurum, Cinnamon, and Ginger Combination).

In people who begin in the lesser yin stage, the disease may turn into lesser yang disease in five or six days or into a sunlight yang disease if the patient has taken an excessive dosage of aconite prescribed by a physician. The disease may also change into greater yang or absolute yin in which case the patient may vomit and have diarrhea, distress within the chest, abdominal aching, cold limbs, and a submerged and minute pulse. At this point *Szu-ni-tang* (Aconite and G. L. Combination) and *Tung-mo-szu-ni-tang* (Aconite, Licorice, and Ginger Pulse Combination) are indicated. Diseases that begin with lesser yin disease change quickly and special attention must be given to their treatment. In the first week, the initial stage of the disease, the patient may suffer from nosebleeds; this is a *Ma-huang-tang* conformation.

As the disease progresses, it changes from lesser yang disease to sunlight yang. In this stage the temperature hovers at 39-40°C and the chills disappear. The illness now becomes a somatic or tidal type fever. The patient has a distended abdomen, constipation or diarrhea, and anorexia; his tongue becomes dry and coated with a yellow fur, or the fur may even become black; or prickles and rhagades grow on the tongue. The patient also becomes delirious. Both the spleen and liver swell. At this time such prescriptions as *Ta-chai-hu-tang* (Major Bupleurum Combination) or *Cheng-chi-tang* are suitable. During this week, the patient may have pityriasis rosea (patches of thin, scaly skin) and tinnitus, or impaired hearing. In most cases the pulse is submerged and comparatively slow. In this stage there may also be intestinal bleeding, a dangerous symptom. However, some patients contrarily improve with bleeding. For this condition, *Huang-tu-tang (Fu-lung-kan* Combination) or *Wen-ching-yin (Tang-kuei* and Gardenia Combination) is indicated.

As the disease enters into the second week, it does not always become a sunlight yang disease. At times it begins and ends in the same stage and does not alter. There also may be diarrhea, abdominal pain, and intestinal bleeding and inflammation of the lining of the digestive organs leading to perforation; cold limbs; and a minute pulse. Subsequently the disease may alter to the absolute yin stage. The patient is then in a very dangerous state.

Delirium mostly denotes a sunlight yang disease and calls for such purgatives as *Cheng-chi-tang*. However, one cannot diagnose sunlight yang disease by merely relying on the symptom of delirium because delirium also occurs in lesser yang or lesser yin disease. Tinnitus and impaired hearing are symptoms of the lesser yang disease. Occasionally bronchitis will occur simultaneously. If the pulse is submerged, slow, and forceful, then purgatives may be employed. If it is submerged and harsh or submerged and minute, the use of purgatives is out of the question despite symptoms of abdominal pain, constipation, and delirium. In some cases purgatives such as *Cheng-chi-tang* should be used, espeically for patients who are having hallucinations, are unconscious, or are in a coma. Other patients need *Sheng-yang-san-huo-tang* (Bupleurum and Ginseng Combination) for the nutritive lubrication and warm supplementation it provides. Deciding the appropriate treatment is difficult and can only be achieved by precise pulse diagnosis.

In the third week some patients may have gone from sunlight yang to lesser yang disease and thus are recovering gradually; others may sink into absolute yin disease exhibiting symptoms that indicate the condition is lifethreatening. On the other hand some patients experience complications which delay recovery. Still others remain in the lesser yang stage without progressing to the sunlight yang stage in the second week and remain there even in the third week.

If the illness proceeds as expected, by the third week the fever begins to decline, the patient's mind also becomes clearer, the tongue fur disappears, and the general condition improves. However, hyperhidrosis may occur as the fever begins to subside. Night sweats arise and occasional sweat papules appear.

In the recuperation stage the body temperature approaches normal but can be elevated by slight physical exercise and the pulse becomes knotty and impeded or fast. For this condition, *Chih-kan-tsao-tang* (Baked Licorice Combination) is indicated.

The above is a brief description of typhoid fever. In mild cases typhoid migrates from the greater yang to the lesser yang disease before being cured. Recovery will be particularly shortened if chloramphenicol is administered at the initial stage. Note: At times the malady is of the *Pai-hu-tang* (Gypsum Combination) conformation, all three yang disease symptoms being present, a condition which is usually erroneously diagnosed and treated.

Chinese Herb Formulas
1. **Ma-huang-tang** 麻黃湯
   (Ma-huang Combination)
   Ko-ken-tang 葛根湯
   (Pueraria Combination)

At the initial stage of the bout a certain diagnosis of typhoid fever cannot be reached, the patient has a headache, low back pain, fever, and chills—the symptoms of a common cold—with a buoyant pulse or a buoyant, fast, and forceful pulse. These formulas are for this stage.

2. **Ma-huang-hsi-hsin-fu-tzu-tang** 麻黃細辛附子湯
   (Ma-huang, Aconite, and Asarum Combination)
   Ma-huang-fu-tzu-kan-tsao-tang 麻黃附子甘草湯
   (Ma-huang, Aconite, and Licorice Combination)

These formulas are suitable for persons whose illness begins as a lesser yin disease, chills and lassitude being the chief complaints. The body temperature is elevated but the patient does not feel any great heat. The pulse is thin and minute, the face is pale, the limbs are cold, and the patient is anorexic. However, if these symptoms are accompanied by diarrhea and abdominal pain, *Chen-wu-tang*

(Vitality Combination) is called for.

3. **Chai-hu-kuei-chih-tang** 柴胡桂枝湯
   (Bupleurum and Cinnamon Combination)
   Hsiao-chai-hu-tang 小柴胡湯
   (Minor Bupleurum Combination)

When the patient has suffered from the disease for a few days and has the combined symptoms of greater yang and lesser yang such as headache, chills, aching limbs, and buoyant pulse, white fur on the tongue, anorexia, nausea and thoraco-costal distress, he should be treated with *Chai-hu-kuei-chih-tang*. On the other hand, if the greater yang symptoms of chills, aching limbs, and buoyant pulse have disappeared, it is the lesser yang disease and *Hsiao-chai-hu-tang* is needed.

4. **Chai-hu-kuei-chih-kan-chiang-tang** 柴胡桂枝乾薑湯
   (Bupleurum, Cinnamon, and Ginger Combination)

With the lesser yang symptoms the patient should take *Chai-hu-kuei-chih-tang* for more than ten days; if the fever remains high, the tongue has white fur, and the thoracic and costal distress still do not disappear, the conformation is still of the lesser yang and if the patient has night sweats, thirst, and signs of weakness, then *Hsiao-chai-hu-tang* is suitable.

5. **Szu-ni-tang** 四逆湯
   (Aconite, Ginseng, and Licorice Combination)
   Chen-wu-tang 眞武湯
   (Vitality Combination)

If the surface symptoms of the lesser yin disease have gone and the disease has sunk into the interior conformational state of diarrhea, vomiting, abdominal pain, cold limbs and a submerged and minute pulse, then *Szu-ni-tang* is indicated. If constipation of greater yang or lesser yang origin is misdiagnosed and mistaken for constipation of the interior firm conformation of sunlight yang disease and treated with a purgative, the condition may change to greater yin disease with diarrhea, vomiting, and abdominal pain; then *Chen-wu-tang* or *Szu-ni-tang* is required. Also, for absolute yin disease with a feverish upper torso, cold lower torso, thirst, intrathoracic distress, and cold limbs or diarrhea, *Szu-ni-tang* is used.

6. Ma-huang-tang　　　　　　　　　　　麻黃湯
   (Ma-huang Combination)
   San-huang-hsieh-hsin-tang　　　　　　三黃瀉心湯
   (Coptis and Rhubarb Combination)
   Tao-ho-cheng-chi-tang　　　　　　　　桃核承氣湯
   (Persica and Rhubarb Combination)

Ma-huang-tang is used for such surface symptoms as buoyant pulse, headache, fever, and nosebleeds. *San-huang-hsieh-hsin-tang* is used for persons without surface symptoms who have a buoyant and big pulse, a flushed face, insomnia, discomforting gas, and nosebleeds. Nosebleeds due to the welling up of stagnant blood usually are accompanied by abdominal cramps, constipation, and delirium. In these circumstances *Tao-ho-cheng-chi-tang* is suitable.

7. Ta-chai-hu-tang　　　　　　　　　　大柴胡湯
   (Major Bupleurum Combination)

This formula is used for the stage when the disease has migrated from a lesser yang to a sunlight yang conformation characterized by the following symptoms: a somatic or tidal type fever, a tongue coated with white fur which then turns yellowish and dry, thirst, distended abdomen, and, in most cases, constipation.

8. Tiao-wei-cheng-chi-tang　　　　　　調胃承氣湯
   (Rhubarb and Mirabilitum Combination)
   Hsiao-cheng-chi-tang　　　　　　　　小承氣湯
   (Minor Rhubarb Combination)
   Ta-cheng-chi-tang　　　　　　　　　　大承氣湯
   (Major Rhubarb Combination)
   Tao-ho-cheng-chi-tang　　　　　　　　桃核承氣湯
   (Persica and Rhubarb Combination)

These formulas are used for patients with sunlight yang disease and resulting constipation. However, in recent years patients suffering from such symptoms are rarely encountered.

Bloody Diarrhea

This illness is known in Chinese medicine as "diarrheal disease" and has a one-week incubation period. It starts with chills, fever, lethargy, and low back pain followed immediately by abdominal cramps and diarrhea. The diarrhea begins with a soft or watery stool. In two or three days the frequency increases and blood, mucus, and pus appear in the stool. Paradoxically, the patient experiences an urgent need to defecate but finds it difficult to do so.

At the onset the body temperature may rise to 39°C or more. However, it drops to below 38°C in two to three days and may even at times be subnormal.

Bloody diarrhea has a great range of symptoms depending on the constitutional strength and age of the patient, the severity of the contagion, and the nature of the epidemic occurring that year. Therapeutic methods vary according to the course of the illness. However, owing to the wide spread use of antibiotics since World War II, the pathological severity of symptoms is no longer as serious as it was.

Symptoms

The illness usually starts abruptly with diarrhea, lower abdominal cramps, and tenesmus (difficulty and straining in urination and defecation). The diarrheal stool shows blood and mucus. Systemic symptoms are fever (in young children, up to 104°F), chills, anorexia and malaise, headache, lethargy, and in the most severe cases, meningismus, unconsciousness, and convulsions. As the illness progresses, the patient grows increasingly weaker and more dehydrated and the abdomen becomes tender. Sigmoidoscopic examination reveals inflamed, engorged mucosa with punctate, and sometimes large, areas of ulceration.

Treatment

Treatment of shock, restoration of blood circulation, and renal perfusion are lifesaving in severe cases. Parenteral hydration and correction of acidosis and electrolyte disturbances are essential for all moderately or severely ill patients. After the bowel has been at rest for a short time, clear fluids are given for two to three days. Avoiding whole milk and high-residue and fatty foods the patient should follow a diet of soft, easy to digest foods taken in small, frequent feedings.

Paregorics provide effective symptomatic relief. Infected stools should be isolated both in the hospital and at home to limit the spread of the infection.

Chinese Herb Formulas

1. Ko-ken-tang 葛根湯
   (Pueraria Combination)

For stalwart young men suffering from bloody diarrhea, this formula is suitable during the initial stage, especially when the symptoms are fever and chills, stiff shoulders, low back pain, diarrhea, and a buoyant but forceful pulse. After sweating profusely, the patient's fever should drop and he will feel weak but better.

2. Hsing-ho-shao-yao-tang 行和芍藥湯
   (Paeonia, Tang-kuei, and Coptis Combination)

This formula is used when the illness has been present for two to three days and the patient has severe tenesmus, bloody stools with mucus, and a fever. At this stage the patient has a dry tongue with yellow fur, a fast pulse, and thirst.

3. Ta-chai-hu-tang 大柴胡湯
   (Major Bupleurum Combination)

This formula is used for conditions similar to that of *Hsing-ho-shao-yao-tang*, that is, severe tenesmus; however, other symptoms present should be a dry tongue with yellow fur, thoraco-costal distress, hardness beneath the heart, and vomiting.

4. Kuei-chih-chia-shao-yao-tang 桂枝加芍藥湯
   (Cinnamon and Paeonia Combination)
   Kuei-chih-chia-shao-yao-ta-huang-tang 桂枝加芍藥大黃湯
   (Cinnamon, Paeonia, and Rhubarb Combination)

The first formula is suitable for mild cases with just a trace of fever, abdominal pain, diarrhea, and tenesmus. If tenesmus is severe, *Kuei-chih-chia-shao-yao-ta-huang-tang* is used.

5. Ta-huang-mu-tan-pi-tang 大黃牡丹皮湯
   (Rhubarb and Moutan Combination)

This formula is used in severe cases when the diarrhea has become gangrenous, the fever is very high, the tongue fur appears dirty brown and dry, and the patient feels extremely thirsty. In addition, tenesmus is severe, there is a frequent urge to urinate, and the stools have a fetid odor resembling rotten meat. The dose of rhubarb may be increased proportionately.

6. Chen-wu-tang   眞武湯
    (Vitality Combination)
    Fu-tzu-li-chung-tang   附子理中湯
    (Ginseng, Ginger, and Aconite Combination)
    Fu-ling-szu-ni-tang   茯苓四逆湯
    (Hoelen, G. L. and Aconite Combination)

The last formula here is used for aged or feeble patients who have suddenly sunk into a prostrated state and have abdominal cramps, an urgent need to defecate, incontinence, cold limbs, and a submerged and weak, or buoyant and weak, pulse. When the symptoms are becoming less severe but the body is still weak and the lower limbs are edematous, *Chen-wu-tang* is recommended.

Malaria

Malaria is an infectious febrile disease caused by protozoa of the genus *Plasmodium*. The bacteria is transmitted through the bites of infected mosquitoes of the genus *Anopheles*. This disease is characterized by attacks of chills, fever, and sweating occurring at intervals which depend on the time required for development of a new generation of parasites in the body. In Chinese medicine, this condition is called "three-day-fever" or "four-day-fever". The intervals between attacks of "three-day-fever" is one day, and "four-day-fever" is two days. Malaria first occurs as an acute attack but it becomes a chronic condition that occasionally relapses.

Chinese Herb Formulas
1. Chai-hu-kuei-chih-tang   柴胡桂枝湯
    (Bupleurum and Cinnamon Combination)

For malaria with recurrent chills and fever, headache, generalized pain, and swelling in the spleen, this combination is prescribed.

2. Hsiao-chai-hu-tang-chia-chang-shan   小柴胡湯加常山
    (Minor Bupleurum Combination with Dichroa)

This combination is effective for malaria.

3. Chai-hu-kuei-chih-kan-chiang-tang   柴胡桂枝乾薑湯
    (Bupleurum, Cinnamon, and Ginger Combination)

This combination is effective for malaria with severe chills, weak pulse, abdominal weakness, and mild fever.

4. **Pai-hu-chia-kuei-chih-tang** 白虎加桂枝湯
   (Gypsum and Cinnamon Combination)

This combination is given for mild malaria with high fever, muscular pain, arthralgia, thirst, nausea, emotional instability, and mild chills.

5. **Ta-chai-hu-tang** 大柴胡湯
   (Major Bupleurum Combination)

This combination is taken for malaria with distention in the chest and beneath the heart due to a swollen spleen, loss of appetite, nausea, vomiting, jaundice, constipation, and a yellow coating on the tongue.

6. **Pu-chung-i-chi-tang-chia-fu-tzu** 補中益氣湯加附子
   (Ginseng and Astragalus Combination with Aconite)
   Shih-chuan-ta-pu-tang 十全大補湯
   (Ginseng and Tang-kuei Ten Combination)

Both combinations are effective for chronic malaria with anemia, coarse skin, diarrhea, loss of appetite, coughing, and a delicate constitution.

Influenza

Influenza occurs as an epidemic and is caused by a virus. Depending on an individual's physical condition and the nature of the prevailing epidemic, the range of symptoms varies greatly from the mild symptoms of a common cold to the most dangerous of conditions.

The typical incubation period for this disease is three to four days. Abrupt chills with high fever and severe aching in the head, joints and loins occur during this time. At the same time the patient will have anorexia; vomiting or thirst, and red, sore eyes or a sore throat; hoarseness; and cough. In most cases the cough is a hacking one and the chest and abdomen ache.

The fever starts at 38°C and rises to 40°C then drops to

below 37°C in about three days. However, after three or four days the same symptoms may recur with the temperature rising to as high as 40°C and subsiding only after four to seven days. In the most dangerous cases, bronchitis develops and turns into bronchial pneumonia. Occasionally the patient suffers from blurred vision and disordered speech and sinks into a comatose state with meningitis-like symptoms.

Influenza attacks essentially the respiratory and the digestive organs. If the latter are attacked there is nausea, vomiting, diarrhea and abdominal pain along with bloody stools with mucus in them.

Treatment

Bed rest to reduce complications is important. Analgesics and a cough sedative are palliative. Antibiotics should be reserved for treatment of bacterial complications.

Chinese Herb Formulas

1. **Ma-huang-tang** 麻黃湯
   (Ma-huang Combination)
   Ko-ken-tang 葛根湯
   (Pueraria Combination)
   Ta-ching-lung-tang 大青龍湯
   (Major Blue Dragon Combination)

When the malady begins with greater yang symptoms such as fever, chills, buoyant and tense pulse, headache, low back pain, arthralgia, and no spontaneous sweating, *Ma-huang-tang* is indicated. When there is tension and aching from the neck down the spine to the loins, then *Ko-ken-tang* is indicated. If *Ma-huang-tang* or *Ko-ken-tang* stimulate sweating, the symptoms will be alleviated. If there is no sweating after administration of these formulas but instead there is aridity, thirst, and a buoyant, tense, and fast pulse, then *Ta-ching-lung-tang* should be administered.

2. **Ma-huang-hsi-hsin-fu-tzu-tang** 麻黃細辛附子湯
   (Ma-huang, Aconite, and Asarum Combination)
   Chen-wu-tang 眞武湯
   (Vitality Combination)
   Szu-ni-tang 四逆湯
   (Aconite, Ginger, and Licorice Combination)

These formulas are used for patients initially affected by lesser yin disease. *Ma-huang-hsi-hsin-fu-tzu-tang* is given to geriatric or feeble patients who have lesser yin symptoms from the beginning even though they may not experience a sensation of heat despite a body temperature from 38-40°C. Other symptoms presented by these patients include paleness, chills, cold limbs, lack of vigor, headache, low back pain, arthralgia, or cough. These patients will also have a submerged and small pulse. A few days after the onset of the disease, if the patients have a buoyant and big but soft and forceless pulse, cold limbs, diarrhea or constipation, and prostration, then *Chen-wu-tang, Szu-ni-tang,* or the like is to be administered.

3. **Chai-hu-kuei-chih-tang** 柴胡桂枝湯
   (Bupleurum and Cinnamon Combination)
   Hsiao-chai-hu-tang 小柴胡湯
   (Minor Bupleurum Combination)

If after administration of *Ma-huang-tang* or *Ko-ken-tang* the patient develops white fur on the tongue, a bitter taste in the mouth, anorexia, vomiting and a residual headache, arthralgia or other surface symptoms, *Chai-hu-kuei-chih-tang* is indicated. If there are no surface symptoms, *Hsiao-chai-hu-tang* is given instead. If after the fever has subsided the patient still has anorexia, an aching chest, and difficulty expectorating, *Hsiao-chai-hu-tang* should be given.

4. **Chai-hsien-tang** 柴陷湯
   (Bupleurum and Scute Combination)

This formula is used for pain in the chest during coughing and difficulty in expectoration.

5. **Chu-ju-wen-tan-tang** 竹茹溫膽湯
   (Bamboo and Ginseng Combination)

This formula is used in the recuperation period when the fever has lowered to normal or near normal but there is still a cough, copious sputum, and insomnia present.

6. **Mai-men-tung-tang** 麥門冬湯
   (Ophiopogon Combination)

This formula is used in the recuperation period when there is only slight sputum clinging to the throat and inhibiting expectoration and the voice is hoarse.

7. Tao-ho-cheng-chi-tang　　　　　　　桃核承氣湯
   (Persica and Rhubarb Combination)
In extremely severe cases the patient has blurred vision, disordered speech, and delirium with accompanying constipation, a dry tongue with blackish-brown fur, and abdominal cramps. Administration of this formula for a few times may bring about defecation and a restoration of lucidity.

Diphtheria

Diphtheria, an acute contagious disease, is caused by the toxigenic bacillus *Corynebacterium diphtheriae*. It affects primarily the membranes of the nose, throat, or larynx and is characterized by the formation of a gray-white false membrane in the air passages. Generally, the illness manifests itself in the form of laryngeal diphtheria or pharyngeal diphtheria. The patient with laryngeal diphtheria shows the symptoms of generalized fatigue, fever, severe chills, headache, difficulty in swallowing, loss of appetite, stomachache, and vomiting. Pharyngeal diphtheria develops from laryngeal diphtheria. The symptoms are severe coughing and hoarseness. It is attended by fever and pain of varying degrees and, in the laryngeal form, by a loss of speech (aphonia) and respiratory obstruction. Myocarditis and cranial or peripheral neuritis are complications resulting from the effects of the toxin released from the diseased site.

Chinese Herb Formulas
1. Ko-ken-tang-chia-chieh-keng-shih-kao　　葛根湯加桔梗石膏
   (Pueraria Combination with Platycodon and Gypsum)
This combination is given in the initial stage of diphtheria when the patient has fever, severe chills, and a floating pulse but good vitality.

2. Chu-feng-chieh-tu-tang　　　　　　　　驅風解毒湯
   (Siler and Forsythia Combination)
If *Ko-ken-tang-chia-chieh-keng-shih-kao* has no effect, the patient given this combination for swelling and pain in the throat and

difficulty in swallowing.

3. Chai-hu-kuei-chih-tang　　　　　　　　　柴胡桂枝湯
    (Bupleurum and Cinnamon Combination)
For the primary stage of diphtheria with stomachache and vomiting the patient is given this combination.

4. Chia-wei-liang-ke-san-chia-chu-yeh　　加味涼膈散加竹葉
    (Forsythia and Gypsum Formula with Bamboo Leaves)
This herbal compound is given for diphtheria when the patient has swelling and suppuration in the larynx.

5. Sheng-lien-tang　　　　　　　　　　　　參連湯
    (Ginseng and Coptis Combination)
This combination is given patients with diphtheria who have a weak heart, pallor, emotional instability, and a weak pulse.

6. Jen-sheng-hu-tao-tang　　　　　　　　　人參胡桃湯
    (Ginseng and Juglans Combination)
This combination is prescribed for diphtheria when there is difficulty in breathing, stridor, and hoarseness.

7. Chieh-keng-pai-san　　　　　　　　　　桔梗白散
    (Platycodon and Croton Formula)
This formula is given for treatment of diphtheria when the false membrane has formed.

Tetanus

Tetanus, an acute infectious disease, is caused by the bacillus *Clostridium tetani*. The incubation of tetanus is about four to fourteen days after sustaining an external injury. Following infection, the patient shows rigid continuous spasmodic contraction of various voluntary muscles, trismus (lockjaw), generalized muscle spasms, aching of the back, shoulder stiffness, and abdominal pain.

Chinese Herb Formulas
1. Ko-ken-tang　　　　　　　　　　　　　葛根湯

(Pueraria Combination)
This herbal is for treating tetanus to relieve muscular tension and stiffness in the shoulders and back, and to normalized floating and tight pulse.

2. **Kua-lu-kuei-chih-tang** 瓜呂桂枝湯
   (Trichosanthes and Cinnamon Combination)
This combination is taken for mild cases of tetanus with a sunken pulse and muscular tension.

3. **Ta-cheng-chi-tang** 大承氣湯
   (Major Rhubarb Combination)
This combination is employed for the treatment of tetanus with severe muscular stiffness of the neck and back, abdominal distention, constipation, and a sunken pulse.

Acute Infectious Jaundice (Weil's Disease)

Weil's disease is an infection due to an organism of the genus *Leptospira*. Its source is contaminated food or water. After five or six days incubation, an infected person develops an abnormal fear of the cold and chills with shuddering as well as fever of 39-40°C. Other symptoms present are headache, muscular pain, low back pain, and lassitude. In severe cases the patient has difficulty rising. Generally the patient has nausea, vomiting, and anorexia for one or two days. The patient also has decreased urine volume, thirst, and constipation or diarrhea. Two or three days later, the conjunctiva becomes congested and the lymph nodes swell. Then toward the sixth or seventh day, the fever begins to subside and jaundice appears. By this time the spleen and liver have become swollen and hemorrhaging is occurring in the subcutaneous tissues, mucous membranes, and viscera. In the most severe cases, the critical symptoms presaging death appear toward the thirteenth or fourteenth day.

Symptoms

A sudden onset of fever to 39-40°C, chills, abdominal pains, vomiting, and myalgia, especially of the calf musle. An extremely severe headache is usually present. The conjunctiva is markedly reddened. The liver may be palpable; and in about 50 percent of the cases, jaundice occurs about the fifth day and may be associated with nephritis. Capillary hemorrhages and purpuric skin lesions may also appear. Meningeal irritation and associated findings of aseptic meningitis may occur. Cases in which the pretibial area is affected show a localized fever and patchy erythema on the skin of the lower legs or generalized erythema.

Complications

Iridocyclitis (inflammation of the iris or ciliary body) may occur. Myocarditis, aseptic meningitis, renal failure, and massive hemorrhage are not common but are the usual cause of death.

Treatment

Antibiotics such as penicillin or tetracyclines should be taken as early as possible and continued for six days. Careful observation for evidences of renal failure are necessary.

Chinese Herb Formulas
1. Pai-hu-chia-kuei-chih-tang　　　　　　　　　白虎加桂枝湯
   (Cinnamon and Gypsum Combination)

According to the author's experience, even though the onset of this disease is evidenced by chills, shivering or a high fever, the greater yang symptoms which call for the use of *Ma-huang-tang* or *Ta-ching-lung-tang* occur rarely. In most cases the symptoms immediately turn into *Pai-hu-chia-kuei-chih-tang* conformation and then into a *Chai-hu* conformation. Thus this formula is given at the initial stage when the patient has a violent headache, myalgia, or low back pain.

2. Hsiao-chai-hu-tang　　　　　　　　　　　　小柴胡湯
   (Minor Bupleurum Combination)
   Ta-chai-hu-tang　　　　　　　　　　　　　　大柴胡湯
   (Major Bupleurum Combination)
   Yin-chen-hao-tang　　　　　　　　　　　　　茵陳蒿湯
   (Capillaris Combination)

If nausea, vomiting, hardness beneath the heart or thoraco-costal distress are present and tongue has fur and aridity, *Hsiao-chai-hu-tang* is administered first. Then if the thoraco-costal distress or hardness beneath the heart is not alleviated and the patient still has nausea and the other symtpoms, *Ta-chai-hu-tang* is given regardless of whether there is diarrhea or constipation. If thirst and reduced urine volume are still conspicuously present, *Ta-chai-hu-tang* in combination with *Yin-chen-hao-tang* or the latter alone is given, it being effective against jaundice also.

3. **Yin-chen-wu-ling-san** 茵陳五苓散
   (Capillaris and Hoelen Five Formula)
   Fu-ling-szu-ni-tang 茯苓四逆湯
   (Hoelen, G.L. and Aconite Combination)

Although anuria (lack of urination) is a symptom of a severe condition, prognosis is good if diuresis can be rendered by these formulas. The first formula, *Yin-chen-wu-ling-san,* is used for a yang conformation while the latter formula is used for a yin conformation.

4. **Tao-ho-cheng-chi-tang** 桃核承氣湯
   (Persica and Rhubarb Combination)
   Kan-chiang-fu-tzu-tang 乾薑附子湯
   (Ginger and Aconite Combination)
   Fu-ling-szu-ni-tang 茯苓四逆湯
   (Hoelen, G.L. and Aconite Combination)

Delirium is a symptom of the *Tao-ho-cheng-chi-tang* conformation which belongs to the sunlight yang firm stage of disease. However, if the patient's voice is barely audible and his pulse weak and limbs cold, then it is a yin-conformation delirium and *Kan-chiang-fu-tzu-tang* or *Fu-ling-szu-ni-tang* or the like must be administered. In a yin conformation, patients need warm enriching tonics, and the erroneous administration of rhubarb purgatives may well hasten death.

5. **Chen-wu-tang** 眞武湯
   (Vitality Combination)
   Fu-tzu-tang 附子湯
   (Aconite Combination)
   Szu-ni-tang 四逆湯
   (Aconite, Ginger, and Licorice Combination)

If senile or feeble patients begin the disease in the yin conformation, the body temperature may not rise appreciably and the symptoms appear light; however, they may easily sink into a dangerous condition at any moment. These formulas are then efficacious. If the illness begins in a yang conformation but is mistreated causing it to turn into a yin conformation, then these formulas are indicated too. Constipation denotes a firm conformation for which the prognosis is always good; diarrhea, on the other hand, is a yin conformation and must be well attended.

6. Chen-wu-tang-ho-sheng-mo-san　　眞武湯合生脈散
    (*Vitality Combination with Ginseng, Schizandra, and Ophiopogon Formula*)
    Chih-kan-tsao-tang　　炙甘草湯
    (*Baked Licorice Combination*)
    Fu-ling-szu-ni-tang　　茯苓四逆湯
    (*Hoelen, G.L. and Aconite Combination*)

These formulas are given to patients with a weak heart and a fast, knotty, or uneven pulse.

Scarlet Fever

Scarlet fever is an acute infectious fever caused by *Hemolytic streptococci*. After three days of incubation the patient shows high fever, headache, sore throat, arthralgia, nausea, and abdominal pain. In children this condition also causes vomiting and spasms. The skin manifests a combination of a generalized flush on the trunk and proximal parts of the extremities and cheeks, and of pinpoint papular eruptions on all parts of the body except the face. The rash may last only a few hours but typically lasts two to three days before fading.

Chinese Herb Formulas
1. Ko-ken-tang　　葛根湯
    (*Pueraria Combination*)
    Ko-ken-chia-pan-hsia-tang　　葛根加半夏湯
    (*Pueraria and Pinellia Combination*)
    Kuei-chih-chia-ko-ken-tang　　桂枝加葛根湯
    (*Cinnamon and Pueraria Combination*)

These formulas are effective for scarlet fever. For floating and strong pulse *Ko-ken-tang* should be used. For nausea and spasms *Ko-ken-chia-pan-hsia-tang* should be used. For floating and weak pulse and sweating *Kuei-chih-chia-ko-ken-tang* should be used.

2. **Chai-hu-kuei-chih-tang** 柴胡桂枝湯
   (Bupleurum and Cinnamon Combination)
   This combination is taken for scarlet fever with abdominal pain, severe chills, and headache.

3. **Hsiao-chai-hu-tang** 小柴胡湯
   (Minor Bupleurum Combination)
   This combination is taken for scarlet fever with coating on the tongue, a bitter taste in the mouth, loss of appetite, bronchitis, and a swollen spleen.

4. **Pai-hu-chia-jen-sheng-tang** 白虎加人參湯
   (Gypsum and Ginseng Combination)
   This combination is taken for scarlet fever with big pulse, high fever, thirst, and stress.

5. **Chu-yeh-shih-kao-tang** 竹葉石膏湯
   (Bamboo Leaves and Gypsum Combination)
   Mai-men-tung-tang 麥門冬湯
   (Ophiopogon Combination)
   Both combinations are used for treating the later stage of scarlet fever when the patient has a fever and coarse skin.

6. **Chu-feng-chieh-tu-tang** 驅風解毒湯
   (Siler and Forsythia Combination)
   This combination is taken for scarlet fever, swollen tonsils, stomatitis (inflammation of the mouth), and swelling in the neck.

Erysipelas

Erysipelas is an infectious disease of the skin and subcutaneous tissue. It is a condition marked by redness and swelling of affected areas and somatic symptoms such as inflammation, slight pain, fever, headache, loss of appetite, insomnia, vomiting, and severe chills; sometimes these symptoms are accompanied by vesicular and bullous lesions. The condition becomes severe if the erysipelas invades the laryngeal membrane.

Chinese Herb Formulas

1. **Shih-wei-pai-tu-san** 十味敗毒散
   (Bupleurum and Schizonepeta Formula)

This formula is to be taken in the initial stage of erysipelas to combat severe chills and fever.

2. **Pai-hu-chia-kuei-chih-tang** 白虎加桂枝湯
   (Gypsum and Cinnamon Combination)

This medicinal combination is for erysipelas with high fever.

3. **Wen-ching-yin** 溫清飲
   (Tang-kuei and Gardenia Combination)
   Lung-tan-hsieh-kan-tang 龍膽瀉肝湯
   (Gentiana Combination)

These formulas are prescribed for erysipelas when the patient has a sensation of heat, swelling, severe chills, and painful urination.

4. **Hsiao-chai-hu-tang** 小柴胡湯
   (Minor Bupleurum Combination)
   Ta-chai-hu-tang 大柴胡湯
   (Major Bupleurum Combination)

Either of these combinations is prescribed for erysipelas with recurrent fever and chills, loss of appetite, nausea, and vomiting.

5. **Huang-lien-chieh-tu-tang** 黃連解毒湯
   (Coptis and Scute Combination)

For erysipelas accompanied by high fever, anxiety, and headache but with no severe chills, this combination is given. In case of loss of consciousness, emotional instability, and excitability, rhubarb should be added.

6. **Tao-ho-cheng-chi-tang** 桃核承氣湯
   (Persica and Rhubarb Combination)

This combination is taken for erysipelas with loss of consciousness, excitability, constipation, and abdominal spasms.

7. Fang-feng-tung-sheng-san　　　　　　防風通聖散
   (*Siler and Platycodon Formula*)

Elderly patients suffering from erysipelas with habitual constipation and a strong constitution are given this formula.

RESPIRATORY DISEASES

Common Cold

This is a common disease, but its symptoms vary according to individual differences and the time of year. Most common colds are infections caused by one of a number of various types of virus. These viruses are spread from person to person by coughing or sneezing. The influenza virus is exceptionally virulent and causes severe symptoms; it should not be ignored. Patients who suspect influenza should seek a doctor's diagnosis.

Symptoms
This is a typical systemic disease. There is mild itching in the nose, sore throat or swollen glands, and, as it progresses, fever, headache, cough, general lassitude, and muscular pain throughout the whole body.

Treatment
Treatment consists of quiet and rest, high fluid intake, nutritious and well-balanced meals, and keeping warm. Antihistamines (which are slightly hypnotic) and aspirin are also effective. It is suggested that those prone to the common cold, rub their body with cold water every day when in good health.

Chinese Herb Formulas

1. Ma-huang-tang 麻黃湯
   (Ma-huang Combination)

To be taken for influenza by those with a strong physique who have severe chills, high fever, and pain in the joints.

2. Kuei-chih-tang 桂枝湯
   (Cinnamon Combination)

To be taken for the common cold by those having a delicate constitution and perspiration. The main herbs of this formula are cinnamon, jujube, and paeonia.

3. Ko-ken-tang 葛根湯
   (Pueraria Combination)

To be taken for the common cold by those with an average constitution who have stiffness in the shoulders and neck.

4. Hsiang-su-san 香蘇散
   (Cyperus and Perilla Formula)

To be taken for the common cold by those with a delicate constitution who have stomach distention. *Kuei-chih-tang* (桂枝湯 , Cinnamon Combination) should be taken first.

5. Hsiao-chai-hu-Tang 小柴胡湯
   (Minor Bupleurum Combination)

To be taken by those having an average constituion and a severe lingering cold, recurrent shaking chills, fever, and gastric disturbances. Those having a delicate constitution should take *Chai-hu-kuei-chih-kan-chiang-tang* (柴胡桂枝乾薑湯 , Bupleurum, Cinnamon, and Ginger Combination).

6. Ma-huang-hsi-hsin-fu-tzu-tang 麻黃細辛附子湯
   (Ma-huang, Aconite, and Asarum Combination)

To be taken for fever accompanied by severe chills, sore throat, and cough.

7. Chen-wu-tang 眞武湯
   (Vitality Combination)

To be taken for a common cold with chills and diarrhea.

8. **Hsiao-ching-lung-tang** 小青龍湯
   (Minor Blue Dragon Combination)
   To be taken for a common cold with sneezing, nasal-drainage, and lacrimation. It is also effective for bronchial asthma.

9. **Wu-ling-san** 五苓散
   (Hoelen Five Herb Formula)
   To be taken by children with a common cold.

10. **Chu-ju-wen-tan-tang** 竹茹溫膽湯
    (Bamboo and Ginseng Combination)
    To be taken for cough with copious sputum and insomnia.

Bronchitis

When a patient suffers from influenza or the common cold, viruses or bacteria will multiply rapidly inside the bronchial tubes causing bronchitis. When the pathogens invade the alveoli of the lungs, they cause bronchopneumonia. This disease easily becomes chronic.

Symptoms

The patient with this disease has the symptoms of fever (over 37°C), sore throat, cough with sputum, chest pain, and difficult respiration. In the primary stage there is watery sputum; when the disease has become chronic, there is sticky sputum.

Treatment

From the onset, the patient should rest in bed, avoid bathing or sports, and use an inhaler or mouthpiece. Antihistamines, antipyretics, and phosphoric codeine may produce good results. In addition, a doctor may prescribe a sulfur agent or antibiotic.

Chinese Herb Formulas
1. **Ma-huang-tang** 麻黃湯
   (Ma-huang Combination)
   To be taken by those suffering from bronchitis with shaking chills, fever, and severe cough.

2. **Ma-huang-hsi-hsin-fu-tzu-tang** 麻黃細辛附子湯
   (Ma-huang, Aconite, and Asarum Combination)
   To be taken by those having bronchitis with fever and severe chills.

3. **Hsiao-chai-hu-tang** 小柴胡湯
   (Minor Bupleurum Combination)
   To be taken by those having bronchitis due to a common cold and accompanied by anorexia and vomiting.

4. **Chai-hu-kuei-chih-kan-chiang-tang** 柴胡桂枝乾薑湯
   (Bupleurum, Cinnamon, and Ginger Combination)
   This formula is for a lingering cold with bronchitis. To be taken by those having a delicate constitution with night sweats and perspiration.

5. **Chai-hsien-tang** 柴陷湯
   (Bupleurum and Scute Combination)
   To be taken for severe cough with difficulty in expectoration and chest pain due to cough.

6. **Hsiao-ching-lung-tang** 小青龍湯
   (Minor Blue Dragon Combination)
   To be taken for persistent cough, stridor, difficult respiration, watery sputum, and edema in the morning.

7. **Ma-hsing-kan-shih-tang** 麻杏甘石湯
   (Ma-huang and Apricot seed Combination)
   To be taken by children suffering from bronchial asthma due to a common cold, with stridor and rapid respiration.

8. **Ling-kan-chiang-wei-hsin-hsia-jen-tang** 苓甘薑味辛夏仁湯
   (Hoelen and Schizandra Combination)
   To be taken by those with a delicate constitution who are suffering from chronic bronchitis with mild stridor, rapid respiration, and a tendency to raise a large amount of sputum.

9. **Kua-lu-chih-shih-tang** 瓜呂枳實湯
   (Trichosanthes and Chih-shih Combination)

To be taken by smokers who have chronic bronchitis with sticky sputum and difficulty in expectoration, mild respiratory distress, and cough.

10. Mai-men-tung-tang 麥門冬湯
   (*Ophiopogon Combination*)
To be taken for persistent bronchitis with severe cough, dry throat, difficulty in expectoration, facial redness, and hoarseness.

11. Tzu-yin-chiang-huo-tang 滋陰降火湯
   (*Phellodendron Combination*)
To be taken for chronic bronchitis with severe, dry cough during the night.

12. Ching-fei-tang 清肺湯
   (*Platycodon and Fritillaria Combination*)
To be taken for chronic bronchitis with copious sputum.

13. Hua-kai-san 華蓋散
   (*Ma-huang and Morus Formula*)
To be taken by small children of delicate constitution who have bronchitis, anorexia, and diarrhea. *Ma-hsing-kan-shih-tang* (麻杏甘石湯, *Ma-huang* and Apricot Seed Combination) should be given first.

14. Pan-hsia-hou-pu-tang 半夏厚朴湯
   (*Pinellia and Magnolia Combination*)
To be taken for cough due to hysteria.

15. Tun-sou-san 頓嗽散
   (*Morus and Platycodon Formula*)
To be taken for whooping cough.

Bronchial Asthma

People have been troubled with this disease since ancient times, and it is still a typical recalcitrant disease. The patient suffers from difficult respiration and pain. This disease is generally caused by allergies, and it is influenced by the environment and the individual's particular constitution and emotional makeup.

Symptoms
The symptoms of this disease are severe cough, wheezing, difficult respiration, pain in the chest, purple fingers and lips (cyanosis), sweat, and chilling of the hands and feet.

Treatment
The patient should take antihistamine under a doctor's guidance. In severe cases, ACTH (Cortisone) is especially effective. In some cases the patient may need to live in a sanitarium during convalescence. Stimulation of the skin, supersonic therapy, anion therapy, finger pressure, or spinal column adjustment therapy may produce good results.

Chinese Herb Formulas
1. Kan-tsao-ma-huang-tang　　　　　　　　　　甘草麻黃湯
   (Licorice and Ma-huang Combination)
   To be taken as a preventive against bronchial asthma.

2. Hsiao-ching-lung-tang　　　　　　　　　　　小青龍湯
   (Minor Blue Dragon Combination)
   To be taken by those having a delicate constitution with watery sputum, difficult respiration, and wheezing.

3. Hsiao-chai-hu-tang-ho-Pan-hsia-hou-pu-tang
   　　　　　　　　　　　　　　　小柴胡湯合半夏厚朴湯
   (Minor Bupleurum Combination with Pinellia and Magnolia Combination)
   To be taken for lingering, recalcitrant bronchial asthma in those of average constitution.

4. Ta-chai-hu-tang-ho-Pan-hsia-hou-pu-tang
   　　　　　　　　　　　　　　　大柴胡湯合半夏厚朴湯
   (Major Bupleurum Combination with Pinellia and Magnolia Combination)
   To be taken by those having an obese constitution with severe wheezing, chest distention, congestion and resistance in the upper abdomen, thirst, and a tendency towards constipation.

5. **Ma-hsing-kan-shih-tang** 麻杏甘石湯
    (Ma-huang and Apricot Seed Combination)

To be taken by those having bronchial asthma with a low resistance to the common cold and a tendency towards ephidrosis. It is also effective for childhood asthma. Those having gastrointestinal weakness should avoid taking this formula.

6. **Ling-kan-chiang-wei-hsin-hsia-jen-tang** 苓甘薑味辛夏仁湯
    (Hoelen and Schizandra Combination)

To be taken by those of delicate constitution who have asthma and pulmonary emphysema, sunken and weak pulse, chills, pallor and edema.

7. **Mu-fang-chi-tang** 木防己湯
    (Stephania and Ginseng Combination)

To be taken for bronchial asthma, stomach distention, pallor, stridor, and wheezing.

8. **Szu-chun-tzu-tang** 四君子湯
    (Major Four Herb Combination)
    Jen-sheng-tang 人參湯
    (Ginseng and Ginger Combination)

To be taken by those having stomach distention, weak abdomen, loss of appetite, nausea, chills, a tendency towards fatigue, pallor, and a weak and sunken pulse.

Pneumonia

Viruses, fungi, or bacteria may invade the alveoli of the lungs and cause pneumonia. There are two categories: primary pneumonia and pneumonia which developes as a complication of a common cold, bronchitis, or influenza. If respiratory disturbance has developed (dyspnea, hemoptysis, etc.), the patient should be careful in dealing with it as it is a very dangerous symptom.

Symptoms

In severe cases there is a productive cough, hemoptysis, high fever, wheezing, chest pain, decrease of appetite, pallor, and rapid respiration. In less serious cases there is a mild productive cough and fever.

Treatment
There is still no specific drug for viral pneumonia. For diplococcus and bacterial pneumonia, antibiotics, sulfur agents, and penicillin are effective. The patient should have good care and rest in a quiet environment, and nutrition should be optimum. Sometimes, application of a moist cloth on the chest or inhalation of oxygen may be effective. The patient should see a doctor as soon as possible. Antibiotics are of no value to viral or senile pneumonia; Chinese herb formulas can be more effective in these cases.

Chinese Herb Formulas
1. **Hsiao-chai-hu-tang**　　　　　　　　　　　　　小柴胡湯
    (Minor Bupleurum Combination)
To be taken for fever, pressure and distention in the chest, bitter taste or white coating on the tongue, loss of appetite, cough, and mild difficulty in respiration.

2. **Chai-hu-kuei-chih-kan-chiang-tang**　　　柴胡桂枝乾薑湯
    (Bupleurum, Cinnamon, and Ginger Combination)
To be taken by those having a delicate constitution with chills, pallor, weak pulse, palpitation at the umbilicus, thirst, sweat on the head, and night sweats.

3. **Pai-hu-chia-jen-sheng-tang**　　　　　　　　白虎加人參湯
    (Ginseng and Gypsum Combination)
To be taken by those having high fever, dry lips, anxiety, thirst, and perspiration.

4. **Chen-wu-tang**　　　　　　　　　　　　　　　　眞武湯
    (Vitality Combination)
To be taken by those lacking vigor who feel chilled but have no fever.

5. **Ta-ching-lung-tang**　　　　　　　　　　　　　大靑龍湯
    (Major Blue Dragon Combination)
To be taken by those of average constitution who have lobar

pneumonia with a floating and tense pulse, pain, severe chills, high fever, thirst, and anxiety. Those having a weak pulse or perspiration should avoid taking this formula.

6. **Chai-hsien-tang** 柴陷湯
   (Bupleurum and Scute Combination)

To be taken by those having lobar pneumonia without shaking chills, but with fever, severe cough, difficulty in expectoration, pain and sensation of pressure in the chest, and difficult respiration.

7. **Ta-chai-hu-tang** 大柴胡湯
   (Major Bupleurum Combination)

To be taken by those of strong constitution who have lobar pneumonia with chest distention, constipation, tea-brown or yellow coating on the tongue, and a strong pulse.

8. **Hsiao-ching-lung-tang** 小青龍湯
   (Minor Blue Dragon Combination)

To be taken for primary lobar pneumonia with severe chills, fever, and cough.

9. **Ma-huang-hsi-hsin-fu-tzu-tang** 麻黃細辛附子湯
   (Ma-huang, Aconite, and Asarum Combination)

To be taken for senile pneumonia with chills, headache, sunken pulse, and fever.

10. **Chu-yeh-shih-kao-tang** 竹葉石膏湯
    (Bamboo Leaves and Gypsum Combination)

To be taken for childhood pneumonia with lingering fever and cough, dry lips, thirst, dry skin, wheezing, anxiety, and dysuria.

11. **Chu-ju-wen-tan-tang** 竹茹溫膽湯
    (Bamboo and Ginseng Combination)

To be taken by those having fever, productive cough, insomnia, nightmares, and nervousness.

12. **Szu-ni-tang** 四逆湯
    (Aconite and G L. Combination)

To be taken for pneumonia of the yin conformation with high

body temperature, weak pulse, chilling of the hands and feet, and diluted urine.

13. Tao-ho-cheng-chi-tang 桃核承氣湯
    (Persica and Rhubarb Combination)
To be taken for lobar pneumonia, high fever, unconsiciousness, constipation, and delirium.

Tuberculosis

Respiratory organs such as the throat, bronchial tubes, and lungs are susceptible to tubercle bacillus. After invading the lungs, the bacilli spread to other organs. Tuberculosis is transmitted in the sputum of an infected patient. Those with arrested tuberculosis have no tubercle bacillus in their sputum; therefore, they are not infectious.

Symptoms
The symptoms are productive cough, mild fever, night sweats, fatigue, wheezing, and loss of weight. Sometimes, in the primary stage of this disease, there are no symptoms of which the patient is aware. Therefore, it is important to have periodic physical examinations.

Treatment
Chemical: Take streptomycin or INH.
Surgical: Lung resection.
Specifics: Although there are many types of antibiotics, the tubercle bacillus is becoming increasingly resistant to them.

Most important is fresh air, quiet, and good nutrition. The best therapy is to increase the resistance of the patient. Sometimes, individual emotions also affect the progress of this disease.

Chinese therapy attempts to increase the vigor of the patient and to help bring about a natural recovery. The patient should choose the proper formula according to his individual requirements.

Chinese Herb Formulas

1. Tzu-yin-chih-pao-tang   滋陰至寶湯
  (Tang-kuei and Lycium Combination)

The main herbs of this formula are *tang-kuei,* paeonia and hoelen. To be taken by those having severe weakness and cough with copious sputum.

2. Chai-hu-kuei-chih-kan-chiang-tang   柴胡桂枝乾薑湯
  (Bupleurum, Cinnamon, and Ginger Combination)

To be taken by those having prolonged fever, severe chills, and loss of appetite.

3. Hsiao-chai-hu-tang   小柴胡湯
  (Minor Bupleurum Combination)

To be taken by those having fever, severe chills, loss of appetite, and weakness.

4. Pu-chung-i-chi-tang   補中益氣湯
  (Ginseng and Astragalus Combination)

To be taken for chronic tuberculosis with lack of vigor, a tendency towards fatigue, loss of appetite, night sweats, and mild cough. It is especially effective for women.

5. Tzu-yin-chiang-huo-tang   滋陰降火湯
  (Phellodendron Combination)

To be taken by those having cough with a small amount of sputum and difficulty in expectoration, dark skin, a tendency towards constipation, and a weak pulse.

6. Mai-men-tung-tang   麥門冬湯
  (Ophiopogon Combination)

To be taken for severe cough, convulsions, difficulty in expectoration, sputum, and facial redness.

7. Chia-wei-hsiao-yao-san   加味逍遙散
  (Bupleurum and Paeonia Formula)

To be taken by women who have headache, fever, facial flushing, irregular menstruation, thirst, night sweats, and cough.

8. Chih-kan-tsao-tang 炙甘草湯
   (Baked Licorice Combination)
   To be taken by those having rapid heart palpitations, wheezing, dry throat, and severe cough.

9. San-huang-hsieh-hsin-tang 三黃瀉心湯
   (Coptis and Rhubarb Combination)
   Huang-chieh-san 黃解散
   (Coptis and Scute Formula)
   To be taken for hemoptysis, emotional instability, and excitability.

10. Hsiang-sha-liu-chu-tzu-tang 香砂六君子湯
    (Cyperus and Cardamon Combination)
    To be taken by those having gastrointestinal weakness, loss of appetite, abdominal distention, fatigue, and a weak pulse.

11. Chen-wu-tang 眞武湯
    (Vitality Combination)
    To be taken by those having intestinal disorders, diarrhea, abdominal distention, low back pain, chills, and a weak pulse.

12. Chuan-szu-chun-tzu-tang 喘四君子湯
    (Magnolia and Citrus Combination)
    To be taken for tertiary tuberculosis with stridor, shallow respiration, and severe gasping.

Lung Gangrene

This disease is caused by an infection from putrefactive bacteria and is characterized by a stench and fetid odor in the patient's sputum and exhaled air, a condition readily detected upon entering the patient's room. First necrosis occurs in the lungs, followed by cavities resulting from the virulent activity of the pathogens which include anaerobes, spindle-shaped bacilli, spirochaeta, Fadenpilz, and ameba.

Similar to lung abscesses and hardly distinguishable from them, lung gangrene happens as a consequence of pneumonia, bronchial pneumonia, bronchitis, bronchiectasis, swallowing of foods or liquid by mistake, pathological change of esophageal cancer, metastasis of suppurative lesions through the blood stream, and injuries of lung tissue by external wounds.

Symptoms

Subjective symptoms are fever, perspiration, fatigue, anorexia, cough, expectoration, and chest pain. The body temperature generally reaches as high as 39-40°C. In the beginning, auscultation and percussion do not reveal the existence of a pathological condition. Gradually a dullness can be heard with decreased breathing sounds due to obstruction of the trachea. Rale is hardly detectable. X-ray examination reveals the same non-localized shade as in lung abscesses, and the cavity is clearly visible. Fluid retention is also exhibited. The lesion periphery has a dark shade and beyond the peripheral shade a comparatively lighter scattered shade can be seen, resembling that of pneumonia infiltration or effusion. The profuse sputum emanates a noxiously fetid odor. When placed in a glass, the sputum will separate into three layers: the upper layer consists of frothing mucous; the middle layer, a dirty serous substance; and the lower layer, a dark brownish or greenish-brown sediment containing rice-grain-sized debris of putrefacted tissue and other kinds of particles. When smeared, these are found microscopically to contain bacteria; long needle-shaped, fatty acid Dittrich's plug; erythrocytes; leucocytes; epidermis; and a lot of elastic fibers which are the enzymatic hydrolysate of the putrefactive bacteria.

Treatment
1. For spirochaeta and spindle-shaped bacilli, Salvasan can be administered in doses of 0.15-0.3g each time.
2. Penicillin can be given intratracheally.
3. Parenteral administration of penicillin, streptomycin, and other antibiotics may be employed.
4. Penicillin, mercuric chloride solution, or phenol may be inhaled.
5. The patient may be injected with his own vaccine.
6. Surgery may be necessary.

Chinese Herb Formulas
1. Chieh-keng-pai-san 桔梗白散
   (Platycodon and Croton Formula)

Owing to the drastic action of this treatment, this formula can only be used in the initial stage when the patient still has abundant body strength. It is used as a one-time drug and must not be taken successively. Four to ten minutes after administration, a thick sputum along with tissue debris from the lesion will be expectorated a couple of times. Thirty to forty minutes later, diarrhea begins which, if incessant, can be stopped simply by taking one glass of cold congee. Afterwards the patient may recover quickly: the body temperature lowers, the sputum reduces, and the general condition improves. However, for a prolonged sufferer having debilitated body strength, this formula is contraindicated.

2. Chai-hu-chih-chieh-tang-chia-ting-li 柴胡枳桔湯加葶藶
   (Bupleurum, Chih-shih, and Platycodon Combination with Lepidium)

This formula can be used lengthily by patients having all the symptoms of lung gangrene, such as chest pain, cough, fetid sputum, and alternating chills and fever.

3. Wei-ching-tang 葦莖湯
   (Phragmites Stem Combination)

This combination is suitable for mild cases. If there is copious sputum and excessive cough, 2.0g of fritillaria and 1.0g each of platycodon, aster, and licorice are added to the formula.

4. Fei-yung-tang 肺癰湯
   (Platycodon and Scute Combination)

During the initial stage, sufferers whose body strength is not strong enough to withstand the use of *Chieh-keng-pai-san* use this formula.

Cough

Chinese Herb Formulas

1. **Ma-huang-tang** 麻黃湯
   (Ma-huang Combination)
   To be taken by those of average constitution who have a common cold with fever and severe cough.

2. **Ko-ken-tang** 葛根湯
   (Pueraria Combination)
   To be taken for productive cough and sore throat accompanying a common cold.

3. **Ma-huang-hsi-hsin-fu-tzu-tang** 麻黃細辛附子湯
   (Ma-huang, Aconite, and Asarum Combination)
   To be taken for a common cold with severe chills, sore throat, and cough.

4. **Hsiao-chai-hu-tang** 小柴胡湯
   (Minor Bupleurum Combination)
   To be taken for a lingering cold with cough.

5. **Chai-hu-kuei-chih-kan-chiang-tang** 柴胡桂枝乾薑湯
   (Bupleurum, Cinnamon, and Ginger Combination)
   To be taken for a lingering cold or for bronchitis with cough. It is effective for those of delicate constitution.

6. **Hsiao-ching-lung-tang** 小青龍湯
   (Minor Blue Dragon Combination)
   To be taken for a moist cough or a cough with wheezing. It is also effective for chronic cough.

7. **Mai-men-tung-tang** 麥門冬湯
   (Ophiopogon Combination)
   To be taken for a severe hacking cough with difficulty in expectoration and emotional instability.

Sputum

Chinese Herb Formulas
1. Hsiao-ching-lung-tang　　　　　　　　小青龍湯
    (Minor Blue Dragon Combination)
    To be taken for sputum that is watery or filled with air bubbles.

2. Tzu-yin-chih-pao-tang　　　　　　　　滋陰至寶湯
    (Tang-kuei and Lycium Combination)
    To be taken by those having tuberculosis or bronchiectasis, a delicate constitution, and cough with copious sputum.

3. Ching-fei-tang　　　　　　　　　　　　清肺湯
    (Platycodon and Fritillaria Combination)
    To be taken for cough due to chronic bronchitis, bronchiectasis, and tuberculosis with copious sputum.

Difficult Breathing

Chinese Herb Formulas
1. Hsiao-ching-lung-tang　　　　　　　　小青龍湯
    (Minor Blue Dragon Combination)
    To be taken for watery sputum, cough, and difficult breathing.

2. Hsiao-chai-hu-tang-ho-Pan-hsia-hou-pu-tang
    　　　　　　　　　　　　　小柴胡湯合半夏厚朴湯
    (Minor Bupleurum Combination with Pinellia and Magnolia Combination)
    To be taken for bronchial asthma and difficult breathing.

3. Mu-fang-chi-tang　　　　　　　　　　木防己湯
    (Stephania and Ginseng Combination)
    To be taken for heart disorders with cough, difficult breathing, pallor, anemia, and edema or dysuria.

Bronchiectasis

The main symptoms of bronchiectasis are severe cough in the

morning, copious sputum, and occasional hemoptysis. In severe cases, the patient may also have difficulty breathing. The proper Chinese formulas should be chosen with regard to the patient's condition and symptoms.

Chinese Herb Formulas
1. **Ching-fei-tang** 清肺湯
    (Platycodon and Fritillaria Combination)
To be taken by those of average constitution who have a productive cough.

2. **Ling-kan-chiang-wei-hsin-hsia-jen-tang** 苓甘薑味辛夏仁湯
    (Hoelen and Schizandra Combination)
To be taken by those of delicate constitution with difficult breathing and sputum.

3. **Tzu-yin-chih-pao-tang** 滋陰至寶湯
    (Tang-kuei and Lycium Combination)
To be taken by those of delicate constitution who have bronchiectasis with tuberculosis, productive cough, loss of appetite, and night sweats.

Lung Cancer

It is very difficult to cure lung cancer completely, but use of Chinese herb formulas can reduce the symptoms of cough, chest pain, and wheezing, thereby helping the patient to feel more comfortable.

Chinese Herb Formulas
1. **Chai-hu-su-kan-tang** 柴胡疏肝湯
    (Bupleurum and Gardenia Combination)
This is effective for severe pain in the chest due to lung cancer. In the abdominal conformation, there is resistant pressure beneath the ribs, abdominal hardness, and heart distention.

2. **Tzu-ken-mu-li-tang** 紫根牡蠣湯
    (Lithospermum and Oyster Shell Combination)

This is effective for malignant tumors and lung cancer.

Pulmonary Emphysema

Pulmonary emphysema begins with chronic bronchitis or bronchial asthma. Some cases are due to job-related or environmental factors.

The symptoms of pulmonary emphysema are productive cough, a feeling of pressure in the chest, and difficult breathing on physical exertion. In severe cases, there is abdominal weakness and a weak pulse. Although it cannot be completely cured, Chinese herb formulas can make the patient feel more comfortable.

Chinese Herb Formulas

1. **Ling-kan-chiang-wei-hsin-hsia-jen-tang** 苓甘薑味辛夏仁湯
   (Hoelen and Schizandra Combination)

To be taken for pallor, productive cough, difficult breathing, weak abdomen and pulse, and edema in the lower limbs.

2. **Hou-pu-ma-huang-tang** 厚朴麻黃湯
   (Magnolia and Ma-huang Combination)

To be taken for mild pulmonary emphysema, abdominal distention, strong pulse and abdomen, cough, and difficult breathing.

3. **Hsiao-chai-hu-tang** 小柴胡湯
   (Minor Bupleurum Combination)

To be taken for pulmonary emphysema with bronchitis and severe wheezing. In cases with anxiety and thirst, gypsum should be added.

4. **Chuan-szu-chun-tzu-tang** 喘四君子湯
   (Magnolia and Citrus Combination)

To be taken by those of delicate constitution with severe pulmonary emphysema, weak pulse, wheezing, rapid respiration, and anxiety.

5. **Fu-ling-hsing-jen-kan-tsao-tang** 茯苓杏仁甘草湯
   (Hoelen, Apricot Seed, and Licorice Combination)

To be taken for difficult breathing, heart palpitations, cough, painful urination, and edema.

Pleuritis

In the majority of cases, this disease is tubercular in origin. The main symptoms are fever, cough, pain in the chest, and difficult breathing. Sometimes pus remains in the pleural cavity due to an abscess.

Chinese Herb Formulas

1. *Hsiao-chai-hu-tang* 小柴胡湯
    (Minor Bupleurum Combination)

To be taken for primary pleuritis, fever, cough, and pain or a sensation of pressure in the chest.

2. *Chai-hsien-tang* 柴陷湯
    (Bupleurum and Scute Combination)

To be taken for symptoms similar to those treated by *Hsiao-chai-hu-tang*, but with severe pain in the chest and severe cough.

3. *Chai-hu-kuei-chih-tang* 柴胡桂枝湯
    (Bupleurum and Cinnamon Combination)

To be taken for pleuritis with peritonitis or resistance of the abdominal wall, and a tense abdomen.

4. *Hsiao-ching-lung-tang* 小青龍湯
    (Minor Blue Dragon Combination)

To be taken for primary moist pleuritis without anemia, night sweats, and loss of appetite.

5. *Chai-hu-kuei-chih-kan-chiang-tang* 柴胡桂枝乾薑湯
    (Bupleurum, Cinnamon, and Ginger Combination)

To be taken by those of delicate constitution who have a weak abdomen, palpitation at the umbilicus, painful urination, thirst, asthma, and night sweats.

6. *Pu-chung-i-chi-tang* 補中益氣湯
    (Ginseng and Astragalus Combination)

To be taken for fever, cough, lack of vigor, a tendency towards fatigue, and night sweats; promotes recovery from illness.

7. Chen-wu-tang 眞武湯
   (Vitality Combination)
To be taken for severe chills, gasping respirations, loss of appetite, fatigue, tendency towards diarrhea, and a weak and sunken pulse.

8. Fu-ling-yin 茯苓飲
   (Hoelen Combination)
To be taken for pleuritis, abdominal congestion, painful urination, and loss of appetite.

Pulmonary Edema

Pulmonary edema is due to heart weakness, stagnant blood in the pulmonary veins, and fluid in the lungs. The patient has difficult breathing, stridor, watery sputum, and insomnia.

Chinese Herb Formulas
1. Ling-kan-chiang-wei-hsin-hsia-jen-tang 苓甘薑味辛夏仁湯
   (Hoelen and Schizandra Combination)
To be taken for mild pulmonary edema, weak pulse, difficult breathing, watery sputum, pallor, and insomnia.

2. Tzu-yuan 紫圓
   (Croton and Hematite Formula)
To be taken for pulmonary edema in those of average constitution.

3. Chuan-szu-chun-tzu-tang 喘四君子湯
   (Magnolia and Citrus Combination)
To be taken for pulmonary edema in tertiary tuberculosis with stridor and rapid breathing.

4. Mu-fang-chi-tang 木防己湯
   (Stephania and Ginseng Combination)
To be taken for cardiac hypertrophy and lung hypertrophy with stridor, difficult breathing, edema, and cyanosis.

DISEASES OF THE CIRCULATORY SYSTEM

Endocarditis

Endocarditis is caused by rheumatic fever or bacteria and is divided into three categories — acute, subacute, and chronic.

The patient with endocarditis from rheumatic fever has the symptoms of heart aching, a pressing sensation in the chest, difficult respiration, petechiae, and mild fever.

The patient with acute bacterial endocarditis has septicemia and is seriously ill. Subacute cases have the symptoms of anemia, fatigue, arthrodynia, enlarged spleen, hemorrhage of mucous membranes, labored breathing, and edema; there is no fever.

After recovery, the patient will still have valvular ailments. During therapy, antibiotics such as penicillin may be used in conjunction with Chinese herb formulas.

Chinese Herb Formulas
1. Chai-hu-chiang-kuei-tang-chia-wu-chu-yu-fu-ling
柴胡薑桂湯加吳茱萸茯苓
(Bupleurum, Cinnamon, and Ginger Combination with Evodia and Hoelen)
To be taken for physical weakness, palpitations, pressure at the chest, anemia, and weak pulse.

2. **Mu-fang-chi-tang** 木防己湯
   (Stephania and Ginseng Combination)
   To be taken for labored breathing, edema, stridor, and distention.

3. **Chih-kan-tsao-tang** 炙甘草湯
   (Baked Licorice Combination)
   To be taken for palpitations, disordered pulse, heated palms, and anemia.

Heart Disease of Obese Individuals
(Fatty Heart)

Fatty heart occurs as a result of the proliferation of lipid tissue on the pericardium of the heart. At times the thickness of the lipid layer may be well over 1 cm. The whole surface of the heart becomes covered making the cardiac muscle invisible. Frequently the lipid tissue infiltrates intramascularly, deep into the endocardium. Fatty heart is one of the results of obesity. Sometimes it seems to be a compensatory enlargement of the lipid tissue to fill the empty space left over by a highly atrophied heart. In the most severe cases, the heart's function is hindered. In a few cases, heart attack may result.

Obese individuals with a fatty heart usually have excessive lipid sedimentation and will experience gasping and palpitation upon the slightest body movement. Those over middle age must be attentive to the danger of the complication of arteriosclerosis.

Treatment
Since this condition is due to obesity, treatment is for obesity.

Chinese Herb Formulas
1. Ta-chai-hu-tang-chia-hou-pu-hsing-jen 大柴胡湯加厚朴杏仁
   (Major Bupleurum Combination with Magnolia Bark and Apricot Seed)

This formula is indicated for distention of the abdomen, especially that of the epigastrium; thoraco-costal distress with palpitations; asthma; and constipation. Administration of this formula will reduce the abdominal distention and thoraco-costal distress; respiration will become regular and comfortable. Palpitation also decreases. In addition, fat and carbohydrates must be restricted in the diet.

2. Chai-hu-chia-lung-ku-mu-li-tang　　　柴胡加龍骨牡蠣湯
  (Bupleurum and Dragon Bone Combination)
This formula is used for the same symptoms as the *Ta-chai-hu-tang* conformation above with the accompanying symptoms of palpitations, asthma, and nervousness.

3. Chiu-wei-pin-lang-tang-chia-wu-chu-yu-fu-ling
　　　　　　　　　　　　　九味檳榔湯加吳茱萸茯苓
  (Areca Seed Nine Combination with Evodia and Hoelen)
This formula is prescribed for obese individuals with loose and flaccid muscles, edematous tendencies, lassitude, palpitations, and asthma. *Ta-cheng-chi-tang* (大承氣湯 Major Rhubarb Combination), and *Fang-feng-tung-sheng-san* (防風通聖散 Siler and Platycodon Formula) may also be given. (See the monogram on obesity.)

Valvular Disease

The valves of the heart may thicken and harden for some particular reason, and then sometimes they will twist and operate (open and close) irregularly, becoming narrow. This is called "valvular disease", and it is divided into two categories — congenital and acquired.

Acquired valvular disease is usually caused by rheumatic fever. Endocarditis, a complication of rheumatic fever, will also induce valvular inflammation. Other causes are syphilis, arteriosclerosis, tonsilitis, and scarlet fever.

Symptoms

In the primary stage of this disease, there are no symptoms of which the patient is aware. The heart will compensate by adjusting its activities automatically to complete its job. This adjustment will cause cardiac hypertrophy. Then when the patient does some exercise or even walks up or down stairs, he will experience palpitation or wheezing due to the heart's loss of efficiency as a pump. In severe cases, the condition will gradually lead to congestive heart failure.

Treatment
Because the cause of rheumatic fever is not clear, there is no perfect therapy. But whether the disease is congenital or acquired, it should be prevented from leading to congestive heart failure. Meanwhile, even influenza should not be allowed to continue. Recently, cardiac surgeons have been able to remove successfully the diseased valves and replace them with artificial ones.

The various categories of valvular disease are classified according to the locations of the valves involved, whether the condition is congenital or acquired, and the extent of the stenosis. However, Chinese therapy is not based on the above differences; it treats according to the patient's complaint and abdominal and pulse conformation.

Chinese Herb Formulas:
1. **Mu-fang-chi-tang** 木防己湯
   (Stephania and Ginseng Combination)
This is the most common formula to be taken for congestive heart failure. In abdominal conformation, there is distention, edema, stridor, rapid respiration, and decrease of urine. In severe cases, add digitalis power (0.1 gm.) each day.

2. **Chih-kan-tsao-tang** 炙甘草湯
   (Baked Licorice Combination)
To be taken for palpitations, gasping, stagnant pulse, thirst, hot palms and feet, anemia, and dry skin. Those having diarrhea or a tendency towards diarrhea should avoid taking this formula.

3. **Pien-chih-hsin-chi-yin** 變製心氣飲
   (Areca and Evodia Combination)
To be taken for difficult urination and edema, palpitations, gasping, heaviness of head, and depression. In the abdominal con-

formation, there is resistance under the heart and hepatomegalia. For cases that do not respond to *Mu-fang-chi-tang,* use this formula, and vice versa.

4. **Chai-hu-chiang-kuei-tang-chia-wu-chu-yu-fu-ling**　　　　柴胡薑桂湯加吳茱萸茯苓
   (Bupleurum and C. G. Combination with Evodia and Hoelen)
To be taken for mild valvular diseases, physical weakness, anemia, palpitation, gasping, abdominal weakness, chilling, and nervousness.

5. **Chai-hu-chia-lung-ku-mu-li-tang**　　　　柴胡加龍骨牡蠣湯
   (Bupleurum and Dragon Bone Combination)
To be taken for mild valvular diseases, palpitation and vertigo, difficult excretion, distention, and fullness in the upper abdomen.

6. **Wu-ling-san**　　　　五苓散
   (Hoelen Five Herb Formula)
It is effective for thirst, difficult urination, palpitations, and edema.

7. **Fu-ling-kan-tsao-tang**　　　　茯苓甘草湯
   (Hoelen and Licorice Combination)
To be taken for difficult urination and edema, palpitation, and chilling of the hands and feet.

8. **Fu-ling-hsing-jen-kan-tsao-tang**　　　　茯苓杏仁甘草湯
   (Hoelen, Apricot Seed, and Licorice Combination)
To be taken for severe valvular diseases, rapid respirations, gasping and coughing, edema, and severe distention at the chest. The effect lasts only a short time.

9. **Tang-kuei-shao-yao-san**　　　　當歸芍藥散
   (Tang-kuei and Paeonia Formula)
It is effective for mild valvular diseases, anemia, palpitation, heaviness of head, and chilling of the hands and feet.

10. **Kuei-chih-fu-ling-wan-chia-che-chien-tzu-mao-ken**
    　　　　桂枝茯苓丸加車前子茅根
    (Cinnamon and Hoelen Formula with Plantago and Imperata)

To be taken for valvular diseases with stagnant blood.

11. Liu-chun-tzu-tang 六君子湯
(Major Six Herb Combination)
To be taken for gastrointestinal and physical weaknesses. If there is anemia, add *tang-kuei* 3.0g and astragalus 2.0g. If there is edema, add magnolia bark 2.0g, cyperus 3.0g, and saussurea 1.0.

Hypertension

As a confined fluid, blood will naturally exert pressure on the blood vessel walls as it circulates in them. The term for this is "blood pressure", and it varies somewhat at different locations of measurement. It will increase with the contraction of the heart and the transport of blood (this is called the maximum or systolic pressure); it will decrease when the heart is relaxing and absorbing blood (this is called the minimum or diastolic pressure).

We can measure the maximum (systolic) and the minimum (diastolic) blood pressure with the mercury pressure gauge. If we say that the blood pressure is "120", it means that the weight of a column of mercury 120 mm. high is equal to the pressure of the stream of blood in the vessels.

From the standpoint of modern medicine, hypertension is an abnormal increase of the internal pressure in the artery. According to the World Health Organization, hypertension exists when the maximum (systolic) blood pressure is over 160 mm. and the minimum (diastolic) is over 95 mm.

Hypertension and hypotension are not good indications. It has been said that an individual's normal maximum (systolic) pressure should be 90 plus his age. Statistical results have shown this dictum to be incorrect. Now, at any age, the ideal maximum (systolic) pressure is considered to be 120 mm., and the minimum (diastolic) pressure, about 70 mm. Hypertension itself is not essentially dangerous, but it may aggravate other conditions such as nephritis, heart disease, and arteriosclerosis.

Symptoms
The common symptoms of which the patient is aware are headache, a feeling of heaviness in the head, shoulder aching,

vertigo, palpitations, gasping, and tinnitus. Often this type of hypertension is caused by overwork, drunkenness, and other external causes. These stress factors increase the blood pressure in most cases, and this increase is called "secondary hypertension." On the other hand, there may be symptoms which can only be detected during a physical examination; the rise in blood pressure accompanying these is called "essential hypertension", the cause of which is unknown.

Treatment

It is very important to treat hypertension early. There are various hypotensive agents to decrease the blood pressure. Unfortunately, the general public often takes these medicines at random, thereby limiting the blood supply to the kidneys and the brain, causing cerebromalacia. For the sake of safety, the patient should be under a doctor's care. However, it is better not to depend on medicines. In order to prevent the diseases accompanying hypertension, it is best to depend on taking good care of oneself daily.

In Chinese formula therapy, hypotensives are not always used to decrease blood pressure. It first adjusts the imbalance in the whole body; then the blood pressure will become normal as a result of the proper balance which has been restored within the body. Therefore, it does not use the common formulas to decrease blood pressure. The patient taking Chinese herb formulas will not suffer from hypotension or side effects, even when the formulas are taken over a long period of time.

Chinese Herb Formulas

There is no specific for hypertension in Chinese herb formulas, but proper prescriptions for its symptoms will make the patient more comfortable and decrease the blood pressure.

1. Ta-chai-hu-tang   大柴胡湯
(Major Bupleurum Combination)

To be taken by those having good structure, vigor, and strength. It is effective for chest fullness, heart distention, lung congestion, a tendency towards fatigue, loss of appetite, abdominal distention, and constipation in the physically tough and strong. The patient generally feels shoulder stiffness and heaviness of the head. If there is constipation, add rhubarb. Prolonged use of this formula can reduce chest fullness and tenseness in the abdomen, after which blood pressure will become normal.

2. **Huang-lien-chieh-tu-tang** 黃連解毒湯
   (Coptis and Scute Combination)

This is effective for congestion, flushed face, anxiety, nosebleed, hemophthalmia, headache, vertigo, tinnitus, and insomnia. If there is constipation, add rhubarb. In the abdominal conformation, there is heart distention without chest fullness or tense abdominal tendons.

3. **Chai-hu-chia-lung-ku-mu-li-tang** 柴胡加龍骨牡蠣湯
   (Bupleurum and Dragon Bone Combination)

To be taken for chest fullness, sensation of fullness at the upper abdomen, palpitation, vertigo, insomnia, nervousness, and a tendency towards emotional excitability. If there is no constipation, rhubarb may be omitted.

4. **Chi-wu-chiang-hsia-tang** 七物降下湯
   (Tang-kuei and Gambir Combination)

This is effective for hypertension, repeated hemophthalmia, spasms in the lower limbs, fatigue, headache, nosebleed, and night sweats. It is also effective for chronic hypertension, elevated diastolic pressure, and hypertension due to nephrosclerosis.

5. **Tiao-teng-san** 釣藤散
   (Gambir Formula)

To be taken for headache in the morning, tinnitus, depression, amnesia, and hypertension due to cerebral arteriosclerosis.

6. **Pa-wei-wan** 八味丸
   (Rehmannia Eight Formula)

To be taken for nephrosclerosis, chronic nephritis, and intermittent trouble walking. It is also effective for nocturia, thirst, hot palms and feet, pain at the waist, and edema in the lower limbs.

7. **Fang-feng-tung-sheng-san** 防風通聖散
   (Siler and Platycodon Formula)

To be taken by those who are obese and physically strong who have fullness at the abdomen and a tendency towards constipation.

8. Pan-hsia-pai-chu-tien-ma-tang 半夏白朮天麻湯
(Pinellia and Gastrodia Combination)
This is effective for gastrointestinal weakness, lack of strength, pallor, chilling, headache, vertigo, and nausea.

Hypotension

Hypotension alone is not necessarily a disease. It is a good health practice to maintain a lower blood pressure after middle age. However, hypotension can signal the various disorders caused by low blood pressure. Usually those having a systolic pressure under 100 mm. are prone to have these disorders. But there are still quite a few people with hypotension who are healthy and free from illness. Therefore, it cannot be positively stated that a systolic pressure below a certain level is "hypotension".

Those having a maximum (systolic) blood pressure under 90 mm. with vertigo, anemia, and loss of appetite should pay special attention to the situation, as should those who have only about 10 mm. difference between their maximum (systolic) and minimum (diastolic) pressure and who show no improvement even after treatment. Also in this category are those who have no symptoms of which they are aware (including those who have a weak pulse).

There are two types of hypotension. One is "natural hypotension" (physical hypotension). This is the type generally referred to in connection with various disorders. Its cause is not yet clear. The other is the "consecutive hypotension" (acute hypotension) caused by heart or endocrine disorders, internal bleeding, and other diseases.

Symptoms
Symptoms consist of a maximum (systolic) blood pressure below 100 mm., a minimum (diastolic) blood pressure which cannot be measured in some cases, occasional vertigo, lassitude, headache, chilled limbs, shoulder stiffness, palpitations, tinnitus,

insomnia, easy fatigability, and pressure at the chest. Occasionally, there is chronic gastrointestinal disorder (loss of appetite, vomiting, constipation, diarrhea).

Treatment
Since it is a chronic disorder, hypotension should be treated with patience while attempting to increase the blood pressure. Hypotension, like hypertension, is greatly affected by mental and emotional factors. Therefore, the patient should attempt to maintain emotional stability. Improvement can be expected if the patient can live in an area of lower atmospheric pressure.

Chinese Herb Formulas
1. Chen-wu-tang　　　　　　　　　　　　　　眞武湯
   (*Vitality Combination*)

To be taken by slender persons who lack vigor and have chills in the limbs, vertigo, unsteadiness, gastrointestinal weakness, pain in the abdomen, diarrhea, palpitations, and ascites. After taking this formula, the patient will have vigor and an increase in appetite; the blood pressure will rise naturally.

2. Chia-wei-hsiao-yao-san　　　　　　　　　加味逍遙散
   (*Bupleurum and Paeonia Formula*)

To be taken by those having physical weakness, vertigo, headache, palpitations, and hypotension.

3. Pan-hsia-pai-chu-tien-ma-tang　　　　　半夏白朮天麻湯
   (*Pinellia and Gastrodia Combination*)

This is effective for the patient having gastroptosis, gastrointestinal weakness, easy fatigability, drowsiness after meals, chilling of the feet, vertigo, headache, and nausea.

Cardioneurosis

The patient with this disease has subjective symptoms and an uneasy feeling. He suffers from palpitations, difficult respiration, and aching at the heart. Any slightly abnormal contraction will cause anxiety and symptoms similar to those of angina pectoris. All of these symptoms will become more severe with each relapse. The patient will have a tendency towards fatigue, headache, insomnia, night sweats, pale or flushed face, vertigo, trembling of the fingers, and absent-mindedness. It can be cured quickly by Chinese herb formulas.

Chinese Herb Formulas

1. **Pan-hsia-hou-pu-tang**   半夏厚朴湯
   (Pinellia and Magnolia Combination)

To be taken for asphyxia-like palpitations due to pressure at the chest and fear of death. In abdominal conformation, there is distention and a watery sound beneath the heart.

2. **Chai-hu-chia-lung-ku-mu-li-tang**   柴胡加龍骨牡蠣湯
   (Bupleurum and Dragon Bone Combination)

To be taken for distention at the chest and heart, nervousness, palpitations, rapid respirations, and aching at the chest. The patient will also suffer from insomnia, shoulder stiffness, vertigo, and constipation. In abdominal diagnosis, there is palpitation in the area of the umbilicus.

3. **Tang-kuei-tang**   當歸湯
   (Tang-kuei Combination)

To be taken for symptoms resembling those of angina pectoris — pain from chest to back and labored breathing, and for chilling in the abdomen, chest, and back. Although there is fullness in the upper abdomen, it is weak and full of gas.

4. **Pen-tun-tang**   奔豚湯
   (Pueraria and Ginger Combination)

This is effective for palpitations, pain in the chest and back, and labored breathing.

Paroxysmal Tachycardia

Paroxysmal tachycardia is the sudden increase of heartbeat to 150-250 followed by gradual restoration to normal. A paroxysm may last from one to two minutes to several hours or several days. The increase is from an extra systolic contraction after an extrasinal stimulation and may occur as an atrial, atrioventricular, or ventricular tachycardia. Atrial type tachycardia commonly occurs in juveniles because of excessive fatigue, drinking of liquor, smoking, G I disturbances, or change of posture, and not generally because of cardiac disease. It may also be caused by acute rheumatism, pneumonia, Graves' disease, pregnancy, or mitral stenosis. Ventricular tachycardia is found mostly in people over middle age and is caused by organic heart disease, especially hypertension, coronary arteriosclerosis, and myocardial infarction.

Symptoms
The patient will have palpitations; quick and short breathing; an insecure sensation; and occasionally the shock symptoms of pallor, cold sweating, nausea, and vomiting. Commonly the heart beat rises to 150-250, gradually becoming irregular; however, the slow and fast irregularity cannot be detected by stethoscopic differentiation. The paroxysm may cease in a few minutes or a few hours and return to normal.

Treatment
Upon having paroxysms, the patient must rest, and then be treated with the following paroxysm-interruption method. First the right side of the carotid sinus, then the left side, finally both the carotid sini are depressed for five to ten seconds each, or the Valsalva test is performed: the patient is directed to close his nose and mouth while forceful expiratory efforts are made. If this paroxysm-interruption method does not work, then quinidine sulfate (1-1.5g divided into three to five doses daily) or digitalis is given in large quantities. For prophylaxis, the inducing factors should be eliminated; in the repeatedly occurring cases, sedatives or quinidine are recommended. If there are signs of heart exhaustion after repetitive paroxysms, digitalis is prescribed.

Chinese Herb Formulas
1. Pan-hsia-hou-pu-tang-ho-kuei-chih-kan-tsao-lung-ku-mu-li-tang
   半夏厚朴湯合桂枝甘草龍骨牡蠣湯
   (Pinellia and Magnolia Combination with Cinnamon, Licorice, and Dragon Bone Combination)
This formula is indicated for patients with paroxysmal tachycardia, an uneasy feeling, and frequent urination with increased volume.

2. **Chih-kan-tsao-tang** 炙甘草湯
   (Baked Licorice Combination)
   This formula is mostly given with the knotty and alternate pulse as its targets. Abdominal diagnosis will reveal hyperfunctional pulsation above the navel in most cases.

3. **Chai-hu-chia-lung-ku-mu-li-tang** 柴胡加龍骨牡蠣湯
   (Bupleurum and Dragon Bone Combination)
   This formula can be used by persons with thoraco-costal distress, hardness and distention beneath the heart, and constipation.

4. **Chai-hu-chiang-kuei-tang-chia-wu-chu-yu-fu-ling**
   柴胡薑桂湯加吳茱萸茯苓
   (Bupleurum, Ginger, and Cinnamon Combination with Evodia and Hoelen)
   This formula is used for a weaker conformation than that of *Chai-hu-chia-lung-ku-mu-li-tang*. The abdomen is toneless, and there is hyperfunctional pulsation at the navel.

Arteriosclerosis

The artery is an important supporting vessel of life. Therefore, its structure is exquisite and delicate. If it bears excessive work and strain, this vessel will have a tendency to deteriorate as happens in arteriosclerosis. Most older people have arteriosclerosis to a greater or lesser extent. As with hypertension, this disease has a high mortality rate.

The following illustrations show the composition of a healthy artery and that of an artery affected by arteriosclerosis:

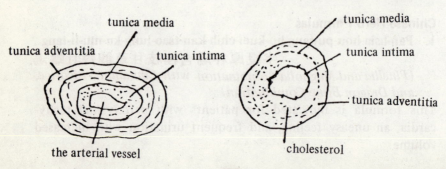

According to the above diagram, the artery is composed of three layers — tunica adventitia, tunica media, and tunica intima, within which the blood circulates. When the tunica intima grows thick or there is cholesterol (a type of lipid) between the tunica intima and the tunica media, calcium salts will be deposited on the inner wall of the blood vessel and harden the vessel. The inner diameter of the blood vessel gradually becomes smaller and a situation occurs which will disturb the blood circulation and eventually cause a blockage. This disease is called "arteriosclerosis".

The general public is aware that metabolic disorders of cholesterol are the probable cause of arteriosclerosis. Nevertheless, there are other causes of this disease such as heredity, the condition of the liver, faulty blood circulation, mental factors, and drugs. In short, arteriosclerosis is directly caused by cholesterol which has built up on the inside wall of the artery, and it will become more serious as the amount of cholesterol in the blood stream increases.

Symptoms

In addition to the general symptoms of arteriosclerosis, there are specific symptoms due to different locations affected. The majority of cases of this disease eventually involve cerebral arteriosclerosis. Cerebral arteriosclerosis is the cause of cerebromalacia and cerebral hemorrhage and is indicated by symptoms of vertigo, paralysis, tinnitus, heaviness of head, and impaired eyesight and hearing. In addition, there are mental disturbances such as decrease of memory and computing power and unstable emotions. In severe cases, there will be speech disturbance, hemiplegia, and difficulty in walking. The patient with coronary arteriosclerosis will have cardiac arrhythmia, angina pectoris, and myocardial infarction. Nephrosclerosis (arteriosclerosis of the kidney) will cause albuminuria and decrease of renal function. Intestinal arteriosclerosis will cause intermittent difficulty in walking and gastralgia. Arteriosclerosis in the legs will cause intermittent claudication and consequent difficulty in walking.

Treatment

The first step is to prevent the progress of arteriosclerosis.

Hypertension, obesity, and diabetes, all of which aggravate arteriosclerosis, must be cured first. The basic treatment for this disease is diet therapy. It is important to lead a regular daily life and maintain mental calmness.

Chinese Herb Formulas

1. **Mu-fang-chi-tang** 木防己湯
   (Stephania and Ginseng Combination)

To be taken by the patient with this disease who has the symptoms of gasping, palpitations, and pressure at the chest. In abdominal conformation, there may be distention at the heart. When perilla 5.0g, morus 3.0g, and ginger 3.0g are added to the drug, the combination may be taken for stridor and dyspnea.

2. **Chai-hu-chia-lung-ku-mu-li-tang** 柴胡加龍骨牡蠣湯
   (Bupleurum and Dragon Bone Combination)

To be taken by the patient with this disease who has nervousness, palpitations, pressure at the chest, insomnia, fullness at the chest and beneath the heart, and constipation.

3. **Chih-kan-tsao-tang** 炙甘草湯
   (Baked Licorice Combination)

A formula for palpitation and stagnant pulse, it is also effective for coronary arteriosclerosis.

4. **Ta-chai-hu-tang-ho-tao-ho-cheng-chi-tang**
   大柴胡湯合桃核承氣湯
   (Major Bupleurum Combination with Persica and Rhubarb Combination)

To be taken for obesity, fullness at the chest, distention in the lower abdomen, and constipation. It is especially effective for women.

5. **Fang-feng-tung-sheng-san** 防風通聖散
   (Siler and Platycodon Formula)

It is effective for the physically strong and obese who have a sensation of fullness at the abdomen, shoulder stiffness, headache, and constipation.

6. Tiao-teng-san　　　　　　　　　　　　　釣藤散
   (Gambir Formula)
   To be taken for headache caused by arteriosclerosis. The headache is not severe, but occurs when one gets up in the morning. It is a disease of senility and will respond rapidly to treatment.

7. San-huang-hsieh-hsin-tang　　　　　　三黃瀉心湯
   (Coptis and Rhubarb Combination)　　黃連解毒湯
   Huang-lien-chieh-tu-tang
   (Coptis and Scute Combination)
   To be taken by the patient with this disease who has symptoms of facial edema, nervousness, vertigo, tinnitus, and insomnia.

8. Pa-wei-wan　　　　　　　　　　　　　　八味丸
   (Rehmannia Eight Formula)
   To be taken for nephrosclerosis, fatigue, nocturnal polyuria, low back pain, weakness in the legs, and intermittent difficulty in walking.

9. Shih-chuan-ta-pu-tang　　　　　　　　十全大補湯
   (Ginseng and Tang-kuei Ten Combination)
   To be taken for physical weakness, pallor, dry skin, retarded motion, and amnesia.

Intermittent Walking Difficulty

Arteriosclerosis in the legs is the cause of this condition. The left leg is more often affected than the right. The patient will feel pain in the legs after walking 100 to 200 meters, and he needs to rest before he can walk again. This is due to the arteriosclerosis in the legs which causes poor blood circulation.

Chinese Herb Formulas
1. Pa-wei-wan　　　　　　　　　　　　　　八味丸
   (Rehmannia Eight Formula)
   The patient will be able to take long walks comfortably after taking this drug for a month. However, this formula should be continued to prevent recurrences.

2. **Pu-yin-tang** 補陰湯
   (Tang-kuei and Rehmannia Combination)
   Pa-wei-wan (八味丸 , Rehmannia Eight Formula) will be effective in most cases; if it isn't, use this formula.

Cardiac Asthma

The onset of difficult respirations is the main symptom of cardiac asthma. The attack may occur either during activity or while at rest during sleep. It begins with labored breathing and cough, clammy perspiration, and a feeling of uneasiness. The attack lasts from ten minutes to two hours, followed by weak or stagnant pulse. At this time, the patient is in danger of death.

Chinese Herb Formulas
1. **Mu-fang-chi-tang** 木防己湯
   (Stephania and Ginseng Combination)
   This formula can be taken for treatment or for prevention. It is effective for distention at the heart, rapid respirations, stridor, and edema.

2. **Pien-chih-hsin-chi-yin** 變製心氣飲
   (Areca and Evodia Combination)
   This formula can be taken for prevention. It is effective for distention at the heart and for edema. Some patients who have used *Mu-fang-chi-tang* without obtaining results may use this formula, and vice versa.

3. **Fu-ling-hsing-jen-kan-tsao-tang** 茯苓杏仁甘草湯
   (Hoelen, Apricot Seed, and Licorice Combination)
   Fu-ling-hsing-jen-kan-tsao-tang-ho-Ma-huang-hsing-jen-kan tsao-shih-kao-tang
   茯苓杏仁甘草湯合麻黃杏仁甘草石膏湯
   (Hoelen, Apricot Seed, and Licorice Combination with Ma-huang and Apricot Seed Combination)
   To be taken by those patients having labored breathing, distention at the chest, stridor, and edema. It may be taken during an attack when *ma-huang* and gypsum are added to *Fu-ling-hsing-jen-kan-tsao-tang*. The combination is called *Fu-ling-hsing-jen-kan-tsao-*

tang and *Ma-huang-hsing-jen-kan-tsao-shih-kao-tang*. *Ma-huang* is effective for bronchial asthma and cardiac asthma.

4. Chih-chuan-i-fang   治喘一方
 (Hoelen, Magnolia, and Apricot Seed Formula)
To be taken during an attack of cardiac asthma; it has a short term effect.

Angina Pectoris

Angina pectoris is a syndrome in which there is paroxysmal pain at the heart. The blood vessel that supplies oxygen and nutrients to the heart is called the "coronaria". When there is a disorder and subsequent blockage of this blood vessel, the resultant stricture causes an insufficient blood supply which results in "angina pectoris" and further leads to myocardial infarction.

Most myocardial infarction patients are male. Those having hypotension also suffer from this disease. Angina pectoris does not occur in other heart diseases.

The majority of patients suffering from hypertension are obese and have a pot belly with a characteristic hard distention beneath the ribs. Their electrocardiogram is normal.

The proposed causes of angina pectoris are coronary arteriosclerosis, clonus (spasm), and syphilis. The suspected immediate factors responsible for an attack are those common to other heart attacks — excessive exercise, careless diet, excitement, sudden contact with cold air. There is also pseudo angina pectoris.

Symptoms

Occasionally, there is a severe pain and a feeling of pressure at the heart. This sensation will extend to the shoulders, back, and left wrist. There is also pallor or clammy perspiration; breathing is normal. At the onset, some of those having a weak heart find the attack unbearable. There will also be depression, fear, and a feeling of despair. The majority of patients will be unable to lie prone, but will squat or pace, holding the chest.

The duration of the attack may last several minutes to about an hour. It usually eases after ten minutes if there is no other disorder. After the initial attack, some may have relapses two or three times a month; others may have only one in several years. Relapses, however, do not necessarily signify advancing heart disease.

Treatment

Either amyl nitrite or nitroglycerin is effective during the attack. Amyl nitrite will work in 5 to 15 seconds, and nitroglycerine in a minute. Because the relapses of this disease are sudden and serious, the patient should consult a doctor and bring his medication along.

The above drugs are for temporary suppression of pain. To avoid toxicity, they should not be taken too often. The patient can lessen the chances of relapse by living a normal life, by avoiding stress inducing situations, and by maintaining emotional stability. The obese should be on a limited diet or taking enzymes with every meal to disperse useless fat. Syphilis should be cured if it is the cause.

Chinese Herb Formulas

Even when the electrocardiogram is normal, if there is a hard and distended feeling beneath the ribs, the patient should take the Chinese herb formulas and try to live a normal life.

1. Chai-hu-chia-lung-ku-mu-li-tang with Coptis 1.5g and Pueraria 5.0g 柴胡加龍骨牡蠣湯加黃連1.5g葛根5.0g
(Bupleurum and Dragon Bone Combination with Coptis 1.5g and Pueraria 5.0g)

To be taken for treatment and prevention of nervousness, distention at the heart, palpitation at the umbilicus, insomnia, and overreaction to stress.

2. Kua-lu-hsieh-pai-pai-chiu-tang 瓜呂薤白白酒湯
(Trichosanthes, Bakeri, and Vinegar Combination)

To be taken by the patient with severe angina pectoris who has aching in the chest and back, stridor, and labored respiration. If it is difficult to drink during the attack, wait and drink when the discomfort eases a little.

3. **Kua-lou-tang** 栝樓湯
   (Trichosanthes Combination)

This is effective for the patient who does not respond to *Kua-lou hsieh-pai-pai-chiu-tang* and whose condition worsens. To be taken for severe pain extending from chest to back accompanied by rapid respirations.

4. **Tang-kuei-tang** 當歸湯
   (Tang-kuei Combination)

More effective for pseudo angina pectoris, this formula is adopted from *Chien chin fang* (Precious Prescriptions), and is to be taken for paroxysmal pain at the heart and abdomen with chilling and distention, severe pain from abdomen to chest and often in the arm as far as the wrist. It is especially suitable for chilling in the upper chest and back.

5. **Pan-hsia-hou-pu-tang** 半夏厚朴湯
   (Pinellia and Magnolia Combination)

To be taken for pseudo angina pectoris.

6. **Kua-lou-chih-shih-tang** 栝樓枳實湯
   (Trichosanthes and Chih-shih Combination)

To be taken for smoker's bronchitis, lung congestion, a sensation of chest pain, difficult respirations, hoarseness, and angina pectoris.

Phlebitis

If a vein is blocked by blood clots, venous thrombosis, inflammation of the vein (phlebitis) will follow, and there will be edema, violent muscle spasm, pain, and difficulty in walking. This occurs more often in the left lower limb. The main causes of this disease are childbirth, abortion, excessive strain, and infections. When there is an attack, Chinese herb formulas should be taken as soon as possible to effect a cure. The longer it is left untreated, the more difficult it will be to cure.

Chinese Herb Formulas
1. **Kuei-chih-fu-ling-wan**　　　　　　　　桂枝茯苓丸
    (Cinnamon and Hoelen Formula)
To be taken for inflammation of the vein (phlebitis).

2. **Ta-huang-mu-tan-pi-tang**　　　　　　大黃牡丹皮湯
    (Rhubarb and Moutan Combination)
To be taken by those of strong conformation with resistance and swelling in the lower abdomen and constipation.

Aneurysm

Dilatation of an artery is called an "aneurysm". When it is small, there are no evident symptoms; as it enlarges, it will put pressure on the neighboring tissues and cause pain in the chest, difficulty in swallowing, coughing, labored breathing, and hoarseness.

Chinese herb formulas cannot completely cure this condition, but they can make the patient comfortable.

Chinese Herb Formulas
1. **Chai-hu-chia-lung-ku-mu-li-tang**　　柴胡加龍骨牡蠣湯
    (Bupleurum and Dragon Bone Combination)
To be taken for palpitations, gasping, pain and pressure in the chest, nervousness, insomnia, fullness in the upper abdomen, and constipation.

2. **Kuei-chih-fu-ling-wan**　　　　　　　　桂枝茯苓丸
    (Cinnamon and Hoelen Formula)
To be taken for aneurysm in the abdomen. In abdominal conformation, there is stagnant blood at the abdomen. Add rhubarb as the case requires.

Quincke's Disease

(Angioneurotic Edema)

Limited to one area of the skin and mucous membrane, this

disease is a paroxysmal edema which moves and disappears. It is a chronic edematous condition which appears on the face or around the joints of the limbs.

Chinese Herb Formula
Wu-ling-san 五苓散
(Hoelen Five Herb Formula)
This is very effective for Quincke's disease.

Raynaud's Disease
(Symmetrical Gangrene)

Young women often suffer from this disease. It is a condition in which the arteries supplying blood to the fingers and toes become temporarily narrowed, reducing the blood flow to the extremities. It most often affects the hands which first become white, then purple. It is very painful and progresses to symmetrical gangrene.

Chinese Herb Formulas
1. **Tang-kuei-szu-ni-chia-wu-chu-yu-sheng-chiang-tang**
 當歸四逆加吳茱萸生薑湯
 (Tang-kuei, Evodia, and Ginger Combination)
This is effective in alleviating spasm of the arterial wall. Continue this formula to stop the pain.

2. **Tang-kuei-nien-tung-tang** 當歸拈痛湯
 (Tang-kuei and Anemarrhena Combination)
To be taken for a tendency towards symmetrical gangrene. This will relieve the symptoms.

Terminal Spasm

The majority of patients with this condition are women. In cold weather the patient will have very pale skin and feel extremely cold.

Chinese Herb Formulas
1. Tang-kuei-szu-ni-chia-wu-chu-yu-sheng-chiang-tang
當歸四逆加吳茱萸生薑湯
(Tang-kuei, Evodia, and Ginger Combination)
This is effective for terminal spasm disease. If the patient wants to be completely cured, she should take this formula for one year (including the summer).

2. Fu-tzu-li-chung-tang   附子理中湯
(Ginseng, Ginger, and Aconite Combination)
To be taken by the patient with terminal spasm disease who has gastrointestinal weakness, loss of appetite, and weak abdomen.

Acromelalgia (Erythromelalgia)

This disease occurs abruptly exhibiting drastic pain and flushing in the skin accompanied by swelling and a rise in temperature at the site of a lesion. The pain is augmented by warmth and exercise and alleviated by cold and rest. It occurs mostly in the toes and feet, and occasionally in the calves, fingers, and hands. It attacks one or more limbs but rarely effects the face. It is found in male and female teenagers after puberty but rarely in children. It takes a chronic proceeding and relapses for years, resulting in atrophy of the skin and subdermic tissues and deformation of bones and nails at the lesion. Besides being complicated by nervous system diseases and syphilis, it occurs independently as a single disease.

Treatment
Treatment is the same as for Raynaud's disease.

Chinese Herb Formulas
See Raynaud's disease.

Apoplexy

Apoplexy is a physical state caused by hemorrhage in a blood vessel of the brain. The patient suddenly loses consciousness and falls, his feet and hands become numb, and he may progress rapidly into a coma and death.

In Taiwan, many people have died as a result of apoplexy; it is one of the ten major causes of death. Obese people over forty-five years of age are most susceptible to this disease.

Apoplexy is divided into three categories: 1) Rupture of a cerebral blood vessel resulting in cerebral hemorrhage; 2) Cerebromalacia in which the cerebral vessel narrows gradually until it becomes obstructed (cerebral thrombus, cerebral thrombosis); 3) Arachnoidea encephali bleeding which occurs very seldom. The incidence of cerebral bleeding and cerebromalacia is almost the same. Those who suffer from apoplexy are usually middle aged (between forty and sixty years of age); those with cerebromalacia are usually elderly.

Apoplectic attacks often occur in the bathroom, during sleep, in times of stress, or during the excitement of a competitive game or other strenuous exercise. On these occasions, the common element is a sudden elevation of blood pressure, a condition which is harmful to the patient. Those having hypertension should take good care of themselves at all times.

The real cause of apoplexy is still not clear. Although hypertension has been thought to be the cause, external stimuli have recently been indicated as contributing factors.

Symptoms

The symptoms of cerebral hemorrhage and cerebromalacia are much alike. There are no signs prior to the onset of cerebral hemorrhage except headache and vertigo. The patient may lose consciousness. In severe cases, the patient will have rapid, non-rhythmic respiration, disordered pulse, and an elevated temperature as high as 40°C. Death may follow immediately. Some patients remain conscious for a week or semi-conscious for a long period of time. In the semiconscious state, the patient exhales with heavy snoring and has a flushed face.

In cerebromalacia, the patient generally has suffered from symptoms of recurrent headache, tinnitus, numbness of hands and feet for several months prior to onset. An attack is the same as that of cerebral hemorrhage. In mild cerebromalacia, the patient remains conscious but experiences temporary vertigo and pallor.

Following the attack, paralysis occurs according to the area of the brain in which the cerebral hemorrhage or cerebromalacia has occurred.

Treatment

Apoplexy, a disease with a sudden onset, should be treated with emergency measures. The patient's clothes should be unbuttoned immediately in order to ease his breathing, and food should be removed from his trachea. His face should be turned to one side and a doctor sent for immediately. In winter, the room should be kept warm to prevent pneumonia. Physical therapy and rehabilitation should begin as soon as possible so that the functions of the paralyzed parts of the body may be restored. Most of the functions will return through the willpower and consistent efforts of the patient.

Chinese Herb Formulas

1. **Hsu-ming-tang**   續命湯
   (Ma-huang and Ginseng Combination)

To be taken for paralysis, language disturbance, inability to turn over, generalized pains, convulsions, and sensory disorders. It is effective for those who have been physically strong.

2. **Hsiao-hsu-ming-tang**   小續命湯
   (Ma-huang and Paeonia Combination)

To be taken by those who have been physically weak with chilling in the limbs. It is effective for sensory confusion, urinary incontinence, and edema. It is also effective for those who have recovered consciousness but still have paralysis and weakness in the hands and legs.

Cerebromalacia

Cerebromalacia is a disease of apoplexy. It is a result of a blood circulation disorder causing degeneration of an area of the brain. In medical science, cerebromalacia is divided into cerebromalacia thrombosis and cerebromalacia thrombus.

Cerebromalacia thrombosis is caused by valvular blockage of some cerebral veins followed by their collapse. Younger people are more susceptible to this disease.

Cerebromalacia thrombus is caused by cerebral arteriosclerosis or by changes in syphilitic blood vessels. It is a disease of old age. Most cases are caused by senile cerebral arteriosclerosis.

Symptoms

Common cerebromalacia thrombus has progressive symptoms of confusion, and motion and language disturbance which begin one or more days before onset. Subsequently, these symptoms will recur and broaden the range of the disorder. The deterioration is usually irreversible and becomes progressively worse.

There are no early symptoms of cerebromalacia thrombosis. Most cases begin with a sudden convulsion. There is a tendency towards paralysis of the left side and occasional language disorder, but eventual recovery can be expected.

Treatment

Heterotherapy is best for this disease. There is still no effective therapy for senile cerebromalacia thrombus. Therefore, it is very important to prevent the disease by sound health practices in daily life. It is better to use the brain to prevent degeneration.

Chinese Herb Formula
Hsu-ming-tang 續命湯
(Ma-huang and Ginseng Combination)
To be taken by those who have recovered consciousness but are still suffering from both paralysis of the body and language disturbance. It is effective for the physically strong. Those who have been physically weak may take *Hsiao-hsu-ming-tang* (小續命湯 , *Ma-huang* and Paeonia Combination).

Anemia

A decrease of hemoglobin in the blood is called "anemia". There are several causes of anemia, the major one being a lack of hematin in the erythrocytes. Since it is a result of iron or protein deficiency, the condition is also called "iron-deficiency anemia". Other types of anemia are pernicious anemia which is due to insufficient hemoglobin production, hemolytic anemia caused by abnormal pancreatic function, and aplastic anemia resulting from damage to the bone marrow by chemical agents such as mercury.

Symptoms
Anemia causes the symptoms of pallor, vertigo, rapid respiration, headache, fever, palpitations, edema of the hands and feet, and a feeling of heaviness in the chest.

Treatment
It is sometimes effective for those having pernicious anemia to take supplements of vitamins, especially B_{12} and E. Those having iron-deficiency anemia should take hematinics or foods rich in iron.

Chinese Herb Formula
Lien-chu-yin 連珠飲
(Tang-kuei and Atractylodes Combination)
To be taken for palpitation, gasping, vertigo, tinnitus, and edema. It is not suitable for those having gastrointestinal weakness and a tendency towards diarrhea. If chlorophyll is added to this Chinese herb formula, it will produce more marked results.

Myocardial Infarction

When there is a blockage in the coronary arteries, the blood cannot circulate in them and the cardiac muscle will be deprived of oxygen. After a period of time, the cardiac muscle will become necrotic. This disease is called myocardial infarction and occurs most often in the elderly. Following an attack of angina pectoris, the heart will gradually become weak.

It is not uncommon in severe cases for the patient to die within several days. An adequate period for recuperation is very important, even in mild cases. It is necessary to allow at least four weeks for complete healing of the necrotic cardiac muscle.

Symptoms
Symptoms of myocardial infarction are more severe and last longer than those of angina pectoris. It produces excessive, viselike pains, a sensation of uneasiness, fear of death, dyspnea, decrease in blood pressure, and petechiae. Nitroglycerin or amyl nitrite are

ineffective as treatment. Sudden death is rather common.

Treatment

After an attack, the patient should be kept as quiet as possible, and a doctor should be sent for immediately. Because there is severe pain, the doctor may use morphine. When the patient is dyspneic, oxygen is usually given. It takes four weeks for necrotic cardiac muscle to heal, and the patient should remain mentally quiet during this period of time.

He should be given high quality food in moderate amounts at each meal, and he should avoid all fats. He should also avoid constipation and take only prescribed anticoagulants. Recovery is most likely for those who follow the doctor's directions and who maintain a positive outlook.

Chinese Herb Formulas

1. **Kua-lou-hsieh-pai-pai-chiu-tang** 栝樓薤白白酒湯
   (Trichosanthes, Bakeri, and Vinegar Combination)
   To be taken for severe pain in the chest and back, cough, and excessive salivation.

2. **Chai-hu-chia-lung-ku-mu-li-tang** 柴胡加龍骨牡蠣湯
   (Bupleurum and Dragon Bone Combination)
   This is effective for those with a weak heart who have a good physique and adequate strength, but who eat an unbalanced diet and are under stress.

Disordered Pulse

The pulse rate can be felt as the heart contracts. In healthy adults this rate is 50 to 70 beats per minute and the intensity and time interval between two beats is regular. Occasionally there is an abnormal situation such as a weakened pulse or an irregular interval. The patient's pulse rate will be 150 to 250 beats per minute and he will have severe palpitations accompanied by an uneasy and unpleasant feeling. In serious cases, there is cyanosis, difficult respiration, vena jugularis dilatation, hepatomegalia, hematuria, and edema.

The cause is usually temporary fatigue or reaction to stress, and recovery is spontaneous. However, if the cause is goiter, arteriosclerosis, or heart disease and the pulse disorder has lasted for a week, the patient should seek a physical examination by a doctor.

Treatment

It is important to cure completely the cause of this disease. If it is a temporarily disordered pulse, adequate sleep and regular living can restore the pulse to normal. If this does not bring results, the patient should try one or more of the following methods during an attack: 1.) Take stair exercises, walking up two stairs in one step. 2.) Insert a finger in the throat to cause vomiting. 3.) Drink a cup of cold water. 4.) Draw a deep breath, close the mouth and nose, and press the abdomen to stimulate the heart.

Chinese Herb Formulas

1. **Pan-hsia-hou-pu-tang-chia-kuei-chih-kan-tsao-lung-ku-mu-li-tang** 半夏厚朴湯加桂枝甘草龍骨牡蠣湯
    (Pinellia and Magnolia Combination with Cinnamon and L. D. O. Combination)
    To be taken for disordered pulse, uneasy feeling, and polyuria.

2. **Chih-kan-tsao-tang** 炙甘草湯
    (Baked Licorice Combination)
    To be taken for stagnant and disordered pulse. In abdominal diagnosis, there is palpitation at the umbilicus.

3. **Chai-hu-chia-lung-ku-mu-li-tang** 柴胡加龍骨牡蠣湯
    (Bupleurum and Dragon Bone Combination)
    To be taken by the patient having disordered pulse, fullness at the chest and heart, and constipation.

4. **Chai-hu-chiang-kuei-tang-chia-wu-chu-yu-fu-ling** 柴胡薑桂湯加吳茱萸茯苓
    (Bupleurum, Cinnamon, and Ginger Combination with Evodia and Hoelen)
    To be taken for weak abdomen and palpitation at the umbilicus in the patient of the weak type.

5. Fu-ling-kan-tsao-chia-lung-ku-mu-li-tang 茯苓甘草加龍骨牡蠣湯
   (Hoelen and L.D.O. Combination)
   To be taken for a hard sensation beneath the ribs and nervousness or uneasiness.

6. Chia-wei-hsiao-yao-san 加味逍遙散
   (Bupleurum and Paeonia Formula)
   To be taken by a woman having physical weakness and nervousness.

Buerger's Disease
(Thromboangiitis Obliterans)

The main symptoms of thromboangiitis obliterans are recalcitrant chilling and severe pain in the limbs. There was a young patient who was advised by the doctor to have the lower limbs amputated. The author, however, advised the patient to stop smoking, eat a vegetarian diet, and take *Kuei-chih-fu-ling-wan* (桂枝茯苓丸, Cinnamon and Hoelen Formula). Finally the disease was cured.

DISEASES OF THE ALIMENTARY SYSTEM

Esophagitis

An inflammation of the esophagus may be caused by either physical, chemical or physiological stimuli. On eating, a painful sensation is felt behind the sternum and along the esophagus.

Petic esophagitis is probably second only to duodenal ulcers as a discernible cause of upper gastrointestinal symptoms. The esophagus is damaged whenever it is exposed to the contents of either the stomach or the small intestine through reflux (back flushing). (Since the condition occurs in the absence of hydrochloric acid in the stomach, and bile is known to be irritating, the "acid-pepsin theory" as the primary cause is apparently not adequate.) The common denominator in the genesis of reflux esophagitis, therefore, is a reflux of either acid or alkaline gastric juice. The lower esophageal sphincter, an important protective mechanism against reflux, functions as a high pressure valve between the stomach and esophagus. The sphincter, which is normally infradiaphragmatic, is responsive to any increase in intragastric pressure induced by elevation of intra-abdomen pressure and thereby creates a barrier between the stomach and the thoracic esophagus. Among conditions which contribute to reflux are (1) hiatus hernia, (2) a short esophagus, (3) pregnancy,

(4) pernicious vomiting, and (5) nasogastric intubation (insertion of tubes through the nose to the stomach).

The esophagus is most severely injured by the ingestion of any corrosive substances. It is most common in children but also occurs in cases of attempted suicide. The substances most commonly swallowed are strong acids (sulfuric or nitric), alkalies (lye or potash), oxalic acid, iodine, bichloride of mercury, arsenic, silver nitrate, and carbolic acid. Gastric changes vary from superficial edema and hyperedemia to deep necrosis and sloughing or even perforation.

Symptoms

Symptoms of milder gastric injuries include a burning sensation (pyrosis), which is often worsened by recumbency and ameliorated by antacids; waterbrash (the combination of regurgitation and increased salivation); and difficulty (dysphagia) and pain (odynophagia) in swallowing. Blood tinged, regurgitated material or occasional vomiting of blood, anemia, and stricture formation are later manifestations.

Symptoms of more serious gastric injuries are corrosion of the lips, tongue, mouth, and pharynx, and pain and dysphagia due to esophageal lesions. Nitric acid causes brown discoloration; oxalic acid causes white discoloration of mucous membranes. Severe epigastric burning and cramping pain, nausea, vomiting, and diarrhea also occur. The vomitus is often blood-tinged. Severe prostration with an appearance of shock may occur, accompanied by thirst. Palpation of the abdomen may show epigastric tenderness or extreme rigidity. An increased leukocyte count (leukocytosis) and protein in the urine (proteinuria) are additional symptoms.

Treatment

Immediate treatment for ingestion of poison is supportive: nasogastric suction, analgesics, intravenous fluids with electrolytes, sedatives, and antacids. Although the specific antidote should be administered immediately, supportive measures must not be neglected. The benefit to be expected from the antidote appears miniscule if a large amount of corrosive has been ingested and of doubtful benefit considering that tissue damage occurs almost immediately. Emetics and washes should be avoided if corrosion is severe because of the danger of perforation. The outcome depends upon the extent of tissue damage. Careful fiberoptic endoscopy (visual examination of the interior by means of an instrument) may serve to determine tissue necrosis. An incision through the abdominal wall (laparotomy) may be indicated to resect the area of gangrene and potential perforation. If alkali has been ingested, 20mg prednisone orally every eight hours started immediately may prevent esophageal stricture. This dose should be tapered down slowly over several weeks. After the acute phase has passed, the patient needs to go on a peptic ulcer regimen. If perforation has not occurred, recovery is the rule.

Successful treatment for reflux esophagitis depends on preventing reflux or ameliorating its effects. Therefore, conditions which predispose the patient to increased intra-abdominal pressure, e.g. tight belts or girdles, should be avoided. Elevation of the head of the bed and frequent administration of antacids are important concomitants of effective therapy. Keeping patients in a sitting position during the course of nasogastric intubation is prophylactically important to avoid reflux and potential constriction. Dysphagia secondary to stricture formation is effectively managed by esophageal dilation, using either Puestow "stringless" dilators or mercury filled bougies. If medical management is not successful, surgical treatment is indicated.

Chinese Herb Formulas

Chih-tzu-shih-tang 梔子豉湯
(Gardenia and Soja Combination)
Chih-tzu-kan-tsao-shih-tang 梔子甘草豉湯
(Gardenia, Licorice, and Soja Combination)

These formulas are very effective for esophagitis. Even acute cases may be cured in two or three days.

Esophageal Stenosis
(Constriction of the Esophagus)

Except in the case of cancer, stricture of the esophagus results from the healing of an inflammatory lesion of the esophagus. Common causes of injuries to the esophagus are peptic esophagitis secondary to gastro-esophageal reflux; Barrett's epithelium and ulcer formation; ingestion of corrosive substances; acute viral or bacterial infectious diseases; and, rarely, damage caused by endoscopes.

Symptoms

The principal symptom is difficulty in swallowing, which may not appear for years after the initial injury. Patients who have swallowed caustics may have an initial difficulty with swallowing caused by edema but it will be short-lived. However, stricture formation can follow weeks or months later. The ability to swallow liquids is maintained the longest.

Pain often accompanies difficult swallowing. The patient's description of the point at which he senses a "hang-up" of food conforms with amazing accuracy to the level of the obstruction.

X-ray is the normal diagnostic procedure used. However, esophagoscopy, biopsy, and cytologic examination are mandatory in all cases to rule out the possibility of malignancy.

Treatment

Dilation using Puestow dilators or mercury-filled (Mahoney or Hurst) bougies to attain a lumen size of 45-60° is the definitive form of treatment. However, both the patient and the physician must be prepared for a continuing program of bougienage, since recurrence of stenosis will invariably ensue if dilation is terminated when swallowing again becomes normal. Monthly use of the largest bougie which the patient can tolerate usually prevents regression. If dilation is unsuccessful, resection of the stricture with esophago-gastrostomy or jejunal or colonic interposition is indicated.

Chinese Herb Formulas

Tang-kuei-yang-hsieh-tang　　　　　　　　當歸養血湯
(*Tang-kuei, Paeonia, and Rehmannia Combination*)
Sheng-chin-pu-hsieh-tang　　　　　　　　生津補血湯
(*Tang-kuei,* Paeonia, and Ophiopogon Combination)

The contents of these two formulas are alike. Both are used for esophagus stenosis and the accompanying difficulty in swallowing and vomiting. The important signal for using these formulas is aridity of the patient's skin and mucous membranes.

Sheng-chin-pu-hsieh-tang was used with great effectivness on a patient who had swallowed a large quantity of oxalic acid, causing esophageal stenosis resulting from the healing scar tissue.

Carcinoma of the Esophagus

In the United States cancer of the esophagus predominantly affects males in their fifties and sixties. Stagnation induced by inflammation such as is seen in achalasia, or esophageal stricture, or chronic irritation induced by the excessive use of alcohol seemingly are causative factors in the development of this growth. Malignant tumors of the distal esophagus usually develop from adenocarcinomas which originate in the stomach and spread toward the head and throat. Conversely, squamous cell (plate-like) carcinoma of the esophagus is rare. An even more unusual growth is esophageal carcinosarcoma. Regardless of cell type, the prognosis for malignancy of the esophagus is usually poor.

Symptoms

Progressive dysphagia, the principal symptom, ultimately prevents the swallowing of even liquids. Anterior or posterior chest pain which is unrelated to eating implies local extension of the tumor, whereas significant weight loss over a short period is an ominous sign.

Barium X-ray shows an irregular, frequently annular, space-occupying lesion, usually localized in the midesophagus. Esophagoscopy, biopsy, and cytologic examination confirm the diagnosis.

The inability of the esophagus to relax can be determined by means of internal examination (endoscopy), by measuring the pressure of liquids and gases (esophageal manometry), and by cinefluorography. Since there is a significant association of stricture with malignancy, any doubts about the diagnosis should be followed by an evaluation with esophagoscopy and biopsy.

Treatment

Although once considered a hopeless disease, dramatic improvements during the last two decades in anesthesia, surgical technics, and radiation therapy have substantially improved the survival rate of patients with esophageal carcinoma. Irradiation generally is the best form of therapy, particularly for lesions in the proximal half of the esophagus. When there is no evidence of metastases, tumors of the lower half of the esophagus may be treated by resection and esophagogastrostomy, jejunal or colonic interpositions. After dilation of tumor-bearing portions of the esophagus, effective palliation can often be accomplished by the use of prosthetic tubes which are inserted by way of the mouth to facilitate swallowing.

A gastrostomy (external opening for feeding) is supposed to improve nutrition but does not prolong survival, and the inability of completely obstructed patients to swallow even saliva makes the operation of questionable value for palliation. Anticancer drugs have not proved to be of value.

Chinese Herb Formulas
1. Li-ke-tang-ho-kan-tsao-kan-chiang-tang 利膈湯合甘草乾薑湯
(Pinellia and Gardenia Combination with Licorice and Ginger Combination)
Li-ke-tang-ho-fu-ling-hsing-jen-kan-tsao-tang 利膈湯合茯苓杏仁甘草湯
(Pinellia and Gardenia Combination with Hoelen, Apricot Seed, and Licorice Combination)
In ancient times people said that *Li-ke-tang* was 100 percent effective against *ke ye, ke ye* being a collective term for diseases such as esophageal or gastric conditions which prohibit the ingestion of foods regardless of whether it is a benign or malignant condition. Unless the patient is extremely weak, these formulas ease swallowing whenever there is difficulty and when vomiting occurs. However, the effect is temporary and cannot persist forever. *Li-ke-tang* alone is effective but will have a better suppressive effect if combined with *Kan-tsao-kan-chiang-tang* or *Fu-ling-hsing-jen-kan-tsao-tang.*

2. Fu-ling-hsing-jen-kan-tsao-tang 茯苓杏仁甘草湯
(Hoelen, Apricot Seed, and Licorice Combination)
This combination is effective for difficulty in swallowing, and for sore throats or coughs. It should be used jointly with *Li-ke-tang.* If the licorice component in *Fu-ling-kan-tsao-tang* is replaced with

morus bark, the formula becomes *Po-kuan-tang,* which is also suitable for sore throats, coughs, and difficulty in swallowing.

Esophageal Neurosis
(Esophageal Spasm)

Esophageal neurosis is a condition of esophageal spasms. It is most often found in neurotic patients, but not exclusively. Spasms occur where the esophagus joins the stomach, thereby hindering the passage of food and causing pain.

The causes of this disease are esophageal ulceration or inflammation, hysteria, neurasthenia, rabies, tetanus, meningitis, strychnine poisoning, abuse of tobacco, and sexual dysfunction.

Symptoms
Symptoms include difficulty in swallowing, a compressed sensation in the chest, labored breathing, cardiac palpitation, and an aching and burning sensation in the esophagus. Passage of a bougie through the esophagus is impossible at first but spontaneously becomes possible. The location of the site where passage of the bougie is hindered will vary. Although the disease can be easily detected upon onset, esophagoscopic examination is necessary to rule out other organic diseases. Prognosis in the neurosis-originated spasm generally is good while that derived from rabies, tetanus and poisoning is poor.

Treatment
First the cause of the disease must be determined, then sedatives are given to the patient and bougienage is employed from time to time. It is also necessary to reassure the patient.

Chinese Herb Formula
Pan-hsia-hou-pu-tang 半夏厚朴湯
(Pinellia and Magnolia Combination)
This formula is effective against esophageal spasms. A woman suddenly began to have chest pains and could not swallow food. She became worried that she might have cancer. She was examined at a university and was told that there was nothing

wrong and that the disease would heal spontaneously in a short while. However, she continued to suffer from attacks periodically and sought Chinese herb treatment. It is recorded in *Chin kuei yao lueh,* "Women who feel as if a piece of barbecued meat was clinging to their throat are treated primarily with *Pan-hsia-hou-pu-tang.*" Hence the formula was given to this woman and it was efficacious. She has had no more incidence of spasms.

Laxity of the Stomach

Laxity of the stomach is due to inadequate muscle tone. A patient with this condition exhibits the following symptoms: a sensation of gastric distention, obstruction of ingested foods in the stomach, belching, nausea, and a loss of appetite. Most patients have a slack and vigorless physique, fatigability and nervousness, and sometimes prolapse of the stomach (gastroptosis). Abdominal examination usually reveals a splashing sound.

Chinese Herb Formulas
1. **Ping-wei-san** 平胃散
   (Magnolia and Ginger Formula)
   Hsiang-sha-ping-wei-san 香砂平胃散
   (Cyperus, Cardamon, and Atractylodes Formula)

The first formula, *Ping-wei-san,* is used for the following symptoms: mild laxity of the stomach, hardness beneath the heart, and a sensation of distention in the abdomen. The second formula is used when one wishes to stimulate the stomach in order to promote its function.

2. **Liu-chun-tzu-tang** 六君子湯
   (Six Major Herb Combination)
   Hsiang-sha-liu-chun-tzu-tang 香砂六君子湯
   (Cyperus and Cardamon Combination)

Liu-chun-tzu-tang is indicated in more serious cases in which the patient has a poor complexion, debilitated vitality, forcelessness in both pulse and abdomen, sleepiness after a meal, lassitude, a heavy head, and vertigo. If the patient has severe discomfort and a painful feeling in the epigastrium in addition to constant mental sullenness, then *Hsiang-sha-liu-chun-tzu-tang* should be used.

3. **Pan-hsia-pai-chu-tien-ma-tang** 半夏白朮天麻湯
    (Pinellia and Gastrodia Combination)

This formula is given to patients having symptoms similar to those of *Liu-chun-tzu-tang* with the additional symptoms of headache, vertigo, and cold feet.

4. **Ling-kuei-chu-kan-tang** 苓桂朮甘湯
    (Hoelen and Atractylodes Combination)

This formula is used for a firmer conformation than that of *Pan-hsia-pai-chu-tien-ma-tang:* the patient has a forceful pulse and abdomen, distention beneath the heart, a feverish feeling, vertigo, cardiac palpitations, and reduced urine volume. Abdominal examination often reveals a splashing sound and a hyperfunctional palpitation at the navel.

5. **Kuei-chih-chia-shao-yao-tang** 桂枝加芍藥湯
    (Cinnamon and Paeonia Combination)
    Hsiao-chien-chung-tang 小建中湯
    (Minor Cinnamon and Paeonia Combination)

The first formula is suitable for persons with tight and tense abdominal muscles, distention in the abdomen, thin subdermal adipose fat, and a thin abdominal wall; it is also good for gastric laxity, stiff shoulders, and stomachaches. In addition to the above symptoms, if the patient's vitality is deteriorating and he has a poor complexion, then *Hsiao-chien-chung-tang* is suitable; if there is an eminent splashing sound, 4.0g of pinellia and 3.0g of hoelen are added to the formula.

6. **Kuei-chih-chia-shao-yao-ta-huang-tang** 桂枝加芍藥大黃湯
    (Cinnamon, Paeonia, and Rhubarb Combination)

This formula is indicated when the patient has not only laxity of the stomach but also of the intestines with resultant constipation and lower abdominal distention. The dose of rhubarb should be adjusted to as low as 0.3-1.0g for best results.

7. **Kuei-chih-chia-shao-yao-su-chiao-jen-sheng-tang**
    桂枝加芍藥蜀椒人參湯
    (Cinnamon with Paeonia, Zanthoxylum, and Ginseng Combination)

This formula is the combination of *Hsiao-chien-chung-tang* and

Ta-chien-chung-tang minus maltose. It is suitable for patients with gastric laxity and constipation who experience stomachaches and discomfort after taking rhubarb preparations. Administration of this formula will ease bowel movements.

8. **Chen-wu-tang** 眞武湯
   (Vitality Combination)

This formula is suitable for patients having a soft and forceless abdomen; a submerged and weak or submerged, weak and slow pulse; a poor complexion; cold limbs, and a tendency toward diarrhea.

9. **Fu-ling-yin** 茯苓飲
   (Hoelen Combination)

This formula is indicated for patients having a strong abdomen and pulse, gastric distention and a sensation of blockage, a splashing sound in the stomach, belching, and regurgitation of gastric fluid into the mouth. If there are burning sensations and excessive belching, then 2.0g of evodia and 3.0g of oyster shell are added.

Hiccups

Hiccups are usually a benign, transient phenomenon, and they occur as a manifestation of many diseases. It is important to assess specific causes such as neuroses, CNS disorders, phrenic nerve irritation, cardiorespiratory disorders, gastrointestinal disorders, renal failure, infectious diseases, or other diseases. Sometimes they are the only symptom of peptic esophagitis.

Treatment

Countless measures have been suggested for interrupting the rhythmic reflex that produces hiccups. None of these are 100 percent successful, however, and the attacks sometimes may be so prolonged and severe as to jeopardize the patient's life. Simple Home Remedies:

The following measures probably work by diverting the patient's attention: distracting conversation, fright, painful or unpleasant stimuli, or procedures such as holding the breath, sipping ice water, or inhaling strong fumes.

Medical Measures

Sedation. Any of the common sedative drugs may be effective, e.g. pentobarbital sodium, 0.1g orally or 0.13g by rectal suppository.

Stimulation of the nasopharynx. A soft catheter can be introduced nasally to stimulate the nasopharynx and pharynx.

Local anesthetics. Viscous lidocaine may be of some use. General anesthesia may be tried in intractable cases.

Antispasmodics. 0.3-0.6g of atropine sulfate may be given subcutaneously.

CO_2 inhalations. Breathing into a paper bag for three to five minutes, or taking 10-15% CO_2 mixture by face mask for three to five minutes may bring relief.

Amyl nitrite inhalations.

Tranquilizers. Chlorpromazine HC1 and promazine HC1 have been used successfully for prolonged or intractable hiccups.

Antacids.

Chinese Herb Formulas

1. **Wu-chu-yu-tang**　　　　　　　　　　吳茱萸湯
    (Evodia Combination)

Whenever hiccups are mentioned, one usually thinks of the persimmon, a commonly known anti-hiccup remedy. However, in a surprisingly large number of cases, *Wu-chu-yu-tang* can cure hiccups with one day's dosage. This formula is suitable for hiccups along with internal chills, submerged pulse, distended abdomen, and stomach gas.

2. **Chu-pi-chu-ju-tang**　　　　　　　　橘皮竹茹湯
    (Aurantium and Bamboo Combination)
    Chu-pi-tang　　　　　　　　　　　　橘皮湯
    (Aurantium Combination)

These two formulas are from *Chin kuei yao lueh*. It says, "For hiccups, *Chu-pi-chu-ju-tang* is primarily indicated. For hiccups accompanied by cold limbs, *Chu-pi-tang* is primarily indicated." Arichi Keiri recommended this formula when he said, "This formula is effective for any hiccups, regardless of the cause, pulse, or abdominal condition." It is also said to be effective for severe hiccups. The *chu-pi*, citrus peels, used today do not have the bitter taste and strong smell which are characteristic of superior quality. Instead, *chen-pi*, stale citrus peels are used which are practically ineffectual. According to the account from *Ku fang yao pin kao* (An Investigation of Ancient Prescriptions) *chu-pi* must be prepared from the orange peel with the endoderm removed. The endoderm is also called the sweet muscle; the removal of the endoderm enhances the bitter flavor. About thirty years ago *chu-pi* processed in this manner was still available. However, nowadays such a processed product is no longer found because crude drug dealers will not undertake such a cumbersome process.

3. Shih-ti-tang   柿蒂湯
    (Kaki Combination)

Among the common people kaki peduncles are used as a drink to cure hiccups. Although they work alone, clove and ginger have been added to the kaki peduncle in this formula. It is effective when *Wu-chu-yu-tang* or *Chu-pi-tang* fails.

4. Hsiao-cheng-chi-tang   小承氣湯
    (Minor Rhubarb Combination)
    Tiao-wei-cheng-chi-tang   調胃承氣湯
    (Rhubarb and Mirabilitum Combination)

These formulas are indicated for hiccups accompanied by constipation. In *Chin kuei yao lueh* there is one sentence which says, "In case of hiccups with abdominal distention, the cure is to purge the part that is obstructed." Another article in *Chien chin fang* reads, "*Hsiao-cheng-chi-tang* treats obstructed stools (constipation), hiccups, and frequent delirium." Hence we can see *Hsiao-cheng-chi-tang* is effective for hiccups. *Hsiao-cheng-chi-tang* eases abdominal distention, constipation, and a forceful pulse. However, this formula is ineffective for hiccups caused by ascites (accumulation of serous fluid in the peritoneal cavity) or peritonitis, even though abdominal distention and constipation are present. This formula contains magnolia bark which relieves muscular spasm and tension. *Tiao-wei-cheng-chi-tang* is used for patients with slight abdominal distention and constipation.

5. Szu-ni-tang   四逆湯
    (Aconite and G.L. Combination)

This formula is effective in curing hiccups caused by severe dysentery, a condition having a poor prognosis. Arimochi Keiri said, "In most cases, *Szu-ni-tang* is suitable for hiccups caused by very severe diseases." Kato Kensai said, "Hiccups after delivery is an adverse symptom for which moxibustion on the *ch'i-men* locus and *Szu-ni-chia-jen-sheng-tang* are suitable."

6. Chinese Taoist Practice

Add lukewarm boiled water to a glass or cup or any container having an open mouth representing the human mouth or throat; cross the glass mouth with two chopsticks or any kind of sticks or two pencils if sticks are unavailable. Drink one mouthful of water from each of the four quadrant openings divided by the two crisscrossed sticks in a sequential order, either clockwise or counter-clockwise. As the last mouthful of water is drunk, the hiccups also disappear.

Ascites

Ascites is the retention of fluid in the abdominal cavity. It results from effusions from diseases such as cardiac disease, nephrosis, or hemastasis of the portal veins, but generally does not include effusions from an inflammatory disease. Commonly, the fluid has a color ranging from pale yellow to yellowish green and contains endemic cells, leukocytes, erythrocytes and, in case of cancer, carcinoma cells. It has a protein content below 3 percent, a specific gravity below 1.015, and a negative Rivalta's reaction.

Ascites can be classified into the following three types: (1) chylous ascites (chyle is a milk-white emulsion that forms in the small intestine during digestion); (2) adiposic ascites as a result of an abdominal carcinoma which releases denatured adiposic cells into the fluid; and (3) mucous ascites due to peritoneal mucous swelling or the rupture of an ovarian tumor. Generally, it is necessary for the ascites to have a volume of fluid of more than one liter in order to be palpated or detected by percussion. Diagnosis of ascites can be done by performing a puncture.

Symptoms

The caput medusae, the subdermal veins of the abdomen,

become visible and the patient will have increased cardiac palpitations and labored breathing as a result of the raised diaphragm caused by the ascites.

Treatment

First one must determine how to treat the ascites by finding the cause and removing it. As a palliative treatment, cardiotonics, diuretics or cathartics may be given in an attempt to discharge the fluid. If the patient has cardiac palpitation caused by excessive ascites, puncture is mandatory.

Chinese Herb Formulas
1. Wu-ling-san   五苓散
    (Hoelen Five Herb Formula)

This combination is effective against ascites caused by nephritis and other pathological diseases of the kidneys. The targets of treatment are thirst and oliguria (decreased amount of urine). (It is also suitable for those with only a minor degree of thirst.)

2. Wu-ling-san-ho-jen-sheng-tang   五苓散合人參湯
    (Hoelen Five Herb Formula combined with Ginseng and Ginger Combination)

This herbal combination is effective for ascites caused by cirrhosis of the liver; it is also adaptable to patients whose ascites has been treated by surgical puncture.

3. Wei-ling-tang   胃苓湯
    (Magnolia and Hoelen Combination)

This combination should be prescribed in the early stage of ascites when the vitality of the patient has not been depleted. It is suitable for patients with oliguria and thirst.

4. Fen-hsiao-tang   分消湯
    (Hoelen and Alisma Combination)

This formula can be given when the strength of the patient still exists, the pulse is sinking and energetic, constipation is usual with a tonic abdominal wall (normal tone and tension), and the shape of the abdomen does not vary with the shift of posture. Mainly it is used for patients who do not show an extremely weak conformation.

5. Pu-chung-chih-shih-tang　　　　　補中治濕湯
   (Ginseng and Akebia Combination)

This combination is for treating edema in a person with a weak conformation. It is especially suitable for patients who have become debilitated because of long suffering from ascites.

6. Kuei-chiang-tsao-tsao-huang-hsin-fu-tang 桂薑棗草黃辛附湯
   (Cinnamon and Six Herb Combination)

This combination has been used to cure patients with ascites caused by splenic hemorrhage. *Chin kuei yao lueh* (Summaries of Household Drugs) states, "Abnormal circulation of *ch'i* causes a hardening below the heart as large as a plate with a margin like that of a turning cup. Such a disease is caused by water stagnation and is primarily treated with *Kuei-chiang-tsao-tsao-huang-hsin-fu-tang*." The application of this combination is according to this statement.

7. Ling-kan-chiang-wei-hsin-hsia-jen-tang　　苓甘薑味辛夏仁湯
   (Hoelen and Schizandra Combination)

Takino Kazuo has released a therapeutic case report about the application of this combination for treating ascites.

8. Ta-ching-lung-tang　　　　　　　　　大青龍湯
   (Major Blue Dragon Combination)

Sato Shogo too has reported on a therapeutic case using this prescription to cure ascites. *Ling-kan-chiang-wei-hsin-hsia-jen-tang* is for persons without any superficial symptoms who have only internal stagnated water, whereas this combination treats people with superficial symptoms and an internal fever accompanied by stagnation of water.

Peritonitis

Localized peritonitis such as that caused by appendicitis can be healed by Chinese herb therapy, but acute suppurative peritonitis lies outside its scope.

Of all chronic peritonitis, tubercular peritonitis is the most common. Peritonitis is further differentiated into the exudative and dry. In the exudative type, the abdomen is distended by the exudated fluid; while in the dry type the abdominal distention is not evident, but there are sites that show pain and resistance when the abdomen is palpated. Diarrhea or constipation and a slight rise in body temperature are common. Though the abdominal pain is not severe, as the coalesced area enlarges, the pain grows and vomiting occurs.

Symptoms

Systemic reactions. Malaise, prostration, nausea, vomiting, septic fever, leukocytosis (increase in the luekocyte count) and electrolyte imbalance are usually seen in proportion to the severity of the process. If infection is not controlled, toxemia is progressive and toxic shock, which can be fatal, may develop.

Abdominal signs. Depending upon the extent of involvement, pain and tenderness may be localized or generalized. Abdominal pain on coughing, resistant tenderness confined to the area of peritonitis, and tenderness to light percussion over the inflamed peritoneum are characteristic. Pelvic peritonitis is associated with rectal and vaginal tenderness.

The muscles overlying the area of inflammation usually become spastic. When peritonitis is generalized (e.g. after perforation of a peptic ulcer), marked rigidity of the entire abdominal wall may develop immediately. Rigidity is frequently diminished or absent in the late stages of peritonitis, in severe toxemia, and when the abdominal wall is weak, flabby, or obese.

Intestinal motility is markedly inhibited by peritoneal inflammation. The cardinal signs are absence of peristalsis and progressive abdominal distention. Vomiting occurs as a result of pooling of gastrointestinal secretions and gas, 70 percent of which is swallowed air.

Abdominal films by Roentgenography show gas and fluid collections in both large and small bowels, usually with generalized rather than localized dilation. The bowel walls, when thrown into relief, may appear to be thickened, indicating the presence of edema or peritoneal fluid.

Treatment

The objectives of treatment are to (1) control infection; (2)

minimize the effects of paralytic ileus; and (3) correct the fluid, electrolyte and nutritional disorders. For tubercular peritonitis, it is necessary to simultaneously employ chemotherapy.

Chinese Herb Formulas

1. **Hsiao-chien-chung-tang** 小建中湯
   (Minor Cinnamon and Paeonia Combination)
   Huang-chi-chien-chung-tang 黃耆建中湯
   (Astragalus Combination)
   Tang-kuei-chien-chung-tang 當歸建中湯
   (Tang-kuei, Cinnamon, and Paeonia Combination)

These formulas are effective for the dry-type peritonitis. They can also be applied to the exudative type if the exudation is slight. The symptoms are abdominal tension and distention with hardening of tissue, or pain on pressure. However, the abdominal wall ought not be tensive and diarrhea is a contraindication. In patients with constipation, administration of these formulas will make the bowel movement smooth. *Huang-chi-chien-chung-tang* is used for patients with excessive sweating. If the peritonitis is primarily situated in the lower abdomen, especially the pelvis, it is suitable to administer *Tang-kuei-chien-chung-tang*. Persons with chronic peritonitis who have a persistent high fever over 38°C should not be regimened solely on *Hsiao-chien-chung-tang*. Note: It is essential to institute an antitubercular chemotherapy at the same time.

2. **Chen-wu-tang** 眞武湯
   (Vitality Combination)

This formula is indicated for peritonitis patients who have a tendency toward diarrhea. The patient may have abdominal distention and abdominal pain and tenderness, areas of induration, and mild symptoms of coalescence. This formula is also suitable for suspected intestinal tuberculosis peritonitis and retention of exudated fluid.

3. **Chai-hu-kuei-chih-kan-chiang-tang** 柴胡桂枝乾薑湯
   (Bupleurum, Cinnamon, and Ginger Combination)

This formula is to be used for dry peritonitis. If there are indurations, paeonia and turtle shell are added to the formula. If there is night sweating, astragalus is added. Patients suited to this formula may not have evident thoraco-costal distress, but they have a stronger abdomen than the *Chen-wu-tang* patients and tend to have palpitations at the umbilicus.

4. **Chai-hu-kuei-chih-tang** 柴胡桂枝湯
   (Bupleurum and Cinnamon Combination)
This formula is used when the condition is mild and the patient's stamina has not yet deteriorated. The conformation for this formula is more firm than that of *Chai-hu-kuei-chih-kan-chiang-tang:* the abdominal wall is wholly tensive, indurations are present around the umbilicus and along the abdominal straight muscles, and pain on pressure is evident.

5. **Tiao-chung-i-chi-tang** 調中益氣湯
   (Ginseng, Astragalus, and Paeonia Combination)
This formula is made by adding hoelen and paeonia to *Pu-chung-i-chi-tang* and is applicable to either dry or exudative peritonitis in patients whose stamina is debilitated because the disease has become chronic and who feel weak, fatigued, and lethargic.

6. **Fen-hsiao-tang** 分消湯
   (Hoelen and Alisma Combination)
This formula is indicated for patients having copious exudate, a distended abdomen, a forceful pulse, a tendency to be constipated, and a firm conformation. They will have retained their stamina.

7. **Hsing-shih-pu-chi-yang-hsieh-tang** 行濕補氣養血湯
   (Ginseng and Lygodium Combination)
This formula is used for patients with exudative peritonitis who have a nutritional deficiency and deterioration in both the circulatory and respiratory systems.

Gastroasthenia

Gastroasthenia is a weak state of the stomach due to the muscular relaxation of the abdominal wall. As a result, the passage of food from the stomach to the intestines is difficult. Patients with a congenitally weak constitution are susceptible to gastroasthenia as well as gastroptosis. In addition, chronic gastritis or gastroxnysis may also induce gastroasthenia.

Symptoms
The primary symptoms of this disease are anorexia and a feeling of stagnation in the stomach. Other subjective symptoms are bloating, belching, nausea, stomachache, stomach discomfort, distress, emotional instability, irritability, impatience, tinnitus, vertigo, insomnia, and nervousness. Patients also have succussion – splashing in the stomach due to the presence of stagnant food. This undigested food may cause recurrent diarrhea and constipation. Thin and nervous people often suffer from these symptoms.

Treatment
For mild cases of gastroasthenia caused by emotional stress, sour foods (such as lemons or prunes) or beverages, to increase the appetite may be an effective cure. Appetizers, acupressure, and moxibustion are also helpful.

In cases of severe or constitutional gastroasthenia, the patient should follow a proper diet that is high in protein and carbohydrates. All foods should be well chewed. A thirty minute rest after meals is very beneficial. In addition a sufficient amount of sleep and regular exercise are important. (Strenuous exercises or riding a bus should be avoided after eating.)

Chinese Herb Formulas
1. **Liu-chun-tzu-tang** 六君子湯
(Major Six Herb Combination)
This formula is effective for patients of delicate constitution with cold arms and legs, pallor, a tendency toward fatigue, lack of vigor, weak abdominal muscles, succussion, anorexia, and a feeling of stagnation in the stomach.

2. **Szu-chun-tzu-tang** 四君子湯
(Major Four Herb Combination)
This formula is used for patients of delicate constitutions and a lack of vitality.

Gastroptosis

Gastroptosis is an abnormal falling of the stomach, usually

accompanied by the displacement of other organs. Normally, the stomach lies above the umbilicus, but in cases of gastroptosis the stomach lies below the umbilicus and may even droop as far as the pelvis. Patients with prolonged illness and delicate constitution, thin people, and middle-aged women who have had several pregnancies all tend to have this condition. Irregular eating habits, emotional instability, and stress are also possible causes of gastroptosis.

Symptoms

On examination, the patient's abdomen seems hollow between the ribs, and there is swelling in the lower abdomen. Other symptoms are heaviness of the head; vertigo due to constipation; headache; insomnia; amnesia; chronic, constitutional fatigue; anxiety; lack of vitality; and nervousness. When gastroptosis is accompanied by gastric disturbance, the patient will experience anorexia and stomachache.

Treatment

While there is no specific cure for gastroptosis, the practice of yoga and correct posture is said to be effective for prolonged conditions. However, a combination of a balanced diet, proper exercise, and herbal formulas will help to cure gastroptosis within a month. Worrying does not help and should be avoided.

Gastroxnysis

Gastroxnysis occurs when the stomach secretes excess hydrochloric acid. Since hyperchlorhydria is one of the symptoms of chronic gastritis, gastric ulcer, and gastric cancer, a patient with this condition should have a thorough laboratory examination. In some cases, gastroxnysis is caused by excessive smoking, drinking, or eating spicy foods. Gastroxnysis is also associated with neurotic disorders.

Symptoms

The primary symptom of this disease is a feverish feeling in the stomach. The patient also experiences chest discomfort, regurgitation of sour fluid, belching, and stomachache. Although these symptoms usually occur before eating (when the stomach is empty), they become even more severe after eating foods with spices, fats, sugar, and salt. Other symptoms are increased appetite, constipation, and diarrhea.

Treatment

Mild cases of gastroxnysis may be cured by making sure that food is chewed slowly or by taking a small amount of sodium bicarbonate (baking soda) to neutralize excess acidity. However even the patient with a temporary condition of gastroxnysis should have a physical examination.

Generally, the stomach secretes gastric juice every three to four hours in preparation for digestion. However, when meal times are irregular or the stomach is empty for a long time, more gastric acids are secreted. As a result the patient feels gastric pain and gastroxnysis. Over a prolonged period, if eating habits are not changed, the stomach will secrete less gastric juice and induce a condition of hypohydrochloria. Both hyperhydrochloria and hypohydrochloria may be cured by eating meals at regular intervals and avoiding spicy foods and excessive drinking.

Recently, medical studies have shown that physical constitution and personality type are predisposing factors for this disease. In 75% of the cases, patients with gastroxnysis are under emotional stress due to professional or family problems. Therefore, the patient with gastroxnysis should try to eliminate the causes of stress and improve his lifestyle.

Gastrectasis

Gastrectasis is a condition of abnormal stomach enlargement and may be either acute or chronic. This type of disease is a form of stomach weakness since a stomach that has poor tonus will relax instead of contract when empty. Possible causes may be obstruction of the pylorus, atony, overeating, congenital weakness, imperfect peristalsis, omental hernia, periduodenal adhesions, or gastroptosis.

Symptoms

The symptoms of gastrectasis are indigestion, abdominal

distention with succussion in the stomach, anorexia, discomfort, nausea, vomiting, thirst, and a sensation of heavy pressure in the stomach. In severe cases, the patient suffers from general fatigue and has dry skin.

Treatment

Succussion in the stomach indicates a deterioration of the gastric function. Mild cases of gastrectasis may be cured without direct specific treatment by eating less food and drinking less fluid (especially water). In severe cases of hypohydrochloria or gastrointestinal weakness, it is important to increase the secretion of gastric juices. Therefore, the patient should eat sour plums, lemon, or vinegar before meals. For patients who crave food all day, gum is a good substitute.

Acute Gastritis

Acute gastritis is a condition of acute inflammation of the mucous lining of the stomach. Possible causes are overeating, excessive drinking (alcohol), food poisoning, and excessive intake of drugs or chemicals. Allergenic foods or drugs may induce gastritis in hypersensitive individuals. Since acute gastritis may deteriorate to a chronic condition, it should be treated as soon as possible.

Symptoms

The symptoms of gastritis are discomfort or stagnation in the stomach, stomachache, vomiting, headache, severe chills, fever, and diarrhea. In severe cases, gastroenteritis may result.

Treatment

The patient with acute gastritis should try to vomit the food from his stomach by placing his fingers in the back of his throat. Afterward, he should be sure to rest and follow a proper diet. If there is fever, a doctor should be consulted.

For mild cases, fasting or following a strict, careful diet for several days is an effective therapy. To break the fast, the patient should first drink fluids. Afterward soft pureed foods and finally whole food may be added to the diet.

Overeating, eating spoiled foods and excessive drinking as well as overwork and mental stress stress should be avoided.

Chronic Gastritis

Chronic gastritis is a condition of chronic inflammation of the mucous lining of the stomach and is the result of persistent acute gastritis. Suppuration is sometimes present.

A physical examination is necessary for diagnosis, since this disease is frequently asymptomatic. Although roentgenograms will show that the patient's stomach is shaped abnormally, a biopsy is essential for diagnosis. Recently, the incidence of chronic gastritis has risen sharply. Although the reasons are not known, stress is no doubt an important factor.

Symptoms

Often chronic gastritis is asymptomatic; yet the symptoms that do appear are different for every individual. One of the main symptoms may be either a feeling of heaviness in the stomach or chest distention. Despite the presence of inflammation, the patient's gastric function is still sound. However, he may have sub-cardiac pain after eating, vomiting, a tendency toward fatigue, or weight loss.

If the above-mentioned symptoms continue for a prolonged period, then the condition of inflammation will deteriorate and cause the secretion of gastric juice to decrease, the abdominal muscles to atrophy, and the gastric function to become impaired.

At this point the patient may develop the following symptoms: anorexia, abdominal pain after eating, diarrhea, halitosis, and gastric bleeding or ulcers. In other cases, the patient may feel abdominal pain (even when the stomach is empty) and have persistent constipation and an abnormal appetite.

Because the subjective symptoms are so varied and because chronic gastritis is associated with other diseases, a physical examination is necessary for correct diagnosis.

Treatment

Although the cause of chronic gastritis may be different in

each case, the patient should adopt a lifestyle that emphasizes proper diet and health care. Careless eating habits, eating spicy foods, insufficient chewing (due to tooth decay or pyorrhea), smoking, excessive drinking, lack of exercise, emotional outbursts, and stress should all be avoided. Instead, the patient should lead a more balanced life and try to maintain regular hours, eat easily digestible foods, and exercise regularly.

Gastrospasm

Gastrospasm is a prickling pain that occurs in the stomach area, caused by muscular spasms of the stomach. (The pain is not considered severe).

Gastrospasm is frequently caused by gallstones, gastric ulcers, acute gastritis, hysteria, neurosis, and allergic reactions to certain foods. Women are more susceptible to gastrospasm than men, and onset may occur before menstruation or as a result of chilling.

Symptoms
This disease is characterized by sudden, severe pain in the upper abdomen which soon then becomes spasmodic. The spasms may be temporary, or they may be come chronic.

Treatment
Analgesics and sedatives are effective for treating the severe pain of gastrospasm. Patients with chronic spasms should avoid stress, overeating, and excessive drinking. A physical examination is essential for diagnosis.

Peptic Ulcer

Peptic Ulcer is an ulceration of the mucous membrane penetrating through the muscularis mucosa. It usually occurs in places where gastric acid or pepsin is secreted, such as the duodenum (duodenal ulcers) or the stomach (gastric ulcers), but may also occur in the areas between the esophagus and the intestines. The patient with peptic ulcers often undergoes periods of spontaneous remission followed by relapse. In severe cases, surgery may be necessary.

The etiology of peptic ulcers is still theoretical. Stress, nervous tension, overwork, emotional instability, and improper diet are all possible causes. The secretion of excess gastric acid or pepsin also seems to play a major role in ulcer formation; however the causative factors are more complex. If the mucousal protective factors such as mucus production, membrane permeability, and cellular lifespan are disturbed in any way, ulcers may result (especially duodenal ulcers, since the duodenum does not secrete protective mucus).

Peptic ulcers vary in size, with diameters ranging from 5 to 20 mm. In some cases the ulcer is small but penetrates deeply into the stomach wall. Suppuration is also common, especially among middle-aged patients.

Symptoms

The main symptoms of gastric and duodenal ulcers are severe stomachache, severe nausea, bloody sputum, dark tarry stools, stomach discomfort, a sensation of stagnation in the stomach, and subcardiac pain. In severe cases, the patient may feel severe pain in the abdomen that radiates to the back.

Treatment

Since hyperfunction of the stomach may be responsible for gastric ulcers, it is important to let the stomach rest so that it can recover. If any medication is prescribed, stimulants for the stomach should be avoided; the stomach can heal itself without much difficulty. In cases of severe gastric ulcers, surgery may be necessary.

Since emotional stress is intimately linked with the formation of gastric ulcers, therapies which alleviate stress such as acupressure, massage, chiropractic therapy, applications of lukewarm water, hot water bottles, hot springs therapy, acupuncture, and moxibustion are all effective treatments for gastric ulcers. In addition, antacids are also effective in relieving excess acidity. Sodium bicarbonate (Baking soda) (1.0g) is one of the best remedies.

By following a careful diet, the patient with peptic ulcers can avoid the aggravation of suppurative ulcers. Spicy foods and foods that are difficult to digest should be eliminated from the diet. According to the findings of recent research, patients with peptic ulcers may eat whole foods instead of soft or pureed foods; however, the quantities should be limited and meals should be eaten regularly (every three hours).

Gastric ulcers are not symptoms of gastric cancer. Therefore the patient has no reason to worry.

Gastric Cancer

In Taiwan, cancer has become one of the ten major causes of death over the past ten years. The majority of these cancer patients have gastric cancer. Gastric cancer is responsible for several thousand deaths each year, and the number continually increases.

Presently, there is no cure for gastric cancer. Surgery is effective for removing tumors and other affected organs; however, about 70% of the patients with gastric cancer suffer a relapse within five years after surgery. After relapse, the prognosis is hopeless. However if the symptoms of gastric cancer are detected early and proper treatment is given, the chances of relapse are substantially reduced.

Symptoms

In general, the initial stages of all cancers are asymptomatic. However, sometimes there are early warning signs which are similar to the symptoms of gastritis such as: weight loss, anorexia, a change in eating habits, stagnation in the stomach, nausea, abdominal pain, chest distention, and vomiting. If the patient vomits blood or has black tarry stools, then the cancer is usually in its advanced stage. Unfortunately, Western physicians do not look for some of these symptoms during the early stages. For preventative medicine, a physical examination is recommended every six months.

Treatment

Once the diagnosis of gastric cancer has been confirmed, surgery is necessary. However, if the patient is unwilling to undergo such radical treatment, alternative treatments such as

X-ray therapy are recommended. Although Chinese herbal formulas cannot completely cure gastric cancer, they do help to supply some of the body's vital needs. Therefore, Chinese formulas are prescribed to relieve some of the existing symptoms and to prevent the development of new ones.

Chinese Herb Formulas

There is no specific Chinese herb formula for treating gastric cancer. Generally, formulas are prescribed according to the different symptoms present.

1. **Liu-chun-tzu-tang**   六君子湯
   (Major Six Herb Combination)

It is effective for treating patients of delicate constitution who have cold limbs, pallor, a tendency toward fatigue, a lack of vigor, weak abdominal muscles, succussion in the stomach, anorexia, and stagnation in the stomach.

2. **Szu-chun-tzu-tang**   四君子湯
   (Major Four Herb Combination)

This formula may be used to treat patients of delicate constitution who lack vigor.

3. **Pan-hsia-hsieh-hsin-tang**   半夏瀉心湯
   (Pinellia Combination)

This formula may be taken for subcardiac distention, anorexia, and nausea.

4. **Li-ke-tang**   利膈湯
   (Pinellia and Gardenia Combination)

It is used to treat profuse vomiting.

Appendicitis

Appendicitis is the inflammation of the veriform appendix. The onset is sudden, and the disease may be acute, subacute, or chronic. According to recent studies, some of the indirect causes of acute appendicitis are overwork, anxiety, insufficient sleep, overeating, and excessive drinking. Acute appendicitis is curable, usually through surgery. However, patients of delicate constitution with acute appendicitis are in danger of developing chronic appendicitis if the disease is not treated as soon as possible.

Symptoms

Patients with acute appendicitis feel sudden, severe pain in the stomach, accompanied by nausea. (This condition is often misjudged as acute gastritis.) After thirty minutes to an hour, the persistent pain becomes localized in the area of the right lower abdomen with tenderness and rigidity over the right rectus muscle or McBurney's point. The following sign is another indication of appendicitis: when the patient stretches his right leg, he feels severe pain and tension and his abdominal muscles become rigid. Other symptoms of acute appendicitis are fever and a tendency toward constipation (no diarrhea).

Chronic appendicitis may follow an acute attack causing a narrowing of the lumen of the appendix or adhesions. The main subjective symptoms are a feeling of stagnation, gastric indigestion, (which may feel like a peptic ulcer or gallbladder attack), pain in the right lower abdomen, diarrhea or persistent constipation, and belching.

Treatment

Appendicitis should be treated as early as possible since rupture will result in peritonitis or possible death.

Sometimes mild cases of acute appendicitis may be cured with medication; however, relapse is still possible. A doctor should be consulted at once if any of the above mentioned symptoms are present. After a diagnosis is made, an appendectomy should be performed. Cathartics are contraindicated. The patient should be kept as comfortable and calm as possible, with cool compresses over the area of pain.

For chronic appendicitis, appendectomy is the most effective cure. The surgical procedure is safe and simple. However, for patients with delicate constitutions who are unable to undergo surgery (poor risks), Chinese herb formulas are recommended.

Gastrointestinal Weakness

Patients of a weak constitution are often prone to gastrointestinal weakness. This disease is usually caused by stress or overwork.

Symptoms
Patients with gastrointestinal weakness are usually thin, lack vitality, and tend to be easily fatigued. Other symptoms are diarrhea, slight abdominal pain, mild vertigo, palpitation, succussion in the stomach, and (sometimes) rigid abdominal walls.

Treatment
For temporary relief, stress-reducing agents are recommended; these are especially effective for diarrhea. In cases of persistent constipation, Biofermin is used. Carthatics, however, are contraindicated except in emergency.

The objective of treatment for gastrointestinal weakness is to improve the digestive function, especially peristalsis. Peristaltic action occurs every fifteen to twenty seconds. However, if no roughage is present to stimulate movement in the stomach and the intestines, digestion becomes sluggish, a sufficient amount of plant fiber in the diet will promote intestinal function. Furthermore, any exercise for the legs and toes will serve to stimulate the nerves (important because the rectum is distal to the automatic nerve center) and improve peristalsis. Walking is therefore an excellent therapy; acupuncture at the *tsu-san-li* (St-36) point is also effective.

In cases of gastrointestinal weakness with diarrhea, the water is absorbed through the intestines and discharged as watery diarrhea through the rectum. Since the body is over 70% water, dehydration is a potential danger. Patients with diarrhea should therefore drink water after a bowel movement. In severe cases hypodermoclysis may be necessary.

Cholelithiasis (Gallstones)

Cholelithiasis is a condition in which calculi are formed in the gallbladder or bile ducts due to the presence of excess cholesterol. While the underlying cause of this disease is still unknown, it is certain that improper diet plays a major role in the development of gallstones.

Symptoms

This disease is characterized by recurrent attacks of severe pain in the upper abdomen. Other symptoms are upper abdominal discomfort, bloating, flatulence, belching, and food intolerance. Foods that are high in animal fats will cause an increase in the production of bile and induce gall-bladder attack or biliary colic (cholecystalglia). As a result the patient will feel severe pain with jaundice, vomiting, and constipation.

Treatment

For patients with continuous pain and jaundice, cholecystecomy is usually necessary. However, patients with "silent stones" are often able to expel them naturally.

For patients who do not undergo surgery, long term dietary therapy is essential. Fat intake should be restricted, since an overconsumption of fats will impede the emulsifying action of the bile. Fried or greasy foods, pastries, and gas-forming vegetables should be eliminated; a vegetarian diet is recommended.

For patients following diets a cholagogue is usually effective during acute gallbladder attacks. Surgery is not required except in an emergency.

Cholecystitis

Cholecystitis is the inflammation of the gallbladder due to the presence of bacteria. In most cases the disease occurs when a gallstone occludes a cystic duct.

Symptoms

Cholecystitis may either be acute or chronic. In cases of acute inflammation the symptoms are sudden, acute fever, and severe pain. In chronic cases, the patient may have prolonged relapsing fever or pain.

Treatment

When a patient suffers from unbearable biliary colic, cholecystectomy may be necessary. However, since the gallbladder is such an important organ in the digestive system surgical removal should be performed only as a last resort.

Antibiotics are an effective treatment for cholecystitis, but a dietary therapy is even more crucial for recovery. A diet that is high in vegetables and low in animal fats is recommended.

Hepatitis

In the majority of cases, when liver disease is accompanied by jaundice, the patient has acute hepatitis. Acute viral hepatitis is classified into two distinct types according to the virus present. Acute infectious hepatitis (hepatitis A) is a communicable disease that is usually transmitted through fecally contaminated food and water. The symptoms of hepatitis A are similar to those of typhoid and dysentery. Serum hepatitis (hepatitis B) is mainly transmitted parenterally through the use of unsterile hypodermic needles (frequent among drug addicts) or by transfusions with contaminated blood. Sometimes transmission is nonparental, through sexual intercourse.

Jaundice, the characteristic symptom of hepatitis, is a result of severe liver inflammation and the destruction of liver cells due to the virus. The patient's liver function therefore, becomes impaired, and he experiences a loss of appetite. If the disease is not cured during its acute stage, it may deteriorate and become chronic persistent hepatitis.

Symptoms

The disease begins suddenly with the onset of fever and flu-like symptoms such as general fatigue, anorexia, nausea, and abdominal pain. After two to three days, the icteric phase begins with the appearance of dark urine, yellowness of the skin, and whiteness of the eyes. The liver is usually enlarged and there is pressure pain below the right ribs. The jaundice reaches a peak in about one to two weeks, then gradually fades within a month. During this recovery period, the patient's appetite gradually increases and the hepatomegaly spontaneously disappears.

Treatment

As far as treatment for hepatitis is concerned, bedrest and complete quiet are essential for recovery as well as sufficient sleep and proper nutrition. If the patient's condition of anorexia does not improve, intravenous feeding may be necessary. Other effective treatments include acupuncture, moxibustion, and (sometimes) fasting.

Pancreatitis

Pancreatitis is classified clinically into two main forms: acute (acute relapsing) or chronic (chronic relapsing). In most cases the patient's condition is acute. Acute pancreatitis is subdivided into three types: edematous, hemorrhagic, and necrotic. Middle-aged, obese patients are often susceptible to this disease.

Symptoms
The onset of acute pancreatitis occurs without warning signs. The patient suddenly feels excruciating pain in the abdomen accompanied by pallor, clammy perspiration, and vomiting. If the condition deteriorates, then the diseased pancreas may discharge some of its enzymes directly into the peritoneum, causing peritonitis. The patient's pulse then becomes rapid and feeble. During the initial stages, acute pancreatitis is difficult to distinguish from gastric ulcer, cholelithiasis, or appendicitis. In gallbladder attacks the pain is confined to the upper quadrant, while in pancreatitis the pain begins in the epigastric region and may radiate to the upper quadrants and even to the back. Another distinction is that patients with pancreatitis show an increase of amylase in the blood; therefore, laboratory examination is essential for diagnosis.

In chronic pancreatitis the pancreas becomes fibrous, scarred, and calcified after repeated attacks. The main symptoms are gradual weight loss and continuous pain around the umbilicus. Nausea and vomiting are also common. Chronic pancreatitis is difficult to diagnose and treat since the symptoms are nonspecific.

Treatment
For acute pancreatitis, bed rest is essential. Since food is forbidden during attacks in order to suppress secretion of pancreatic fluids, the patient is fed intravenously. Meperidine is used as an analgesic; morphine and codeine are contraindicated. Between attacks a diet that is high in carbohydrates and low in fats and protein is recommended. Heavy meals and alcohol should

be avoided. Surgery may be necessary if the disease is complicated by gallstones.

For chronic pancreatitis, the replacement of pancreatic enzymes is the standard procedure. Bed rest is essential. Fluid balance is maintained intravenously, and a diet high in carbohydrates and easily digestible food is prescribed. In some cases surgery is recommended.

Hemorrhoids

Hemorrhoids occur when the veins around the anus or inside the rectum become varicosed. Complications such as anal fissure, hemorrhage, fistula, proctoptosis, and peri-proctitis may result.

Symptoms
Generally, the patient feels slight pain or a strange sensation in the rectum. Sometimes the pain is severe especially if the inflamed hemorrhoidal mass or swollen vein and tissue have prolapsed outside the rectum. Rectal bleeding is common.

Treatment
Patients with hemorrhoids should avoid straining in order to move the bowels. Application of hot, wet packs, ointments, or suppositories is also effective. Proper hygiene is important after evacuation. In severe cases, surgery is necessary.

Parasitic Infections

Roundworms, hookworms, pinworms, and tapeworms are all examples of parasitic infections that invade the human body. Patients with these diseases are generally unaware of their condition since the symptoms are nonspecific. Generally, the patient experiences gradual weight loss, abdominal pain, or diarrhea of unknown cause.

Symptoms
The symptoms of intestinal parasitic infections vary according to the parasite involved.

1. Ascariasis (roundworms): The main symptom of this disease is migrating, colicky pain in the abdomen. Other symptoms are urticaria, polyphagia or anorexia, vomiting, diarrhea, constipation, coughing, headache, convulsion, or bronchial symptoms. Sometimes the patient's fingernails or tongue may change shape.

2. Ancylostomiasis (hookworms): The main symptom of this disease is anemia. Other symptoms are weakness, a tendency toward fatigue, vertigo, tinnitus, pallor, and thin, abnormally-shaped fingernails.

3. Enterobiasis (pinworms): The main symptom of this disease is perianal and perineal pruritus. During sleep (after the first half hour or hour), the female pinworm emerges from the anus and lays her eggs around the anus and rectum (10,000 at a time); this severe itching. Other symptoms include insomnia, nervousness, a tendency toward fatigue, and anorexia due to itching.

4. Taeniasis (tapeworms): Symptoms of this infection are anorexia or increase in appetite, a sensation of abdominal heaviness, headache, vertigo, convulsion, and anemia.

Treatment

An appropriate parasiticide should be prescribed by a physician, and the patient should continue to examine his own stools.

Vomiting

Vomiting is a symptom which appears in numerous diseases and is usually accompanied by nausea. Among the digestive disorders with vomiting are food poisoning, gastritis, peptic ulcer, stomach cancer, worms, intestinal obstruction, and appendicitis. Vomiting may also be induced by emotional distress and nervous conditions such as hysteria and migraine. Antinausea medicines or antiemetics are prescribed for treatment.

Abdominal Pain

Abdominal pain may be caused by chilling, external stress, constipation, diarrhea, food poisoning, gallstones, and appendicitis. Since there are different degrees of pain, it is important to evaluate its onset, quality, frequency, the areas involved, and the circumstances of occurrence (as well as the other associated symptoms) before prescribing treatment.

Stomachache

Stomachache may be caused by various diseases. Therefore, it is necessary to evaluate the accompanying symptoms in order to make a proper diagnosis and prescribe an appropriate treatment.

Constipation

Constipation is a condition of suppressed or difficult evacuation of the bowels and is usually caused by insufficient exercise, improper diet, or external stress. Other possible causes are intestinal contriction, enteroplegia, megacolon, and enterostenosis.

Bloating

Bloating or abdominal distenstion is caused by chilling, improper diet, (especially overindulging in foods that are difficult to digest), and gastrointestinal weakness.

Chinese Herb Formulas
1. Kuei-chih-chia-shao-yao-tang　　　　　　桂枝加芍藥湯
    (Cinnamon and Paeonia Combination)

It is a combination of *Kuei-chih-tang* (Cinnamon Combination) and *Paeonia*. It is effective for bloating due to chills.

2. Chen-wu-tang　　　　　　　　　　　　眞武湯
    (Vitality Combination)

It is used to treat patients of delicate constitution with severe chills.

Diarrhea

There are various forms and degrees of diarrhea. In some

cases, the patient may defecate soft, muddy stools once or twice each day; in other cases, the patient may defecate watery stools between twenty and thirty times each day. Generally, acute cases are more severe than persistent ones.

Chinese Herb Formulas
1. Pan-hsia-hsieh-hsin-tang　　　　　　半夏瀉心湯
    (Pinellia Combination)
It is recommended for patients of average build with diarrhea.

2. Chen-wu-tang　　　　　　　　　　　眞武湯
    (Vitality Combination)
It is effective for patients of delicate constitution with diarrhea.

Jaundice

Jaundice is caused by the presence of bile pigments that result from a condition of excess bilirubin in the blood (hyperbilirubinemia). Characterized by yellowness of the skin and the mucous membranes and whiteness of the eyes, jaundice usually indicates that disorders of the liver, pancreas, or gallbladder are present.

Anorexia

The symptom of anorexia or loss of appetite often appears in disorders of the digestive system, especially the stomach. It may also be caused by stress, anxiety, fear, and emotional problems. In older patients, anorexia is especially dangerous.

Treatment.
Stomachics are usually effective for anorexia.

Acute Enteritis

Acute enteritis is a condition of intestinal inflammation.

Although diarrhea is generally the main symptom, the symptoms vary depending on which parts of the intestines are affected. Young children and older patients are especially susceptible to severe conditions of enteritis. These patients usually become very weak after several days.

Symptoms

In cases of inflammation in the small intestine, diarrhea may not appear, but abdominal pain and borborygmus are common. If there is inflammation in the colon, the patient may have intestinal colic. If the inflammation is limited to the rectum, the patient may have tenesmus.

Treatment

No specific treatment for this disease is known; however, Chinese herb formulas are effective in relieving some of the symptoms of acute enteritis.

Intestinal Obstruction and Intestinal Constriction

There are many possible causes for the condition of intestinal constriction. This condition is potentially dangerous and requires hospital treatment, usually emergency surgery. However, Chinese herb formulas may also be effective in relieving the symptoms of this disorder.

Symptoms

The main symptoms are constipation or diarrhea, vomiting, abdominal pain, borborymus, and succussion in the stomach.

Ulcerative Colitis

Ulcerative colitis is a nonspecific, chronic, ulcerous inflammation of the colon. The patient with this condition usually has bloody diarrhea, anorexia, weight loss, and anemia.

Treatment

Treatment varies according to the severity of the patient's

condition.

Chinese Herb Formulas
1. Chai-hu-kuei-chih-tang　　　　　　　　柴胡桂枝湯
    (Bupleurum and Cinnamon Combination)
It is used to treat ulcerative colitis.

2. Wei-feng-tang　　　　　　　　　　　　胃風湯
    (Atractylodes and Setaria Combination)
It is effective for treating rectal ulcers with tarry stools, abdominal pain, and diarrhea.

Rectal Cancer

The symptoms of rectal cancer are similar to those of rectal ulcers and hemorrhoids including constipation, tenesmus, diarrhea, and tarry stools. During the early stages of this disease, the best treatment for the patient is surgical removal of tumors. However, even though there is no specific Chinese herb formula for treating rectal cancer, the formulas listed below may be effective for the patient who refuses to undergo surgery.

Chinese Herb Formulas
1. Tzu-ken-mu-li-tang　　　　　　　　　紫根牡蠣湯
    (Lithospermum and Oyster Shell Combination)
It is recommended of patients with malignant tumors.

2. Jun-chang-tang　　　　　　　　　　　潤腸湯
    (Linum and Rhubarb Combination)
It is used to treat constipation alternating with tarry stools.

3. Wei-feng-tang　　　　　　　　　　　　胃風湯
    (Atractylodes and Setaria Combination)
It is effective for diarrhea, tarry stools, and tenesmus.

DISEASES OF THE KIDNEYS

Acute Nephritis

Abnormal glomeruli and capillaries of the kidneys cause acute nephritis. Seventy to eighty percent of the cases of this disease are preceded by influenza, tonsillitis, and angina. Acute nephritis often occurs after the patient has suffered from tonsillitis for ten days to two weeks. Other causes are pneumonia, otitis media, scarlet fever, para-rhinitis, and endocarditis. The detailed process of infection is not yet clear. It is now thought that the glomerular or capillary degeneration and inflammation is caused by pyogenic pneumococci and streptococci.

Symptoms

The patient has a sore throat and fever. After 10 to 20 days, the above symptoms disappear but the patient remains tired and has low back pain, a tendency towards fatigue, thirst, and loss of appetite. In acute nephritis, there is albuminuria, hematuria, and sometimes edema. When there is edema, the volume of urine decreases, but the blood pressure increases and is accompanied by headache and nausea. If the patient has facial edema (especially about the eyes) upon arising in the morning, it will spread to the whole body; at the same time, the blood pressure will decrease and there may be albuminuria or hematuria or a sudden decrease in the volume of urine.

Treatment

In order to prevent acute nephritis from becoming chronic, the patient should remain completely calm and keep the kidneys well protected. It is better for the patient to stay in the hospital and accept a special diet of low-sodium, high-protein foods. He should drink at least six to eight glasses of water daily.

Chinese Herb Formulas

1. Wu-ling-san　　　　　　　　　　　　　　　　　五苓散
   (Hoelen Five Herb Formula)
   This is effective for oliguria after drinking due to thirst of the patient with or without edema.

2. Hsiao-ching-lung-tang　　　　　　　　　　　　小青龍湯
   (Minor Blue Dragon Combination)
   This is effective for fever, oliguria, and edema due to acute nephritis. The patient will have the symptoms of muscular tension at both sides of the umbilicus and a watery sound when the stomach is tapped.

3. Hsiao-chai-hu-tang-chia-huang-lien-fu-ling
   　　　　　　　　　　　　　　　　　　小柴胡湯加黃連茯苓
   (Minor Bupleurum Combination with Coptis and Hoelen)
   The patient without edema but with fever, nausea, loss of appetite, and pressing sensation at the heart should take *Hsiao-chai-hu-tang* (小柴胡湯 , Minor Bupleurum Combination). For subacute or chronic nephritis which is mild or without edema, hoelen 3.0g and coptis 1.5g should be added.

4. Ta-ching-lung-tang　　　　　　　　　　　　　大青龍湯
   (Major Blue Dragon Combination)
   To be taken by the patient with acute nephritis who has severe edema, headache, anxiety, and rapid respiration. It is also effective for acute uremia.

5. Pu-chung-chih-shih-tang　　　　　　　　　　　補中治濕湯
   (Ginseng and Akebia Combination)

To be taken by those of delicate constitution with lingering edema.

6. **Chai-hu-chia-lung-ku-mu-li-tang**　　　柴胡加龍骨牡蠣湯
   (Bupleurum and Dragon Bone Combination)
   To be taken by the patient without edema, but with high blood pressure, decreased urine, constipation, palpitation, and a sensation of pressure in the chest. The patients are usually obese and have chest and abdominal distention.

Chronic Nephritis

This disease is divided into two categories — chronic nephritis following acute nephritis and typical chronic nephritis. The cause of this disease is the same as that of acute nephritis, probably streptococcus infection.

Symptoms
In the primary stage, typical chronic nephritis is without any symptoms of which the patient is aware. When he is sick or weak, the patient will have edema. Some patients have only albuminuria without edema. As the disease progresses, there is an increase in blood pressure, pallor, blurred eyesight, palpitations, gasping respirations, and nocturia. In severe cases, uremia and death will follow.

Treatment
Patients with mild symptoms who do not have high blood pressure and edema may remain in good condition with proper care. But the patient with high blood pressure should pay special attention to it. Chronic nephritis is a typical recalcitrant disease and should be carefully treated from the onset. It is very important to select a proper therapy.

Chinese Herb Formulas
1. **Hsiao-chai-hu-tang-chia-fu-ling-huang-lien**

   　　　　　　　　　　　　　　　　小柴胡湯加茯苓黃連
   (Minor Bupleurum Combination with Hoelen and Coptis)
   This is effective for chronic nephritis with albuminuria, but

without edema. Usually ginger is omitted beofre use.

2. **Pa-wei-wan** 八味丸
   (Rehmannia Eight Formula)
This is effective for fatigue from the waist to the legs, nocturia, albuminuria, and hypertension with or without edema. Those having gastrointestinal disorders should avoid taking this formula.

3. **Mu-fang-chi-tang** 木防己湯
   (Stephania and Ginseng Combination)
To be taken for chronic nephritis with edema, rapid breathing, cardiac hypertrophy, stridor, and a resistant sensation in the lower heart.

4. **Chi-wu-chiang-hsia-tang** 七物降下湯
   (Tang-kuei and Gambir Formula)
This is effective for chronic nephritis in women with mild or no edema, constipation, headache, vertigo, high blood pressure, and abdominal conformation with stagnant blood.

5. **Tao-ho-cheng-chi-tang** 桃核承氣湯
   (Persica and Rhubarb Combination)
To be taken for chronic nephritis in the female with mild or no edema, constipation, headache, vertigo, high blood pressure, and abdominal conformation with stagnant blood.

Degenerative Nephritis

Recent research indicates that this disease is due to a variety of causes such as abnormal metabolism, allergies, and especially the storage of lipids, lipoids, and aminoids in the renal tubules and glomeruli. Although this disease is different from nephritis, both often occur simultaneously.

Symptoms
Degenerative nephritis is a chronic disease causing loss of appetite and other complications. The patient has albuminuria, decrease in urinary output, and more marked edema than that of

nephritis. In some patients this disease may be due to a chronic external ulcer.

Treatment
The treatment of this disease should include a low-sodium diet. If the patient shows a loss of appetite because of the decreased salt, every effort should be made to encourage him to eat a balanced diet and regular meals. In addition, he should use diuretics to dispel the edema and decrease the workload of the heart.

Chinese Herb Formulas
1. Mu-fang-chi-tang 木防己湯
   (Stephania and Ginseng Combination)
To be taken for gasping, palpitations, labored breathing, severe edema due to atelocardia, and oliguria.

2. Fen-hsiao-tang 分消湯
   (Hoelen and Alisma Combination)
This is effective for the primary symptoms of this disease and for a swelling sensation at the abdomen.

3. Yin-chen-hao-tang 茵陳蒿湯
   (Capillaris Combination)
This is especially effective for degenerative nephritis with edema and abdominal and chest distention.

Pyelitis

The renal pelvis, a part of the kidneys; is shaped like a bag. It collects the urine from the kidneys and transports it to the bladder. Pyelitis occurs when the renal pelvis is infected by bacteria such as *Escherichia coli,* staphylococci, or streptococci which move from the urethra, bladder, and ureter to the renal pelvis. It is more common in women than men.

Pyelitis has a tendency to become a chronic disease and should be cured as soon as possible after the diagnosis is made. When it becomes chronic, it will spread to both kidneys becoming pyelonephritis and causing chronic renal malfunction.

Symptoms
The onset is sudden with severe chills and shivering, fever (38-40°), dull pain at both sides of the abdomen, frequent and increased urination, turbid urine, and albuminuria. The fever drops after two or three days. If the patient does not receive immediate, proper treatment, he will suffer relapses of fever and an aggravation of the condition.

Treatment
The patient should remain calm, cool the area in acute pain, and avoid alcohol and highly seasoned foods.

Chinese Herb Formulas
1. Chu-ling-tang   猪苓湯
    (Polyporus Combination)
    To be taken for pyelitis, strangury, sensation of urine remaining after voiding, ardor urinae, and hematuria.

2. Wu-ling-san   五苓散
    (Hoelen Five Herb Formula)
    It is effective for pyelitis, turbid urine, and thirst.

3. Chai-hu-kuei-chih-tang   柴胡桂枝湯
    (Bupleurum and Cinnamon Combination)
    To be taken for fever and for pain on both sides of the abdomen.

4. Hsiao-chai-hu-tang   小柴胡湯
    (Minor Bupleurum Combination)
    This is good to treat recurrent fever and chills, white coating on the tongue, bitter taste, nausea or vomiting, and loss of appetite.

5. Ta-huang-mu-tan-pi-tang   大黃牡丹皮湯
    (Rhubarb and Moutan Combination)
    Kuei-chih-fu-ling-wan   桂枝茯苓丸
    (Cinnamon and Hoelen Formula)
    When there is a pressing pain in the kidneys, swelling, and constipation, take *Ta-huang-mu-tan-pi-tang*. If there is no constipation, the patient may try *Kuei-chih-fu-ling-wan*.

6. Ta-chai-hu-tang　　　　　　　　　　大柴胡湯
    (Major Bupleurum Combination)
To be taken for the similar conformation of *Hsiao-chai-hu-tang*, but with abdominal pain, constipation, and yellow coating on the tongue.

7. Ta-huang-fu-tzu-tang　　　　　　　　大黃附子湯
    (Rhubarb and Aconite Combination)
To be taken for acute abdominal pain, severe chills, cold feet, and constipation.

8. Ching-hsin-lien-tzu-yin　　　　　　　清心蓮子飲
    (Lotus Seed Combination)
To be taken for chronic pyelitis with the symptoms of mild fever, gastrointestinal weakness, loss of appetite, nausea, and a tendency towards diarrhea.

9. Tzu-yin-chiang-huo-tang　　　　　　滋陰降火湯
    (Phellodendron Combination)
To be taken for subacute pyelitis, lingering fever, thirst, palpitation at the umbilicus, and turbid urine.

Urethral Calculi

Urethral calculi or stones are differentiated into renal calculi, ureteral calculi, and vesical calculi. Renal and ureteral calculi can bring about drastic paroxysmal abdominal pain. The abdominal pain starts from the side of the kidney and radiates toward the bladder, the urethra, and the thighs. The progression is accompanied by nausea and vomiting.

Vesical calculi cause pain on urination and frequency of urination or, at times, a complete stoppage of urination. The urine is turbid and somtimes bloody. The symptoms can be aggravated by physical exercise.

Chinese Herb Formulas
1. Chu-ling-tang　　　　　　　　　　　猪苓湯
    (Polyporus Combination)
This formula is used to help discharge the stones if contractions to

expel them are not occurring. The formula reduces thirst and decreases urination, urinary stuttering, and hematuria. These symptoms are sometimes not very obvious. The formula is more often used for vesical calculi.

2. **Kuei-chih-fu-ling-wan** 桂枝茯苓丸
   (Cinnamon and Hoelen Formula)
   Ta-huang-mu-tan-pi-tang 大黃牡丹皮湯
   (Rhubarb and Moutan Combination)
   Tao-ho-cheng-chi-tang 桃核承氣湯
   (Persica and Rhubarb Combination)

These formulas are intended to treat the abdominal symptom of stagnated blood. Urethral calculi become resistant, the patient experiencing pain in the lower abdomen when palpated. For these symptoms *Kuei-chih-fu-ling-wan* plus 10g of coix is administered. The taking of this formula must be continued even when there is no muscle contraction, so that all the calculi will be excreted. When there are resistance and pain in the lower abdomen as well as a tendency toward constipation, then *Ta-huang-mu-tan-pi-tang* is indicated. In case of abdominal cramps, pain, and constipation, *Tao-ho-cheng-chi-tang* is indicated. These formulas are also prescribed for severe contractions caused by urethral calculi.

3. **Ta-chien-chung-tang** 大建中湯
   (Major Zanthoxylum Combination)

This formula is used during the time of clonus (contractions). It is effective against the violent abdominal pain and the distress caused by tight distention of the abdomen because of gas in the stomach and intestines. In such cases, the above formulas usually cannot be taken by the patient. The author had experience with administering *Ta-chai-hu-tang* to one patient whose symptoms included thoraco-costal distress, abdominal distention, and constipation. The abdominal pain became even more violent, and the drug was vomited so the patient was shifted to *Ta-chien-chung-tang*. Thirty minutes later, the abdominal pain was alleviated and the patient fell asleep. Soon one stone the size of a red bean and another half that size were excreted. The patient has not had a recurrence of urethral calculus for nearly thirty years.

4. Shao-yao-kan-tsao-tang　　　　　　　芍藥甘草湯
    (Paeonia and Licorice Combination)
This formula is used as a one dose medication for tense abdominal muscles and the extreme pain caused by muscle contractions.

5. Ta-huang-fu-tzu-tang　　　　　　　　大黃附子湯
    (Rhubarb and Aconite Combination)
This formula is also used for clonus with a tense and chordal pulse, and lateral pain at the ribs (right or left abdomen). It is taken by patients having a firm conformation similar to that of *Ta-chien-chung-tang*.

6. Fang-feng-tung-sheng-san　　　　　　防風通聖散
    (Siler and Platycodon Formula)
This formula is used for patients with a stalwart physique, abdominal distention, and constipation.

7. Pa-wei-wan　　　　　　　　　　　　八味丸
    (Rehmannia Eight Formula)
This prescription is indicated for patients with frequent clonus who have had low back pain or a fatigued sensation in the back and waist area. It should be taken lengthily.

Urethral Tuberculosis

Urethral tuberculosis rarely occurs and is usually not found until it appears in the form of cystitis. It occurs more frequently in males than in females in the form of intratubular infection due to renal or prostatic tuberculosis. It seldom causes anterior urethritis but usually causes posterior urethritis with frequent and painful urination as the main complaint. The urine is turbid, usually containing pus and occasionally blood. The patient may have low back pains and swelling and pain in the kidney.

The methods of examination are external palpation, catheterization, urethroscopy, and urethrography. The prognosis is not good since usually it results in urethral stricture causing the retention of the tuberculous urine which leads to a multiple and spreading infection.

Treatment
Treatment is carried out with chemotherapy along with the following formulas. If detected in the initial stage, a complete cure is expected. For those on whom surgery may not be performed, these formulas may alleviate the symptoms.

Chinese Herb Formulas
1. **Szu-wu-tang-ho-chu-ling-tang**　　　　　四物湯合猪苓湯
   (Tang-kuei Four Combination with Polyporus Combination)

This formula is indicated for frequent and incontinent urination, discomfort on urination, urinary stuttering, and the sensation of residual urine. It is also efficacious for the pain at the site of the kidney and the pain disseminating through the urinary bladder and thighs.

2. **Tao-ho-cheng-chi-tang**　　　　　桃核承氣湯
   (Persica and Rhubarb Combination)

This formula is used for patients having colicky pain disseminating from the lower abdomen to the urethra, or for those suffering from abrupt urine retention or urethral stenosis (constriction). The formula may be used singularly or in combination with *Pa-wei-wan*. If there is cramping and pain in the lower abdomen, this formula should be used immediately without hesitation.

3. **Chiung-kuei-chiao-ai-tang**　　　　　芎歸膠艾湯
   (Tang-kuei and Gelatin Combination)
   Wen-ching-yin　　　　　溫清飲
   (Tang-kuei and Gardenia Combination)

These are used for the constant appearance of blood in the urine (hematuria).

4. **Chu-ling-tang**　　　　　猪苓湯
   (Polyporus Combination)

Mostly rehmannia-containing preparations are indicated for renal tuberculosis. However, these preparations sometimes cause gastrointestinal disturbances such as diarrhea and a decreased appetite. For patients having urinary bladder troubles, this formula is suitable.

5. **Wu-lin-san** 五淋散
   (Gardenia and Hoelen Formula)
   This formula may be given to a patient who has bloody urine following nephrectomy (kidney removal) when other treatments have been ineffective.

6. **Ching-hsin-lien-tzu-yin** 清心蓮子飲
   (Lotus Seed Combination)
   This formula is suitable for patients with a poor G I system and thirst, insomnia, and loss of appetite, in addition to difficulty in urinating.

7. **Vespae Nidus** 露蜂房
   (Bee's Hive)
   This drug is taken in powder form along with other decoctions in daily doses of 6g; it has the effect of clarifying the urine.

8. **Luan-fa-shuang** 亂髮霜
   (Human Hair Formula)
   When used in daily doses of 6g along with other decoctions, it has diuretic and hemastatic effects.

9. **Pa-wei-wan** 八味丸
   (Rehmannia Eight Formula)
   This formula is used for polyuria, urinary incontinency, discomfort during urination, urinary stuttering, and the sensation of residual urine. It is also effective for pain in the kidney area and pain that radiates toward the urinary bladder and thighs.

10. **Shih-chuan-ta-pu-tang** 十全大補湯
    (Ginseng and Tang-kuei Ten Combination)
    This formula is used for excessively anemic people who tend to become more and more debilitated or for those who have had a nephrectomy and have not yet regained their normal vitality.

Kidney Stones

Kidney stones are calculi which remain at the renal pelvis. The constituents of the stones are uric salt, oxalic acid, carbonate, and other minerals. Although the definite cause is still unknown, it is presumed to be the condensate of various precipitates in the urine. Usually the stones are found in only one of the kidneys; however, they may be in both. There may be a number of small stones or one or two larger ones.

Symptoms

The severe pain is due to the increased inner pressure in the renal pelvis. The paroxysmal pain at the lower abdomen is called nephrocolic. In severe cases, the patient will exude fatlike sweats accompanied by occasional vomiting and a swollen abdomen. Nephrocolic will last about 30 minutes and then subside.

If there are kidney stones, the patient will suffer from relapses of pain and hematuria.

Treatment

When the kidney stones are small, the patient should drink water freely in order to increase urine volume and encourage passage of the calculi. If the stones are not passed, the patient should undergo surgery for their removal.

Chinese Herb Formulas

1. **Ta-chien-chung-tang** 大建中湯
    (Major Zanthoxylum Combination)

This is effective for severe pain in the lower abdomen, weak abdominal muscles, kidney stones, and swelling of the abdomen.

2. **Shao-yao-kan-tsao-tang** 芍藥甘草湯
    (Paeonia and Licorice Combination)

To be taken for sudden and severe nephrocolic.

3. **Pa-wei-wan** 八味丸
    (Rehmannia Eight Formula)

This is effective for occasional mild nephrocolic and nocturnal polyuria.

4. **Chu-ling-tang** 猪苓湯
    (Polyporus Combination)

To be taken by the patient with kidney stones who has albuminuria, thirst, and difficult urination.

5. Kuei-chih-fu-ling-wan 桂枝茯苓丸
   (Cinnamon and Hoelen Formula)
   Ta-huang-mu-tan-pi-tang 大黃牡丹皮湯
   (Rhubarb and Moutan Combination)
   Tao-ho-cheng-chi-tang 桃核承氣湯
   (Persica and Rhubarb Combination)

All are effective for stagnant blood. When there is resistent pressing pain in the lower abdomen, *Kuei-chih-fu-ling-wan* with coix 10.0g should be taken. Those with the above symptoms and a tendency towards constipation should take *Ta-huang-mu-tan-pi-tang*. For acute abdominal pain with constipation, take *Tao-ho-cheng-chi-tang*.

6. Ta-huang-fu-tzu-tang 大黃附子湯
   (Rhubarb and Aconite Combination)

To be taken for tense pulse and abdominal pain. It is effective for the strong conformation similar to that of *Ta-chien-chung-tang*.

7. Fang-feng-tung-sheng-san 防風通聖散
   (Siler and Platycodon Formula)

To be taken by those of obese physique with swelling abdomen and constipation.

Nephroptosis
(Wandering Kidneys)

Nephroptosis is a common condition in women, young men, and very thin people. It is generally known as "wandering kidneys". Since the kidneys are not fixed, but kept in a normal position by blood vessels, fatty pads surrounding them, and the pressure of abdominal organs, they wander more or less when a person stands up or sits down. However, it is only when they drop a rather large distance that the condition is called "wandering kidneys".

Those having a long congenital arteria renalis, weak supporting muscles near the kidneys, or recent loss of a considerable amount of weight often suffer from this problem. Pregnancy, childbirth, or surgery in the area near the kidneys may cause the abdominal pressure to change suddenly, resulting in this condition.

Symptoms
The condition is characterized by a sensation of heaviness or pain at both sides of the abdomen which occurs after standing for a long time and is relieved by bed rest. The other symptoms are low back pain, hematuria, and a tendency towards vomiting.

Treatment
In severe cases, surgery should be performed to anchor the kidneys. In some cases, a kidney belt alone may produce good results.

Those having hypotension, anemia, and physical weakness will be very susceptible to this condition. Therefore, improvement of the physical constitution by exercise such as Yoga, a well-balanced diet, and other good health practices can produce good results.

Chinese Herb Formulas
1. Chiung-kuei-chiao-ai-tang　　　　　　　　芎歸膠艾湯
   (Tang-kuei and Gelatin Combination)
   To be taken for hematuria.

2. Liu-chun-tzu-tang　　　　　　　　　　　　六君子湯
   (Major Six Herb Combination)
   Hsiao-chien-chung-tang　　　　　　　　　　小建中湯
   (Minor Cinnamon and Paeonia Combination)
   These are effective for "wandering kidneys" with gastroptosis.

3. Tang-kuei-shao-yao-san　　　　　　　　　當歸芍藥散
   (Tang-kuei and Paeonia Formula)
   Tang-kuei-chien-chung-tang　　　　　　　當歸建中湯
   (Tang-kuei, Cinnamon, and Paeonia Combination)
   To be taken by the woman with "wandering kidneys", chilling, and physical weakness. They are also used to increase vigor.

Renal Atrophy

Renal atrophy is a hardened and atrophic state of the kidneys. The kidneys are reduced to between one-third and one-fourth of their normal size. This condition is most often caused by a sudden exacerbation of untreated chronic nephritis or by renal arteriosclerosis due to hypertension. Because the blood which flows to the kidney is decreased and renal function is lowered, some cases will lead to uremia and death.

Symptoms

The function of the kidneys is decreased and only dilute rather than turbid urine is passed. Occasionally the patient will have frequent urination, albuminuria, edema, tinnitus, and pallor due to anemia. In severe cases, angina pectoris and gasping breath will also occur. Whenever there is increased urination and a tendency towards fatigue in a person of middle age, he should seek a medical examination to determine whether or not the cause is diabetes and renal atrophy.

Treatment

Prophylaxis is better than therapy. The patient should be cured of chronic nephritis and hypertension.

Chinese Herb Formula
Tzu-shen-tung-erh-tang
(Scute Combination)
To be taken for tinnitus due to renal atrophy.

滋腎通耳湯

Cystitis

When the bladder is infected by bacteria, the disease is known as "cystitis". Various bacteria such as *Escherichia coli*, streptococci, gonococci, staphylococci, bacilli, and tubercle bacilli are responsible. The infection often begins when the patient is cleaning the anus after defecation and the colon bacteria invade the urethra. Since the urethra of the female is shorter than the male's (its average length in an adult female is about 4 cm.), women suffer more frequently from this disease, especially in summer. After several relapses, it will become chronic. Therefore it should be completely cured in the beginning.

Symptoms

The main symptoms of this disease are pain, strangury, and turbid urine. During or at the completion of urination, there is severe pain. The mucous membrane of the bladder is irritated by the bacteria; the capacity of the bladder decreases and causes strangury and a sensation of residual urine. Turbid urine is due to the pus excreted from the mucous membrane of the bladder and mixed in the urine. The spasmodic contraction of constrictor muscles causes stagnation of the urine and a frequent urge to void, but with oliguria. In severe cases, the patient will have fever. When the bladder lining is bleeding, the urine is reddish in color. In some cases, bacterial infection, bladder stones, a tumor, or other causes may initiate a relapse. Symptoms of chronic cystitis are milder than those of acute cystitis.

Treatment

Sulfa drugs are effective for this disease. Since women are greatly affected by the autonomic nervous system, tranquilizers and steroids may be of use in treatment. It is helpful to remain calm at home, to place a hot-water bottle on the bladder and lower abdomen, and to avoid ingestion of alcohol and highly-seasoned food.

Chinese Herb Formulas

1. **Chu-ling-tang** 猪苓湯
   (Polyporus Combination)

This is effective for acute and chronic cystitis, strangury, a tendency towards dribbling after urination, painful urination, and occasional hematuria.

2. **Pa-wei-wan** 八味丸
   (Rehmannia Eight Formula)

To be taken for acute and chronic cystitis, unpleasant feeling or sensation of residual urine, increased urination, and frequent low back pain.

3. **Ching-hsin-lien-tzu-yin** 清心蓮子飲
   (Lotus Seed Combination)

This is effective for pallor, unpleasant feeling during urination, turbid and residual urine, loss of appetite, and general fatigue.

The woman with pallor, soft muscles, and physical weakness will be susceptible to having the above symptoms.

4. **Wu-ling-san** 五苓散
   (Hoelen Five Herb Formula)
   To be taken for moderate symptoms of frequent urination, turbid urine, and thirst.

5. **Lung-tan-hsieh-kan-tang** 龍膽瀉肝湯
   (Gentiana Combination)
   To be taken for severe inflammation with painful urination.

6. **Ta-huang-mu-tan-pi-tang** 大黃牡丹皮湯
   (Rhubarb and Moutan Combination)
   To be taken by those of hearty constitution with constipation and painful urination.

Edema

Edema is an abnormal amount of fluid stored in cells and tissues. When it is the result of cardiac insufficiency, it appears at the hands and feet; nephrotic edema occurs in the eyelids and face. In the final stage of kidney disease, edema occurs in the back, feet, and eyelids.

Physiologically, sitting for a long period of time will cause edema of the feet; insufficient sleep will cause edema of the face. If there is edema of the eyelids that continues for more than three or four days, it may be a warning of nephritis. Edema should not be ignored. It should be brought under control immediately, even if it is at the hands and feet.

Treatment

It is important to cure the causes of edema as the first step. Generally, the patient should maintain calmness, avoid taking foods containing too much salt and water, and eat only a moderate amount of rice or bread.

Chinese Herb Formulas
1. **Wu-ling-san**   五苓散
   (Hoelen Five Herb Formula)
   This formula is a typical diuretic for edema.

2. **Pa-wei-wan**   八味丸
   (Rehmannia Eight Formula)
   This is effective for edema in the lower body.

3. **Mu-fang-chi-tang**   木防己湯
   (Stephania and Ginseng Combination)
   This is effective for cardiac and nephrotic edema.

4. **Fen-hsiao-tang**   分消湯
   (Hoelen and Alisma Combination)
   This is effective for edema of the abdomen.

Frequent Urination

An average person urinates five to seven times during the day and not more than once during the night. A greater number is called frequent urination. Nervousness is one cause, but it can also be a result of polyuria, a decrease in bladder capacity due to senility, prostatomegaly, and a narrow opening in the urethra.

Treatment
The best treatment is sleep, as sound sleep reduces the speed of urine accumulation. Avoid taking too much tea, coffee, or wine between dinner and bedtime. If the frequent urination is due to another disease, cure that disease first.

Chinese Herb Formulas
1. **Chu-ling-tang**   猪苓湯
   (Polyporus Combination)
   To be taken for frequent urination and oliguria.

2. **Pa-wei-wan**   八味丸
   (Rehmannia Eight Formula)
   This is effective for frequent urination at night.

METABOLIC DISEASES

Obesity

Obesity is a complex disorder which may be defined as an increase of 10% or more in weight above "normal," due to generalized deposition of fat. It is important to differentiate between weight increase resulting from fat deposits and an increase resulting from body water. However, "normal" weight is difficult to determine; clinically, standard age, height, and weight tables are ordinarily used for practical purposes, although they are not always reliable. Body build, musculature, familial tendencies, and socioeconomic factors must be taken into consideration. Social factors have a marked influence on the prevalence of obesity, and situational determinants have a great effect on the eating habits of obese persons. Research technics for evaluating total body fat are available but are not practical for clinical purposes. The measurement of skinfold thickness (triceps fat fold) has been reported to be a simple and reliable method to identify obesity among individuals in the medium range of body size. About 40-50% of the adult population of the United States is considered to be overweight.

From a metabolic point of view, all obesity has a common cause: intake of more calories than are required for energy metabolism. The differences in the food intake vs. energy utilization vary for individuals—which makes it possible for one person to utilize his calories more "efficiently" than another. It has been suggested that the intestines absorb foodstuffs more effectively in obese individuals than in lean subjects. Many clinicians feel that the metabolic changes of obesity are a result of obesity itself rather than a cause of it. Obese patients have been found to have an increased number of fat cells as well as an increase in size of fat cells. Weight reduction in obese patients may decrease the size of fat cells, but the total number remains constant.

Although most cases of obesity are due to simple overeating which is often a consequence of emotional, familial, metabolic, and genetic factors, a few endocrine and metabolic disorders are known to lead to specific types of obesity (e.g. Cushing's syndrome and hypothalamic lesions). Compulsive overeating is similar in some respects to the addiction to tobacco or alcohol. It is particularly difficult to explain the phenomena of fluid retention and fat mobilization and storage. Hypothyroidism is rarely a cause of obesity.

The association of obesity with increased morbidity and mortality is well known. Hypertension, diabetes mellitus, gallbladder disease, gout, and possibly coronary atherosclerosis are frequently associated with obesity. Obesity presents special hazards in pregnancy and in surgery. The psychological and cosmetic implications of obesity are also significant factors.

Treatment

"Specific" weight-reducing chemical agents and hormones (including the currently popular chorionic gonadotropin), singly or in combination, are either ineffective or hazardous and have no place in the treatment of obesity. Juvenile obesity is often very difficult to treat, but it is important to institute a therapeutic program as early as possible.

Diet is the most important factor in the management of obesity. Preventive education about diet should be started during the formative years at a time when eating habits are being established. There are a number of points involved.

1. Calories: an intake of 500 calories per day less than the required calories should lead to a weight loss of approximately one pound a week. A daily caloric intake of 800-1200 calories is

satisfactory for a modest reducing diet.

2. Protein: a protein intake of at least 1g/kg body weight should be maintained.

3. Carbohydrate and fat: after the protein requirements have been met, the remaining calories may be half carbohydrate and half fat.

4. Vitamins and minerals: most reducing diets are likely to be deficient in vitamins but adequate in minerals. Therefore, vitamins should be used to supply the average daily maintenance requirements during the time of weight reduction.

5. The intake of sodium should be restricted.

6. Starvation regimen: total starvation has again been advocated as a weight reduction regimen. Although rapid loss of weight can be achieved by this means, the method may be quite hazardous and must be carried out in a hospital setting with strict supervision.

7. Shunt operation: jejuno-ileal shunt is being performed on selected patients whose massive obesity (i.e. two to three times ideal weight) has failed to respond to all conservative measures and is considered to be a hazard to physical, psychological, and socioeconomic well being.

Medication can include appetite suppressants and drugs to speed up metabolism. Although exercise increases the energy output, extreme exercise is necessary to significantly alter weight. Overeating is largely a matter of habit and may be associated with varying degrees of emotional problems. Once significant obesity has been established, many secondary psychological reactions occur relating to altered body image and changes in interpersonal relationships. Weight reduction is therefore essential for general psychological, as well as physical, well being.

Note: Sudden weight reduction in emotionally unstable persons may cause severe psychic consequences (e.g. anorexia nervosa or psychotic reaction).

Chinese Herb Formulas
1. Ta-chai-hu-tang   大柴胡湯
    (Major Bupleurum Combination)

This formula is indicated for patients having an obese, stalwart physique, firm and tight musculature, thoracocostal distress, subcardiac hardness and distention, constipation, and stiff shoulders. The dose of rhubarb is so adjusted as to render one to two bowel movements each day. Employment of this formula will result in subsidence of the distention, making the turning and movement of the body light and easy. When patients have hypertension, this formula also will bring about a drop in blood pressure.

2. **Fang-feng-tung-sheng-san** 防風通聖散
   (Siler and Platycodon Formula)

This formula is used for abdominal distention without thoraco-costal distress.

3. **Ta-cheng-chi-tang** 大承氣湯
   (Major Rhubarb Combination)

This formula is prescribed for high extent distention in the abdomen with resistance and elasticity and severe constipation. *Ta-chai-hu-tang* aims at the epigastric distention as the primary target, while this formula centers on the umbilicus. Obstructed menses in obese patients will flow easily again after administration of this formula.

4. **Chai-hu-chia-lung-ku-mu-li-tang** 柴胡加龍骨牡蠣湯
   (Bupleurum and Dragon Bone Combination)

In addition to the symptoms resembling those of *Ta-chai-hu-tang*, this formula may be employed for palpitations, fast and impetuous breathing, vertigo, insomnia, and reduced libido.

5. **Fang-chi-huang-chi-tang** 防己黃耆湯
   (Stephania and Astragalus Combination)

Most obese patients have a firm conformation and are thus treated with laxative-containing formulas which, however, are at times contraindicated. For women with white skin; soft and flaccid muscles or the so-called "watery plumpness" state; hidrosis, fatigability and edema after exercise, this formula is suitable. It can also be applied to the condition of erosion in the lower abdomen or thighs due to sweating in the summer.

6. **Chia-wei-pan-hsia-tang-chia-chih-hsiao-tou**
   加味半夏湯加赤小豆
   (Pinellia, Citrus, and Polyporus Combination plus Phaseolus)

This formula is to be used for obese patients after middle age with the symptoms of flushing up and vertigo.

7. Ta-huang-mu-tan-pi-tang　　　　　　　大黃牡丹皮湯
   (Rhubarb and Moutan Combination)
   Tao-ho-cheng-chi-tang　　　　　　　　桃核承氣湯
   (Persica and Rhubarb Combination)
   Kuei-chih-fu-ling-wan　　　　　　　　桂枝茯苓丸
   (Cinnamon and Hoelen Formula)

Scantiness or retardation of menses in obese middle-aged women is generally caused by blood occlusion. If abdominal diagnosis identifies blood occlusion conformation, these formulas may be used.

Leukemia

Leukemia, a progressive and malignant disease effecting the bone marrow, spleen, liver and the blood, is characterized by abnormal proliferation and development of leukocytes and their precursors in the blood and bone marrow. It is classified clinically on the basis of (1) duration and character of the disease, acute or chronic; (2) the type of cells involved, myeloic or lymphatic; and (3) increase or non-increase in the number of abnormal cells in the blood, leukemic or aleukemic.

Acute leukemia can affect all ages and races while acute myeloblastic leukemia is a disease of adults and chronic leukemia is rare under the age of thirty or among Orientals.

Acute leukemia (lymphatic or myelocytic) is characterized by massive proliferation of abnormal primitive white cells in the bone marrow. Chronic leukemia involves distorted white cell proliferation and infiltration to specific parts of the body, causing local symptoms. However, it is inevitably fatal. Massive accumulation of small lymphocytes, which originate in lymph nodes and have a long life span of several years, characterizes chronic lymphatic leukemia with a strikingly low mitotic rate.

Symptoms

General symptoms of leukemia are weakness, facial pallor, anemia, lassitude, fever, malaise, anorexia, leukocytosis or lymphocytosis, and purpura. Enlargement of the spleen, liver, or lymph nodes may also occur.

Treatment
Acute Lymphatic Leukemia. It is believed that unless every leukemic cell in the body is destroyed, the residual cells will multiply and cause a relapse. Hence multiple agents are employed to destroy all leukemic cells in an attempt to cure the disease:
1. Vincristine, 0.05mg/kg (2mg/sq m) IV once a week for four weeks plus Prednisone, 1mg/kg (40mg/sq m) orally daily.
2. Methotrexate, 15mg/sq m orally twice a week.
3. Radiation to cerebrospinal axis, 2400 R.
4. Mercaptopurine, 2.5mg/kg daily orally, or methotrexate, 15mg/sq m twice a week orally, or cyclophosphamide, 200mg/sq m weekly orally.

Acute Myeloblastic Leukemia. The objective of therapy is prolonged remission since cure is not possible at the present. The drugs generally used are cytarabine, thioguanine, vincristine, and "COAP" (acronym for Cytoxan, Oncovin, Ara-C and Prednisone).

Chronic Myelocytic Leukemia.
1. General measures: the aim of therapy is palliation of symptoms and correction of anemia. Life-long treatment and periodic observation are necessary.
2. Irradiation: X-ray therapy.
3. Chemotherapy: Busulfan (Myleran), an alkylating agent, is used. 2mg are administered two to four times daily.

Chronic Lymphatic Leukemia
1. General measures: unless clinical manifestation appears or hematologic complication develops, generally no therapy is applied.
2. Irradiation: therapy is carried out as for myelocytic leukemia.
3. Chemotherapy: Chlorambucil is widely used, 0.1-0.2mg/kg daily. Cyclophosphamide, 50-100mg is taken orally one to three times daily. Initially, 40mg of corticosteroids are given daily until a response occurs. 10-20mg every two

days are needed for maintenance.

Chinese Herb Formula
Chia-wei-kuei-pi-tang-chia-tzu-ken　　加味歸脾湯加紫根
(Bupleurum, Ginseng, and Longan Combination plus Lithospermum)
This formula is indicated for the symptoms of bleeding, anemia, fatigue, lassitude, swollen spleen, and swollen liver. Lithospermum is added at the dosage rate of 10g daily because it always treats malignancies.

Purpura

Purpura is a group of disorders characterized by purplish or brownish-red skin discoloration. The malady is caused by hemorrhages in the skin, a condition which is easily visible. Skin petechiae, ecchymoses, and easy bruisability may be caused by thrombocytopenia, qualitative platelet disorders, or vascular defects.

Idiopathic thrombocytopenia purpura, a disease common in children, is a disorder of increased platelet destruction. In this case the platelet survival is only one to three days or even less compared to the normal eight to ten day life span. The cause of this destruction may be the presence of an anti-platelet factor, an antibody, in the plasma. However, the disorder may be post-infectious or due to isoimmunity following transfusions. At times it may develop in diseases with autoimmune manifestations, or result from using certain drugs (e.g. quinine, thiazide). The spleen, while not enlarged, sequesters the damaged platelets and manufactures some antibodies. At onset chronic thrombocytopenic purpura, a disease affecting all ages and especially common among females, is hard to distinguish from the acute form.

Disorders with qualitative platelet defects are another cause of purpura. The platelet counts may be normal, or slightly low in this case, but the platelets look abnormal on the blood smear. Depending on the defects they may be small (Wiskott-Aldrich syndrome), large (May-Hegglin amonaly) or fail to aggregate (Glanzmann's disease, preferably known as thrombasthenia, which is an autosomal recessive disorder in which the platelets appear isolated on the blood smear).

Purpura caused by vascular defects may be acquired (Henoch-Schonlein syndrome) or inherited (hereditary hemorrhagic telangiectasia). The acquired hemorrhagic disorder is characterized by general vasculitis involving multiple organ systems. The inherited vascular abnormality involves primarily the veins; vessels are dilated and their walls are thin.

Thrombotic thrombocytopenic purpura, a severe, acute illness with poor prognosis, is another form of purpura characterized by fragmented red blood cells, renal abnormalities and, at times, local manifestations, especially vascular lesions located at arteriocapillary junctions.

Von Willebrand's disease is a disorder resembling hemophilia in that it causes prolonged bleeding, particularly after oropharyngeal surgery or trauma. It is characterized by low values of Willebrand factor activity, factor VIII antigen, and factor VIII activity. The lack of Willebrand factor is responsible for poor adherence of platelets and prolonged bleeding.

Symptoms

Symptoms of acute idiopathic thrombocytopenic purpura include the sudden onset (at times) of petechiae (small purplish spots); nosebleeds; bleeding in the gums, vagina, or GI tract; and hematuria. Bleeding is prolonged and clot retraction is poor.

Symptoms of purpura resulting from disorders with qualitative platelet defects involve skin lesions after minor trauma, dependent petechiae, mucocutaneous bleeding, easy bruising, and prolonged bleeding.

Purpura resulting from vascular defects has the symptoms of abdominal pain, inversion of the intestine, gastrointestinal bleeding, hematuria (bloody urine), proteinuria (protein in the urine), inflammatory kidney disease, arthralgia (joint pain), red muscular lesions on the body, and epistaxis.

Treatment

General measures. Patients should avoid trauma, contact sports, elective surgery, tooth extraction, and all unnecessary medications.

Corticosteroids. Corticosteroids are warranted in patients

with moderately severe purpura of short duration, especially in gastrointestinal or genitourinary bleeding. Prednisolone (or equivalent) is usually required to control bleeding, 10-20mg four times daily. Dosage is continued until platelet count returns to normal.

Splenectomy. Splenectomy is indicated for patients with well-documented thrombocytopenic purpura of more than one year's duration or for relapsing purpura which does not respond to corticosteroids.

The above measures are warranted in general purpura. However, there is no cure for hereditary hemorrhagic telangiectasia (irondextran injection, 5-10ml IV once weekly may be applied to remedy serious bleeding). The bleeding in Von Willebrand's disease can be compensated by AHF (antihemophilic globulin) concentrates to correct the level of factor VIII. At times local pressure is applied to accessible bleeding sites, or topical hemostatic agents may be used.

Chinese Herb Formulas
1. **Chai-hu-kuei-chih-tang** 柴胡桂枝湯
   (Bupleurum and Cinnamon Combination)

According to *Chin kuei yao lueh*, this combination is indicated for cardiac and acute abdominal pain. Its effect was proven by a clinical case years ago. It also treats bleeding in the nose, mouth, or skin.

2. **Yueh-pi-chia-chu-tang** 越婢加朮湯
   (Atractylodes Combination)

This combination is given in the initial stage of the disease when the patient's physical strength has not yet been weakened; otherwise *Chai-hu-kuei-chih-tang* (Bupleurum and Cinnamon Combination) is to be taken instead.

3. **Hsiao-chien-chung-tang** 小建中湯
   (Minor Cinnamon and Paeonia Combination)
   Kuei-chi-chien-chung-tang 歸耆建中湯
   (Tang-kuei, Astragalus, and Paeonia Combination)

The combination *Hsiao-chien-chung-tang* is indicated for extremely tired and exhausted children who are suffering from lingering purpura. The habitual bleeding in purpura is also this formula's major target. *Kuei-chi-chien-chung-tang* is given to patients with more severe anemia and weakness than that of the former combination.

4. **Shu-ching-huo-hsieh-tang** 疏經活血湯
   (Clematis and Stephania Combination)
   Slight but lingering rheumatic purpura, especially in women, is an indication of this combination.

5. **Chiung-kuei-chiao-ai-tang** 芎歸膠艾湯
   (Tang-kuei and Gelatin Combination)
   Wen-ching-yin 溫清飲
   (Tang-kuei and Gardenia Combination)
   These formulas aim at stopping bleeding but usually are not very effective for purpura.

6. **Kuei-chih-chia-fu-tzu-tang** 桂枝加附子湯
   (Cinnamon, Jujube, and Aconite Combination)
   This formula is indicated for simple purpura with slight but prolonged bleeding, limb chills, and fatigue.

7. **Chia-wei-kuei-pi-tang** 加味歸脾湯
   (Bupleurum, Ginseng, and Longan Combination)
   This combination is given to persons who experience abrupt fits, incessant bleeding, and a swollen spleen.

Basedow's Disease (Graves' Disease)

Thyrotoxicosis is one of the most common endocrine disorders. Its highest incidence is in women between the ages of twenty and forty. When associated with ocular signs or ocular disturbances and a diffuse goiter, it is called Graves' disease. This term, however, is commonly used to mean all forms of hyperthyroidism. Instead of a diffuse goiter, there may be a nodular toxic goiter, or all the metabolic features of thyrotoxicosis may occasionally be present without visible or palpable thyroid enlargement. The latter form is quite common in the elderly, who may even lack some of the hypermetabolic signs (apathetic Graves' disease) but may have a refractory cardiac illness. Lastly, a poorly understood syndrome of marked eye ulcerations, often without hypermetabolism, may precede, accompany, or follow treatment of thyrotoxicosis, and has been termed hyperexophthalmic Graves' disease, exophthalmic ophthalmoplegia, and malignant (progressive) exophthalmos (infiltrative ophthalmopathy). A rare cause of clinical hyperthyroidism is struma ovarii (pathological tissue in the ovary) or hydatidiform mole (placenta transformed into cysts), although asymptomatic elevation of T_4 may be seen in chorionic tumors, presumably due to ectopic production of TSH (thyroid stimulating hormone).

Symptoms

Restlessness, nervousness, irritability, easy fatigability, especially toward the latter part of the day, and unexplained weight loss in spite of ravenous appetite are often the early features. There is usually excessive sweating and heat intolerance, quick movements with incoordination varying from fine tremulousness to gross tremor. Less commonly, the patient's primary complaint is difficulty in focusing his eyes; pressure from the goiter; diarrhea; or rapid, irregular heart action.

The patient is quick in all motions, including speech. The skin is warm and moist and the hands tremble. A diffuse or nodular goiter may be visible or heard by auscultation with thrill or bruit. The eyes appear bright, may stare, and have at times periorbital edema. Commonly there is lid lag, lack of accommodation, protruding eyeballs, and even double vision. The hair and skin are thin and silky. At times there is increased pigmentation of the skin, but white spots may also occur. Spider angiomas (tumors) and gynecomastia (excessive tissue of the mammary in males) are common. Cardiovascular manifestations vary from rapid heartbeat, especially during sleep, to paroxysmal atrial fibrillation and congestive failure of the "high-output" type. At times a harsh pulmonary systolic murmur is heard (Means' murmur). Disease of the lymph nodes and an enlarged spleen may be present. Wasting of muscle and bone are common features, especially in long-standing thyrotoxicosis. Occasionally one finds nausea, vomiting, and even fever and jaundice in which case the prognosis is poor. Mental changes are common, varying from mild exhiliration to delirium and exhaustion progressing to severe depression.

Associated with severe or malignant exophthalmos (protruding eyeballs) is, at times, a localized, bilateral, hard, nonpitting, symmetric swelling ("pretibial myxedema") over the shins and dorsum of the feet (infiltrative dermopathy). At times there is a thickening and swelling of the fingers (acropachy). It often subsides spontaneously.

X-ray findings. Barium tests may demonstrate low or intrathoracic goiter. Skeletal changes include diffuse demineralization, or at times resorptive changes (osteitis). Hypertrophic osteoarthropathy with proliferation of periosteal bone may be present, especially in the hands (acropachy).

ECG findings. ECG may show rapid heartbeat, atrial fibrillation, and P and T wave changes.

Treatment

Treatment is aimed at halting excessive secretion of the thyroid hormone. Several methods are available; the method of choice is still being debated and varies with different patients. The most widely accepted method in the past has been subtotal removal after adequate preparation. There is a greater tendency toward trying long term medical treatment with antithyroid drugs to achieve remission of the disease and to use radioactive iodine therapy rather than surgery except for large multinodular glands.

Chinese Herb Formulas
1. Chih-kan-tsao-tang 炙甘草湯
   (Baked Licorice Combination)
Although the effectiveness of this formula for Basedow's disease is not definite in the male, it is effective in most females. It will normalize and stabilize the pulse, dissolve the goiter, restore the eyes, and alleviate all symptoms. It must be taken continuously for one to three years. The symptoms treated are knotty and alternate pulse and cardiac hyperfunction. However, it may also be used by patients without knotty and alternate pulses.

2. Pan-hsia-hou-pu-tang-ho-kuei-chih-kan-tsao-lung-ku-mu-li-tang 半夏厚朴湯合桂枝甘草龍骨牡蠣湯
   (Pinellia and Magnolia Combination plus Cinnamon, Licorice, and Dragon Bone Combination)
Some patients may have GI disturbances after taking rehmannia-

containing preparations such as *Chih-kan-tsao-tang,* and cannot continue such a formula. If the additional symptoms of nervousness with cardiac hyperfunction and quick pulse are present, then this formula may be used.

3. **Chai-hu-chia-lung-ku-mu-li-tang** 柴胡加龍骨牡蠣湯
   (Bupleurum and Dragon Bone Combination)

This formula is indicated during the initial stage of the disease for people with some stamina, thoraco-costal distress, and abdominal distention and, in addition, the symptoms of excitability, fatigability, palpitations, and insomnia.

4. **Chia-wei-hsiao-yao-san** 加味逍遙散
   (Bupleurum and Paeonia Formula)

After the onset of Basedow's disease, menses will become irregular and climacteric neurosis will appear. This formula is suitable for such women with the symptoms of vertigo, stiff shoulders, palpitation, tinnitus, flushing up, chilled feet, and heavy headedness.

5. **Kan-tsao-hsieh-hsin-tang** 甘草瀉心湯
   (Pinellia and Licorice Combination)
   Sheng-ling-pai-chu-san 參苓白朮散
   (Ginseng and Atractylodes Formula)

This formula is used for Basedow's disease patients with diarrhea.

Banti's Disease

This disease, also called Banti-Senator disease, has a precedent symptom of an enlarged spleen as described by Banti in 1899. The disease takes a chronic proceeding. In the early stage the patient may have the chief symptom of anemia followed by a hemorrhagic constitution, general poor health, and finally death. Later, Senator pointed out that this disease may be accompanied by cirrhosis of the liver in some cases. Thus it has become controversial among pathologists whether this disease is to be regarded as an independent disease or just a syndrome. From the standpoint of hypersplenism, the suppression of the maturation of bone marrow cells (e.g. anemia or leukopenia) is not a specific phenomenon of this disease and the question of whether the enlarged spleen is a causative factor of hepatic disorder remains unanswered. Calling it splenic intoxication, Tomoda found that some factor existed in the serum of this disease which would suppress the bone marrow and cause hepatic disturbance. Meanwhile, Kono had determined the structure of hepatic tissue from the cirrhotic liver and the enlarged spleen due to arterial congestion. These findings are the most positive evidences of this disease.

Treatment
Treatment for this disease is a splenectomy or iron supplement therapy.

Chinese Herb Formulas
1. Kuei-pi-tang   歸脾湯
   (Ginseng and Longan Combination)
This formula will relieve the serious symptoms and cure mild cases of the disease.

2. Kuei-chih-chu-shao-yao-chia-ma-huang-hsi-hsin-fu-tzu-tang
   桂枝去芍藥加麻黃細辛附子湯
   (Cinnamon, Ma-huang, Aconite, and Asarum Combiantion)
A female patient suffering from Banti's disease whose abdomen was swollen with ascites (abdominal fluid) and who could not go to the toilet by herself was cured by this formula. Her ascites was resolved and she could move about freely. The treatment was based on a formula from *Chin kuei yao lueh*, which reads: "For patients with a *ch'i* (vapor) ailment and a hardness beneath the heart, the hardness being as large as a pan with the edge of it feeling like a turning cup, which has been caused by water stagnation, *Kuei-chih-chu-shao-yao-chia-ma-huang-hsi-hsin-fu-tzu-tang* is indicated."

DISEASES OF THE JOINTS AND NERVOUS SYSTEM

Arthrosis Deformans of the Knee

Among the various kinds of arthritis deformans, this type is the most frequently found, especially in women over fifty. In mild cases the patient experiences dull pain and swelling during exercise and has difficulty sitting down. In severe cases water is retained within the joint; there is no inflammation present. Deformation is due to the simultaneous occurrence of degradative and proliferative changes of the joint. It happens more often to the large joints of the knee, femur, and elbow and to persons who are physically active or are frequently exposed to the elements because of their jobs. There is no special cause, the common cause being essentially due to the individual's physique. The joint becomes deformed as a result of degeneration. The disease may also be congenital or acquired through external injuries, diseases, and metabolic abnormalities.

Symptoms

This disease takes a latent proceeding. Initially the joint aches when exercising or lifting heavy weights. Gradually the range of movement and flexibility of the joint lessens. Mild contraction and mild swelling of the synovial bursa occur. However, there is no change in the skin or the subdermal tissue at this stage. As the disease advances, conspicuous friction and cracking sounds can be heard. Generally no somatic fever is found. X-ray reveals a gradual sharpening of the edge of the joint, the formation of bone pricks, a narrowing of joint clefts, and a darkening of the subcartilage layer of the joint.

Treatment
1. Pharmaceutical therapy: salicylates, sex hormones.
2. Physical therapy: massage, X-ray irradiation, steam baths, very short heat waves, warm baths.
3. Traction.
4. Surgery: plastic surgery.

Chinese Herb Formulas
1. Fang-chi-huang-chi-tang 防己黃耆湯
    (*Stephania and Astragalus Combination*)

After intake of this formula, swelling and pain are eliminated in most cases. Occasionally *ma-huang* must be added to the formula. Generally it is taken for one month.

2. Yueh-pi-chia-chu-tang 越婢加朮湯
    (*Atractylodes Combination*)

Most cases of this disease may be cured by *Fang-chi-huang-chi-tang* or *Fang-chi-huang-chi-tang* plus *ma-huang*. However, occasionally both formulas fail to cure. This formula may then be used, and, depending on the condition, *Fang-chi-huang-chi-tang* may be used jointly.

3. Kuei-chih-fu-ling-wan-liao-chia-i-yi-jen
    桂枝茯苓丸料加薏苡仁
    (*Cinnamon and Hoelen Formula with Coix*)

This formula once cured an old woman with a mildly deformed knee which had been aggravated by a contusion sustained in falling down. The knee was painful and swollen.

Spondylosis Detormans

This disease is also called spondylitis deformans. In England and the United States, it is known as osteoarthritis, even though there is no inflammation. It is a wasting disease with the pathological change being essentially of a retrogressive, degenerative nature. Deformation happens on the edge of the vertebra, especially the superior-anterior and inferior edge, where the form changes from strongly labial and spike form to the bridge form, and involves the intervertebral joint and the spinous process. The occurrence of this disease is related to the individual physique and to some extent age. (It worsens with age.) In a broad sense injury to the vertebra or the intervertebral disc which then causes abnormal curving of the spine and disturbs the static balance may hasten the deformation and cause the neck-wrist syndrome and paralysis of the spine. The complaint common to this disease is aching on awakening in the morning, which lessens after exercise, and aching and fatigue again in the evening after the day's activity. The mechanism is still unknown.

Treatment

A corset can be worn to relieve the load on the spine. Other ways to alleviate discomfort are a warm bath, massage, or a corticoid steroid hormone injected intervertebrally. Tranquility and analgesics are helpful. However, rigid fixation with a corset or brace may promote muscle spasm and the reappearance of complaints.

Chinese Herb Formulas

1. Pa-wei-wan   八味丸
   (*Rehmannia Eight Formula*)

Although total cure of the deformed part is difficult, this formula may alleviate the condition, hence it is worth trying.

2. Huang-chi-chien-chung-tang   黃耆建中湯
   (*Astragalus Combination*)

A woman having very severe pain in the back and great difficulty in carrying on the activities of daily living was cured by this formula.

Neuralgia

Neuralgia is an acute pain radiating along the course of a

nerve and its branches. It may occur either persistently or paroxysmally with occasional exacerbations. This disease is due to faulty nerve nutrition or it is a complication of other diseases. Sometimes the cause is unknown. At times chills and fatigue induce the onset of this disease.

Among various kinds of neuralgia encountered in daily life are trigeminal neuralgia, sciatic neuralgia, intercostal neuralgia, and brachial neuralgia. The trigeminal nerve of the face has three branches. Depending upon which branch is affected, the site of neuralgia will differ. The pain may occur anywhere from the left or right lower eyelid down the cheeks and beneath the nose or even in the upper jaw causing a toothache, which sometimes results in mistaken tooth extraction as treatment. Sciatic neuralgia affects the thigh down to the lower extremities; intercostal neuralgia, the chest; and brachial neuralgia, the upper arm. Although all of these belong to the same disease, neuralgia, Chinese herbal treatment uses different formulas for the different conditions.

Chinese Herb Formulas
1. Ko-ken-tang　　　　　　　　　　　　　　葛根湯
(Pueraria Combination)
This formula is used at the onset of trigeminal neuralgia as a means of treating a forceful pulse in a patient with good muscle tone. It is also effective against brachial neuralgia. Occasionally 4.0g of atractylodes and 1.0g of aconite must be added to the formula.

2. Wu-ling-san　　　　　　　　　　　　　　五苓散
(Hoelen Five Herb Formula)
Essentialy this formula is indicated for thirst and oliguria (insufficient urination). If these symptoms are not prominent in trigeminal neuralgia, this formula will have a great effect. It is also worth trying when other formulas are ineffective.

3. Kuei-chih-chia-ling-chu-fu-tang　　　桂枝加苓朮附湯
(Cinnamon and Atractylodes Combination)
This formula is indicated for trigeminalgic patients who have a forceless abdomen and pulse and exhausted stamina, a condition implying a cold conformation.

4. **Ching-shang-chuan-tung-tang** 清上蠲痛湯
   (Ophiopogon and Asarum Combination)

This is for headaches of all kinds and so is good for stubborn trigeminalgia.

5. **Shao-kan-huang-hsin-fu-tang** 芍甘黃辛附湯
   (Licorice, Asarum, and Rhubarb Combination)

This is used for sciatica when the patient has chills in one of his legs coupled with dragging, convulsive pain and a tendency toward constipation.

6. **Tang-kuei-szu-ni-chia-wu-chu-yu-sheng-chiang-tang** 當歸四逆加吳茱萸生薑湯
   (Tang-kuei, Evodia, and Ginger Combination)

This formula is prescribed for the kind of sciatica which ancient people called "hernia" ache, a condition in which the patient has a cold conformation and pain from the waist down to the lower extremities. This combination is frequently used for intervertebral disc hernia or following abdominal operations. It is especially for women with gynecological problems who have sciatica.

7. **Shu-ching-huo-hsieh-tang** 疏經活血湯
   (Clematis and Stephania Combination)

This formula is also for sciatica. It is found in *Wan ping huei chuen* where it says: " . . . treats the mobile pain that moves about like a spike all over the body. The aching is especially severe in the left leg, because the left side belongs to the domain of blood. Ν patients suffer from this disease as the result of injury caused by excessive wine and carnal pleasure or from contraction of "wind," "cold moistness," and "heat" that is encapsulated by the cold, resulting in pain and injury to the muscles. Such problems can be suitably treated by formulas that activate the blood and remove the moistness. The above mentioned condition is not that of *pai hu li chieh feng* (白虎歷節風 rheumatic arthritis)." Sciatica is not necessarily restricted to the left leg; this formula is also effective for sciatica of the right leg.

8. **Kuei-chih-fu-ling-wan** 桂枝茯苓丸
   (Cinnamon and Hoelen Formula)
   Tao-ho-cheng-chi-tang 桃核承氣湯

(*Persica and Rhubarb Combination*)
These compounds are used for neuralgia caused by external wounds, especially contusions. They are also suitable for sciatica brought on by menoxenia or the relapse of gynecological diseases. Attention must be paid to the symptom of blood stagnancy in the abdomen.

9. Pa-wei-wan   八味丸
   (*Rehmannia Eight Formula*)
This formula is suitable for diabetic patients having sciatica, or old men having a loss of strength from the waist down, vigorlessness, intolerable pain, and traces of numbness.

10. Ching-shih-hua-tan-tang   清濕化痰湯
    (*Pinellia and Arisaema Combination*)
This herbal combination is indicated for intercostal neuralgia resulting from "water toxin." The pain is not restricted to the chest only, but moves. It is widely used by people with lax stomachs or gastroptosis. A chilly sensation in the back is one of the main indications of this formula but not the necessary one.

11. Jen-sheng-tang   人參湯
    (*Ginseng and Ginger Combination*)
Among the abdominal symptoms of *Jen-sheng-tang*, one is a soft and forceless abdomen, and another is an abdomen as hard as plywood. If the patient has the latter condition and has intercostal neuralgia then *Jen-sheng-tang* is indicated. Patients needing this formula have weak G I tracts, cold fingertips, and weak pulses. The pain is not necessarily confined to the chest but may occur in the arms and legs and lumbar region.

12. Chai-hu-shu-kan-san   柴胡疏肝散
    (*Bupleurum and Gardenia Formula*)
This formula is indicated for intercostal neuralgia in patients with inflammation complicated by swelling and ulcers. The formula is similar to *Szu-ni-san*, hence it has the same abdominal conformation.

13. Wu-chi-san   五積散
    (*Tang-kuei and Magnolia Formula*)

This formula is used for patients with mild, chronic pain in the legs, waist, and back. The symptoms treated are a cold, submerged and weak pulse and abdominal weakness.

14. Fang-feng-tung-sheng-san   防風通聖散
    (Siler and Platycodon Formula)

This formula is used for chronic brachial neuralgia in patients having full stamina, a distended abdomen, and constipation.

15. Ma-huang-fu-tzu-hsi-hsin-tang   麻黄附子細辛湯
    (Ma-huang, Aconite, and Asarum Combination)

This is a formula for headaches caused by chills. It is used for the combined condition of lesser yin disease and surface symptoms in which the patient has trigeminal neuralgia and posterior headache. The patient's head feels cold a condition which may be relieved by warm cloths. In most cases the patient has a submerged and thin pulse and a poor complexion.

Parkinsonism (Paralysis Agitans)

Parkinson's syndrome is a group of neurological disorders characterized by involuntary tremors, hypokinesia (decreased muscular movement), and rigidity; the person's mental powers are usually not affected. Usually it occurs in later life and its etiology is still undetermined; however, a juvenile form has been described. The disease occurs as a complication of epidemic encephalitis and has been known to occur in vascular disorders, neurosyphilis, and following head trauma. Reversible reactions including paralysis agitans with gait and postural abnormalities, rigidity, tremors, salivation and similar symptoms, may follow the use of tranquilizers such as the phenothiazines. However, most cases are attributed to degeneration of the cells and tracts of the striate bodies, globus pallidus, and substantia nigra.

Symptoms

Paralysis agitans is a disease characterized by a blank, immobilized face, and a characteristic tremor originating in rigidity of the waist or feet which alters into slight tremor and spreads throughout the muscles of the whole body. Consequently the arms and legs begin to feel stiff and heavy. A stopping posture is common with arms at the sides, elbows slightly flexed, and fingers abducted. "Pill-rolling" tremor is minimal at rest but emotional tension and fatigue are apt to aggravate the tremors. Turning is difficult and some patients, usually slow in body movement, may break into a festinating gait. Patients may also have difficulty getting out of a chair, so that several efforts or attempts to rise have to be made. The voice tends to become weak, low in volume and monotonous, and oculogyric crises may occur.

Treatment

Drugs. Treatment is mainly symptomatic and multiple drugs are used in combination to obtain the optimal palliative result. Trihexyphenidyl and diphenhydramine three times daily may be used initially. Many antiparkinsonism drugs are available.

Newer drugs. Levodopa (Dopar, Larodopa) is effective against the akinesia and rigidity of parkinsonism. Capsules (250mg) are given three to four times daily (maximum daily dose 4-8g). Optimal clinical response may be obtained by a combination of carbidopa with minimum levodopa dosage. Amantadine hydrochloride (symmetrel) in daily dosages of 200mg (100mg twice daily) is effective. Both of the above drugs induce several side effects.

Surgical measures. In carefully selected patients, surgical destruction of portions of the globus pallidus or the ventrolateral nucleus of the thalamus has proved highly beneficial.

General measures. Physical therapy should include massage, stretching of muscles, and active exercise when possible. Reassurance and psychological support are necessary.

Chinese Herb Formulas
1. Hsiao-cheng-chi-tang-ho-shao-yao-kan-tsao-tang
小承氣湯合芍藥甘草湯
(Minor Rhubarb Combination with Paeonia and Licorice Combination)
Taken three to four times with an ordinary dose of magnolia bark, this formula will stop tremors and relax muscle stiffness. The quantity of rhubarb is adjusted according to the condition of bowel movement.

2. I-kan-san-ho-shao-yao-kan-tsao-tang-chia-hou-pu
抑肝散合芍藥甘草湯加厚朴
(Bupleurum Formula with Paeonia and Licorice Combination plus Magnolia)
This combination is for persons with irritability, debilitating anxiety, and insomnia. Ozawa Kats reported that one person had been cured with the single herb magnolia.

Behcet's Syndrome

The cause of this disease has not as yet been determined. Some doctors believe it is the result of viral infection, an allergic reaction caused by bacteria, or a collagen disease. The disease has the chief symptoms of (1) accumulation of pus in the eyes (uveitis) and inflammation of the iris (iritis); (2) painful mouth ulcers (aphthous stomatitis); and (3) ulcers on the external genitalia and skin rashes. These symptoms occur repeatedly and take a chronic proceeding. Similar symptoms also occur, such as Stevens-Johnson syndrome with ulcers forming on the inside of the lips and muco-cutaneous-ocular syndrome. Generally the prognosis is good, but in most cases of ocular involvement the prognosis is poor.

The symptoms are more severe in men and the ratio of sufferers among men and women is 2:1. The disease rarely occurs in children and middle-aged people. It occurs most frequently in patients around age twenty. If the disease manifests all the symptoms mentioned above, it is a complete type. Manifestation of only a few symptoms is considered to be an incomplete type. Visceral changes are not seen. Sometimes symptoms appear in major joints, the alimentary tract (especially the intestines), the nervous system, and the circulatory system but more often the symptoms are generalized. About 20% of the cases are of a neurotic origin with neuro-Behcet's syndrome as the chief manifestation. It is to be noted that a very large proportion of patients with neurosis have a high rate of marked spinal fluid abnormality: elevated spinal fluid pressure, cell proliferation, increased globulin, etc. In addition, there are abnormalities in serum globulin, serum protein, increases in mucoprotein, and an elevated ESR (erythrocyte sedimentation rate).

Treatment

Antihistaminics, antibiotics and steroidal hormones are employed but a definite result is hard to secure.

Chinese Herb Formula
　　Wen-ching-yin　　　　　　　　　　　　　　溫清飲
　　(Tang-kuei and Gardenia Combination)

This formula is indicated for most cases of this disease. After lengthy intake the disease can be cured completely although the symptoms may fluctuate during therapy. In the case of uveitis, this formula can stop the progression of the suppuration. If the formula is used at an early stage, the disease can be cured without any residual visual problems.

Migraine

Migraine is characterized by paroxysmal attacks of headache often preceded by psychological or visual disturbances and sometimes followed by drowsiness. It affects about 8% of the population, is more frequent among women than men, and occurs more commonly among persons with a background of inflexibility and shyness in childhood and with perfectionistic, rigid, resentful and ambitious character traits in adult life. Commonly a history of migraine runs in families.

Migraine headache is believed to result from vascular changes. An initial episode of cerebral meningeal and extra-cranial arterial vasoconstriction is believed to occur (accounting for the visual and other prodromal phenomena), followed by dilation and distention of cranial vessels, especially of the external carotid artery. Increased amplitude of pulsation is said to cause the throbbing nature of the headache. Rigid, pipe-like vessels result from persistent dilation, and the headache becomes steady. A phase of painful muscle contraction is believed to follow.

Migraine often begins in childhood; about half of the migraine patients report their initial attack occurred before the age of fifteen. Characteristically the headache is accompanied by gastrointestinal or visual symptoms (nausea, vomiting, impaired vision, sensitivity to light (photophobia), blindness in one-half of the visual field (hemianopsia), or blurred vision).

Treatment

Treatment of Acute Attack
Ergotamine tartrate 0.25-0.5mg IM is administered as early in the attack as possible. It is never repeated more often than once weekly.

Dihydroergotamine 1.0mg IM or IV taken every hour if necessary.

Ergotamin with caffeine or atropine is taken orally in tablet form or rectally in suppositories, which is sometimes more effective and requires a smaller total dose.

Pressure on the external carotid artery or one of its branches relieves the pain.

Oxygen, 100%, by nasal mask may relieve acute attacks.

General Measures. Until the drug begins to relieve the headache, have the patient rest in a chair. After the headache has subsided he should rest in bed for at least two hours in a quiet, darkened room without food or drink. This will promote relaxation and is necessary to prevent another attack from occurring immediately.

Aborting an Attack. When the patient feels a migraine coming on he should relax and rest in bed in a quiet, darkened room. The following drugs may help: pentobarbital, 0.1g orally; ergotamine tartrate, 3.0-4.0mg sublingually; or even aspirin, with or without codeine. An ergotamine inhaler may also be effective.

Chinese Herb Formulas
1. Wu-chu-yu-tang 吳茱萸湯
(Evodia Combination)

This formula is suitable for most recurring migraines. At onset of the attack, the unilateral contraction of the neck muscle causes stiffness from the shoulders to the neck; abdominal diagnosis exhibits distention beneath the heart. In addition, the patient is aware of gastric distention and fullness. This symptom is called epigastric adverse distention and is different from thoraco-costal distress. As the attack progresses, the limbs become cold and the pulse, submerged and slow. The patient is in a distressed, agitated, restless condition, and frequently rises up and lies down. In severe cases, the patient may vomit. For this condition *Wu-chu-yu-tang* can be used. It not only suppresses the onset but also prevents paroxysms from recurring if lengthy administration is carried out.

2. **Wu-ling-san** 五苓散
   (Hoelen Five Herb Formula)

The difference in the application of this formula from the preceding one is that *Wu-ling-san* is used for patients with thirst and reduced urine. Theoretically, *Wu-chu-yu-tang* is to be used for patients with a yin conformation and *Wu-ling-san* for those with a yang conformation. The former have a submerged and slow pulse and the latter a buoyant and quick pulse. However, there are exceptions; hence if diagnosis indicated *Wu-chu-yu-tang* but use of it fails to take effect, then *Wu-ling-san* may be used in its place.

3. **Tao-ho-cheng-chi-tang** 桃核承氣湯
   (Persica and Rhubarb Combination)

This formula is for women with a stalwart physique, good muscle tone, a tendency to constipation, and abdominal cramping. Frequently the migraine results from abnormal menstruation (menoxenia) and scanty flow (oligomenses).

4. **Chia-wei-hsiao-yao-san** 加味逍遙散
   (Bupleurum and Paeonia Formula)

This formula is suitable for women with menoxenia and stiffness in the shoulders who have a weaker physique than that of *Tao-ho-cheng-chi-tang* and a cold and nervous temperament. (These symptoms are what people commonly call climacteric headache and are not a real migraine.)

Insomnia

In Chinese herb medicine there is no drug equivalent to the so-called hypnotics of modern Western medicine. Chinese herbal treatment for insomnia is based on an individual's conformation. If the patient responds well to the formula, i.e. if the prescribed drug is appropriate for the patient's condition, the patient will sleep well, free from the worry of any side effects or habituation.

Factors contributing to insomnia include: (1) situational

problems such as transient stress, job pressures, and marital discord; (2) medical disorders which inevitably include pain and physical discomfort; (3) drug-related episodes, including withdrawal from alcohol or sedatives; and (4) psychological conditions, particularly major mental illnesses such as schizophrenia and primary affective disorders. Schizophrenics vary markedly in the degree of sleep disturbance they experience. In acute episodes the disruption is severe, even to the point of total insomnia. The chronic schizophrenic or the patient in remission often does not have any complaints, and his EEG pattern is not remarkably abnormal.

Treatment

Antipsychotic drugs have minimal effect on EEG sleep tracing but are clinically helpful. Sedating phenothiazines such as chlorpromazine, given at bedtime, obviate the need for sedatives in the schizophrenic with sleep problems. Antidepressants decrease REM sleep and have varying effects on slow wave sleep. Use of the more sedating tricyclic antidepressants such as amitriptyline, given at bedtime in full dosage, frequently eliminates the need to use a sedative. Barbituates and nonbarbituate sedative-hypnotics, such as glutethimide, are initially effective and reduce REM sleep only slightly, but tolerance develops quickly and there is a return to baseline levels by the end of one week. Chronic use of multiple doses of these drugs produces a more marked decrease of both REM and slow wave sleep, with rebound increase of both types of sleep when the drug is withdrawn. For transient sleep difficulties, a sedative such as flurazepam is relatively safe, effective, and not prone to abuse or tolerance.

All of the commonly abused drugs affect sleep. Narcotics substantially reduce REM sleep, but tolerance and a return to normal baseline levels develop in several days. Stimulants effect a moderate reduction in REM sleep and the same quick tolerance. Alcohol and meprobamate are similar to barbituates in their effect on sleep. While the proper use of medication may provide symptomatic relief for insomnia over the short term, the clinician must be attuned to the possibility of underlying problems, particularly severe depression. This is of major importance in early and effective treatment since the majority of suicide victims see their physician in the month prior to the suicide and tend to use the drugs prescribed, particularly sedatives, to commit the act.

Chinese Herb Formulas
1. Huang-lien-chieh-tu-tang　　　　　　　黃連解毒湯
    (Scute and Coptis Combination)
    San-huang-hsieh-hsin-tang　　　　　　三黃瀉心湯
    (Coptis and Rhubarb Combination)

These formulas are for insomnia in people who have a good complexion, "up-flaming fire" tendency, an agitated and uneasy mood, and ready excitability. They are also used for the insomnia caused by hypertension and climacteric disturbances. If constipation occurs, then use *San-huang-hsieh-hsin-tang* or *Huang-lien-chieh-tu-tang* plus rhubarb.

2. Wen-tan-tang　　　　　　　　　　　　溫膽湯
    (Bamboo and Citrus Combination)

This formula is used for patients who, after a dangerous disease or hard work, have become very nervous and oversensitive to trivial things or have melancholic moods. Occasionally 1.0g of coptis and 5.0g of sour zizyphus kernel must be added.

3. Kan-tsao-hsieh-hsin-tang　　　　　　　甘草瀉心湯
    (Pinellia and Licorice Combination)

This formula is indicated for hardness and pain beneath the heart, gas, and diarrhea, as well as this disease which is noted in *Chin kuei yao lueh*: "The devil-charmed disease has symptoms similar to those of *shang han* (cold and feverish diseases); patients suffering from such disease will become wordless and somnolent, have restless eyes, and an uneasy way of living. For such disease *Kan-tsao-hsieh-hsin-tang* is indicated." According to this instruction, this formula may be used for insomnia.

4. Chia-wei-kuei-pi-tang　　　　　　　　加味歸脾湯
    (Ginseng, Longan, and Bupleurum Combination)

This formula is suitable for anemic patients with amnesia, nervousness, and insomnia. The use of this formula is not limited only to the aged. It can also be used by patients having a weak stomach and intestines, poor complexion, and a forceless pulse and abdomen. The combination treats sullen and melancholic moods and the resultant insomnia.

5. Chu-ju-wen-tan-tang 竹茹溫膽湯
   (Bamboo and Ginseng Combination)

This formula is suitable for patients having copious sputum and much coughing. For example, pneumonia patients have much sputum and can't sleep easily after the fever has subsided.

6. Suan-tsao-jen-tang 酸棗仁湯
   (Zizyphus Combination)

It is recorded in *Chin kuei yao lueh:* "For wasting phthisis (tuberculosis) and "weakness vexation" leading to insomnia, *Suan-tsao-jen-tang* is indicated." Thus this formula is suitable for insomnia caused by mental and physical fatigue. It is also suitable for chronic and geriatric patients who cannot sleep at night.

7. Ching-hsin-lien-tzu-yin 清心蓮子飲
   (Lotus Seed Combination)
   Chu-ling-tang 豬苓湯
   (Polyporus Combination)

These formulas are suitable for persons with a weak stomach and intestines, night emission, spermatorrhea (involuntary discharge of sperm), urethral discomfort or urinary stuttering, and inability to fall asleep.

8. San-wu-huang-chin-tang 三物黃芩湯
   (Scute Three Herb Combination)

This formula takes the vexatious fever in the limbs as the target of treatment and is quite effective for persons with feverish arms and legs who cannot sleep at night. *Lueh chu fang kuang yi* states: "It treats patients having fever and discomfort in the palms and soles each summer; the symptom gets more violent at night, causing insomnia."

9. Chai-hu-chia-lung-ku-mu-li-tang 柴胡加龍骨牡蠣湯
   (Bupleurum and Dragon Bone Combination)

Some persons may look strong and obese, but they cannot go to sleep because of nervous hypersensitivity. If the patient also has epigastric distention, thoraco-costal distress, palpitation of the navel and a tendency toward constipation, he can be treated with this formula.

258

10. **Kuei-chih-chia-shao-yao-ta-huang-tang**　桂枝加芍藥大黃湯
    (Cinnamon, Paeonia, and Rhubarb Combination)
This formula is used for persons with abdominal distention and insomnia.

11. **Chu-sha-an-shen-wan**　　　　　　　硃砂安神丸
    (Cinnabar Formula)
This formula is to be taken in combination with decocted preparations for the treatment of insomnia.

Vertigo

The terms "vertigo" and "dizziness" are synonymously used to denote the subjective sensation of rotatory movement, either of the individual (subjective vertigo) or of his environment (objective vertigo), and imply an inability to orient the body in relation to surrounding objects. Vertigo is mainly found in diseases involving the labyrinths (the vestibular portion of the eighth cranial nerve) and their nuclei or connections. True vertigo is usually manifested by nystagmus (oscillatory movement of the eyes), falling to one side, and abnormal reaction to tests of vestibular function. Among the more common causes are Meniere's syndrome; acute labyrinthitis; organic brain damage involving the vestibular nerve, its end organs or connections, or the cerebellum; and drug and chemical toxicity.

Symptoms

A "spinning" sensation of surrounding objects or of the patient himself, which appears to throw the patient off balance, are the principal symptoms. Brief loss of consciousness may happen occasionally.

Treatment

Treatment is based upon accurate diagnosis of the underlying disorder.

Chinese Herb Formulas
1. **Ling-kuei-chu-kan-tang**　　　　　　　苓桂朮甘湯
   (Hoelen and Atractylodes Combination)

This formula is suitable for patients with a sensation of dizziness usually accompanied by water stagnation and distention below the heart, oliguria, and also palpitation. A common symptom of dizziness in the head, the so-called static vertigo, is the main indication for this formula.

2. **Pan-hsia-hou-pu-tang** 半夏厚朴湯
   (Pinellia and Magnolia Combination)

For the dizziness experienced by restless, neurotic patients who also have paroxysmal cardiac palpitation and a sensation of something blocking the throat, this formula is indicated.

3. **Pan-hsia-pai-chu-tien-ma-tang** 半夏白朮天麻湯
   (Pinellia and Gastrodia Combination)

This combination is for cases of vertigo with gastroptosis and stomach laxness, usually with headache. In this instance, the insecure sensation appears less marked than that of *Pan-hsia-hou-pu-tang,* and the abdominal conformation is also weaker.

4. **Chen-wu-tang** 眞武湯
   (Vitality Combination)

This combination is indicated for hypotensive vertigo in patients having a tendency to tire easily; diarrhea; and a chill conformation with a submerged, small and weak or a submerged and slow pulse.

5. **Tang-kuei-shao-yao-san** 當歸芍藥散
   (Tang-kuei and Paeonia Formula)

Vertigo of pregnancy or postpartal vertigo, and that caused by nephritis, are the indications of this formula. The patient usually has a sensation of heavy-headedness and feels dizzy. Most chill-conformational patients have a poor complexion.

6. **Chia-wei-hsiao-yao-san** 加味逍遙散
   (Bupleurum and Paeonia Formula)
   Nu-shen-san 女神散
   (Tang-kuei and Cyperus Formula)

These formulas are indicated for climacteric neuroses and menopausal disturbances.

7. **Tse-hsieh-tang** 澤瀉湯
   (Alisma Combination)

This formula is indicated for abruptly aroused vertigo, and for those who feel dizzy even when they lie in bed. It is composed of two herbs only, namely, alisma and atractylodes. As a rule, most simple formulas which contain only a few herbs are suitable for abruptly occurring and violent-symptom diseases. The ancient people named them "a direct approach measure."

8. **Hsieh-hsin-tang** 瀉心湯
   (Coptis and Rhubarb Combination)
   Huang-lien-chieh-tu-tang 黃連解毒湯
   (Coptis and Scute Combination)

These herbs are used for vertigo caused by the "flushing up" congestion of "fire-*ch'i*" on the occasions of cerebral hemorrhage; hypertension; and menopausal disturbances where the patient has a red facial complexion, anxiety, uneasiness, and sometimes insomnia.

9. **Chai-hu-chia-lung-ku-mu-li-tang** 柴胡加龍骨牡蠣湯
   (Bupleurum and Dragon Bone Combination)

This formula is indicated for patients with vertigo who have a strong and obese physique, epigastric distention, and thoracocostal distress. The vertigo is a consequence of their nervousness and excitability.

Facial Nerve Paralysis

(Bell's Palsy)

Bell's palsy is the paralysis of the muscles on one side of the face. A typical facial appearance develops due to the lesion of the peripheral nerves. Sometimes it is precipitated by exposure, chill, or trauma. It may occur at any age but is slightly more common in the age group from twenty to fifty.

Symptoms

The patient has a typical distorted facial appearance with one side of the face and its mimic muscles paralyzed. The frontal folds disappear. The eyes are not able to close properly nor is the mouth. The mouth is dragged toward the side, thus distorting its shape. When eating, food may drip off the lips; when talking, the tongue is tied and tangled so that clear articulation is impossible; and the taste sense is lost. At times deafness may result.

Treatment

Assure the patient that recovery usually occurs in two to eight weeks (or up to one to two years in older patients). The face should be kept warm and away from further exposure, especially to wind and dust. If necessary, protect the eye with a patch and support the face with tape or wire anchored at the angle of the mouth and looped about the ear. Electric stimulation (every other day after the fourteenth day) may be used to help prevent muscle atrophy. Gentle upward massage of the involved muscles for five to ten minutes two to three times daily may help to maintain muscle tone. Heat from an infra-red lamp may hasten recovery. Prednisone therapy (40mg daily for four days and tapering to 8mg in eight days) is effective for this disease.

Chinese Herb Formulas

1. Ko-ken-tang　　　　　　　　　　　　　　　　葛根湯
    (Pueraria Combination)

This formula is applied in the initial stage of the disease, especially after a cold. It is for patients with good muscle tone.

2. Kuei-chih-chia-ling-chu-fu-tang　　　　　桂枝加苓朮附湯
    (Cinnamon and Aconite Combination)

In comparison with the preceding combination, this one is for external weakness conformation while the first formula is indicated for the externally firm type. Patients with a weak pulse, chills, and lack of strength should be advised to take this formula.

3. Chia-wei-pa-hsien-tang　　　　　　　　　　加味八仙湯
    (Siler and Chiang-huo Combination)

This formula aims at the numbness conformation. Persons with such symptoms as paralysis of the arms and legs, particularly the upper arms, and of the tongue are advised to take this formula.

4. Huang-chi-keui-chih-wu-wu-tang　　　　黃耆桂枝五物湯
    (Astragalus and Cinnamon Five Combination)
   Shen-hsiao-huang-chi-tang　　　　　　　神效黃耆湯
    (Astragalus and Vitex Combination)
   Both of these formulas are indicated for the symptoms of pale complexion and generalized edema in women.

5. Hsiang-chuan-chieh-tu-chi　　　　　　　香川解毒劑
    (Smilax and Akebia Combination)
   This formula is indicated for syphilitic facial paralysis and is sometimes used in combination with *Kuei-chih-chia-ling-chu-fu-tang*.

6. Hsu-ming-tang　　　　　　　　　　　　續命湯
    (Ma-huang and Ginseng Combination)
   This combination is taken during the lingering period following an acute episode of the disease with no symptoms other than paralysis.

7. Kuei-chih-fu-ling-wan　　　　　　　　　桂枝茯苓丸
    (Cinnamon and Hoelen Formula)
   This formula is indicated for patients with abdominal blood stagnation conformation.

Myelitis

Myelitis, an inflammation of the spinal cord, is classified into two types: leukomyelitis and poliomyelitis. The former is the inflammation of the white substance of the spinal cord, while the latter is the inflammation of the spinal cord caused by infectious poliomyelitic virus. In the latter, three antigenically distinct types of virus (I, II, and III) are recognized in the throat washings and stools of the infected subjects. Since the introduction of an effective, oral live virus vaccine (Sabin), the disease has become rare in developed areas of the world.

The incubation period of the virus is from five to thirty-five days (usually seven to fourteen days). Contagiousness is maximal during the first week. Infection can be acquired by the respiratory droplet route or by ingestion. The family or other contacts of diagnosed cases may become "transient carriers" and excrete virus in the absence of symptoms.

Poliomyelitis is further divided into three types: abortive, nonparalytic, and paralytic poliomyelitis.

Symptoms

The symptoms of myelitis vary with the location of the lesion and generally involve pain in the back, girdle sensation, hyperesthesia, formication, anesthesia, motor disturbance, paralysis, increase of reflexes, paralysis of the sphincters, decubitus ulcers and, in later stages, spasmodic contraction of the paralyzed limbs. The diagnostic symptoms for poliomyelitis are muscular weakness, headache, stiff neck, fever, nausea, vomiting, sore throat, and lower motor neuron lesion with decreased deep tendon reflexes and muscle wasting.

Treatment

Prevention. Vaccination by oral live virus vaccine (Sabin) is essential for primary immunization of all infants.

Basic Treatment. Early detection of cranial nerve involvement, particularly difficulty in swallowing saliva and weakness of respiratory muscles, is important. Polio bed, hot moist packs, and other means may be applied to relieve the pain. Low calcium diet (maximum 0.5g daily) is recommended. In case of bulbar poliomyelitis or when there is weakness of respiratory muscles, patients require intensive care. Attention must be focused on maintaining a clear airway, handling secretions, preventing respiratory infection, and maintaining adequate ventilation.

Convalescence and Rehabilitation. Rehabilitation should begin as early as possible; active exercise under skilled direction. However, during the febrile period, exercise should be avoided, and only motion exercise and position change on the bed are recommended.

Chinese Herb Formulas
1. Pa-wei-wan 八味丸
(Rehmannia Eight Formula)
There is an increasing number of reports on the curative effect of this formula in myelitis patients who have been disabled and crippled.

2. Kuei-chih-chia-ling-chu-fu-tang　　桂枝加苓朮附湯
    (Cinnamon and Atractylodes Combination)
This combination is effective for patients with weak digestive organs, a condition the above formula doesn't suit.

3. Shih-chuan-ta-pu-tang　　十全大補湯
    (Ginseng and Tang-kuei Ten Combination)
This combination is applied when the disease has lingered for quite a long time and the patient is exhausted in both the blood and the *ch'i*.

Tabes Dorsalis

Tabes dorsalis, a type of neurosyphilis, is a chronic progressive degeneration of the parenchyma (essential tissue) of the posterior columns of the spinal cord and of the posterior sensory ganglia and nerve roots. This disease is due to the infection of the central nervous system by *Treponema pallidum*. Infection occurs most frequently during sexual contact through minor skin or mucosal lesions. The organism is extremely sensitive to heat and drying but can survive for days in fluids. However, it may be transmitted via the placenta from mother to fetus after the fifth month of pregnancy (known as congenital syphilis). The disease occurs mostly after middle age and is more frequent in males. It is also known by the terms Duchenne's disease, locomotor ataxia, and syphilis posterior spinal sclerosis.

Symptoms

The disease, a tertiary (or late) form of syphilis, is marked by paroxysms or crises of intense pain, which include gastric crises, laryngeal crises, rectal and anal crises, impairment of proprioception and vibration, Argyll-Robertson pupils, and muscular hypotonia and hyporeflexia (reduced reflexes). Impairment of proprioception results in a wide-based gait and inability to walk in the dark. Paresthesias, analgesia, or sharp recurrent pains in the muscles of the leg may occur. It is also accompanied by various atrophic disturbances, especially of the bones and joints, incontinence or retention of urine, and failure of sexual power.

Treatment

It is most important to prevent neurosyphilis by prompt diagnosis, adequate treatment, and follow-up on early syphilis.

Treatment consists of procaine penicillin G, 60,000 units IM daily to a total of 12 million units or more. A second course of penicillin therapy may be given if necessary.

However, all patients must have spinal fluid examinations at three month intervals for the first year and every six months for the second year following completion of antisyphilis therapy.

Chinese Herb Formulas

1. Wei-cheng-fang-chia-fu-tzu　　　　　　　　痿證方加附子
   (Eucommia and Achyranthes Formula with Aconite)

Paralysis in the motor and sensory nerves from below the waist indicates the use of this formula. Besides this formula, *Pa-wei-wan* and *Ching-shih-tang* may also be used to cure the disease.

2. Tao-ho-cheng-chi-tang　　　　　　　　桃核承氣湯
   (Persica and Rhubarb Combination)

This formula has been applied successfully to a patient in the initial stage of the disease with the additional symptoms of hypogastrium cramps and constipation.

Cerebral (Spinal) Syphilis

The disease, a late (tertiary) syphilis, is characterized by meningeal involvement or changes in the vascular structures of the brain or both. The symptoms are usually detected three years after initial infection; more often they turn severe at night. Sometimes it may involve the cranial nerve and nerve roots and gives rise to various neurological symptoms. Lesions in the spinal cord may bring about several symptoms in the body, depending of the site of infection, such as spinolegia and paresis of the lower limbs. Combinations of various forms of neurosyphilis (especially tabes and paresis) are not uncommon.

Symptoms

Generally, the symptoms vary according to the sites of infection or lesion. The disease may bring about headache, vomiting, vertigo, spasms, memory loss, lethargy, somnolence or the eruption of mania. Vascular cerebral syphilis may develop according to lesion sites with symptoms of cerebral dysfunction, headache, dysarthria, memory loss, emotional change, etc.; the spinal lesions can bring about general symptoms such as spinalegia, pain and paresis in the lower limbs.

Treatment

It is most important to prevent spinal syphilis by prompt diagnosis, adequate treatment, and follow-up of early syphilis.

Treatment consists of procaine penicillin G, 60,000 units IM daily to a total of 12 million units or more. A second course of penicillin therapy may be given if necessary.

However, all patients must have spinal fluid examinations at three month intervals for the first year and every six months for the second year following completion of antisyphilis therapy.

Chinese Herb Formulas

1. **Hsiang-chuan-chieh-tu-chi** 香川解毒劑
   (Smilax and Akebia Combination)

This is a popular formula for syphilis. It works for cerebrospinal syphilis too.

2. **Fan-pi-chiao-kan-tan-liao** 反鼻交感丹料
   (Hoelen and Viper Formula)

This formula is applied when syphilis is getting quite serious and the patient shows signs of insanity.

3. **Tou-feng-shen-fang** 頭風神方
   (Smilax and Gastrodia Formula)

This formula is indicated for cerebrospinal syphilis with headache and tinnitus.

4. **Tao-ho-cheng-chi-tang** 桃核承氣湯
   (Persica and Rhubarb Combination)

Patients with awkwardness and dullness in speech, multiplicity of hallucinations, and excitability can be given this formula if they also have constipation and lower abdominal cramp.

5. Yang-hsieh-tang 養血湯
    (Tang-kuei and Eucommia Combination)
Cerebrospinal syphilis with aching limbs and motor nerve paralysis are indications for this combination.

6. Pa-wei-wan 八味丸
    (Rehmannia Eight Formula)
This formula is applied to cases with lower limb paralysis and urinary bladder disturbances.

7. Wei-cheng-fang-chia-fu-tzu 痿證方加附子
    (Eucommia and Achyranthes Formula with Aconite)
    Ta-fang-feng-tang 大防風湯
    (Major Siler Combination)
These formulas are indicated for patients with akinesia resulting from cerebral syphilis.

Schizophrenia

Schizophrenia includes a group of mental disorders which are characterized by the following variables:

Biogenetic: a genetic disposition with variable penetrance, probably affecting catecholamine metabolism through a number of poorly understood biochemical mechanisms. The so-called induced psychoses (e.g. psychedelic and amphetamine psychoses) along with the most recent twin concordance studies lend credence to this concept.

Psychological: a result of childhood and developmental experiences revolving around family communications and behavioral patterns.

Environmental: threshold of the various stresses which the individual withstands to his biological limits. Studies with sensory deprivation, drugs, and high anxiety indicate that breakdown is a function of the person's ability to withstand stress. Amphetamines and other stimulants used in various "diet pills" commonly precipitate psychotic symptoms in schizophrenics who are not known to be clinically ill when the drugs are prescribed.

Classification

Acute schizophrenia: characterized by a precipitous psychotic episode preceded by good adjustment. Remission is prompt, and subsequent reconstitution is well phased to lead to normal life again.

Chronic schizophrenia: usually includes a long-standing history of chaotic psychotic symptoms. Age of onset is from sixteen through twenty-four years.

Paranoid schizophrenia: characterized by delusions of grandeur or persecution, often accompanied by hallucinations.

Schizo-affective schizophrenia: a sub-type of schizophrenia with prominent mood changes, either manic or depressive, and indeterminable psychoses that are in the early stages and cannot be placed in any of the established categories.

Symptoms

Primary Symptoms: Bleuler's Four A's, which may not be evident early in the disorder.
1. Disturbances in affect (emotional response), either inappropriate or flattened.
2. Loose association, wandering from topic to topic with little relevancy.
3. Autistic thinking or involvement in fantasy material, often completely absorbed in ideas of reference to self.
4. Ambivalence, often not quickly apparent, characterized by conflicting and simultaneous positive and negative feelings toward another person.

Secondary Symptoms
1. Erratic behavior, often day-night reversal
2. Anhedonia
3. Anger and frustration
4. Dependence
5. Depression
6. Pathological coping devices, or attempts to "explain" what is happening
7. "Boundary" problems, or inability to separate oneself (both self and body) as an entity distinct from others
8. Feelings of markedly enhanced or muted sensory awareness

9. Reports of "racing thoughts"
10. Mental exhaustion
11. Deficiencies in focusing attention and concentration

Treatment
Medication
1. Acute schizophrenia. Hospitalization is needed for a short period. Antipsychotics are the treatment of choice during the acute phase. Chlorpromazine, 50-100mg orally, or haloperiodal, 5mg orally, can be given.
2. Chronic schizophrenia. Medical treatment is the major ongoing need in this type of illness. Intermittent hospitalization is usually required, and antipsychotics must be given indefinitely under supervision of the physician for long-term effects. For the acute phase, 500-600mg orally per day of chlorpromazine or thioridazine is given as a sedative. As the symptoms subside, a piperazine drug may be gradually substituted. An injectable long acting preparation such as fluphenazine enanthate is helpful when given in a dosage of about 25mg (1ml) every two weeks.

Psychological therapy. Individual eclectic therapy is helpful in assisting the patients of acute schizophrenia to cope with day-to-day events. Psychotherapy offering insight into problems will prove helpful to patients of both acute and chronic phases in recognizing the sources or antecedents of their stresses. However, for chronic schizophrenics, psychopharmacological agents are the primary mode of treatment. Other Psychological treatments involve social and behavioral measures, both useful in reestablishing the patients' adaptations to their environment.

Chinese Herb Formulas
1. San-huang-hsieh-hsin-tang　　　　　　三黃瀉心湯
   (Coptis and Rhubarb Combination)
   Huang-lien-chieh-tu-tang　　　　　　　黃連解毒湯
   (Coptis and Scute Combination)

Persons who hallucinate and fantasize, or who are often mentally disordered and have restlessness and constipation, should take either of these combinations.

2. Chai-hu-chia-lung-ku-mu-li-tang　　　柴胡加龍骨牡蠣湯
   (Bupleurum and Dragon Bone Combination)
   This combination is given to obese patients who are usually in an excited state with symptoms of headache, dizziness, insomnia, stiff shoulders, and constipation. Sometimes 2.0g of coptis and 3.0g of paeonia are added.

3. Tao-ho-cheng-chi-tang　　　桃核承氣湯
   (Persica and Rhubarb Combination)
   Patients with mental disorders and paranoia (or fear of being killed), with hypogastrium cramps as an abdominal symptom, should be advised to take this combination.

4. Ta-cheng-chi-tang　　　大承氣湯
   (Major Rhubarb Combination)
   Stout patients who tend to become mad and cruel should be advised to take this combination.

5. Lung-ku-tang　　　龍骨湯
   (Dragon Bone Combination)
   This combination cures amnesia, depression, cramps, insomnia, excessive talking, and hysteria.

Melancholia Agitans

Melancholia or depression is an unhappy emotional state with abnormal inhibition of mental and bodily activity. It is theoretically classed into four models: (1) the "agression turned inward" type, in which the patients express anger at themselves; (2) the "loss" model, which postulates that depression is a reaction to loss of some favored object; (3) the "interpersonal relationship" model, in which patients tend to use their depression as a means of controlling others (including doctors); and (4) the "biogenic amine" hypothesis, which holds that biochemical derangements cause a depletion of biogenic amines.

Melancholia agitans, or manic-depressive illness, is an illness belonging to one of the three major groups of depression, the depression of primary affective disorders. Besides this classification the other two categories are the reactive group of depression and the depressions secondary to underlying diseases.

There are two subtypes of primary affective disorders: (1) unipolar, where the patient has either recurrent attacks of depression or manic phases; or (2) bipolar, in which both depressive and manic phases are present, frequently alternating and persisting for variable periods of time.

Studies of twins indicate that a genetic factor plays a role in this disorder. However, patients with the unipolar variety tend to be older at onset (often in the forties), and have lower frequency of attack than the bipolar type, who have peak age of onset at twenty-five and a high recurrent frequency.

Mania is a phase of mental disorder characterized by the following features: (1) flight of ideas; (2) hyperactivity, including motor and social activity; (3) elation; (4) easy distractibility; (5) behavior change from quiet and cooperative to excited and aggressive; and (6) a personal or family history of mood disorders.

Symptoms

The symptoms may vary from mild sadness to the opposite extreme of agitation. However, symptoms such as observed restlessness, retarded movement, and somatic concerns to the point of somatic delusions (psychotic depressions) are more evident in these disorders. The patient may also have deep feelings of guilt, loneliness, and hopelessness, with a restricted affective range and a loss of interest in daily activities. The problems of anorexia; weight loss; constipation; delusional ideas of sin, guilt, and ill health; and insomnia (particularly early morning awakening) are often present. Suicide attempts are not unusual for patients with deep gloom or in the presence of a secondary reinforcement after long term depression.

Treatment

Medical. Hospitalization with precautions against suicide is required when the patient is suicidal or seriously incapacitated. If the suicide risk is high, ECT (electro-convulsive therapy) should be considered as a treatment of choice. Tricyclic antidepressants such as Tofranil, desipiramine, phenelzine and doxepin are effective if administered in adequate dosage and duration. An example would be imipramine, 100mg daily to start, increased by 25mg daily every several days until remission occurs or until 300mg daily are being given. Lithium may be helpful in decreasing the recurrent rate of depressions, particularly the bipolar type (mania and depression). Manic states are treated with haloperiol, 5mg orally or IM every several hours. Lithium carbonate may be given based on prior laboratory tests.

Psychological, social and behavioral. Psychological and behavioral technics are useful mainly in ancillary problem areas. Social structuring such as day hospitalization, and family and work counseling are helpful, particularly for recurrent episodes.

Chinese Herb Formulas

1. San-huang-hsieh-hsin-tang　　　　　　　三黃瀉心湯
   (Coptis and Rhubarb Combination)
   Huang-lien-chieh-tu-tang　　　　　　　　黃連解毒湯
   (Coptis and Scute Combination)

Patients who tend toward a manic state and are unstable and easily agitated may be given either of these combinations.

2. Ta-cheng-chi-tang　　　　　　　　　　　大承氣湯
   (Major Rhubarb Combination)

Patients who tend to be manic usually have an obese physique. This combination is indicated for these persons with constipation and a tendency to brutality.

3. Tao-ho-cheng-chi-tang　　　　　　　　　桃核承氣湯
   (Persica and Rhubarb Combination)

Manic persons that have hypogastrium cramps, mostly with constipation and irregular menstrual cycles, may be treated by this combination.

4. Lung-ku-tang　　　　　　　　　　　　　龍骨湯
   (Dragon Bone Combination)

This combination is indicated for persons with melancholia.

5. Fan-pi-chiao-kan-tan-liao　　　　　　　　反鼻交感丹料
   (Hoelen and Viper Formula)

Melancholic persons with a depressive mood may be given this formula.

6. Pan-hsia-hou-pu-tang 半夏厚朴湯
   (Pinellia and Magnolia Combination)
This combination is for melancholic persons who are pessimistic and depressed.

CHILDREN'S DISEASES
(Pediatric Diseases)

Measles (Rubeola)

Measles is an acute, highly contagious viral infection, characterized by an extensive eruption of small, red macules. A newborn infant whose mother has had measles receives transplacental passive immunization, so the baby is usually immune during the first six months after birth. The age of greatest susceptibility to measles is from two to six years old. Spring and autumn are the most likely seasons in which to get the disease, especially early spring. The invading rubeola virus affects the nose and the throat. Once the infection subsides, the patient usually has lifetime immunity.

Symptoms

The incubation period of measles is ten to twelve days. The primary symptoms are similar to those of the common cold, such as fever, sneezing and coughing. The three stages of measles are as follows:
1. Prodromic period. This period lasts three to four days after the onset of sickness. The patient has a variety of symptoms including fever, conjunctivitis, ophthalmia (inflammation of the eye), lacrimation (excessive tearing), rhinitis (inflamma-

tion of the nasal mucous membranes), sneezing, coughing, and sputum. Small red spots with bluishwhite centers appear on the mucous membranes of the mouth shortly before the appearance of the chief symptom—Koplik's spots (measles rash).
2. Eruption period. Eruption starts at the back of the ears, neck, and face and then spreads to the whole body. The primary eruption consists of red, grain-like spots, which gradually enlarge and spread over the body. The symptoms at this stage are more serious than during the prodromic period. Duration is between four and five days.
3. Resumptive period. The eruptions subside and the fever lessens. The areas of eruption remain more or less pigmented. If the patient suffers from measles for several more days and maintains a high fever, he or she probably has some other condition in addition to the measles.

Treatment

The patient with measles has little resistance to other diseases. If complications ensue (pneumonia, inflammation of the middle ear, bronchitis, or eye ailments), the illness is compounded. Pneumonia is especially dangerous to children during this period. The patient should rest and keep warm to avoid catching a cold. An ice pillow should be used when the patient has a high fever. Antipyretics, antitussives, and sedatives may be taken under doctor's guidance to prevent complications. Sulfonamides and penicillin are effective too.

For preventive medicine, a patient may be immunized with recently developed vaccines, either 20-30g measles serum (gamma globulin) or live attenuated vaccine.

Chinese Herb Formulas
1. **Sheng-ma-ko-ken-tang** 升麻葛根湯
   (Cimicifuga and Pueraria Combination)

The main herbs in this formula, pueraria and cimicifuga, are effective for primary measles.

2. **Ko-ken-tang** 葛根湯
   (Pueraria Combination)

The main herbs in this formula, *ma-huang* and jujube, are taken for measles with high fever when there is no sweating.

3. **Hsiao-chai-hu-tang** 小柴胡湯
   (Minor Bupleurum Combination)
This formula is for measles with lymphadenitis colli (inflammation of the lymph nodes) or bronchitis. For cases complicated by otitis media, platycodon and gypsum should be added.

4. **Ko-ken-huang-lien-huang-chin-tang** 葛根黃連黃芩湯
   (Pueraria, Coptis, and Scute Combination)
This is for measles with high fever, spasm, cough, and diarrhea.

5. **Chu-yeh-shih-kao-tang** 竹葉石膏湯
   (Bamboo Leaves and Gypsum Combination)
This formula is for measles with fever, thirst, dysuria, cough, hoarseness, emotional instability, and stress.

6. **Chen-wu-tang** 眞武湯
   (Vitality Combination)
   Szu-ni-tang 四逆湯
   (Aconite and G. L. Combination)
Both formulas are effective in treating measles.

7. **Hsiao-ching-lung-tang-chia-ma-hsing-kan-shih-tang**
   小青龍湯加麻杏甘石湯
   (Minor Blue Dragon Combination with Ma-huang and Apricot Seed Combination)
This formula is for measles with bronchitis, bronchopneumonia, coughing, and dyspnea (difficulty in breathing).

8. **Erh-hsien-tang** 二仙湯
   (Scute and Paeonia Combination)
This formula is used to treat the dyspnea and stress of pneumonia or cerebral disease contracted as a result of the measles attack.

Whooping Cough

Whooping cough is a contagious respiratory disease caused

by the bacteria *Bordetella pertussis* and transmitted by airborne droplets. In the newborn, whooping cough is a serious infection, since there is no passive immunization from the mother; it is often responsible for an infant's death. Once the patient recovers, he will have active immunity. The greatest incidence is during winter or spring.

Symptoms

Incubation is one to two weeks. During incubation, there are symptoms similar to the common cold: rhinitis (inflammation of the nasal mucous membranes), conjunctivitis, and coughing. This state lasts at least one week, and then the patient experiences marked recurrent paroxysms of violent coughing and sticky sputum. This particular coughing results in edema and ophthalmia (eye inflammation) for one hundred days. Afterward, the condition subsides.

Treatment

The DPT vaccine is routinely given as preventive medicine. Antitussives can help restore vigor. Whooping cough may be easily complicated by bronchitis or pneumonia which endangers the patient's life.

Chinese Herb Formulas

1. **Hsiao-ching-lung-tang** 小青龍湯
   (Minor Blue Dragon Combination)

The main herbs of this formula—*ma-huang,* paeonia, and ginger—are taken for whooping cough with coughing, ophthalmia, facial edema, and bronchitis.

2. **Hsiao-chai-hu-tang-chia-pan-hsia-hou-pu-tang**
   小柴胡湯加半夏厚朴湯
   (Minor Bupleurum Combination with Pinellia and Magnolia Combination)

The main herbs of this formula are bupleurum, pinellia, and scute. It is taken by children for whooping cough accompanied by nervousness, emotional instability, loss of appetite, and coughing.

3. **Ma-hsing-kan-shih-tang-chia-pan-hsia-fu-ling-chen-pi-sheng-chiang** 麻杏甘石湯加半夏茯苓陳皮生薑

(Ma-huang and Apricot Seed Combination with Pinellia 4.0, Hoelen 4.0, Citrus 3.0, and Ginger 1.0)
This formula is taken for whooping cough with sputum.

4. Mai-men-tung-tang   麥門冬湯
    (Ophiopogon Combination)
This formula is taken for whooping cough by children who have coarse skin, hoarseness, dryness of the throat, severe coughing spasms, redness of the face due to coughing, and who are vomiting.

5. Kan-mai-ta-tsao-tang   甘麥大棗湯
    (Licorice and Jujube Combination)
This formula is taken for whooping cough with frequent bouts of acute, severe coughing.

6. Tun-sou-tang   頓嗽湯
    (Morus and Platycodon Combination)
This formula is for whooping cough.

Mumps

Mumps is an acute, contagious viral disease that usually attacks during childhood. It is characterized by swelling of the parotid and other salivary glands. The disease is transmitted by droplet infection. Once the infection subsides, the patient has active immunity to the disease.

Symptoms
The incubation period of this disease is two to three weeks. The patient has mild fever, headache, and edema in one or both ears. The patient feels pain and swelling while chewing. Occasionally, fever will rise to 40°C. After two weeks, the swelling disappears completely. Sometimes the mammary glands and ovaries of girls or the testicles of boys are also affected. Some cases are complicated by encephalitis or splenitis.

Treatment
While there is no specific medical treatment for viral diseases,

this condition will not endanger the patient's life. The patient should rest comfortably during the fever stage and moist cloths changed every four hours should be applied to the areas of swelling.

Chinese Herb Formulas
1. Ko-ken-tang   葛根湯
   (Pueraria Combination)

This formula is effective for primary mumps with severe chills, headache, and fever.

2. Hsiao-chai-hu-tang-chia-chieh-keng-shih-kao

   小柴胡湯加桔梗石膏

   (Minor Bupleurum Combination with Platycodon and Gypsum)

This formula may be taken by children with swollen parotid glands, a white coating on the tongue, anorexia (loss of appetite), and fever.

3. Chai-hu-kuei-chih-tang   柴胡桂枝湯
   (Bupleurum and Cinnamon Combination)

This formula is used to treat mumps accompanied by testitis or ovaritis.

Varicella
(Chickenpox)

Varicella is a highly contagious children's disease characterized by skin eruptions that appear in crops. Chickenpox is spread by direct contact with someone who has the disease or by infected droplets from the nose or mouth.

Symptoms
The incubation period of the varicella is eleven to twelve days. Following a slight fever, small, reddish lesions appear over the whole body. Later, blisters develop in the central parts. Scars will remain for several days on the infected areas. The eruptions

consist of macules, papules, vesicles, and crusting, and characteristically occur in crops.

Treatment
There is no specific medical treatment for viral diseases. The patient should rest comfortably during the fever stage. After one to two weeks the eruptions disappear completely.

Chinese Herb Formulas
1. Wu-ling-san   五苓散
   (Hoelen Five Herb Formula)
This formula is taken for varicella with severe itching and thirst.

2. Kuei-chih-chia-huang-chin-tang   桂枝加黃芩湯
   (Cinnamon and Astragalus Combination)
This formula is for mild cases of varicella.

Muguet (Thrush)

Thrush, an infection of infants caused by the fungus *Candida albicans*, is candidiasis of the mucous membrane of the mouth. Muguet is much more frequent today because of the intake of broad spectrum antibiotics which kill off beneficial as well as harmful bacteria and thus leave the field free for fungus infection.

Symptoms
Slightly raised white patches that look like milk curds appear inside the cheeks and lips and on the gums, tongue, and soft palate. These patches eventually become shallow ulcers. Thrush is often accompanied by fever and gastrointestinal irritation.

Treatment
Treatments include swabbing the mouth with a 1 percent solution of gentian violet, sucking Bradisol lozenges, or rinsing the mouth with washes containing Ziphiran. With supplementing multivitamins, the condition usually clears in a week.

Chinese Herb Formulas
1. San-huang-hsieh-hsin-tang   三黃瀉心湯

(Coptis and Rhubarb Combination)
This prescription is taken frequently in small quantities by infants suffering from muguet and constipation. It is essential that the child have good stamina in order to take this medication.

2. **Chien-shih-pai-chu-san** 錢氏白朮散
(Atractylodes and Pueraria Formula)
This formula is indicated for those who have suffered from thrush for several days and are becoming rather feeble.

3. **Folk Formulas** 民間方
Phellodendron is pulverized, mixed with borax and wrapped up in linen, and then held in the mouth. The raw arisaema may be peeled, ground into paste, and applied to the sore.

Stomatitis

Stomatitis (canker sores), a frequently seen pediatric disease, is inflammation of the mouth. There are many types of stomatitis, three of which are catarrh stomatitis, aphtha stomatitis, and ulcerative stomatitis.

Symptoms
A. Catarrh stomatitis occurs on the oral mucous membrane or on the tongue. It exhibits swelling, pain, halitosis, and slobbering.
B. In aphthous stomatitis painful ulcers form on the mucous lining of the mouth and grow into small yellow spots with reddening at the periphery. This form is very painful.
C. Ulcerative stomatitis is the most severe condition. The whole mouth becomes swollen and covered with a white coat; sometimes pustulation occurs. The pain is severe, and there is an accompanying high fever.

Treatment
Anesthetic cough drops or lozenges may be helpful in relieving the pain. A mouthwash several times a day of a solution of 10 percent Na_2CO_3 in warm water is soothing. High potency vitamin B complex has on occasion shortened the duration of the

sores and prevented their recurrence. Bland mouth rinses and hydrocortisone antibiotic ointments reduce pain and encourage healing. Hydrocortisone in an adhesive base is particularly useful. Systemic antibiotics are usually contraindicated. However, systemic corticosteroids in high doses for a short period of time may be very helpful for severely debilitating recurrent attacks.

Chinese Herb Formulas
1. Tiao-wei-cheng-chi-tang 調胃承氣湯
   (Rhubarb and Mirabilitum Combination)
This prescription is for catarrh stomatitis with constipation that has lasted for a couple of days and cannot be purged by an enema. It effects defecation and promotes healing in most cases.

2. Liang-ke-san 涼膈散
   (Forsythia and Rhubarb Formula)
This formula is used for *Tiao-wei-cheng-chi-tang* sufferers who have more severe inflammation and in whom the reddening and swelling in the mucous membrane of the oral cavity is very serious; the maxillary lymph nodes also become swollen and ache severely. These symptoms always occur with fever and constipation.

3. San-huang-hsieh-hsin-tang 三黃瀉心湯
   (Coptis and Rhubarb Combination)
This combination is taken during the initial stage of stomatitis when the patient is thirsty and has a dry tongue and a tendency to be constipated. If there is no constipation, *Huang-lien-chieh-tu-tang* is indicated.

4. Kan-tsao-hsieh-hsin-tang 甘草瀉心湯
   (Pinellia and Licorice Combination)
This combination is indicated for patients with slight stomatitis who have distention and rigidity under the heart, nausea, anorexia, or diarrheal gastroenteritis.

Dyspepsia

Dyspepsia (upset stomach) can be brought on by badly cooked or unpalatable foods; hasty eating; insufficient food; extended constipation; diseases of the mouth, heart, liver, or kidneys; and prolonged mental strain and anxiety. It is rarely found in breast-fed infants but quite frequently found in formula-fed infants. The condition can become very serious.

Symptoms

Upon suffering dyspepsia, infants will have diarrhea, vomiting, and anorexia. They become vigorless, inactive, and uncomfortable. Reduced body weight and emaciation occur while the abdomen swells and fills with gas and borborygmus. In serious cases, the infant vomits profusely. Hematemesis (vomiting blood), oliguria (decrease in urine), and poor complexion also occur. Additionally there is a high fever with a weak and feeble pulse. In advanced stages, the dangerous conditions of intoxication, convulsion, coma, and even the possibility of death occur. Dyspepsia is often accompanied by flatulence, which is gas or air in the stomach or intestines relieved by belching or passing wind.

Treatment

Meal time must be leisurely and pleasant and ingested food not waterlogged.

Chinese Herb Formulas

1. **Wu-ling-san** 五苓散
   (Hoelen Five Herb Formula)

During the comparatively early stage, the baby is severely thirsty but vomits the liquid immediately after drinking it. Simultaneously he experiences diarrhea, anorexia, and oliguria. This formula quenches thirst and halts vomiting and diarrhea. It is best to give the remedy as early as possible.

2. **Jen-sheng-tang** 人參湯
   (Ginseng and Ginger Combination)

This combination is given to feeble and vigorless babies with poor complexions, weak abdomens and pulses, ceaseless diarrhea, and vomiting.

3. **Sheng-ling-pai-chu-san** 參苓白朮散
   (Ginseng and Atractylodes Formula)

This formula is indicated when the vomiting has stopped but the diarrhea continues, there is flatus in the abdomen, and the patient still experiences discomfort.

4. Fu-ling-szu-ni-tang 茯苓四逆湯
   (Hoelen, G. L. and Aconite Combination)
This combination is taken for high fever, oliguria, edema, feeble pulse, diarrhea, continuous vomiting, and symptoms of intoxication. For the convulsions and comatose condition caused by intoxication, this formula may be palliative.

Autointoxication

Autointoxication or endogenous toxicosis in a broad sense means the following: (1) the poisonous substances among the metabolites produced by metabolism are normal in quantity but owing to some unknown cause are accumulating in the body and being hindered from excretion; (2) poisonous substances are being physiologically generated in excess; (3) a non-destructive disturbance in local or general metabolism that normally produces metabolites is causing them to not disassociate into harmless substances; and (4) the function of a particular organ has changed or stopped with the result that poisonous substances are entering the blood stream and are not being neutralized. Children with a nervous constitution easily develop this condition.

Symptoms
The onset of symptoms is sudden: recurrent vomiting, headache, vertigo, somnolence, an increase or decrease in cardiac function, frequent vomiting that occurs repetitively sometimes with black blood, heavy breathing, a quick pulse, and signs of a dangerous condition. Vomiting is accompanied by great thirst. However, immediately after drinking, the water is vomited. The vomitus smells like acetone. Prognosis is good. The patient may recover within two to seven days. This disease may occur repetitively but heals spontaneously by school age.

Chinese Herb Formulas
To prevent the occurrence and to assure a complete cure,

the following Chinese formulas may be administered.

1. **Wu-ling-san**   五苓散
   (Hoelen Five Herb Formula)

This formula ameliorates vomiting, thirst, and oliguria and can be used at the moment of relapse. It is best taken in powder form along with rice starch rather than in the decocted form. After taking this formula, there will be no more vomiting or thirst.

2. **Ling-kuei-kan-tsao-tang**   苓桂甘棗湯
   (Hoelen, Licorice, and Jujube Combination)

This ancient formula used to be given for "rushing hog," the Chinese equivalent of today's hysteria. I similarly have obtained outstanding results using this formula for cases of infantile hysteria brought on by autointoxication.

3. **Kuei-chih-jen-sheng-tang**   桂枝人參湯
   (Cinnamon and Ginseng Combination)

This formula is efficacious for weakness in the stomach and intestines, poor appetite, and poor complexion if taken at the onset.

Infectious Diarrhea

Infectious diarrhea is actually infantile diarrhea, especially when accompanied by the very severe condition of intoxication.

Onset of the disease is abrupt. Infants that are lively and active suddenly become spiritless, sleepy, and yawn frequently. A temperature as high as 39-40°C occurs. The eyeballs may turn upward and the four limbs cramp, or the whole body may cramp. The pulse is weak and the abdomen soft and forceless. Stools are normal with the first one or two defecations but gradually become infiltrated with mucous or water and finally become white or greenish-gray in color. Tenesmus and abdominal pain are rare. The younger the infant is the higher the mortality rate.

Symptoms

The illness usually starts abruptly with diarrhea, lower abdominal cramps, and sometimes tenesmus. The stool is often mixed with blood and mucus. Systemic symptoms are fever (up to 40°C), chills, anorexia and malaise, headache, lethargy, and, in the most severe cases, meningismus, coma, and convulsions. As the illness progresses, the infant becomes progressively weaker and more dehydrated. The abdomen is tender. Sigmoidoscopic examination reveals an inflamed, engorged, punctuated mucosa and sometimes large areas of ulceration. In recent years this disease is not seen as frequently as before.

Treatment
A. The treatment of shock, restoration of circulating blood volume, and renal perfusion are lifesaving for severe cases. The current antimicrobial agent of choice is ampicillin,100mg/kg/day orally in four divided doses for five to seven days. The drug should not be continued longer if there is clinical improvement even if stool cultures remain positive, because ampicillin-resistant strains of Shigella are increasing in frequency. Tetracycline, chloramphenicol, and kanamycin may also be effective; however, since the majority of cases are mild and self-limited, one cannot justify the use of even mildly toxic antibiotics.
B. General measures include correction of acidosis and electrolytic disturbances by intravenous feeding of water solutions. This is essential in all moderately or severely ill patients. After the bowel has been at rest for a short time, clear fluids are given for two to three days. The food should then be soft easily digestible, and given in small, frequent feedings, avoiding whole milk and high-residue and fatty foods. A paregoric provides effective symptomatic relief; atropine sulfate (or tincture of belladonna) is helpful when cramps are severe. Diphenoxylate with atropine (Lomotil) controls moderate diarrhea in adults. The patient should be placed on effective stool isolation precautions both in the hospital and in the home to limit the spread of the infection.

Chinese Herb Formulas
1. Ko-ken-huang-lien-huang-chin-tang　　葛根黃連黃芩湯
   (Pueraria, Coptis, and Scute Combination)
This compound is to be taken during the initial stage of the malady. It is for sudden high fever, spasms, and diarrhea.

2. **Wu-ling-san** 　　　　　　　　　　　　　　　五苓散
    (Hoelen Five Herb Formula)
This formula is used when the administration of the above formula has led to increased thirst and caused a feeling of nausea.

3. **Jen-sheng-tang** 　　　　　　　　　　　　　人參湯
    (Ginseng and Ginger Combination)
This formula is indicated for patients without thirst who may or may not have vomited, but have diarrhea, a forceless abdomen that is as soft as cotton, cold limbs, and a weak pulse. Patients suffering from this illness usually have internal coldness, another indication for this formula.

4. **Fu-ling-szu-ni-tang** 　　　　　　　　　　茯苓四逆湯
    (Hoelen, G. L. and Aconite Combination)
This formula is for a submerged pulse, unconsciousness, copious diarrhea, or unconscious urine incontinence. Patients can be cured by this formula if their limbs are still warm. For infants with cold limbs and pale facial complexion with cyanosis, this formula does not work. Patients with spasms, unconsciousness, or exceedingly cold limbs after convulsion at the very beginning of the illness are generally incurable. However, there are cases that have been cured after taking this formula.

5. **Shen-ling-pai-chu-san-szu-chun-tzu-tang**
　　　　　　　　　　　　　　　　　　　參苓白朮散・四君子湯
    (Ginseng and Atractylodes Formula, Four Major Herb Combination)
This herbal is recommended for management of the infection at a later stage when the disease has retreated and the fever has subsided.

Debilitated Children

In this section I will collectively discuss children of various kinds of constitutions: the effusive constitution, the thymus-lymphatic constitution, and the neuro-arthritic constitution.

An effusive constitution is mostly found in children under the age of two. They look obese and healthy but are in fact not being of the water toxin type. The skin and muscle are not firm and tight but soft, flabby, and whitish. These children catch cold easily. Once they catch cold they readily suffer from stridor, eczema, or rashes.

The thymus-lymphatic constitution is found in children between the ages of three or four to seven or eight. They are more likely to have swelling in the tonsils, lymph nodes, and thymus gland. Children of this constitution can be either of the obese type or the emaciated type. Both types are likely to contract diseases and usually react sensitively to drugs.

The neuro-arthritic constitution appears mostly in children around the age of ten. They are nervous and easily have headaches, stomachaches, and limb aches of unknown cause with a persistent slight fever. They easily become victims of asthma or rheumatic fever.

Treatment

Treatments are mostly palliative. However, the following Chinese herb formulas are very effective in bringing about a change in constitution.

Chinese Herb Formulas

1. Huang-chi-chien-chung-tang　　　　　　　　黃耆建中湯
   (Astragalus Combination)

This combination is for children with an effusive constitution. It tightens and firms muscles, increases resistance to colds, and improves the general health.

2. Ma-hsing-kan-shih-tang　　　　　　　　　　麻杏甘石湯
   (Ma-huang and Apricot Seed Combination)

This combination is very appropriate for the children with an effusive constitution who have persistent asthma or stridor once they catch cold. The asthma usually results in bronchitis.

3. Wu-ling-san　　　　　　　　　　　　　　　五苓散
   (Hoelen Five Herb Formula)

This formula is extremely effective for infantile rashes, hence it is frequently given to children with effusive constitutions.

4. Ta-chiung-huang-tang　　　　　　　　　大芎黃湯
   (Major Cnidium and Rhubarb Combination)
   This combination is suitable for infants with effusive constitutions who often suffer from eczema, referred to as "embryo toxin" by many people in China.

5. Hsiao-chai-hu-tang　　　　　　　　　　小柴胡湯
   (Minor Bupleurum Combination)
   This formula alters a thymus-lymphatic constitution or reduces swelling of the tonsils and lymph nodes.

6. Chai-hu-kuei-chih-tang　　　　　　　　柴胡桂枝湯
   (Bupleurum and Cinnamon Combination)
   Indicated for people with neuro-arthritic constitutions, this formula not only can cure headaches, abdominal pain, or aching of the arms and legs but also can prevent the patients from suffering from asthma or rheumatic fever.

7. Liu-chun-tzu-tang　　　　　　　　　　六君子湯
   (Six Major Herb Combination)
   This combination is to be used by those with gastrointestinal problems, anorexia, poor complexion, and vigorlessness.

Rachitis (Rickets)

This condition is caused by Vitamin D deficiency. Those who are rarely exposed to sunshine and those with dark skin often need supplementation of Vitamin D, which is essential for the metabolism of phosphorus and calcium thus maintaining the normal growth of bones and teeth.

Symptoms

In infants rickets is characterized by restlessness, joylessness, liability to perspiration, softening and thinning of the skull, and weakness of bones throughout the body noted by knockknees, bowlegs, and pigeon breast. The teeth are also malformed. At the appropriate age, the infant can neither walk, sit, nor stand. Later, children with rickets develop kyphosis (curvature of the spine).

Treatment
Vitamin D plus additional calcium and phosphorus must be administered. Remember though that very large doses of Vitamin D can be toxic.

Chinese Herb Formulas
1. I-kan-san 抑肝散
   (Bupleurum Formula)

This formula is suitable for the uneasy spirit, frequent crying, and spasms. It not only calms down the spirit but also improves physical development.

2. Huang-chi-chien-chung-tang 黃耆建中湯
   (Astragalus Combination)

This combination is given to someone suffering from malnutrition, a poor complexion, hyperhidrosis (excessive sweating), night sweating, and polyuria (excessive urination).

3. Liu-chun-tzu-tang 六君子湯
   (Six Major Herb Combination)

This combination is taken for a slight case of rickets with normal nourishment.

Poliomyelitis

Poliomyelitis is a viral infection caused by one of three distinct types of polio virus that attack the central nervous system, often causing muscle paralysis.

Symptoms
The onset is signaled by abrupt high fever, severe headache, sore throat, and fretfulness on the first day. The victim then develops a stiff neck, deep muscle pain, severe weakness, prostration tremors and twitching of the muscles, and paralysis in the arms, legs, and body.

Treatment
Once the disease has taken hold, there is no specific treatment. In the paralytic form there are some procedures that can

lessen the damage to muscles, such as the use of hot water packs on the affected muscles and early physical therapy.

Chinese Herb Formulas
1. **Hsiao-chai-hu-tang** 小柴胡湯
   (Minor Bupleurum Combination)

During the initial stage of the disease very few people resort to Chinese medicinal treatment. However, this formula is for the fever, vomiting, and poor appetite which occur at this stage.

2. **Kuei-chih-chia-ling-chu-fu-tang** 桂枝加苓朮附湯
   (Cinnamon and Atractylodes Combination)

This combination should be taken to lessen paralysis after the fever has subsided.

3. **Shih-chuan-ta-pu-tang** 十全大補湯
   (Ginseng and Tang-kuei Ten Combination)

This combination is taken for anemia and poor nutrition that develops in patients having difficulty or a disability in walking. This prescription is used for months or years after the occurrence of the disease.

Spasm of Mimic Muscles (Tic)

Tics are a neurotic symptom frequently found among school children. The condition is characterized by loud nasal breathing, a distorted mouth, frequent blinking and neck retraction, poor facial control and a sour facial expression, and the habitual action of one portion of the mimic muscles. The condition is very difficult for the sufferer to correct himself.

Chinese Herb Formula
I-kan-san-chia-shao-yao 抑肝散加芍藥
(Bupleurum Formula with Paeonia)

This formula is used for most cases and brings about a comparatively simple cure. However, recurrence is very possible, hence it must be administered continuously from the beginning for a period of time. This formula is also effective for the neurotic symptom in children called the "nodding spasm" which is characterized by a reciprocal anterior-posterior or left-right nod of the head.

Night Crying, Night Terrors

This is one of the pediatric neuroses. The symptoms and treatment are as follows.

Symptoms
A. Night terrors: The child abruptly springs up at night, runs about in a disorderly manner, and cries loudly. The next morning, he has no memory about what happened during the night.
B. Night crying: Once the night comes on the infant gets angry and cries, or cries with an uneasy or panicky expression and can't sleep.

Chinese Herb Formulas
1. **Kuei-chih-chia-lung-ku-mu-li-tang**　　　桂枝加龍骨牡蠣湯
    (Cinnamon and Dragon Bone Combination)
This compound should be given to children having night terrors, uneasiness, and a scared expression.

2. **I-kan-san**　　　抑肝散
    (Bupleurum Formula)
This formula is given to children who cause unreasonable trouble and get angry easily.

3. **Shao-yao-kan-tsao-tang**　　　芍藥甘草湯
    (Paeonia and Licorice Combination)
One dose of this formula can stop the night crying due to abdominal pain and bring the child to a sound sleep. It is specifically effective here.

4. **Kan-mai-ta-tsao-tang**　　　甘麥大棗湯
    (Licorice and Jujube Combination)
This combination is given for hysteric crying.

Bedwetting

Involuntary urination while asleep, nocturnal enuresis, may occur several times every night or only one to two times each week. Some children may have polyuria while others have dysuria. Some children have incontinence even during the day. Ninety percent of the time bedwetting is attributable to psychological disturbances. Emotional conflicts of some type cause the nervous disorders and hence the bedwetting.

Treatment

Nervous children are susceptible to this condition. Treatment should aim at improving relations between the parents and child. Tranquilizers, moxibustion, and acupuncture are effective. A urinal near the bed or an alarm clock is also helpful. The child should be encouraged to drink little water during dinner and not be scolded after bedwetting.

Chinese Herb Formulas

(These formulas should be cut to one-half or one-third the amount prescribed for an adult.)

1. **Hsiao-chien-chung-tang** 小建中湯
    (Minor Cinnamon and Paeonia Combination)

    This formula is for children with a delicate constitution, a tendency toward fatigue, pallor, bedwetting, and polyuria.

2. **Pai-hu-chia-jen-sheng-tang** 白虎加人參湯
    (Ginseng and Gypsum Combination)

    This formula is for children with a healthy body structure who suffer from thirst, ephidrosis, and bedwetting.

3. **Chai-hu-kuei-chih-tang** 柴胡桂枝湯
    (Bupleurum and Cinnamon Combination)

    This formula is for bedwetters who are very nervous.

4. **Pa-wei-ti-huang-wan** 八味地黃丸
    (Rehmannia Eight Formula)

    This formula is for obese children with anorexia (loss of appetite), pallor, thirst, and bedwetting.

5. Ko-ken-tang　　　　　　　　　　　　　　葛根湯
    (Pueraria Combination)
This formula is for bedwetting.

Nervous Vomiting

The main cause of severe neurotic vomiting in a child is either an autonomic nervous disorder or nervous tension. This is a common pediatric disorder.

Symptoms
The patient experiences loss of appetite, discomfort, and ensuing severe recurrent vomiting. In especially severe cases, the patient even vomits gastric and gall juice with blood. Because of the severe vomiting, there is a loss of fluid in the body, as well as rapid breathing, a fast pulse, thirst, unconsciousness, and convulsions. Generally, there is no fever unless tonsillitis is present. The patient has an acetone odor, sudden spasms of pain, and fearfulness. Children two to ten years old are usually most susceptible, with relapses occurring several times each year.

Treatment
The patient should be kept comfortable. Fasting is recommended after severe vomiting. The patient should drink small amounts of water (tea, boiling water, and sugar water) and eat easy to digest foods after the vomiting is over. To prevent dehydration during severe vomiting, hypodermoclysis may be necessary. Tranquilizers should be used only under a doctor's guidance. Acupressure and a balanced diet are effective for this condition. Prevention is the best treatment.

Chinese Herb Formulas
1. Wu-ling-san　　　　　　　　　　　　　　五苓散
    (Hoelen Five Herb Formula)
This formula is taken for nervous vomiting with thirst and polyuria (excessive urination).

2. Ling-kuei-kan-tsao-tang　　　　　　　　苓桂甘棗湯
    (Hoelen, Licorice, and Jujube Combination)

The main herbs of this formula are hoelen and cinnamon. It is used to treat hysteria and thereby is also effective for neurotic vomiting.

3. Kuei-chih-jen-sheng-tang　　　　　　　　　桂枝人參湯
   (Ginseng and Cinnamon Combination)

This formula is given to patients with gastrointestinal weakness, anorexia (loss of appetite), pallor, and cyclic vomiting.

Children's Hysteria

Children's hysteria is a neurotic disorder.

Symptoms
　　　The causes of this condition are complex, but essentially it is due to emotional disturbances. Hysterical children will exhibit mental and emotional instability, uncontrollable crying, and fearfulness.

Treatment
　　　The underlying causes of this condition need to be treated to assure the child's emotional well-being and adjustment.

Chinese Herb Formulas
1. I-kan-san　　　　　　　　　　　　　　　　　抑肝散
   (Bupleurum Formula)

The main herbs of this formula are *tang-kuei,* cnidium and hoelen. It is given for children's hysteria and especially for emotional instability and irritability.

2. Kuei-chih-chia-lung-ku-mu-li-tang　　　桂枝加龍骨牡蠣湯
   (Cinnamon and Dragon Bone Combination)

The main herbs of this formula are cinnamon, paeonia, dragon bone, and oyster shell. It is recommended for children's hysteria when the main symptoms are emotional instability and fearfulness.

3. Shao-yao-kan-tsao-tang　　　　　　　　　芍藥甘草湯
   (Paeonia and Licorice Combination)

This formula is for children with hysteria who have abdominal pain because of fear of the dark.

Children's Asthma

Children's asthma is a little different from bronchial asthma. Bronchial asthma usually relapses at night causing severe difficulty in breathing whereas the child with asthma breathes with a wheezing sound. His overstimulated mucous membrane secretes abundant fluid, which causes a constriction in his trachea. Thus when he breathes, a wheezing sound follows. Children's asthma usually does not occur after the age of four to five years old.

Asthma is due to intrinsic or extrinsic causes. Food allergins, hereditary susceptibility, stress, or environmental factors such as weather and temperature are responsible for this condition.

Symptoms

The patient has all the symptoms of a common cold along with wheezing and labored breathing.

Treatment

As a general treatment for bronchial asthma, antibiotics are effective.

Chinese Herb Formulas
1. Hsiao-ching-lung-tang　　　　　　　　　小青龍湯
    (Minor Blue Dragon Combination)
This formula is for children's asthma with sneezing, rhinitis, polyuria, and increasing difficulty in breathing.

2. Hsiao-chai-hu-tang-chia-pan-hsia-hou-pu-tang
　　　　　　　　　　　小柴胡湯加半夏厚朴湯
    (Minor Bupleurum Combination with Pinellia and Magnolia Combination)
This formula is for children's asthma with anorexia (loss of appetite). It should be taken frequently.

3. Ma-hsing-kan-shih-tang　　　　　　　　麻杏甘石湯
    (Ma-huang and Apricot Seed Combination)

The main components of this formula are *ma-huang*, apricot seed, licorice, and gypsum. It is used to treat children's asthma with ephidrosis, eczema, and bedwetting.

Clonus

Clonus is a form of muscular spasm in which contraction and relaxation rapidly alternate. Habitual relapse is one of the characteristics of clonus. In some cases, clonus is caused by a high fever (39-40°C) and called febrile clonus. In severe cases, an electroencephalogram should be taken to determine whether encephalitis or cerebral disorders are present. Clonus in children may also be caused by emotional instability of the mother, sour foods, or a calcium reduction in the blood.

Treatment

Generally, clonus does not endanger the patient's life. The patient should rest quietly and avoid stimulation. During an attack something should be placed between the patient's jaws to prevent him from biting his tongue. The convalescent's room should receive plenty of fresh air.

Chinese Herb Formula
Ko-ken-tang 葛根湯
(Pueraria Combination)
This formula is taken by children with clonus due to a common cold and high fever.

SURGICAL DISEASES

Contusion

A contusion is an injury to the subdermal tissue or to organs, in which there is almost no damage to the skin — in other words, a bruise. In ancient times punishment was carried out by means of bamboo-beating. In China, therefore, the treatment for any contusion was the same as the treatment for injuries incurred by this punishment. Recently traffic accidents are causing more and more incidences of contusion and whiplash, a type of contusion.

Symptoms
Generally the surface and border of a contusion are irregular and uneven. The surrounding tissue and wounded area are broadly damaged and can easily become gangrenous. A contusion is accompanied by intratissue bleeding and tumidity. The blood vessels are also damaged but they seldom rupture. However, bacterial infection occurs easily.

Treatment
Generally a serious contused wound is circumcised, the cavity cleaned and sutured, and a drainage tube inserted. If the injury is treated within six hours, contamination will be kept to a

minimum. A secondary treatment is necessary for accompanying open wounds.

Chinese Herb Formulas
1. San-huang-hsieh-hsin-tang　　三黃瀉心湯
　　(Coptis and Rhubarb Combination)
This formula has sedative and hemostatic properties and can promote the healing of a contused wound received by a fall from a high place or a sudden blow, or a concussion resulting from a traffic accident. Additional complications also treated by this remedy are the fear, uneasiness, horror, and excitement that follow an accident; flush-up; regurgitation; and mental distress; or even a coma.

2. Tao-ho-cheng-chi-tang　　桃核承氣湯
　　(Persioa and Rhubarb Combination)
This combination is taken for severe pain, the swelling of a contusion, the subepidermal bleeding caused therefrom, and a tendency towards constipation. It also calms emotional excitement and agitation. It is especially effective for a contusion at the perineum that has resulted in urine retention. It is also suitable for patients with a firm fever occlusion of blood and unstrained stamina.

3. Tung-tao-san　　通導散
　　(Tang-kuei and Carthamus Formula)
This formula is taken for subepidermal bleeding caused by a heavy beating as in the ancient corporal punishment mentioned above. It also slows increased heartbeat caused by nervousness.

4. Chi-ming-san　　雞鳴散
　　(Areca Seed and Chaenomeles Formula)
This formula lessens severe swelling from a contusion and should be taken right after sustaining the injury.

5. Chih-ta-pu-i-fang　　治打撲一方
　　(Cinnamon and Nuphar Formula)
This formula is applied externally on painful muscles and bones to relieve swelling following contusion, especially when these symptoms have continued for a long time.

6. Tang-kuei-hsu-san 當歸鬚散
   (Tang-kuei and Lindera Formula)
   This formula is for the chest pain or abdominal pain resulting from a contusion. It is very effective for extravasated blood and the resistant pain when touched of a contusion that has lasted for a long time, especially one in the chest, ribs, abdomen, or loins.

7. Kuei-chih-fu-ling-wan 桂枝茯苓丸
   (Cinnamon and Hoelen Formula)
   This pill is for subdermal bleeding which has become enlarged in scope and purpuric and for swelling in the lower extremities resulting from thrombosis. It is also widely employed for slight injuries caused by whiplash.

8. Yang-po-san 楊柏散
   (Myrica and Phellodendron Formula)
   For pain resulting from a contusion, this formula is mixed with vinegar and egg white to form a putty and then applied to the wound. It can accelerate absorption, mollify the pain, and promoted recovery. For those whose skin is sensitive and likely to erupt in macules as a reaction to the vinegar, the amount applied must be small or the vinegar deleted and only the egg white or wheat flour with water mixed with the *Yang-po-san.*

9. Folk Remedies 民間方
   a. Apply a condensed decoction of chrysanthemum and carthamus as a warm compress onto the contusion. Contusion swelling that has become dark violet may subside in two to three days.
   b. Drink a decoction of the leaf and stalk of the banana plant. It is effective for all contusions.
   c. Mix the ground meal of a small, deboned crucian carp with sugar and apply it to the wound. As the fluid comes out of the mixture, the wound is cured.
   d. On the occasion of suffocation or pseudodeath (unconsciousness) resulting from a contusion due to falling from a high place, open the victim's mouth and pour in urine; the patient will regain consciousness.

Carbuncles and Furunculosis (Boils)

A furuncle (boil) is a deep-seated infection (abscess) involving the entire hair follicle and adjacent subcutaneous tissue. The most common sites of occurrence are the hairy parts of the body exposed to irritation and friction, pressure, or moisture, or to the plugging action of oil based ointments. Because the lesions are autoinoculable, they are often multiple. Thorough investigation usually fails to uncover a predisposing cause, although an occasional patient may have uncontrolled diabetes mellitus, nephritis, or another debilitating disease.

A carbuncle is several furuncles that develop in adjoining hair follicles and coalesce to form a conglomerate. It is a deeply situated mass with multiple drainage points.

Symptoms

The extreme tenderness and pain are due to the pressure on nerve endings, particularly in areas where there is little room for swelling of the underlying structures. The pain, fever, and malaise are more severe in carbuncles than in furuncles. A follicular abscess is either rounded or conical. It gradually enlarges, becomes fluctuant, and then softens and opens spontaneously after a few days or one to two weeks to discharge a core of necrotic tissue and pus. The inflammation occasionally subsides before necrosis occurs.

A carbuncle is much larger than a boil. Instead of having only one core, it will have two or more.

Treatment
1. Systemic anti-infective agents are indicated. Sodium cloxacillin or erythromycin, 1.0g daily by mouth, is usually effective.
2. Bacterial recolonization with a harmless staphylococcus may be tried for recurrent furunculosis.
3. The inflamed area should be immobilized and overmanipulation avoided. Moist heat helps larger lesions to localize. Surgical incision, epilation, or debridgement is done after the lesions are mature. Do not incise deeply. Anti-infective ointment with a bandage should be loosely applied to the area during drainage.
4. The disease is often caused by acidosis as a result of excessive

ingestion of meat or sweets, hence dieting is a good alternative treatment.
5. Chinese herbs are best accompanied by antibiotics; however, for those patients who have severe side effects owing to an allergic constitution, the Chinese prescriptions are the only way of healing.

Chinese Herb Formulas

1. Ko-ken-tang   葛根湯
   (Pueraria Combination)
   Shih-wei-pai-tu-tang   十味敗毒湯
   (Bupleurum and Schizonepeta Combination)

At the beginning stage of the carbuncle or furuncle, there will be reddening, swelling, aching, chills, and fever—all the manifestations of a superficial condensation of fever. These must be dispersed by taking *Ko-ken-tang* for one to two days followed by *Shih-wei-pai-tu-tang* for two to four days. The formulas detoxicate and expel the toxin and comfort the patient.

2. Tuo-li-hsiao-tu-yin   托裏消毒飲
   (Gleditsia Combination)
   Chien-chin-nei-tuo-san   千金內托散
   (Astragalus and Platycodon Formula)

When there is a sign of suppuration rendered by the preceding two formulas, then either *Tuo-li-hsiao-tu-yin* or *Chien-chin-nei-tuo-san* is to be used. *Tuo-li-hsiao-tu-yin* has maturation and detoxication effects while *Chien-chin-nei-tuo-san* acts mainly to maturate the suppuration. Suppuration takes place five to six days after the onset of the disease. That is when these prescriptions are to be taken to disperse or dissipate the lesions or to maturate the pus and produce an opening for the drainage of pus in order to hasten healing. If there is a tendency toward somatic pyemia or cellulitis, *Tuo-li-hsiao-tu-yin* is suitable.

3. Po-chou-san   伯州散
   (Eriocheir and Viper Formula)

This prescription localizes suppurative inflammation, promotes the formation of abscesses, and thus prevents pyemia. It also can augment pus excretion ability, promote granulation, and sometimes bring about an earlier disappearance of suppuration. Thus it is commonly referred to as a "surgery collapser" meaning whenever this drug is at hand there is no more need of a surgeon. But this prescription may aggravate the inflammation, congestion, and aching when it is used during the initial stage of suppuration. This fact must be noted. It is better to use this prescription when suppuration is near culmination and after *Chien-chin-nei-tuo-san* has been used.

4. Tso-tu-kao 左突膏
   (Asphalt Ointment)

This prescription is used at a stage when the abscess has ripened and ruptured or has been incised and the pus is draining. This plaster sucks out the pus and cleans away the rotten tissue. When the pus and the rotten tissue are gone and new granulation appears, then *Tzu-yun-kao* is used, all the while continuing to take *Chien-chin-nei-tuo-san*.

5. Tzu-yun-kao 紫雲膏
   (Lithospermum Ointment)

This ointment promotes granulation; thus healing where there is the loss of tissue which occurs after an abscess treatment. Most carbuncles and furuncles can be cured by using all the processes of treatment mentioned above. In addition there are other prescriptions that supplement the former ones. They are as follows:

6. Nei-shu-huang-lien-tang 內疏黃連湯
   (Coptis and Saussurea Combination)

Patients treated with the preceding prescriptions for carbuncles or furuncles who have severe symptoms of a persistent high fever, dry mouth and tongue, abdominal distention, delirium, and constipation should take this prescription. It is also suitable for patients having cellulitis or an inclination toward pyemia.

7. Shen-kung-nei-tuo-san 神功內托散
   (Tang-kuei, Atractylodes, and Jujube Formula)

Generally *Chien-chin-nei-tuo-san* alone can render the formation of thick pus. If the formation of pus is retarded owing to debility in constitution, the pulse is weak, and there is a strong chill feeling; this prescription is indicated.

8. Kuei-chi-chien-chung-tang 歸耆建中湯
    (Tang-kuei, Astragalus, and Paeonia Combination)
   Shih-chuan-ta-pu-tang 十全大補湯
    (Ginseng and Tang-kuei Ten Combination)
These formulas treat the same symptoms as *Chien-chin-nei-tuo-san*. If the patient cannot recover his stamina and tires easily after the healing of carbuncles or furuncles and there is night sweating, then *Kuei-chi-chien-chung-tang* is appropriate. If the condition has lasted for a long time, then it is suitable to take the second formula.

9. Ta-chai-hu-tang 大柴胡湯
    (Major Bupleurum Combination)
For patients with a strong physique who have severe tension beneath the heart, thoraco-costal distress, and a carbuncle or furuncle on the upper torso, this prescription is effective.

10. Ta-huang-mu-tan-pi-tang 大黃牡丹皮湯
    (Rhubarb and Moutan Combination)
This prescription is suitable for patients with a strong physique and constipation who have carbuncles or furuncles on the hips or in the perianal area. Carbuncles or furuncles in these areas signal a severe condition.

11. Fang-feng-tung-sheng-san 防風通聖散
    (Siler and Platycodon Formula)
When taken continuously, this prescription corrects and improves the physique and constitution of stalwart and obese patients who have hypertension, habitual constipation, and repetitive recurrence of carbuncle or furuncles, especially at the back of the neck or the back of the head.

12. Pai-nung-san 排膿散
    (Platycodon and Chih-shih Formula)
This prescription dissipates or promotes early rupture and healing of localized suppuration when it is slight in severity.

13. Huang-po-mo 黃柏末
    (Phellodendron Powder)
In the beginning stage of the growth of a carbuncle or furuncle

when suppuration is just taking place, a solution of phellodendron powder can be used externally to promote suppuration and localize the inflammation.

14. Ku-sheng-tang 苦參湯
(Sophora Combination)

When the reddening, swelling, and aching of a carbuncle or furuncle are very severe, a decoction of 6.0g of Sophora may alleviate the suffering. It is applied to the lesion in the form of a wash and a cold compress.

15. Folk Medicine: Vespae Nidus 民間藥：露蜂房
(Bee's Nest)

Vespae Nidus or honeycomb, especially that from mountain bees which has been exposed to the sun, rain, and dew in the wild, is widely used for carbuncles, furuncles, and various suppurative diseases. Directions for preparing this medicinal are as follows:
Divide the nest into two halves. Bake one half and keep the other half fresh; pulverize each half individually and mix together equal amounts from each half. The mixture can be taken orally; the daily dose is 2.0-4.0g. The mixture can also be mixed with vinegar and applied to the lesion. It is effective not only for carbuncles or furuncles but also for acute lymphadenitis, mammitis, subdermal tumors, gingivitis, etc., when they do not respond to penicillin therapy. About thirty minutes after administration of this medicinal, the pain is alleviated. For lighter cases, the disease can be diminished solely by taking this medicinal; for severer cases the inflammation is centralized to the core and an opening for pus drainage will form to prompt granulation. Unlike *Po-chou-san,* this medicinal can be used even for the acute stage of severe inflammation.

Frigorism

When the skin is exposed to cold air, the blood vessels contract, the blood condenses, and numbness follows. This phenomenon is known as frigorism.

Most susceptible are those who are also prone to chilblain and who have not taken proper care of themselves. But the hands, toes, and ears of those with glandular diseases, anemia, chilling in the limbs, and kidney diseases are also prone to frigorism.

Symptoms

At first, there is anemia and violet-red skin (first degree). Then blisters appear (second degree). In severe cases, the skin will crack (third degree). Usually, the first degree of this condition is called chilblain; the second and third degrees, frigorism.

Treatment

Patience is necessary in the treatment of this condition. Foods rich in Vitamins C and E (oranges, sweet potatoes, pumpkins, bean sprouts, grains) should be eaten freely. It is also important to exercise the skin. Local massage of the body areas most susceptible to frigorism makes the blood flow more smoothly. Infrared light and sunlight therapy are also effective.

Chinese Herb Formula
Tang-kuei-szu-ni-chia-wu-chu-yu-sheng-chiang-tang
當歸四逆加吳茱萸生薑湯
(Tang-kuei, Evodia, and Ginger Combination)
This is very effective for frigorism. To be taken for chilling of the hands and feet, weak pulse, and tense abdomen.

Acute Suppurative Lymphadenitis

This disease is a manifestation of bacterial infection usually caused by the hemolytic streptococcus. It arises in an area of cellulitis, generally at the site of an infected wound, or occurs as a complication of other suppurative diseases. The wound, which may be very small and superficial or an established abscess, feeds bacteria into the lymphatics.

Symptoms

The involvement of the lymphatics is indicated by a red streak in the skin lined in the direction of the affected lymph nodes which are, in turn, tender and enlarged. Systemic manifestations include fever, chills, and malaise. The infection may progress rapidly, often in a matter of hours, and lead to bacteremia or septicemia and even death. Clinically, throbbing pain is usually present in the area of cellulitis at the site of bacterial invasion. Malaise, anorexia, sweating, chills, and fever (37.8-40°C) develop rapidly. Pain or discomfort is felt in the affected nodes. The red streak, when present, may be definite or it may be very faint and easily missed. It is not usually tender or indurated, as is the area of cellulitis. The involved lymph nodes may be enlarged two to three times their normal size and are often acutely tender. The pulse is usually rapid.

Treatment

Rest, splinting, elevation of the area, heat, and symptomatic treatment of local pain and systemic reaction are helpful. Antibiotic therapy should always be instituted when local infection becomes invasive, as manifested by cellulitis and lymphangitis. Drainage of pus from an infected wound should be carried out, generally after the above measures have been instituted but only when it is an initial infection.

Chinese Herb Formulas
1. Ko-ken-tang 葛根湯
   (Pueraria Combination)
   Shih-wei-pai-tu-tang 十味敗毒湯
   (Bupleurum and Schizonepeta Combination)

At the beginning of the infection when there are only chills and fever or no fever, *Ko-ken-tang* is taken as a dispersant followed by *Shih-wei-pai-tu-tang* as a dispersant and detoxifier.

2. Hsiao-chai-hu-tang-chia-shih-kao 小柴胡湯加石膏
   (Minor Bupleurum Combination plus Gypsum)

If the preceding two formulas fail to cure and the swelling does not go down, this formula may be used to attack the disease from inside. If the incidence is simple, generally only three potions are needed to effect a cure.

3. Tuo-li-hsiao-tu-yin 托裏消毒飲
   (Gleditsia Combination)
   Chien-chin-nei-tuo-san 千金內托散
   (Astragalus and Platycodon Formula)

As the disease advances to the suppuration stage, *Chien-chin-nei-*

tuo-san is to be taken. If the condition of the disease is so severe as to show empyema (presence of pus), then *Tuo-li-hsiao-tu-yin* should be used. Both prescriptions have an internal dissipation effect.

4. Po-chou-san   伯州散
   (*Eriocheir and Viper Formula*)
   Tso-tu-kao   左突膏
   (*Asphalt Ointment*)
   Tzu-yun-kao   紫雲膏
   (*Lithospermum Ointment*)

If administration of *Chien-chin-nei-tuo-san* along with *Po-chou-san* does not bring about internal dissipation, then one must wait until the lesion ruptures at which time *Tso-tu-kao* is applied to draw out the pus. After the pus is gone and only the damaged tissue remains, an application of *Tzu-yun-kao* promotes granulation of the tissue.

5. Folk Medicine: Vespae Nidus   民間方
   (*Bee's Nest or Honeycomb*)

Which has been exposed and unsheltered is used for this purpose. Daily dose is 2.0-4.0g.

Tuberculous Lymphadenitis

This disease, commonly called scrofula, is caused by the tubercle bacillus and occurs mostly in the cervical lymph nodes, tracheobronchial lymph nodes, mesenteric lymph nodes, and only sometimes in the armpit lymph nodes and inguinal lymph nodes. Clinically tuberculosis of the lymph node is classified as either benign or malignant. Histologically it begins with the formation of a tubercle which gradually enlarges and becomes a caseous lesion or a localized lesion resulting in a proliferation of the granulated tissue. The commonly called scrofula belongs to the malignant type. In mesenteric tuberculous lymphadenitis the nodes coalesce into a big mass called tabes mesaraica. Mostly it appears in the small intestinal mesentery in children or in the ileoceum in the adult. The invasion route of the cervical lymphadenitis is through the pharyngeal lymphatic ring, caries, tonsils, mouth, or nasal mucous membrane. It most often occurs in juveniles or those entering puberty who have a poorly built physique and poor nutrition. Tuberculosis of the tracheobronchial lymph nodes occurs as an initial infection from the primary lesion of pulmonary tuberculosis in 80-90 percent of the cases.

Symptoms
A. Tuberculosis of the Tracheobroncial Lymph Nodes
   Generally it is several weeks after the initial infection before the lymph nodes begin to swell. The clinical symptoms appear only after four to six months of infection. In older children the symptoms are imperceptible; in infants there will be fever and cough. As the swelling of lymph nodes becomes severe, the vague nerve and afferent nerve are compressed and the trachea and bronchia attacked, resulting in hiccup-like paroxysms, dyspnea, stridor during respiration, pallor, and a rale caused by tracheal stenosis.
B. Tuberculous Cervical Lymphadenitis
   In this type of tuberculosis, one, two or three lymph nodes usually swell on both sides, in the inferior mandibula, on the lateral side of the neck, inside the cheek, and on the superior recess of the clavicle. Sometimes the inflammation occurs in a host of scattered nodes. The size of the swelling varies and ranges from as small as a bean to as big as an egg. At the beginning the gland looks like a compressed ball or oval having either rigidity or elasticity or even elastic tenderness, but as it becomes caseous, the rigidity gradually softens. As suppuration occurs, a waving movement can be seen. In the initial stage there is no coalescence; the skin and the base being moveable. As the disease advances, perinodal inflammation occurs, the perinodal tissue coalesces, and the motility disappears. As a consequence of the internodal coalescence, the skin becomes wavy, and swollen tumors of uneven rigidity form. Next the skin becomes reddened and thin; then a rupture occurs resulting in an indomitable tuberculous fistula and a residual ulcer. Such skin change is called scrofuloderma.
C. Mesenteric Lymphadenitis
   First there is an acute onset of abdominal pain in the right lower quadrant of the periumbilical area. The pain is generally

steady from the onset rather than colicky. Nausea, vomiting, and anorexia result. Diarrhea often occurs. The abdominal tenderness is mild to severe and usually greatest in the right lower quadrant; localization of pain is unusual while peritoneal irritation and right vault rectal tenderness are mild or absent. A fever to 37.8-39.5°C is usually present.

Treatment

Chinese medical prescriptions are chosen on the basis of the symptoms of the disease; however, the best treatment combines them with Western medical chemotherapy and antibiotics such as INAH, PAS, Streptomycin, Ethambutol, or Rifamycin.

Chinese Herb Formulas

1. **Hsiao-chai-hu-tang** 小柴胡湯
 (Minor Bupleurum Combination)

In the book *Main Indications,* the chapter on *Hsiao-chai-hu-tang* lists tuberculosis lymphadenitis indications as thoraco-costal distress, distention, stiffness and stuffiness under the ribs, or a rigid and stiff neck which implies occluded and obstructed fever within the lymph nodes of the neck or the armpit. The addition of gypsum to *Hsiao-chai-hu-tang* can disperse the slight fever and dissolve the nodal swelling.

On occasion *Hsiao-chai-hu-tang* is used with 2.0g each of prunella, fritillaria, oyster shell and trichosanthes root added.

2. **Hsiao-yao-san-chia-chien-fang** 逍遙散加減方
 (The Modified Prescription of Bupleurum and Tang-kuei Formula)

When *Hsiao-chai-hu-tang* and its modified prescription fail to cure and the patient is suffering from malnutrition and debility, especially female patients, then 2.0g each of prunella, fritillaria, oyster shell, and trichosanthes root are added to *Hsiao-yao-san* as a modified prescription for scrofula.

3. **Chai-hu-ching-kan-san** 柴胡清肝散
 (Bupleurum and Rehmannia Formula)

This formula can be used lengthily as a tonic by patients whose skin has darkened and whose condition calls for *Hsiao-chai-hu-*

tang. The abdominal wall will be thick and completely tensive.

4. **San-chung-kuei-chien-tang** 散腫潰堅湯
   (Forsythia and Laminaria Combination)
When all the foregoing formulas fail to cure and the lesion is a big, malignant tumor that does not show any tendency to diminish, this formula may be taken lengthily.

5. **Kuei-chi-chien-chung-tang** 歸耆建中湯
   (Tang-kuei, Astragalus, and Paeonia Combination)
This formula is suitable for prolonged intake by patients having a weak physique and a lyphadenoma that has turned into a fistula.

6. **Po-chou-san** 伯州散
   (Eriocheir and Viper Formula)
This formula is used as an auxillary treatment for patients with somatic debility and tuberculous fistulas.

7. **I-chi-yang-jung-tang** 益氣養榮湯
   (Ginseng, Tang-kuei, and Cyperus Combination)
   Kuei-pi-tang 歸脾湯
   (Ginseng and Longan Combination)
   Shih-chuan-ta-pu-tang 十全大補湯
   (Ginseng and Tang-kuei Ten Combination)
This is the formula of choice for debilitated and anemic patients whose conditions have been caused by prolonged suffering and an incessant discharge of pus.

8. **Tsing-fu-tang** 淨腑湯
   (Bupleurum and Pinellia Combination)
This formula treats inflamed posterior peritoneal lymph nodes and mesenteric lymph nodes that have caused completely rigid and tensive distention beneath the heart. The lymph nodes have undergone coalescence when patients have alternating chills and fever, thirst, and red and obstructed urine.

9. **Hsiao-kan-yin** 消疳飲
   (Cinnamon and Apricot Seed Combination)
Infantile splenic helminthiasis (a disease caused by parasitic worms) of ancient times is actually mesenteric lymphadenitis;

this is also the so-called *pi-chi* disease. This formula is indicated for patients who have passed through the *Tsing-fu-tang* stage, because the disease has now become chronic. The patient has emaciated limbs, a mummy-like face, no fever, debility, a distended belly like a frog, and an abnormally large appetite.

Tuberculosis of the Bone

This disease rarely occurs as a primary infection but rather results as a secondary, circulatory infection from a remote tuberculous lesion in the body or from a continuous invasion of nearby infected tissue. It affects mostly the ends or middle portion of long bones and the short bones. Bone marrow involvement is very frequently encountered in juveniles. The tuberculous lesion forms in the bone marrow and destroys the surrounding bone tissue, a condition leading to bone gangrene and the formation of cold abscesses. Periosteum tuberculosis occurs mostly in adult patients. Here the tuberculosis destroys the fibrous membrane covering the bone, and the lesion invades the marrow causing a caries state. The beginning stage is almost symptomless, but as the lesion progresses toward the soft tissue, vivid and percussive pain appears.

Symptoms

Symptoms are generally the same as for tubercular arthritis. x-ray revelation of the lesion will show later than the clinical symptoms. The bone shadow is light and slow destruction and erosion are evident. Osteohyperplasia occurs at a later stage during recuperation.

Treatment

It is important to improve the general health and get sufficient bed rest. Chemotherapy is needed to heal the local lesions and arrest the disease. The Chinese herb formulas recommended below are designed to improve the tubercular physique. They generally are effective if used in accordance with the stage and progress of the disease.

Chinese Herb Formulas

1. **Kuei-chi-chien-chung-tang**　　　　　　歸耆建中湯
   (Tang-kuei, Astragalus, and Paeonia Combination)

This formula is made by adding *tang-kuei* and astragalus to *Hsiao-chien-chung-tang*. It treats somatic fatigue; exhausted stamina; a big but forceless pulse or a submerged, minute and thin pulse; and the exhaustion of both *ch'i* and blood internally and externally. When ginseng, atractylodes, and rehmannia are added to this formula, it becomes *Shih-chuan-ta-pu-tang*. Tuberculosis sufferers mostly have underdeveloped bones and muscles, malnutrition, an emaciated build, a narrow angle of the epigastrium, and a bulging but weak abdominal wall. This formula taken for a long period ameliorates tuberculosis of bones by strengthening the body.

2. **Shih-chuan-ta-pu-tang**　　　　　　十全大補湯
   (Ginseng and Tang-kuei Ten Combination)

This formula is indicated for patients who are totally weak, inside and out, in *ch'i* and blood or in yin and yang. Some people become so excessively weak all over their bodies that the G I activity is also weakened. Then the patient will show conspicuous anemia and aridity of the skin but no fever. This formula augments vitality and promotes nutrition; thus it can cure the disease radically.

3. **Kuei-pi-tang**　　　　　　歸脾湯
   (Ginseng and Longan Combination)

If *Shih-chuan-ta-pu-tang* causes an obstructed feeling in the chest and a loss of appetite, this formula is appropriate. In addition it is also very effective in relieving neurotic symptoms and insomnia.

4. **Kua-tzu-jen-tang-chia-chieh-keng**　　　　瓜子仁湯加桔梗
   (Benincasa Combination plus Platycodon)

This formula is for when the body strength has not diminished but the patient has cold abscesses in the lower abdomen and a fistula with continuously draining pus.

5. **Huang-lien-hsiao-tu-yin**　　　　　　黃連消毒飲
   (Coptis and Stephania Combination)

This formula is used to prevent the formation of fistulas that continuously discharge pus. It is taken for a long time by people who are still rather vigorous but have suffered from the disease for a period of time.

6. **Kuei-pan-tang** 龜板湯
    (Tortoise Shell Combination)
    This combination is for spinal bone gangrene and paralysis in the lower torso making the patient unable to walk. It is suitable only for patients with a good and healthy stomach and intestines. The combination is formed by adding 3.0g each of turtle shell and Haliotidis Concha to *Szu-ni-tang*.

7. **Po-chou-san** 伯州散
    (Eriocheir and Viper Formula)
    This formula purges pus and detoxifies. It is also a warm tonic and can be used as a complementary medicine for tuberculosis of the bones.

Acute Serous Arthritis

This disease occurs as a consequence of articular contusion, excessive physical activity, or the transmigration of either rheumatism, gonorrhea, influenza, or an acute infectious disease which causes secondary infection.

Symptoms
External traumas or contusions may cause a primary or secondary inflammatory congestion in the synovial membrane which becomes enlarged after healing. In arthritis serofibrinosa, the synovial bursa fills with turbid fluid, and a fibrous pseudomembrane clogs the inner wall of the joint bursa.

Treatment
In the acute stage a cold compress is generally applied as a palliative treatment, and the patient is kept at rest and medicated with the following formulas.

Chinese Herb Formulas

1. Ma-hsing-i-kan-tang-chia-chu   麻杏薏甘湯加朮
 (Ma-huang and Coix Combination with Atractylodes)
Originally this formula was used for individuals who were frequently subjected to the wind while sweating or for those who suffered from diseases incurred from a long-term common cold. The prescription works against internal water and swelling and pain occurring in the muscles or joints. It is often taken for the swelling and pain of serous arthritis during the initial stage.

2. Yueh-pi-chia-chu-tang   越婢加朮湯
 (Atractylodes Combination)
This formula is found in the book *Shui Ch'i Ping* (Water Moisture Diseases). It is for tumidity as a result of the internal water overflowing and floating, along with sweating and oliguria. Hence it is suitable for edematous swelling and pain in the joints of the lower extremities at the onset of arthritis.

3. Fang-chi-huang-chi-tang   防己黃耆湯
 (Stephania and Astragalus Combination)
The indications for this formula are water toxin on the surface, superficial weakness, and circulatory disturbance between the *ch'i* and blood in the lower extremities which has caused swelling and pain in the knee joint. People for whom this formula is suited have white skin, flaccid muscles, a tendency to tire easily, hyperhidrosis (excessive sweating), oliguria, and a soft and flabby lower abdomen; in other words, this formula is indicated for weak conformational arthritis in so-called "water-obese" individuals.

4. Shu-ching-huo-hsueh-tang   疏經活血湯
 (Clematis and Stephania Combination)
When the muscles or joints of the lower limbs are aching severely because of occluded blood, water toxin, or wind and chills, this formula frees the occluded blood and disperses the wind and moisture. It is good for serous arthritis. When all the foregoing formulas are no longer applicable and the disease has become chronic, this formula is especially efficaceous.

5. Hsu-ming-tang   續命湯
 (Ma-huang and Ginseng Combination)

This formula is for arthritis or rheumatism in a person with a *Yueh-pi-tang* conformation and a tendency toward anemia.

6. Kuei-shao-chih-mu-tang 桂芍知母湯
    (Cinnamon and Anemarrhena Combination)

This formula is good for articular rheumatism or arthritis that causes swelling and pain. It is especially good for knee joint swelling and muscular atrophy in the muscles above and beneath the knee resulting in "crane-knee" deformity. It is also effective for akinesia (loss of or impaired motor function) and dysesthesia (impairment of the senses) of the lower limbs.

7. I-yi-jen-tang 薏苡仁湯
    (Coix Combination)

This combination is effective for subacute and chronic articular rheumatism and serous arthritis or tuberculous arthritis.

Acute Pyogenic Arthritis

Pyogenic means "pus-producing." Primarily pyogenic arthritis comes from a fissure or wound in the joint. Other causes can be nearby pyogenic osteomyelitis or periostitis or cellulitis. Oftentimes the pyogenic bacteria is carried in the blood stream.

This pyogenic cocci (gonococcus, meningococcus, staphylococcus, pneumococcus, and streptococcus), *Haemophilus influenzae,* and gram-negative bacilli are the usual causes of this form of arthritis. The organisms enter the joints directly through a local trauma or injection, or from an adjacent bone, or from the blood stream. In recent years this type of disease has become more common as a result of the development of resistant strains of organisms, the increase in therapeutic use of intra-articular injections, and the decrease in the mortality of premature infants in whom the incidence of septic arthritis is relatively high. Worldwide increase of gonococcal infections, particularly anti-biotic-resistant strains, poses a special problem. Pathologic changes of pyogenic arthritis include varying degrees of acute inflammation with synovitis, effusion, abscess formation in synovial or subchondral tissues, and, if treatment is not adequate, articular destruction.

Since this disease involves cellulitis or somatic infection the following Chinese herb formulas are recommended. However, it is always best to combine them with antibiotic therapy.

Symptoms

The onset of the disease is usually sudden; the joint becomes acutely painful, feverish, and swollen, and chills and fever are often present. In gonococcal infections, disseminated infections may be seen in individuals whose primary infection was asymptomatic. The large weight-bearing joints and the wrists are the most frequently affected. Although only one or two joints are affected, there may be a prodromal period of migratory arthralgia lasting for several days. This condition is especially true during the period of bacteremia (bacteria in the blood).

Special attention needs to be called to the systemic manifestations of gonococcal infection. Disseminated infection is seen commonly in individuals whose proctogenital or throat infection was asymptomatic. Dissemination in females usually occurs during pregnancy or menstruation. The initial bacteremic stage may persist for weeks and be characterized not only by migratory arthralgia but also by chills and fever or normal temperature and skin lesions. The latter are commonly tiny red papules of petechiae vesicular, pustular, and bullous stages. The infecting organism may be extracted from these lesions. Tenosynovitis (inflammation of the tendon sheath) is commonly observed. Less common systemic complications are liver function abnormalities, myocarditis or pericarditis, meningitis, and endocarditis.

Treatment

Prompt systemic antibiotic therapy should be given based on the best clinical judgement of the causative organism arrived at by the results of a smear and culture of the joint fluid, blood, urine, or specific sites of infection. If the organism cannot be determined clinically, treatment should be started with bactericidal antibiotics effective against staphylococci, pneumococci, gonococci, and gram-negative organisms. Cultures for gonococci require immediate inoculation of Thayer-Martin medium.

Frequent (even daily) local aspiration is sometimes indicated. Incision and drainage are rarely required. Local hot compresses and immobilization of the joint with a splint or traction (or both) relieves pain. Rest, immobilization, and elevation of the affected part are sued at the onset of treatment. Subsequent motion exercises within the limits of tolerance will hasten recovery.

Chinese Herb Formulas
1. Kan-tsao-fu-tzu-tang　　　　　　　　　　甘草附子湯
   (Licorice and Aconite Combination)
This formula is used primarily for acute rheumatism that aches violently. However, whether it is acute or chronic rheumatism, this prescription always works. The formula takes as its targets the struggle between wind (including externally incurred diseases and bacterial infections) and moisture (including all internal water toxins) that have aroused the drastic arthritic symptoms of articular swelling, aching, anemophobia, spontaneous sweating, and oliguria. The pulse is generally buoyant, weak, and quick.

2. Huang-chi-chien-chung-tang　　　　　　黃耆建中湯
   (Astragalus Combination)
This combination is used for lingering swelling and aching that is becoming chronic, weakness inside and out, persistent night sweats, and somatic weakness. It is also suitable for long lasting suppuration which has fatigued the patient.

3. Tuo-li-hsiao-tu-yin　　　　　　　　　　托裏消毒飲
   (Gleditsia Combination)
This combination is for purulent conditions in the fourth to the seventh day. It dissipates the pathogen, prevents toxicity of pus and the occurrence of toxemia, reinforces body strength, and arrests inward invasion of the toxin. It can also accelerate pus discharge and healing. In minor cases this formula may dissipate the pyogenesis internally.

4. Chien-chin-nei-tuo-san　　　　　　　　千金內托散
   (Astragalus and Platycodon Formula)
This combination is to be used by individuals in whom suppuration has been on-going, reducing body stamina and worsening fatigue and weakness. It increases stamina and disperses the toxin. Toxin in milder cases is internally dissipated by this formula.

5. **Po-chou-san** 伯州散
   (Eriocheir and Viper Formula)
   This formula is used as a complement to *Tuo-li-hsiao-tu-yin* or *Chien-chin-nei-tuo-san*. It dissolves pus and quickens healing.

6. **Folk Medicine** 民間方
   2.0-4.0g Vespae Nidus (bee's nest) taken daily.

Tuberculous Arthritis

This disease is a secondary infection of *Mycobacterium* tuberculosis that attacks young men in the knee and femur joints. Articular bruises, contusions, and overwork are the inducing and hidden causes. In ancient times this disease was called *her-hsi-feng* meaning "crane-knee wind." Clinically it is divided into tuberculous edema, granuloarticular tuberculosis, and tuberculous pyoarthritis.

Infections of the musculoskeletal system are commonly caused by the blood circulating the bacteria of a primary lesion in the respiratory or gastrointestinal tract. Thus tuberculosis of the thoracic or lumbar spine usually comes from an active lesion of the genitourinary tract. A disease of childhood, it occurs most commonly before puberty. Adult infection is uncommon except in debilitated geriatric patients.

Symptoms

The onset of symptoms is generally insidious, not showing alarming general manifestations of fever, sweating, toxicity, or prostration. Pain in the region of an involved joint may be mild at onset and accompanied by a sensation of stiffness. The pain is commonly accentuated at night. Limping is a mechanism to protect a weight-bearing joint. Restriction of joint motion during the early phase of the infection is another protective mechanism. As the disease progresses, limitation of joint motion becomes fixed because of muscle contractures and organic destruction of the joint.

Local findings during the early stages may be limited to tenderness, soft tissue swelling, joint effusion, and an increase in skin temperature about the involved area. If the disease progresses without treatment, muscular atrophy and deformity occur. Abscesses with spontaneous external drainage lead to sinus or canal formation. Progressive destruction of bone in the spine, especially in the thoraco-lumber region, may cause a humped back. X-ray manifestations are not predictable or especially helpful, there being a latent period between the onset of symptoms and the initial positive x-ray finding. The earliest changes of tuberculous arthritis are soft tissue swelling and distention of the capsule of effusion. Subsequently, bone atrophy causes a thinning of the trabecular pattern, a narrowing of the cortex, and an enlargement of the medullar canal. As the disease progresses in a joint, destruction of cartilage narrows the joint cleft and erodes the articular surface, especially at the margins.

Treatment

The modern treatment of tuberculosis of the skeletal system comes in three parts: general care, surgery, and chemotherapy.
A. General Measures. Especially important when prolonged recumbency is necessary is skillful nursing care, adequate diet, and appropriate treatment of the associated lesions (pulmonary, genitourinary, etc.).
B. Surgical Treatment. No rigid recommendations can be made for the operative treatment of tuberculosis because the stage of the infection and the character of the lesion are the determinants. In acute infections where synovitis is the predominant feature, treatment can be conservative, at least initially. Immobilization by splint or plaster, aspiration of the abscess, and chemotherapy may suffice to control the infection. Various types of operative treatment are necessary for chronic or advanced tuberculosis of the bones and joints depending upon the location of the lesion and the age and general condition of the patient.
C. Chemotherapy. Modern chemotherapy of tuberculosis is based essentially on the systematic administration of drugs to which the strain of pathogen is likely to be susceptible as indicated by *in vitro* testing. Resistant strains are likely to emerge during administration of single drugs. Therefore, combinations of antituberculosis agents are recommended. Although isoniazid (INH) plus aminosalicylic acid (PAS) with or without streptomycin have been used widely in the

past, combinations of isoniazid and ethambutol or rifampin and ethambutol are now employed more frequently. Other useful but more toxic drugs include viomycin, capreomycin, pyrazinamide, cycloserine, and ethionamide.

Chinese Herb Formulas

1. **Ma-hsing-i-kan-tang-chia-chu** 麻杏薏甘湯加朮
   (Ma-huang and Coix Combination plus Atractylodes)

This compound is often used for tuberculous edema which may be treated in a way similar to serous arthritis. According to the patient's physique and disease condition, *Yueh-pi-chia-chu-tang, Fang-chi-huang-chi-tang,* or *I-yi-jen-tang* may be used respectively.

2. **Ta-fang-feng-tang** 大防風湯
   (Major Siler Combination)

This combination is for granular arthritis, the so-called *her-chi-feng* mentioned above. It is manifested by the swelling being in a spindle form and the skin surface being glossy and tensive like white wax. The criterion for administration of this formula is no fever and a weak conformation.

3. **Kua-tzu-jen-tang-chia-chieh-keng** 瓜子仁湯加桔梗
   (Benincasa Combination plus Platycodon)

This combination is also used for bone tuberculosis. On the occasion of tuberculous arthritis with suppuration, this formula may halt the progression of the disease and bring about a cure.

4. **Kuei-chi-chien-chung-tang** 歸耆建中湯
   (Tang-kuei, Astragalus, and Paeonia Combination)

When there is fistula formation and the patient has a tubercular, weak physique, the prolonged intake of this formula may strengthen the body. It is more efficaceous when used in combination with *Po-chou-san*.

5. **Shih-chuan-ta-pu-tang** 十全大補湯
   (Ginseng and Tang-kuei Ten Combination)

Suppuration and a fistula with pus discharging causes deterioration in body strength and anemia. If these symptoms appear, this formula should be taken lengthily At the same time, *Po-chou-san* may be taken and *Tso-tu-kao* applied to the lesion. When the pus lessens and the fistula is still open, the plaster of *Tso-tu-kao* is replaced with *Tzu-yun-kao*.

Hernia

Hernia is the protrusion of an organ or part of an organ, such as the intestine, through an opening in the wall surrounding it. Inguinal hernia and umbilical hernia are the types of hernia most often found in infants.

Symptoms
An inguinal hernia may develop from crying, from straining at stools, or from carrying heavy objects. The side of the thigh becomes swollen. Boys may develop scrotal hernia.

Treatment
For mild cases, a hot towel applied to the site of the hernia or a truss belt will correct and ease the condition. In severe cases, surgery is necessary.

Chinese Herb Formulas
1. Hsiao-chien-chung-tang　　　　　　　　　小建中湯
   (Minor Cinnamon and Paeonia Combination)
This formula is for a hernia in children with a delicate constitution; it should be taken frequently.

2. Kuei-chih-chia-shao-yao-tang　　　　　　桂枝加芍藥湯
   (Cinnamon and Paeonia Combination)
This formula is for children with a hernia and abdominal pain.

Periproctal Abscess

An abscess sometimes develops around the anus and rectum as a result of periproctitis. The abscess is one of two types: acute purulent periproctal abscess or tubercular periproctal abscess. Anatomically the abscess is differentiated according to its location: superficial subdermal abscess, submucous abscess, abscess at the sciatico-rectal recess under the anal elevating muscle, and abscess at the sciatico-rectal cavity above the anal elevating muscle. Acute purulent abscess is mostly caused by streptococcus, streptomyces, or *E. coli* infection of the rectal mucus, while the tubercular periproctal abscess is caused by tuberculosis bacillus. Tubercular periproctal abscesses occur alone or in combination with the purulent periproctal abscesses.

Symptoms

At the beginning an emanating pain from the perianus and a sensation of strong pressure are felt, accompanied by a rise in body temperature. Local swelling, necrosis, pain when touched, and reddening are evident; in addition, the superficial abscess has obvious undulation. In a pure tuberculosis infection symptoms are lacking except for the local undulating swelling. Rarely will "self-collapse" or spontaneous healing take place in the beginning. The symptoms appear only after acute purulent periproctitis has also taken over along with the tuberculosis periproctal abscess.

Treatment

In case of pustulation, the abscess is incised and the pus purged. The symptoms then disappear immediately, and the illness is cured. Occasionally a fistula is formed and remains. In tubercular abscess, regardless of whether it is a self-collapsed or incised abscess, complete recovery is rare. In most cases a fistula will remain. In a combined infection, incision of the abscess relieves the patient of the suffering but does not prevent fistulation.

Chinese Herb Formulas

1. **Ta-huang-mu-tan-pi-tang** 大黃牡丹皮湯
   (Rhubarb and Moutan Combination)

This formula is taken during the initial stage when the swelling and pain are very apparent, and there is high fever, constipation, and retention of urine. After taking this formula, the swelling usually subsides quickly and there is no need to undergo an operation.

2. **Teng-lung-tang** 騰龍湯
   (Moutan and Persica Combination)

This combination is a modified formula used in conditions similar to the above. Generally it is used when the abscess is proceeding slowly or has lasted a number of days and is becoming chronic. According to the condition, the doses of rhubarb and mirabilitum are adjusted.

3. **Tuo-li-hsiao-tu-yin** 托裏消毒飲
   (*Gleditsia Combination*)
   Chien-chin-nei-tuo-san 千金內托散
   (*Astragalus and Platycodon Formula*)

These two formulas are for people with a tubercular or emaciated physique who cannot take the previous two formulas. These formulas are also taken in cases where the pus is discharging and the abscess is progressing chronically, or where a fistula with thin pus has formed.

4. **Shih-chuan-ta-pu-tang** 十全大補湯
   (*Ginseng and Tang-kuei Ten Combination*)

If a fistula forms that oozes pus incessantly, the patient grows anemic and somatically weak. This formula is for such a situation. It and the preceding two are the most effective when combined with *Po-chou-san*.

5. **Tso-tu-kao** 左突膏
   (*Asphalt Ointment*)
   Tzu-yun-kao 紫雲膏
   (*Lithospermum Ointment*)

A severely swollen and aching abscess with suppuration but no opening for the discharge of the pus needs to be encouraged to form an opening. This plaster applied topically does this. If a fistula has been formed, application of *Tzu-yun-kao* will promote granulation of the wound.

Anal Fistula

A fistula is an abnormal tube-like passage or opening from a normal cavity to an opening in the skin or to another cavity. An anal fistula goes from the rectum to an opening in the skin near the anus, serving as another anus without the benefit of a sphincter.

Symptoms

The fistula discharges intermittently causing soiling of clothing and a constant unpleasant odor from the fecal substance. The rectum is usually sore rather than painful.

Treatment

Treatment is always surgical. The fistula is either closed or completely removed. A fistula never heals by itself.

Chinese Herb Formulas

1. Tang-kuei-lien-chiao-tang 當歸連翹湯
(Tang-kuei and Forsythia Combination)

This formula is to be taken by persons with an anal fistula and a darkening of their skin. The skin is also arid, harsh as sand paper, and glossless. It is a brownish color. This formula is to be taken for a long time.

2. Chin-chiu-fang-feng-tang 秦艽防風湯
(Chin-chiu and Siler Combination)

This formula is to be taken by patients with a firm physique, a tendency toward constipation, pain during bowel movement, and frequent pustulation. It is also suitable for hemorrhoidal pain and bleeding. The rhubarb can be increased or reduced depending on the severity of the constipation.

3. Fang-feng-tung-sheng-san 防風通聖散
(Siler and Platycodon Formula)

This formula is for patients with an obese and firm constitution who have syphilitic or non-tuberculosis anal fistula and frequent constipation. The purgative detoxification caused by this formula ameliorates the condition.

4. Tuo-li-hsiao-tu-yin 托裏消毒飲
(Gleditsia Combination)
Chien-chin-nei-tuo-san 千金內托散
(Astragalus and Platycodon Formula)

This formula may be used along with *Po-chou-san* for an anal fistula with persistent pustulation causing the sufferer to become fatigued and weakened. *Chien-chin-nei-tuo-san* is especially suitable for patients who have suffered from the illness for a long time and have become weakened.

5. Kuei-chi-chien-chung-tang   歸耆建中湯
    (Tang-kuei, Astragalus, and Paeonia Combination)
    Kuei-pi-tang   歸脾湯
    (Ginseng and Longan Combination)
    Shih-chuan-ta-pu-tang   十全大補湯
    (Ginseng and Tang-kuei Ten Combination)

Kuei-chi-chien-chung-tang and *Kuei-pi-tang* are for chronic cases with ceaseless suppuration which is leading to anemia and somatic feebleness. It is best to use this combination with *Po-chou-san* and to apply *Tzu-yun-kao* externally. At the culmination of anemia it is necessary to switch to *Shih-chuan-ta-pu-tang*.

Prolapse of the Anus and of the Rectum

There are two kinds of anal prolapse, namely, hemorrhoidal and true anal prolapse. The former most frequently occurs at the time of bowel movement. The latter rarely occurs, but when it does, is found only in children who have had continued and prolonged diarrhea or in the aged when the anal and rectal muscle layer has noticeably atrophied. According to the severity, anal prolapse is divided into three classes, namely, (1) anal mucosa prolapse; (2) prolapse of the whole segment of anus; and (3) anorectal prolapse, a true anal prolapse, in which the anus along with part of the rectal ampulla is involved.

In rectal prolapse the rectal wall falls outside the anal ring; a prolapsed rectum cannot be returned to its normal position. Narrowly defined, then, rectal prolapse refers to the prolapse of the rectum per se, but broadly defined it refers to prolapse of the anus also. Anal prolapse indicates only the prolapse of anal mucosa. The scope of rectal prolapse covers prolapse of the peritoneal portion of Douglas pouch in which the abdominal viscera have also slipped from place. This is called rectal hernia and is found mostly in pediatric and geriatric patients.

Symptoms

Rectal prolapse is easily recognized by the many long transverse recesses at the upper center portion of the rectal mucosa. Slight pressure on the abdomen will cause discomfort, pain, and even hemorrhaging.

Treatment

In children the prolapsed organ may be returned to place and the anus compressed with a heavy pad of gauze to prevent subsequent prolapse. In adults an operation is necessary to cut out the hemorrhoids or the prolapsed anal mucosa or to repair the area by means of Thiersch anal plastic surgery. Pagre analplasty can also simply and successfully cure it. For severe rectal prolapse a more complex and intricate operation is necessary. A detailed description is beyond the scope of this work.

Chinese Herb Formulas

1. Wang-yiu-tang　　　　　　　　　　　　　　忘憂湯
    (Licorice Combination)

When it is difficult to return the prolapsed part to its original place and it aches painfully, the area should be washed with a concentrated decoction of licorice or covered with warm compresses to soften the mucosa. Next the mucosa is gently rubbed with some emolient oil and then put little by little into place. Gradually, it may be completely returned. Often it is better returned by forcing it in form around the external side of the prolapsed mucosa instead of in the center.

2. Pu-chung-i-chi-tang　　　　　　　　　　　補中益氣湯
    (Ginseng and Astragalus Combination)
    Chih-shih-chih-tang　　　　　　　　　　　赤石脂湯
    (Kaolin Combination)

Anal prolapse generally is caused by a slackening of tissues other than in the anus. These formulas are given to people with flaccid skin and muscles and a weak constitution for an extended period to strengthen the muscle tissue thus preventing prolapse.

3. Ti-kang-san　　　　　　　　　　　　　　　提肛散
    (Tang-kuei and Kaolin Formula)

This is the two above formulas combined, so it has a similar effect. Made in powder form, it is suitable for prolonged use.

4. Tang-kuei-shao-yao-san　　　　　　　　　當歸芍藥散
    (Tang-kuei and Paeonia Formula)

This formula is efficaceous for women with a cold conformation who have anemia, anal prolapse, "blind piles," and aching.

5. Tang-kuei-chien-chung-tang　　　　　　　當歸建中湯
   (Tang-kuei, Cinnamon, and Paeonia Combination)
This formula is for patients who tend to be anemic and have proctal prolapse with violent pain.

6. Liu-chun-tzu-tang　　　　　　　　　　　六君子湯
   (Major Six Herb Combination)
Those who suffer from anal prolapse with persistent hemorrhoidal bleeding and resultant severe anemia and weakened vitality can take this formula for a long time if the other hematonics cause a sensation of chest obstruction and anorexia.

7. Ma-hsing-kan-shih-tang　　　　　　　　麻杏甘石湯
   (Ma-huang and Apricot Seed Combination)
This combination is most suitable for patients who have anal prolapse due to hemorrhoids; drastic pain, distention, and suppression in the lower abdomen; and painful defecation.

8. Moxibustion on Pai-huei Point　　　　　　百會之灸

In patients with a weak physique, the anal prolapse may be difficult to cure. However, moxibustion applied to the *pai-huei* point with ten to twelve moxa sticks may prove helpful.

Felon (Panaris)

This illness is defined broadly by some doctors as acute purulent inflammation of the hand while others restrict it to acute purulent inflammation of the fingertips. Generally, then, it refers to acute purulent inflammation of the fingers and toes, especially the former. The typical presentation is subcutaneous cellulitis of the finger or the terminal segment of the finger because this part is anatomically different from the other parts. Subcutaneous tissue consists of numerous tough and resilient connective tissue fibers. When fingers become infected, the inflammation can barely enlarge sideways. As a consequence, the inflammation has a strong tendency to go inward until it reaches the bone. Moreover, the fluid, entrapped in cysts, exerts strong pressure on the tissues causing the sensory nerves, which are abundantly distributed at the end of the finger, to ache violently. The blood vessels that supply nutrition to the fingertip eventually die. Felon is classified according to the site of inflammation: intradermal felon, tendon felon, bone felon, and articular felon. If the fingernail is involved, it is divided into peripheral felon (panaritium panrunguate) or subnail felon (paronychia). Since tendon felon has continuous purulent osteomyelitis and periostitis or purulent arthritis, some doctors treat it as an individual disease.

Symptoms

The typical felon exhibits severe topical pain with swelling, reddening of the skin, a feverish sensation, and pain when touched.

Treatment

In most cases it is necessary to make a complete and thorough incision in the felon during the initial stage. For subnail felon partial removal of the nail is mandatory. The nail regrows in about three months. For tendon felon, the incision is made at the knuckle, avoiding the central line. In bone felon the eroded bone is removed. For articular felon, incision and fixation of the joint are necessary. If anesthesia is called for, Oberst conduction blocking anesthesia is mostly employed. When both the bone and joint are infected, it takes a longer time to heal. For the soft tissue it generally takes three to four weeks. Internal medical therapy with Chinese herbs is effective for mild cases. For felon with cellulitis or necrosis, prognosis is unpredictable.

Chinese Herb Formulas
1. **Wu-wu-ta-huang-tang**　　　　　　　　　　五物大黃湯
   (Rhubarb Five Herb Combination)
   Raw Egg Therapy　　　　　　　　　　　　生卵療法

These two treatments are for mild, beginning cases. They are combined in the following manner:
1. Immerse the infected finger into a cold decoction of *Wu-wu-ta-huang-tang*.

2. Perforate an egg just large enough for the finger to be plunged inside at one end.
   3. Insert the infected finger into the egg and raise the finger to eye level. Hold in that position for several minutes.
   4. Alternately do the two treatments for about an hour. Most mild cases can be cured by this method.

2. **Pai-nung-tang** 排膿湯
   (Platycodon and Jujube Combination)
   Pai-nung-san 排膿散
   (Platycodon and Chih-shih Formula)

At the onset of mild cases when pustulation has not yet occurred and there is no apparent rigid bulge, *Pai-nung-tang* relieves the pain and cures the felon in no time. If pustulation has occurred, the finger aches violently, the lesion is tensive and hardened, the blood and *ch'i* are stagnant, and inflammatory infiltration is very deep. *Pai-nung-san* not only can prevent further pustulation but can also purge the pus.

3. **Chien-chin-nei-tuo-san** 千金內托散
   (Astragalus and Platycodon Formula)

This formula is suitable for mild felon in which pustulation has been going on for a period of time, the pus being continuously excreted.

4. **Chung-huang-kao** 中黃膏
   (Curcuma and Phellodendron Ointment)

This formula promotes the absorption of pus or the formation of an opening in the abscess to discharge the pus.

5. **Tzu-yun-kao** 紫雲膏
   (Lithospermum Ointment)

This formula applied topically heals the abscess hole which rarely closes by itself.

Gangrene

The causes of gangrene of the lower limbs are many. The representative ones are arteriosclerosis and diabetes mellitus.

Symptoms
Gangrene is one kind of necrosis in which the dead and collapsed tissue turns brown to black in color because of denatured hemoglobin at the external surface.

Treatment
For severe cases surgical procedures are necessary. In Chinese treatments, the following four countermeasures are employed: (1) treatment of arteriosclerosis according to the physique; (2) employment of prescriptions, chiefly purgatives; (3) treatment to allay the pain; and (4) prescriptions for extreme chill.

Chinese Herb Formulas
1. Ta-chai-hu-tang　　　　　　　　　　　　　　大柴胡湯
   (Major Bupleurum Combination)
   Tao-ho-cheng-chi-tang　　　　　　　　　　桃核承氣湯
   (Persica and Rhubarb Combination)
   Ta-huang-mu-tan-pi-tang　　　　　　　　　大黃牡丹皮湯
   (Rhubarb and Moutan Combination)
   These prescriptions treat arteriosclerosis.

2. Fang-feng-tung-sheng-san　　　　　　　　防風通聖散
   (Siler and Platycodon Formula)
   This formula is given to persons of an obese and firm physical conformation who have a tendency toward arteriosclerosis, suffer from constipation because of dietary habits, and have poor blood circulation in the extremities where gangrene occurs.

3. Kuei-chih-fu-ling-wan　　　　　　　　　　桂枝茯苓丸
   (Cinnamon and Hoelen Formula)
   This prescription mitigates the beginning symptoms of coldness in the four limbs resulting from occluded blood circulation.

4. Ti-tang-tang　　　　　　　　　　　　　　　抵當湯
   (Rhubarb and Leech Combination)
   This prescription is applicable to gangrene caused by stale extravasated blood that disturbs terminal circulation.

5. Tang-kuei-szu-ni-chia-wu-chu-yu-sheng-chiang-tang
   　　　　　　　　　　　　　　　　　　當歸四逆加吳茱萸生薑湯

(Tang-kuei, Evodia, and Ginger Combination)
This formula is indicated for extreme coldness in the four limbs when the patient has a thin and small pulse.

6. **Kan-tsao-fu-tzu-tang** 甘草附子湯
    (Licorice and Aconite Combination)
   Kuei-chih-chia-fu-tzu-tang 桂枝加附子湯
    (Cinnamon and Aconite Combination)
   Wu-tou-kuei-chih-tang 烏頭桂枝湯
    (Wu-tou and Cinnamon Combination)

These formulas are taken by patients having vicious pain, vigorous anemophobia, and perspiration.

7. **Kuei-chiang-tsao-tsao-huang-hsin-fu-tang** 桂薑棗草黃辛附湯
    (Cinnamon and Six Herbs Combination)

This prescription is effective against various diseases that have been regarded as indomitable and non-accessible to other prescriptions. It channels the yin *ch'i* and the yang *ch'i* that are obstructed and separates them from each other, making them harmonious with each other.

8. **Shih-chuan-ta-pu-tang** 十全大補湯
    (Ginseng and Tang-kuei Ten Combination)

This formula is taken for somatic weakness by people who have a strong tendency to be anemic, who are of a weak conformation, and who are experiencing pain.

9. **Po-chou-san** 伯州散
    (Eriocheir and Viper Formula)
   Tzu-yun-kao 紫雲膏
    (Lithospermum Ointment)

If effusion is present at the surface of the ulcer, the best treatment is to use *Po-chou-san* internally and *Tzu-yun-kao* externally.

10. **Folk Medicine** 民間方
    Green Juice Therapy 青汁療法

This is a therapy for gangrene that has prevailed as a folk remedy. Powdered tea is supposedly effective for diabetes mellitus; hence perhaps it is effective for gangrene caused by diabetes mellitus. Chlorophyll is effective for arteriosclerosis. It can be applied to any kind of gangrene. (Most gangrenous patients will incur acidosis.) Thus green juice from three to five kinds of vegetables or grass that contains chlorophyll flavored with fruit juice, drunk in doses of 20-40ml daily, hastens prompt healing of gangrene.

Wryneck

The term "wryneck" means convulsions in the neck area. Thus when the patient turns his head, he experiences a binding sensation. This spasm, the main symptom, is called retrocollis. Wrynecks can be of dermatologic, mascular, osseous, neural (convulsive or paralytic), or arthritic origin. There are also lymphatic, aural, and ophthalmic wrynecks. The most frequently found type is innate muscular wryneck, the wryneck caused by innate shortage and shrinkage in sternocleidomastoid muscle whereby the head tilts toward the affected side when turned. Wryneck is accompanied by irregularity of the scalp and a laterally bent spine. There are many theories about the underlying causes of wryneck, such things as untrauterine compression, muscle inflammation, and congenital embryonic deformities. However, osseous wryneck is directly caused by a congenital lateral inflection in the neck; arthritic wryneck is due to intervertebral inflammation; neural wryneck (of the nerves) is due to inflammation along the corpus striatum and spasmodic paralysis in the muscles of the neck; lymphatic wryneck is due to lymphadenitis in the deeper part of the neck causing convulsions and rigidity in the upper front muscles; aural wryneck is due to pathological changes in the three semicircular canals of the ear; and ophthalmic wryneck is due to the enforced position of the head because of paralysis in the eye muscles.

Treatment
Wryneck can be treated by either conservative correction —massage—or surgical operation that corrects by removing certain muscles.

Chinese Herb Formulas
1. **I-kan-san-chia-shao-yao-kan-tsao**　　　抑肝散加芍藥甘草
   (Bupleurum Formula plus Paeonia and Licorice)

This formula is for patients having neural wryneck whose abdominal conformaton is manifested by rigidity beneath the heart, tension in the abdominal rectus muscle, and sensitivity in the abdominal muscles at both sides. The formula treats muscle cramping and brings about amelioration of the wryneck; however, it has to be taken lengthily.

2. Chai-hu-kuei-chih-tang　　　　　　　　　柴胡桂枝湯
    (Bupleurum and Cinnamon Combination)
The abdominal conformation and symptoms are similar to the preceding formula's, except that this conformation is firmer. If the preceding formula fails, this one may work. Also if there is a conspicuous thoraco-costal distress conformation, this formula may be used.

OPHTHALMIC DISEASES

Hordeolum

The symptoms are swelling and inflammation in the eyelids, hard sores around the eye rims, and, after several days, suppuration. It is often accompanied by edema in the conjunctiva, pain, and marked pressing pain at the hard sores. In general, the suppuration is a natural discharge and the condition clears up in about one week. However, habitual relapses are characteristic of hordeolum.

Treatment
Lack of sufficient sleep or mental fatigue is the main cause of this disease. Rubbing the eyes with dirty hands can cause severe complications. The direct home therapy is the application of antibiotic ointment on the infected area; however, the best treatment is oral medication. A word of caution: precipitous operations or failure to keep the eyes clean can have disastrous results.

Chinese Herb Formulas:
1. Ko-ken-tang   葛根湯
   (Pueraria Combination)

Ko-ken-tang-chia-chuan-chiung-ta-huang 葛根湯加川芎大黃
(*Pueraria Combination with Cnidium and Rhubarb*)
Chiung-huang-san 芎黃散
(*Cnidium and Rhubarb Formula*)

The inflammation, swelling, and pain in the primary stage of hordeolum should be treated with *Ko-ken-tang*. For patients with a tendency towards constipation, cnidium and rhubarb is added or *Chiung-huang-san* used.

2. Po-chou-san 伯州散
    (*Eriocheir and Viper Formula*)

This formula is to be taken for hordeolum accompanied by suppuration.

3. Tiao-wei-cheng-chi-tang 調胃承氣湯
    (*Rhubarb and Mirabilitum Combination*)
    Fang-feng-tung-sheng-san 防風通聖散
    (*Siler and Platycodon Formula*)

Both of these formulas are effective for hordeolum.

4. Kuei-chih-fu-ling-wan 桂枝茯苓丸
    (*Cinnamon and Hoelen Formula*)
    Tao-ho-cheng-chi-tang 桃核承氣湯
    (*Persica and Rhubarb Combination*)
    Ta-huang-mu-tan-pi-tang 大黃牡丹皮湯
    (*Rhubarb and Moutan Combination*)

All of these formulas are effective for hordeolum for those with stagnant blood.

5. Shih-wei-pai-tu-san 十味敗毒散
    (*Bupleurum and Schizonepeta Formula*)

This formula is also effective for hordeolum.

Blepharitis Marginalis

A glandular constitution, staphylococcic infections, dacryocystitis, upward-migrating rhinitis, chronic conjunctivitis, and trachoma are all causes of blepharitis marginalis, inflammation of the eyelids. There are two types, blepharitis squamosa (nonulcerative) and blepharoulcer (ulcerative). It may be followed by a loss of the eyelashes or eyebrows or inversion of the eyelashes. Some cases are caused by round worms. This is a persistent disease. In Chinese therapy, a glandular constitution is regarded as being due to womb toxication (congenital). Also, people who are subject to suppuration usually have stagnant blood. Therefore, the patient should choose formulas that will improve his constitution.

Chinese Herb Formulas
1. Ko-ken-tang-chia-chuan-chiung-ta-huang-huang-chin-chieh-keng-shih-kao　　葛根湯加川芎大黃黃芩桔梗石膏
  (Pueraria Combination with Cnidium, Rhubarb, Scute, Platycodon, and Gypsum)
This formula is to be taken for blepharitis marginalis.

2. Shih-wei-pai-tu-san-chia-lien-chiao　　十味敗毒散加連翹
  (Bupleurum and Schizonepeta Formula with Forsythia)
This formula is to be taken by those with a glandular constitution, furunculosis, or an allergic constitution.

3. Tzu-yuan　　紫圓
  (Croton and Hematite Formula)
This formula is effective for childhood womb toxication accompanied by eczema on the scalp and severe poison in the abdomen.

4. Kuei-chih-fu-ling-wan　　桂枝茯苓丸
  (Cinnamon and Hoelen Formula)
This formula is to be taken for blepharitis marginalis by those who have stagnant blood.

5. Tao-ho-cheng-chi-tang　　桃核承氣湯
  (Persica and Rhubarb Combination)
This formula is to be taken for blepharitis marginalis by those with stagnant blood and constipation.

6. Hsiang-chuan-chieh-tu-chi　　香川解毒劑
  (Smilax and Akebia Combination)
This formula is to be taken for skin diseases due to syphilis.

This formula should be used frequently.

Acute and Chronic Dacryocystitis

Dacryocystitis is an inflammation of the tear sac, usually accompanied by severely painful swelling and a discharge of pus. Those with narrow lacrimal ducts who beocme infected by the suppurative and tuberculous bacteria tend to contract chronic dacryocystitis. Active bacteria in the subcutaneous tissue cause acute dacryocystitis.

Chinese Herb Formulas
1. Ko-ken-tang-chia-chuan-chiung-ta-huang 葛根湯加川芎大黃
   (Pueraria Combination with Cnidium and Rhubarb)
This formula is to be taken for dacryocystitis accompanied by painful swelling.

2. Shih-wei-pai-tu-san-chia-lien-chiao 十味敗毒散加連翹
   (Bupleurum and Schizonepeta Formula with Forsythia)
This formula is to be taken for chronic dacryocystitis.

3. Ling-kuei-chu-kan-tang-chia-che-chien-tzu
   苓桂朮甘湯加車前子
   (Hoelen and Atractylodes Combination with Plantago)
This formula is to be taken by those having a weak conformation with stagnant water in the abdomen, vertigo, palpitations, congestion, headache, chronic dacryocystitis, excessive lacrimation, and sunken pulse.

4. Wu-ling-san 五苓散
   (Hoelen Five Herb Formula)
This formula is to be taken for eye ailments, chronic dacryocystitis, congestion, nausea, excessive salivation, headache, thirst, dysuria, and floating pulse.

5. Yueh-pi-chia-chu-tang 越婢加朮湯
   (Atractylodes Combination)
This formula is to be taken for dacryocystitis with sunken pulse.

6. **Hsiao-ching-lung-tang** 小青龍湯
   (Minor Blue Dragon Combination)
This formula is to be taken for dacryocystitis accompanied by frequent tearing of the eyes, inflammation, and pain.

7. **Shou-lei-yin** 收淚飲
   (Schizonepeta and Scute Combination)
This formula is to be taken for chronic dacryocystitis with continual tearing.

Conjunctivitis

This is an inflammation of the mucous membrane which lines the eyelid and covers the front part of the eyeball. Congestion in the whites of the eyes causes exudation and asthenopia. Overstimulation, overwork, bacteria and/or a virus can cause conjunctivitis, which can in turn become chronic.

Treatment

Conjunctivitis is often treated by the use of steroid ointment. However, it is most important to keep the eyes clean. The patient should be sure to use separate towels and wash cloths each time that he washes, in order not to infect others or reinfect himself.

Chinese Herb Formulas:
1. **Ko-ken-tang-chia-chuan-chiung-ta-huang** 葛根湯加川芎大黃
   (Pueraria Combination with Cnidium and Rhubarb)
This formula is effective for conjunctivitis.

2. **Yueh-pi-chia-chu-tang** 越婢加朮湯
   (Atractylodes Combination)
This formula is to be taken for conjunctivitis accompanied by suppuration, swelling, congestion, pain, secretion, tearing, floating pulse and dysuria.

3. **Hsiao-ching-lung-tang** 小青龍湯
   (Minor Blue Dragon Combination)
This formula is to be taken for conjunctivitis accompanied by congestion, severe tearing, and a tendency towards floating pulse.

4. Ma-huang-hsi-hsin-fu-tzu-tang　　　　　麻黃細辛附子湯
   (Ma-huang, Aconite, and Asarum Combination)
This formula is to be taken for conjunctivitis by those who have a delicate constitution with a weak and sunken pulse.

5. Ching-shang-fang-feng-tang　　　　　清上防風湯
   (Siler Combination)
This formula is to be taken for conjunctivitis accompanied by congestion, darkening of the skin, and acne.

Trachoma

Trachoma is a contagious viral disease characterized by the formation of hard, granular excrescences on the conjunctive of the eyelids along with inflammation of the lining.

The patient will experience an uncomfortable feeling of dryness in the eyeball, sensitivity to light, a sensation of heavy pressure on the eyelids, asthenopia, and a secretion of lipids. This disease can cause trachomatous pannus, corneal ulcer, conjunctival amyloid, xerosis conjunctivae, trichiasis, and lid ectropion. It is difficult to cure. The use of Chinese herb formulas in conjunction with Western antibiotics produces good results.

Chinese Herb Formulas
1. Ko-ken-tang　　　　　葛根湯
   (Pueraria Combination)
This formula is to be taken by those having inflammation, congestion, secretion, distension in the upper body, and stiffness in the shoulders. For patients with constipation, add cnidium and rhubarb.

2. Yueh-pi-chia-chu-tang　　　　　越婢加朮湯
   (Atractylodes Combination)
This formula is to be taken for inflammation, severe congestion, excessive secretion, trachomatous pannus, corneal ulcer, sensitivity to light, tearing, sunken pulse, and difficulty in urination and elimination.

3. Hsiao-ching-lung-tang 小青龍湯
    (Minor Blue Dragon Combination)

This formula is to be taken for severe inflammation and congestion, tearing, and sunken pulse. In severe cases of corneal ulcer, use *Ta-ching-lung-tang* (大青龍湯, Major Blue Dragon Combination)

4. Ma-huang-hsi-hsin-fu-tzu-tang 麻黃細辛附子湯
    (Ma-huang, Aconite, and Asarum Combination)

This formula is to be taken by those having a delicate constitution with chills and sunken pulse.

5. Ta-chai-hu-tang 大柴胡湯
    (Major Bupleurum Combination)

This formula is to be taken for chronic trachoma with chest distension.

6. Fang-feng-tung-sheng-san 防風通聖散
    (Siler and Platycodon Formula)

This formula is to be taken by those with an obese constitution, abdominal fullness, and constipation.

7. Kuei-chih-fu-ling-wan 桂枝茯苓丸
    (Cinnamon and Hoelen Formula)

This formula is to be taken by those women who have resistant pressure at the umbilicus and stagnant blood.

Phlyctenular Conjunctivitis

Patients who have a glandular constitution can easily contract phlyctenular conjunctivitis and suffer from relapses. This disease is related to tuberculous infections. The patient experiences a severe sensitivity to light, lacrimation, spasms in the eyelids, severe congestion in the conjunctiva and in the corneal rim. Small blisters containing watery or serous fluid form on the cornea. These blisters split, become ulcerous, and then heal themselves.

Chinese Herb Formulas

1. **Ko-ken-tang** 葛根湯
   (Pueraria Combination)

   This formula is to be taken for primary or mild phlyctenular conjunctivitis. For patients with constipation, add 2.0g cnidium and 1.0 rhubarb.

2. **Yueh-pi-chia-chu-tang** 越婢加朮湯
   (Atractylodes Combination)

   This formula is to be taken for the severe symptoms of sunken pulse, sensitivity to light, lacrimation, and congestion.

3. **Hsiao-ching-lung-tang** 小青龍湯
   (Minor Blue Dragon Combination)

   This formula is to be taken for the severe symptoms of sensitivity to light, lacrimation, congestion, and floating pulse.

4. **Ling-kuei-chu-kan-tang** 苓桂朮甘湯
   (Atractylodes and Hoelen Combination)

   This formula is to be taken for stagnant water in the abdomen, water toxin, and gastroptosis.

5. **Wu-ling-san** 五苓散
   (Hoelen Five Herb Formula)

   This formula is to be taken for thirst, fatigue, and dysuria during the summer.

6. **Tang-kuei-shao-yao-san** 當歸芍藥散
   (Tang-kuei and Paeonia Formula)

   This formula is to be taken by women who have a weak constitution with chills, mild anemia, and abnormal menstruation.

7. **Kuei-chih-fu-ling-wan** 桂枝茯苓丸
   (Cinnamon and Hoelen Formula)

   This formula is to be taken by women who have congestion in the eyes due to stagnant blood and experience resistant pressing pain at the umbilicus.

8. **Tao-ho-cheng-chi-tang** 桃核承氣湯
   (Persica and Rhubarb Combination)

This formula is also to be taken by women who have congestion in the eyes due to stagnant blood and experience resistant pressing pain at the umbilicus.

9. **Hsiao-chai-hu-tang** 小柴胡湯
   (Minor Bupleurum Combination)
This formula is to be taken for chest distension.

10. **Chai-hu-ching-kan-tang** 柴胡清肝湯
    (Bupleurum and Rehmannia Combination)
This formula is to be taken for chest distension, tense abdomen, and darkening of the skin.

11. **Hsiao-chien-chung-tang** 小建中湯
    (Minor Cinnamon and Paeonia Combination)
This formula is to be taken by children who have a scrofulous, delicate constitution; pale skin; tense abdomen; frequent urination; and a tendency towards fatigue. This should be taken over an extended period of time.

Keratitis

The majority of cases of inflammation of the cornea are caused by syphilis, especially congenital syphilis. A few cases between six and thirty years of age are caused by tubercle bacillus. This disease is divided into two categories, vascular keratitis and keratitis.

The symptoms of vascular keratitis are sensitivity to light, lacrimation, severe inflammation, and pain. Sometimes, Hutchinson's teeth, a partial hearing loss, saddlenose, and cracked and dry lips are also present.

Chinese Herb Formulas
1. **Yueh-pi-chia-chu-tang** 越婢加朮湯
   (Atractylodes Combination)
This formula is especially effective for vascular keratitis. It is to be taken for the primary symptoms of inflammation, sensitivity to light, lacrimation, pain, and sunken pulse.

2. Hsiao-ching-lung-tang 小青龍湯
    (Minor Blue Dragon Combination)
    Ta-Ching-lung-tang 大青龍湯
    (Major Blue Dragon Combination)

For those having a strong constitution with congestion, headache, inflammation, sensitivity to light, lacrimation, pain, and strong and sunken pulse, *Hsiao-ching-lung-tang* is recommended. For severe cases accompanied by stress, use *Ta-ching-lung-tang*.

3. Hsi-kan-ming-mu-tang 洗肝明目湯
    (Gardenia and Vitex Combination)

This formula is to be taken for keratitis accompanied by chest distension, hard abdomen, and resistance beneath the ribs.

4. Hsiao-chai-hu-tang 小柴胡湯
    (Minor Bupleurum Combination)

Sclerosing Keratitis

Young women are prone to suffer from this disease. The overt symptoms are sensitivity to light, a sensation of foreign matter in the eyes, pain, lacrimation, and visual disturbance. Congestion and turbidity in the sclera, which are difficult to cure, may also be present.

Chinese Herb Formulas
1. Hsi-kan-ming-mu-tang 洗肝明目湯
    (Gardenia and Vitex Combination)

This formula is to be taken for sclerosing keratitis with resistance beneath the ribs on the right side of the body.

2. Yueh-pi-chia-chu-tang 越婢加朮湯
    (Atractylodes Combination)

This formula is to be taken for sensitivity to light, the sensation of foreign matter in the eyes, pain, and lacrimation.

3. Hsiao-chai-hu-tang 小柴胡湯
    (Minor Bupleurum Combination)

This formula is to be taken by those having a tuberculous constitution with a tendency towards constipation and chest distension.

4. Ming-lang-yin 明朗飲
    (Hoelen, Licorice, and Plantago Combination)
This formula is to be taken for chronic sclerosing keratitis, sensitivity to light, tearing, and the general uncomfortable feeling which accompanies this disease. It is effective for a weak conformation with palpitations, vertigo, and sunken pulse.

5. Kuei-chih-fu-ling-wan 桂枝茯苓丸
    (Cinnamon and Hoelen Formula)
This formula is to be taken for prolonged congestion and menstrual irregularities. In cases of constipation, add rhubarb or use *Chiung-huang-san* (芎黃散, Cnidium and Rhubarb Formula)

Iritis

The bacteria from within the body may invade the iridic vessel, causing iritis. Syphilis, bodily injuries, and systemic diseases such as rheumatism, tuberculosis, gout, skin ailments, diabetes, gonococcus, and sympathetic iritis are the causes of this disease.

Symptoms of congestion around the cornea, swelling in the iris, miosis, suppuration in the cornea, severe headache, especially in the early evening hours, visual disturbance, sensitivity to light, and lacrimation are manifested. In severe cases fever, nausea, vomiting, and weakness are present.

Chinese Herb Formulas
1. Ko-ken-tang 葛根湯
    (Pueraria Combination)
This formula is to be taken for the primary symptoms of congestion in the cornea, mild headache, sensitivity to light, and lacrimation.

2. Yueh-pi-chia-chu-tang 越婢加朮湯
    (Atractylodes Combination)
This formula is to be taken for congestion, sensitivity to light, excessive lacrimation, and sunken pulse.

3. **Hsiao-ching-lung-tang** 小青龍湯
   (Minor Blue Dragon Combination)
   This formula is to be taken for severe inflammatory congestion, headache, sensitivity to light, and floating pulse. In severe cases, use *Ta-ching-lung-tang* (大青龍湯 , Major Blue Dragon Combination)

4. **Pai-tu-san** 敗毒散
   (Bupleurum and Tuhuo Formula)
   This formula is to be taken for the severe inflammatory congestion of iritis.

5. **Fang-feng-tung-sheng-san** 防風通聖散
   (Siler and Platycodon Formula)
   This formula is to be taken by those having an obese constitution and strong pulse with an eye ailment due to syphilis or a painful inflammation.

6. **Hsiao-chien-chung-tang** 小建中湯
   (Minor Cinnamon and Paeonia Combination)
   This formula is to be taken by those having tuberculous iritis with a delicate constitution, weak conformation, a tendency towards fatigue, and little or no inflammatory congestion.

7. **Hsiao-chai-hu-tang** 小柴胡湯
   (Minor Bupleurum Combination)
   This formula is to be taken for tuberculous iritis with chest distension and inflammatory congestion.

8. **Ta-chai-hu-tang** 大柴胡湯
   (Major Bupleurum Combination)
   This formula is to be taken for chronic iritis by those having a strong constitution with chest distension.

9. **Tang-kuei-shao-yao-san** 當歸芍藥散
   (Tang-kuei and Paeonia Formula)
   This formula is to be taken by those having chills and anemia.

10. **Kuei-chih-fu-ling-wan** 桂枝茯苓丸
    (Cinnamon and Hoelen Formula)

This formula is to be taken for iritis with stagnant blood, resistant pressure at the umbilicus, and congestion.

11. Tao-ho-cheng-chi-tang   桃核承氣湯
    (Persica and Rhubarb Combination)
This formula is to be taken for iritis with purplish stagnant blood.

12. Ta-huang-mu-tan-pi-tang   大黃牡丹皮湯
    (Rhubarb and Moutan Combination)
This formula is to be taken for resistant pressure at the umbilicus by those with a tendency towards constipation.

Pterygium

As recorded in ancient books, the Chinese have a disease named *nu zou pan tsing* which literally means "a bulging flesh clinging to the eye," the equivalent of pterygium in modern western medicine. The disease is described in *Yi tsung chin chien* (Handbook of Chinese Medicine): "This disease starts on the nasal side of the cornea. At first it attacks the conjunctiva only, but gradually it spreads and covers the pupil." This is the same condition which modern medicine describes as a triangular fold of membrane in the interpalpebral fissure extending from the inner side of the conjunctiva to the cornea and slowly growing toward the rim of the pupil until it finally hinders vision.

The cause of this disease is unknown. However, it occurs most commonly in laborers who are frequently exposed to a combination of wind, sun, sand, and dust.

Symptoms
Symptoms are congestion, tearing, a sensation of a foreign body in the eye, and visual impairment.

Treatment
The growth may be removed by ophthalmic surgery but recurrence is common.

Chinese Herb Formulas
1. Yueh-pi-chia-chu-tang　　　　　　　越婢加朮湯
    (Atractylodes Combination)

The so-called "*zou chi*" in *Chin kuei yao lueh* (Summaries on Household Remedies) from where this formula comes is equivalent to cataracts, nebula of the cornea, or pterygium, and the symptoms of congestion, tearing, a sensation of a foreign body in the eye. Other formulas used for keratitis or conjunctivitis can also be used depending on the condition. This formula when taken continuously for a long time will cure most cases.

2. Ta-chai-hu-tang　　　　　　　　　　大柴胡湯
    (Major Bupleurum Combination)

This formula is indicated for pterygium accompanied by thoracocostal distress. It is prescribed in accordance with abdominal symptoms. At times *Hsiao-chai-hu-tang* (小柴胡湯 Minor Bupleurum Combination) is suitable also.

Cataracts

Symptoms

Cataracts occur when the protein of the lens or cornea becomes turbid and obstructs vision. The person with cataracts experiences visual disturbance: night blindness, day blindness, and partial or total blindness. There are two types of cataracts, congenital and senile. Injuries to the pupils of the eyes and diabetes can also cause cataracts.

Treatment

Chinese formula therapy is directed toward diabetic and senile cataracts in the primary and unripened stage. When the cataract becomes ripe, surgery may be recommended. The taking of vitamin E is sometimes also effective.

Chinese Herb Formulas
1. Ko-ken-tang　　　　　　　　　　　　葛根湯
    (Pueraria Combination)

This formula is to be taken for cataracts in the primary stage accompanied by stiffness in the shoulder or back.

2. **San-huang-hsieh-hsin-tang** 三黃瀉心湯
    (Coptis and Rhubarb Combination)

This formula is to be taken by those who have cataracts but also experience facial redness, congestion, headache, and habitual constipation.

3. **Fang-feng-tung-sheng-san** 防風通聖散
    (Siler and Platycodon Formula)

This formula is to be taken by those having an obese constitution with abdominal distention, food or water poisoning, and constipation.

4. **Chai-hu-chia-lung-ku-mu-li-tang** 柴胡加龍骨牡蠣湯
    (Bupleurum and Dragon Bone Combination)

This formula is to be taken for cataracts by those patients who experience nervousness, chest distension, palpitations, and insomnia.

5. **Ling-kuei-chu-kan-tang** 苓桂朮甘湯
    (Hoelen and Atractylodes Combination)

This formula is to be taken for cataracts by those who have water stagnancy in the abdomen, vertigo, and palpitations.

6. **Chu-yang-huo-hsieh-tang** 助陽活血湯
    (Tang-kuei, Siler, and Astragalus Combination)

This formula is to be taken for diabetic or senile cataracts by those having senile or delicate constitutions.

7. **Tzu-shen-ming-mu-tang** 滋腎明目湯
    (Chrysanthemum Combination)

This formula is effective for eye disorders and cataracts. It is recommended for diabetic and senile cataracts.

8. **Fu-ling-yin** 茯苓飲
    (Hoelen Combination)

This formula is to be taken by those having cataracts who also have gastric distention.

9. **Pa-wei-ti-huang-wan** 八味地黃丸
    (Rehmannia Eight Formula)

This formula is very effective for diabetic and senile cataracts.

10. **Tang-kuei-shao-yao-san** 當歸芍藥散
    (Tang-kuei and Paeonia Formula)
This formula is to be taken by those having a delicate constitution and anemia; mild chills; fatigue; headache; tinnitus; and visual disorders.

Glaucoma

The cause of glaucoma is unknown, but the majority of those who suffer from this disease are post-menopausal women who are elderly and have hyperopia. It is considered to be due to a circulatory disturbance or other eye diseases.

Acute glaucoma exhibits the symptoms of sudden pain in the eyes, severe headache and vomiting, unclear vision, congestion in the conjunctiva, turbidity in the corneas, mydriasis, and hardening of the eyeball. These symptoms are relapsable.

Chinese Herb Formulas
1. **Yueh-pi-chia-chu-tang** 越婢加朮湯
    (Atractylodes Combination)
This formula is to be taken for turbidity in the cornea, congestion, headache, and as a mild stimulant.

2. **Ta-ching-lung-tang** 大青龍湯
    (Major Blue Dragon Combination)
This formula is to be taken for chronic glaucoma with mild inflammative congestion and a tense abdomen. The formula may be used frequently.

3. **Ling-yang-chiao-san** 羚羊角散
    (Antelope Horn Formula)
This formula is to be taken for glaucoma with congestion and severe pain.

4. **Chai-hu-chia-lung-ku-mu-li-tang** 柴胡加龍骨牡蠣湯
    (Bupleurum and Dragon Bone Combination)
This formula is to be taken for glaucoma accompanied by nervous-

ness, insomnia, palpitations, emotional instability, and palpitations in the abdomen.

5. Tao-ho-cheng-chi-tang 桃核承氣湯
   (Persica and Rhubarb Combination)
This formula is to be taken for iritis and glaucoma with stagnant blood.

6. Chu-lan-shui 除爛燧
   (Tang-kuei, Coptis, and Schizonepeta Combination)
This formula is recommended for glaucoma in general.

7. Pa-wei-ti-huang-wan 八味地黃丸
   (Rehmannia Eight Formula)
This formula is to be taken for glaucoma by the chronic and elderly who experience fatigue, tiredness, and weakness beneath the umbilicus.

Nyctalopia

The nyctalopia patient suffers from blindness in dark places. This disease is divided into two categories, congenital and acquired nyctalopia. Congenital nyctalopia is inherited and difficult to cure. Acquired nyctalopia is due to malnutrition, especially a deficiency of Vitamin A. In a few cases, nyctalopia is a complication of jaundice. It is frequently seen in conjunction with xerosis conjunctivae of the cornea. Acute nyctalopia is treated with liver oil. In Chinese therapy, oil from chicken or ox livers and eels is used to supplement Vitamin A.

Chinese Herb Formulas
1. Wu-ling-san 五苓散
   (Hoelen Five Herb Formula)
This formula is to be taken for nyctalopia which occurs in the summer, accompanied by thirst, tiredness, dysuria, and floating pulse.

2. Yin-chen-wu-ling-san 茵陳五苓散
   (Capillaria and Hoelen Formula)

This formula is to be taken for nyctalopia caused by jaundice.

3. Ling-kuei-chu-kan-tang   苓桂朮甘湯
   (Atractylodes and Hoelen Combination)
This formula is to be taken for nyctalopia, accompanied by xerosis corneas, sensitivity to light, lacrimation, stagnant water in the abdomen, and a floating pulse.

Chronic Ophthalmoneuritis

A Vitamin B_1 deficiency can cause ophthalmoneuritis and beriberi, especially in young people. It is often confused with myopia, but its symptoms are neurasthenic.

Its apparent symptoms are visual disturbance, sensitivity to light, hemeralopia, asthenopia, headache, heaviness in the head, emotional instability, vertigo when raising the head, a tendency towards fatigue, palpitations, excessive perspiration, loss of appetite, asthma, insomnia, tinnitus, nausea, congestion, dry throat, and motion sickness. In Chinese therapy, the above symptoms are classified as "water toxin," and similar to the *Ling-kuei-chu-kan-tang* conformation.

Chinese Herb Formulas   苓桂朮甘湯
1. Ling-kuei-chu-kan-tang
   (Atractylodes and Hoelen Combination)
This formula is to be taken for stagnant water in the abdomen, vertigo, heaviness in the head, palpitations, and myopia.

2. Tang-kuei-shao-yao-san   當歸芍藥散
   (Tang-kuei and Paeonia Formula)
This formula is to be taken by those having chills and an anemic constitution.

3. Kuei-chih-fu-ling-wan   桂枝茯苓丸
   (Cinnamon and Hoelen Formula)
This formula is to be taken for chronic stagnant blood. In cases with constipation, add 0.5 to 1.0g rhubarb.

4. Tao-ho-cheng-chi-tang　　　　　　　　　　桃核承氣湯
   (Persica and Rhubarb Combination)
This formula is to be taken for severe stagnant blood with constipation.

5. Hsiao-chai-hu-tang　　　　　　　　　　　　小柴胡湯
   (Minor Bupleurum Combination)
This formula is to be taken by those with an average constitution with chest distension. Sometimes, it is combined with *Ling-kuei-chu-kan-tang* (苓桂朮甘湯 , Atractylodes and Hoelen Combination).

Haemophthalmos

Haemophthalmos refers to a bleeding in the larger part of the retina of which visual defects are a result. Severe bleeding can cause blindness and is difficult to cure. Though in some cases the bleeding is due to an outside injury, the majority of cases are caused by other diseases, especially repeated tuberculosis in young people, syphilis in middle-aged people, and hypertension in the elderly. Other causes are diabetes, renal diseases, leukemia, and anemic reticulosis, as well as Behcet's syndrome.

Chinese Herb Formulas
1. San-huang-hsieh-hsin-tang　　　　　　　　三黃瀉心湯
   (Coptis and Rhubarb Combination)
This formula is to be taken for haemophthalmos due to hypertension, accompanied by congestion, facial redness, and emotional instability.

2. Huang-lien-chieh-tu-tang　　　　　　　　　黃連解毒湯
   (Coptis and Scute Combination)
This formula is to be taken for the rather mild symptoms resembling *San-huang-hsieh-hsin-tang* conformation.

3. Wen-ching-yin　　　　　　　　　　　　　　溫清飲
   (Tang-kuei and Gardenia Combination)
This formula is to be taken for chronic haemophthalmos.

4. Hsi-kan-ming-mu-tang 洗肝明目湯
   (Gardenia and Vitex Combination)
   This formula is to be taken for chronic haemophthalmos caused by an outside injury.

5. Kuei-chih-fu-ling-wan 桂枝茯苓丸
   (Cinnamon and Hoelen Formula)
   This formula is to be taken for chronic haemophthalmos with stagnant blood.

6. Tao-ho-cheng-chi-tang 桃核承氣湯
   (Persica and Rhubarb Combination)
   This formula is to be taken for haemophthalmos by those with constipation and stagnant blood.

7. Hsiao-chai-hu-tang 小柴胡湯
   (Minor Bupleurum Combination)
   This formula is to be taken for tuberculous haemophthalmos.

8. Hsiao-chien-chung-tang 小建中湯
   (Minor Cinnamon and Paeonia Combination)
   This formula is to be taken for haemophthalmos by those with a weak conformation, a tendency towards fatigue, and tense abdominal tendons.

Centralis Retinitis

The main causes of this disease are tuberculosis, syphilis, or the excessive stimulation caused by frequent contact with bright lights. It mostly occurs in males in their 40's. It often affects one eye only and causes visual disturbance, astigmatism, and hyperopia.

Chinese Herb Formulas
1. Hsiao-chai-hu-tang 小柴胡湯
   (Minor Bupleurum Combination)
   This formula is to be taken for tuberculous retinitis. It should be used frequently.

2. **Ta-chai-hu-tang** 大柴胡湯
   (Major Bupleurum Combination)
   This formula is to be taken by those having a strong constitution, habitual constipation, and chest distension.

3. **Kuei-chih-fu-ling-wan** 桂枝茯苓丸
   (Cinnamon and Hoelen Formula)
   This formula is to be taken by women who have abnormal menstruation and chronic stagnant blood in the abdomen.

4. **Tao-ho-cheng-chi-tang** 桃核承氣湯
   (Persica and Rhubarb Combination)
   This formula is to be taken by women who have a markedly abnormal menstruation, severe, chronic stagnant blood, and constipation.

5. **Tang-kuei-shao-yao-san** 當歸芍藥散
   (Tang-kuei and Paeonia Formula)
   This formula is to be taken by women who have chills, mild anemia, or a tendency towards fatigue.

Pseudomyopia

Pseudomyopia is unclear vision when the patient is looking at objects at a great distance. It is due to inelasticity of the eye muscles and the lens (crystalline lens). This disease should only be diagnosed by a physician. The use of the eyes in fine work, such as reading or tailoring, over a long period of time can result in this disease.

Treatment

Pseudomyopia can be cured by the patient's own efforts. The patient should rest his eyes for ten minutes every hour and should avoid fixing his gaze on anything. Physical exercise to improve his general health is necessary, as well as eye exercises. Sufficient sleep is also important. It is best that the patient not wear glasses.

Chinese Herb Formulas

1. **Hisao-chai-hu-tang** 　　　　　　　　　　小柴胡湯
   (Minor Bupleurum Combination)
   This formula is to be taken for primary pseudomyopia in children who have delicate constitutions.

2. **Ling-kuei-chu-kan-tang** 　　　　　　　苓桂朮甘湯
   (Atractylodes and Hoelen Combination)
   This formula is to be taken for pseudomyopia by those patients who experience vertigo when standing.

3. **Wu-ling-san** 　　　　　　　　　　　　　五苓散
   (Hoelen Five Herb Formula)
   This formula is to be taken for pseudomyopia accompanied by thirst. It is especially recommended for children and teenagers.

Asthenopia

Succinctly, asthenopia is a nervous state of the eyes. In mild cases, the patient experiences vertigo and spasms in the eyelids. In severe cases, the patient not only has asthenopia but also experiences pain in the forehead and inner parts of the eyes and a decrease in the clarity of his vision.

Treatment

The main causes of asthenopia are mental fatigue and emotional stress. The immediate therapy is to get some rest, especially a good night's sleep. Whenever a person experiences a disorder in his eyes, he should loosen his clothes, lie down, and rest. If the circumstances are such that he cannot lie down, he should wash his face and eyes with cool water. Once the patient has relaxed and rested, baths, exercise, and a little wine are also therapeutic.

Chinese Herb Formulas

1. **Chia-wei-hsiao-yao-san** 　　　　　　　加味逍遙散
   (Bupleurum and Paeonia Formula)
   This formula is to be taken by those women who are nervous and have a tendency towards fatigue, headache, and insomnia.

2. **Chai-hu-chia-lung-ku-mu-li-tang**　　柴胡加龍骨牡蠣湯
(Bupleurum and Dragon Bone Combination)
This formula is to be taken by men who have a strong constitution and a tendency towards fatigue, resistance beneath the ribs, and hypertension.

NOSE AND THROAT DISEASES

Hearing Losses

Hearing losses or hearing difficulties may occur at any age producing disability dependent upon the degree of loss, the age of occurrence, and whether one or both ears are affected.

Many factors can be attributed to this hearing defect which at times ends up in a complete loss of hearing ability—deafness. Hearing defects can be classified in several categories according to the cause of the defect: sensorineural, conductive, mixed, or functional. Any defects, disorders, or malfunctions in the external ear channel, the middle ear, or the inner ear is likely to impair hearing ability. These impairments may be congenital or affected. Such things as birth trauma, malformation of the inner ear, vascular disorders, bacterial or virus infections, inflammatory middle ear diseases like otitis media and prolonged exposure to a loud sound either singly or in combination may cause hearing loss.

The tuning fork test, audiometric test, labyrinth test, or spoken and whispered voice test are of value in determining the degree of defects and the causes or sites of the defects. Electronystagmography (ENG) sometimes is a useful aid in identifying, recording, and interpreting nystagmus, especially in response to labyrinthine tests.

Treatment
Any sign of hearing loss should be examined and treated promptly so as to revive the hearing ability in the early stage before it is not too late to do so.

Chinese Herb Formulas
1. Hsiao-chai-hu-tang　　　　　　　　　　小柴胡湯
(Minor Bupleurum Combination)
Hardness of hearing induced by colds, fevers and continuous coughing; otitis media; or accompanied by an adenoidal swelling usually manifest the conformation of this combination, the common symptoms of which are thoraco-costal distress, hardness and tension below the heart and near the liver. The occluded fever should be removed to cure the disease. This formula along with 7.0g gypsum is indicated for a severe occluded fever with thirst.

2. Ta-chai-hu-tang　　　　　　　　　　大柴胡湯
(Major Bupleurum Combination)
This formula is given to patients having a yang firm conformation, a strong physique with obstruction and hardness below the ribs and the heart, and apparent thoraco-costal distress. The rhubarb should be removed if there is no constipation. Hardness of hearing can be alleviated by relieving the obstruction and distension beneath the heart no matter what the etiology is.

3. Chai-hu-chia-lung-ku-mu-li-tang　　　柴胡加龍骨牡蠣湯
(Bupleurum and Dragon Bone Combination)
This formula is indicated for a conformation that falls between the Major and Minor Bupleurum conformations and for thoraco-costal distress, resistance and distension below the heart, palpitation beside and above the navel, and the neurotic symptoms of flush-up, insomnia, and mental distress caused by the overfunctioning of the abdominal arteries.

4. Ling-kuei-wei-kan-tang　　　　　　　苓桂味甘湯
(Licorice, Schizandra, and Hoelen Combination)
This formula is for patients with a slightly weak conformation, an ascending *ch'i* that brings about facial flushing and the ap-

pearance of drunkness and hardness of hearing.

5. **Hsieh-hsin-tang** 瀉心湯
    (Coptis and Rhubarb Combination)
This combination is effective for patients with facial reddening caused by the ascending *ch'i*, irritability, restlessness, obstruction and distension beneath the heart, and difficulty in breathing. In this case the patient has a firm conformation, a strong pulse, and a tendency toward constipation.

6. **Fang-feng-tung-sheng-san** 防風通聖散
    (Siler and Platycodon Formula)
Patients having an obese build, a tendency toward constipation, and water or food toxin can be given this formula. Hardness of hearing caused by syphilis can also be cured by this formula.

7. **Man-ching-tzu-san** 蔓荊子散
    (Vitex Formula)
Hardness of hearing in the elderly that has resulted from blood dryness, from fevers occluded in the upper part of the body that have caused tinnitus, or from pus flowing out of the ear can be cured by this formula. This formula also relieves hardness of hearing resulting from chronic otitis media.

8. **Che-ku-tsai-tang** 鵤鴣菜湯
    (Digenea and Rhubarb Combination)
Ascarids in children can cause hearing impairment. Anthelmintics are given for therapy.

9. **Moxibustion** 灸法
Apply moxibustion to the bulging veins or rigid spot on the area from the bottom of the ears to the base of the neck; the more units of moxa applied, the better. This method may be used for all ear diseases.

Tinnitus

Tinnitus is due to a malfunction of the auditory nerve which causes a ringing, rushing, or buzzing sound in the ear. Otitis, otitis media, ototoxicity, labyrinthitis or a foreign object lodged in the external ear canal may cause tinnitus. Arteriosclerosis, anemia, or menopausal disturbances can also cause tinnitus, as can a partial loss of hearing caused by excessive and prolonged noise such as may be found in some factories. The majority of cases of persistent tinnitus are difficult to alleviate. Otosclerosis is especially resistant to treatment. Vertigo often occurs with tinnitus. In severe cases, there is a loss of hearing. In Chinese therapy, tinnitus is considered to be a water toxin disease.

Chinese Herb Formulas
1. **Ling-kuei-chu-kan-tang** 苓桂朮甘湯
   (Atractylodes and Hoelen Combination)
This formula is to be taken for the nervousness that accompanies tinnitus and the vertigo which occurs when standing.

2. **Hsiao-chai-hu-tang** 小柴胡湯
   (Minor Bupleurum Combination)
This formula is to be taken for tinnitus caused by otitis media, by otitis due to the common cold, or by other auditory disorders.

3. **Tang-kuei-shao-yao-san** 當歸芍藥散
   (Tang-kuei and Paeonia Formula)
This formula is to be taken by women with tinnitus, anemia, and chills in the hands and feet.

4. **Pa-wei-ti-huang-wan** 八味地黃丸
   (Rehmannia Eight Formula)
This formula is effective for tinnitus and/or hearing loss in the elderly.

5. **Ling-kuei-wei-kan-tang** 苓桂味甘湯
   (Hoelen, Schizandra, and Licorice Combination)
This formula is effective for patients with chronic otitis media who have a hearing loss. It is also recommended for tinnitus, sunken and weak pulse, chills in the feet, flushing of the face, nausea, a feeling of heaviness in the head, and dysuria.

6. **Fu-ling-yin** 茯苓飲
   (Hoelen Combination)

This formula is to be taken for tinnitus due to stagnant water in the stomach accompanied by gastroptosis or gastric distention. It is also recommended for those of weak conformation who have a tendency towards anemia, weak pulse, and a feeling of heaviness beneath the heart.

7. Fang-feng-tung-sheng-san　　　　防風通聖散
    (Siler and Platycodon Formula)

This formula is to be taken for tinnitus caused by hypertension and arteriosclerosis. It is recommended for obese patients who have a strong pulse and abdomen, and food or water toxin. It also helps relieve constipation, headache, shoulder stiffness, and a feeling of heaviness in the head.

8. Hsiao-chai-hu-tang-ho-hsiang-su-san　　小柴胡湯合香蘇散
    (Minor Bupleurum Combination with Cyperus and Perilla Formula)

This formula is to be taken for tinnitus caused by chronic otitis media and for stuffy noses due to otitis.

9. Ta-chai-hu-tang　　　　大柴胡湯
    (Major Bupleurum Combination)

This formula is recommended for those having a strong constitution and abdomen, chest distention, constipation, and tinnitus due to cerebral hemorrhage.

10. Chih-kan-tsao-tang　　　　炙甘草湯
    (Baked Licorice Combination)

This formula is to be taken for tinnitus due to Meniere's disease. It is also effective for patients with heart disease who have palpitations and poor circulation.

11. Chai-hu-chia-lung-ku-mu-li-tang　　柴胡加龍骨牡蠣湯
    (Bupleurum and Dragon Bone Combination)

This formula is to be taken for tinnitus due to nervous exhaustion, stress, hysteria, or emotional instability. It is also effective for palpitations, insomnia, vertigo, palpitations in the abdomen, and chest distention.

12. Shih-chuan-ta-pu-tang 十全大補湯
   (Ginseng and Tang-kuei Ten Combination)
This formula is to be taken by those of weak conformation who have tinnitus due to severe anemia.

13. Tzu-shen-tung-erh-tang 滋腎通耳湯
   (Scute Combination)
This formula is to be taken for tinnitus and temporary deafness due to kidney disorders.

Otitis Externa

Gram-negative rods such as *Staphylococcus aureus, E. coli*, or *Proteus vulgaris* may infect the external ear canal and cause painful swelling and inflammation. The condition is aggravated by chewing or talking.

If this condition occurs in the front of the ear canal, it will usually cause swelling near the jawbones and of the parotid gland, cheeks, and eyelids. When this condition occurs in the back of the ear canal, it will cause mastoiditis, hearing loss, and abscess in the ear. Usually, the condition will clear spontaneously after several days of purulent discharge.

Chinese Herb Formulas

1. Ko-ken-tang 葛根湯
   (Pueraria Combination)
This formula is to be taken in the first stage of otitis externa for severe chills, fever, and pain due to swelling.

2. Shih-wei-pai-tu-san 十味敗毒散
   (Bupleurum and Schizonepeta Formula)
This formula is to be taken in the first stage of otitis externa for mild fever, chills, and suppuration.

3. Hsiao-chai-hu-tang 小柴胡湯
   (Minor Bupleurum Combination)
This formula is to be taken for otitis externa of several days duration.

4. Tuo-li-hsiao-tu-yin　　　　　　　　托裏消毒飲
    (Gleditsia Combination)
This formula is to be taken for otitis externa accompanied by severe suppuration and mastoid edema.

5. Nei-tuo-san　　　　　　　　　　　　內托散
    (Astragalus and Platycodon Formula)
This formula is to be taken for otitis externa accompanied by suppuration.

Meniere's Syndrome

Meniere's syndrome is a disorder of the labyrinth of the ear characterized by recurrent attacks of vertigo, nausea, vomiting, and sometimes tinnitus or a partial loss of hearing. The syndrome indicates an imbalance in the body.

This condition is precipitated by poor blood circulation in the labyrinth and is accompanied by lymphedema. The major causes are disorders of the autonomic nervous system, maladjustment of the circulatory system, metabolic disturbances, and allergies. In Chinese medicine, this is classified as an abnormal condition of water toxin or stagnant blood with flushing.

Chinese Herb Formulas
1. Chai-hu-chia-lung-ku-mu-li-tang　　柴胡加龍骨牡蠣湯
    (Bupleurum and Dragon Bone Combination)
This formula is to be taken for Meniere's syndrome accompanied by flushing, insomnia, and stress.

2. Kuei-chih-fu-ling-wan　　　　　　　桂枝茯苓丸
    (Cinnamon and Hoelen Formula)
This formula is to be taken for Meniere's syndrome accompanied by stagnant blood, resistant pressure in the lower abdomen, and facial flushing.

3. Pan-hsia-pai-chu-tien-ma-tang　　　半夏白朮天麻湯
    (Pinellia and Gastrodia Combination)
This formula is to be taken for Meniere's syndrome. It is recommended for those having gastrointestinal weakness, stagnant

water in the abdomen, vertigo, vomiting, and headache.

4. **Kou-teng-san** 鈎藤散
   (Gambir Formula)

This formula is to be taken by those past middle age who have vertigo, headache, shoulder stiffness, flushing up, autonomic nervous system disorders, or anxiety.

5. **Chen-wu-tang** 眞武湯
   (Vitality Combination)

This formula is to be taken by those with a delicate constitution who have Meniere's syndrome, vertigo, palpitations, and vomiting.

Acute Mastoiditis

This condition develops from untreated acute otitis media. Generally, stagnant pus in the middle ear causes this condition. Discharge usually occurs along with painful swelling in the mastoids. In severe cases, meningitis and cerebral ulcer will follow. If after one week the patient still has pain, swelling, and fever, surgery is required. The use of Chinese herb formulas with chemical therapy may produce good results.

Chinese Herb Formulas

1. **Ko-ken-tang-chia-chuan-chiung-ta-huang** 葛根湯加川芎大黃
   (Pueraria Combination with Cnidium and Rhubarb)

This formula is to be taken during the initial stage of acute mastoiditis in which there is fever, swelling, and pain.

2. **Hsiao-chai-hu-tang-chia-chieh-keng-shih-kao** 小柴胡湯加桔梗石膏
   (Minor Bupleurum Combination with Platycodon and Gypsum)

This formula is to be taken for white coating on the tongue, fever, severe chills, chest distention, and loss of appetite.

3. Ta-chai-hu-tang-chia-shih-kao　　　大柴胡湯加石膏
   (Major Bupleurum Combination with Gypsum)
   This formula is to be taken by those with a strong constitution who have a tendency towards constipation.

4. Ching-chieh-lien-chiao-tang-chia-chan-shui-man-ching-tzu
   　　　　　　　　　　　　　荊芥連翹湯加蟬蛻蔓荊子
   (Schizonepeta and Forsythia Combination with Cicada and Vitex)
   This formula is to be taken for acute mastoiditis.

5. Tuo-li-hsiao-tu-yin　　　　　　　托裏消毒飲
   (Gleditsia Combination)
   This formula is to be taken by those of delicate constitution who have acute mastoiditis and suppuration.

6. Kuei-chih-chia-huang-chi-tang　　　桂枝加黃耆湯
   (Cinnamon and Astragalus Combination)
   This formula is to be taken for mastoiditis with seropurulent discharge.

7. Kuei-chih-fu-ling-wan-chia-i-yi-jen　桂枝茯苓丸加薏苡仁
   (Cinnamon and Hoelen Formula with Coix)
   This formula is to be taken for acute mastoiditis by those who have stagnant blood.

8. Po-chou-san　　　　　　　　　　伯州散
   (Eriocheir and Viper Formula)
   This formula is to be taken for chronic mastoiditis.

Otitis Media

Otitis media is a middle ear inflammation caused by a bacterial infection. It is divided into acute and chronic otitis media. Acute otitis media is a frequent complication following a common cold or diphtheria. A few cases follow external injury of the eardrum. Chronic otitis media begins during childhood when respiratory infections are recurrent.

Symptoms
Acute otitis media causes earache, tinnitus, aurula, and fever. Children with this condition have a high fever. As the earache becomes severe, the eardrum breaks and suppurates. Chronic otitis media has malodorous suppuration, otorrhoea, and hearing loss, and predisposes the person to mastoiditis. If not cured immediately, it will result in partial or total deafness. Everyone should be aware that purulent discharge is a signal of a serious condition.

Treatment
Antibiotics can cure acute otitis media. If the proper treatment is not given in the primary stage, this disease will become chronic. Therefore, the patient should be advised that strict adherence to the doctor's orders is essential. He should also be forewarned that treatment is lengthy and patience will be needed. In severe cases, surgical operation may be necessary.

Chinese Herb Formulas

1. **Ko-ken-tang** 葛根湯
   (Pueraria Combination)

This formula is taken in the primary stage of acute otitis media for fever, earache, headache, and aching in the shoulders.

2. **Hsiao-chai-hu-tang** 小柴胡湯
   (Minor Bupleurum Combination)

This formula is recommended when *Ko-ken-tang* has had no effect. It should be taken frequently.

3. **Huang-chi-chien-chung-tang** 黃耆建中湯
   (Astragalus Combination)
   Kuei-chih-chia-huang-chi-tang 桂枝加黃耆湯
   (Cinnamon and Astragalus Combination)

These formulas are recommended for those with otitis media who have a delicate constitution and a continuous purulent discharge. Frequent use is recommended.

4. **Ta-chai-hu-tang** 大柴胡湯
   (Major Bupleurum Combination)

This formula is recommended for persons of strong conformation who have headache, severe chills, strong and sunken pulse, abdominal distention, and a tendency towards constipation. In cases exhibiting anxiety and thirst, add 0.5g gypsum.

5. **Liang-ke-san-chia-shih-kao** 涼膈散加石膏
    (Forsythia and Rhubarb Formula with Gypsum)
This formula is recommended for otitis media accompanied by fever, constipation, hematuria, severe thirst, and marked, white coating on the tongue.

6. **Ching-chieh-lien-chiao-tang** 荊芥連翹湯
    (Schizonepeta and Forsythia Combination)
This formula is recommended for those with earache, abundant secretions, and fever.

7. **Fang-feng-tung-sheng-san** 防風通聖散
    (Siler and Platycodon Formula)
This formula is recommended for patients with an obese and strong constitution who have abdominal fullness, a tendency towards constipation, persistent purulent otorrhea, and food and water toxin.

8. **Tuo-li-hsiao-tu-yin** 托裏消毒飲
    (Gleditsia Combination)
This formula is recommended for chronic otitis media with continuous purulent discharge. It should be used frequently. In cases of weak conformation, the patient should take *Chien-chin-nei-tuo-san* (千金內托散, Astragalus and Platycodon Formula)

9. **Po-chou-san** 伯州散
    (Eriocheir and Viper Formula)
This formula is recommended for those with a tendency towards chronic otitis media accompanied by continuous purulent discharge.

Chronic Rhinitis

Chronic rhinitis is an on-going inflammation of the mucous membrane of the nose. It is caused by recurrent acute rhinitis, common colds, swelling of the nasal passages due to smoking, sticky nasal drainage, and temporary nasal mucous membrane disorders. Circulatory disturbances, over indulgence in alcohol and nicotine, sinusitis, enlargement of the tonsils, as well as chronic pharyngitis and tonsillitis, will also cause this condition. It is often found in conjunction with sinusitis.

Symptoms

The symptoms are chronic inflammation of the nasal mucous membranes, accompanied by purulent discharge, a narrow nasal cavity, difficulty in breathing, snoring during sleep, headache, and temporary amnesia.

Treatment

The patient should keep the nasal cavity clean by not allowing any nasal discharge to remain. If washing the nasal cavity and injections of nasal medicine do not cure the condition, surgery or electrotherapy will be necessary. It is best to avoid surgery and most important that measures be taken to improve the general health of the patient.

Chinese Herb Formulas

1. **Hsiao-chai-hu-tang** 小柴胡湯
    (Minor Bupleurum Combination)

This formula is effective for chronic rhinitis which has developed from acute rhinitis.

2. **Shih-wei-pai-tu-san** 十味敗毒散
    (Bupleurum and Schizonepeta Formula)

This formula is to be taken for rhinitis accompanied with copious secretions. It should be taken frequently.

3. **Ma-huang-tang** 麻黃湯
    (Ma-huang Combination)

This formula is to be taken for rhinitis with nasal stuffiness.

4. **Ko-ken-tang** 葛根湯
    (Pueraria Combination)

This formula is to be taken for rhinitis accompanied by headache, fever, severe chills, stuffy nose, and nasal drainage. In cases involing constipation, 3.0g cnidium and 0.5-1.0g rhubarb should be added to this formula.

5. Hsiao-ching-lung-tang　　　　　　　　　小青龍湯
   (Minor Blue Dragon Combination)
This formula is to be taken for rhinitis accompanied by continual nasal drainage, malodorous watery secretions, and a floating pulse.

6. Ching-chieh-lien-chiao-tang　　　　　　　荊芥連翹湯
   (Schizonepeta and Forsythia Combination)
This formula is to be taken for rhinitis accompanied with suppurative secretions, a darkening of the skin, and tense abdominal walls.

Allergic Rhinitis

Allergic rhinitis, a reversible hypersensitivity, is a nasal disorder characterized by obstruction of the nasal passages by a watery discharge. It is accompanied by sneezing and itching eyes and nose. Rhinitis produces the same antibodies found in bronchial asthma. Infections, constant use of irritating inhalants, cold air, excessive exercise, and emotional upsets probably are the cause of nearly half of all allergic cases. However, the onset is often seasonal as in hay fever. Usually the allergens are pollen, dust, animal hair, irritating odors, meat, milk, or eggs. More recent research suggests that the main mechanism of the non-immunologic allergy is a reaction of the parasympathetic nervous system triggered by the irritant receptors of the nose.

Symptoms
The principal symptoms are nasal congestion; a profuse, watery nasal discharge; itching of the nasal mucosa leading to paroxysms of violent sneezing; and itching, burning eyes with involuntary crying. The nasal mucosa becomes blue and moist with occasionally the presence of polyps. The conjunctiva (the mucous membrane covering the eyeball and inner eyelid) is often red and swollen.

Treatment

There is no specific remedy for allergic rhinitis, but a skin test may be of aid in the detection of the allergens. Antihistamines are most commonly used, sometimes in combination with ephedrine, to relieve the attacks.

Chinese Herb Formulas

1. **Hsiao-ching-lung-tang**　　　　　　　　　　　　小青龍湯
   (Minor Blue Dragon Combination)

Water stagnation beneath the heart accompanied by an exterior toxin, frequent sneezing, and profuse nasal drainage from the ascension of the stagnated water sometimes with crying and slobbering, are the usual indications for this combination.

2. **Mai-men-tung-tang**　　　　　　　　　　　　　麥門冬湯
   (Ophiopogon Combination)

A sensation of irritation and dryness in the throat plus a convulsive cough because of the adverse ascension of *ch'i* are the indications for this combination. The conformation difference between this and the preceding one is not readily apparent, but the nasal drainage manifested in this conformation is much less.

3. **Ko-ken-tang**　　　　　　　　　　　　　　　　葛根湯
   (Pueraria Combination)

Patients having an inflammatory congestion of the face, back, or neck areas with stiffness or inflammatory congestion in the eyes, ears, and nose should be given this combination. It is good for severe stiff shoulders, frequent sneezing, and a susceptibility to catch cold.

4. **Tang-kuei-szu-ni-chia-wu-chu-yu-sheng-chiang-tang**
   　　　　　　　　　　　　　　　當歸四逆加吳茱萸生薑湯
   (Tang-kuei, Evodia, and Ginger Combination)

This combination is effective in treating allergic rhinitis patients who have chills, easily catch cold, or have frostbite.

5. **Kan-tsao-fu-tzu-tang**　　　　　　　　　　　　甘草附子湯
   (Licorice and Aconite Combination)

People susceptible to colds with symptoms of frequent sneezing, chills in the back, thin nasal drainage, headaches and ascending *ch'i* should take this combination.

6. **Ma-huang-fu-tzu-hsi-hsin-tang**　　　麻黃附子細辛湯
   (Ma-huang, Aconite, and Asarum Combination)
   Yin type rhinitis is cured by this combination.

7. **Shih-chuan-ta-pu-tang**　　　十全大補湯
   (Ginseng and Tang-kuei Ten Combination)
   Patients who tend toward weakness and anemia, dry skin, dry nasal mucosa, and frequent sneezing are given this combination.

8. **Chia-wei-hsiao-yao-san**　　　加味逍遙散
   (Bupleurum and Paeonia Formula)
   The lengthy use of this formula can improve the physique of patients who have only slight symptoms of the disease.

Ozena Genuina

Atrophic rhinitis, an illness characterized by its stench, still remains without a clearly established etiology. It occurs most often in young girls who have a broad face. Syphilis or tuberculosis may also cause similar symptoms; those caused by syphilis are called ozena.

Objectively the illness has three major symptoms, namely, intranasal atrophy, the formation of scabs, and a putrid odor. Subjectively the patient has a stuffy nose, an unpleasant dry sensation at the bridge of the nose, a loss of smelling ability, an open nasal sound, dull pain in and around the eye sockets, an upset stomach, and a general nervousness.

The secretion is a dull, green color that becomes a yellowish green scab which clings to the whole inner wall of the nasal cavity. The noxious, putrid odor comes from the dried secretion and smells like putrefied cheese or like the intolerable stench of a smashed bedbug. It cannot be detected by the sufferer himself owing to his or her loss of sense of smell.

This illness is a recalcitrant disease and can be alleviated by Chinese herb formulas after lengthy administration in accordance with the corresponding conformaton.

Chinese Herb Formulas

1. Chia-wei-pa-mo-san　　　　　　　　加味八脈散
   (Hoelen, Polyporus, and Alisma Formula)

This prescription is frequently prescribed by Asada Dohaku and his followers. According to their record, "This formula is indicated for the putrid odor of ozena genuina that lasts for years; also it is for a stuffy nose that renders the patient unable to smell." Thus this formula has been frequently used for ozena genuina, syphilitic ozena, and loss of the sense of smell, and often alleviates both subjective and objective symptoms. In this formula rehmannia is employed to moisten or lubricate the aridity resulting from the drying up of the nasal membrane, atrophy and the formation of scabs.

2. Chia-wei-hsiao-yao-san-chia-ti-huang　　加味逍遙散加地黃
   (Bupleurum and Paeonia Formula with Rehmannia)

Although similar to the preceding formula, this one is used for weak phthiasis in young females for improvement of the physique and has to be administered for a long period of time.

3. Ching-chieh-lien-chiao-tang　　　　荊芥連翹湯
   (Schizonepeta and Forsythia Combination)

This formula is suitable for syphilitic ozena for patients who have a strong physique and dark skin indicative of a firm fever conformation.

4. Shih-chuan-ta-pu-tang　　　　　　十全大補湯
   (Ginseng and Tang-kuei Ten Combination)

This formula is for patients with poor nutrition, dry skin, and anemia. These people understandably tire easily. Their condition will improve if their blood and vitality are enriched and restored.

5. Chih-kan-tsao-tang　　　　　　　　炙甘草湯
   (Baked Licorice Combination)

This formula is used for patients that are not as weak as the preceding one but have the same symptoms: poor nutrition, dry skin, lack of energy, annoying fever in the limbs, dry mouth, constipation, and cardiac hyperfunction.

6. **External Remedy** 外用藥

Consisting of equal parts of scute and apricot kernel pulverized and blended well with sesame oil, the mixture is applied to the inside of the nasal cavity. It may mollify the sensation of dryness.

Paranasal Sinusitis

Paranasal sinusitis is an inflammation, either purulent or nonpurulent, of the paranasal sinuses, which include the ethmoidal, frontal, maxillary and sphenoidial sinuses. The infection may be either acute or chronic, depending on its etiology. Most acute paranasal sinusitis follows an acute upper respiratory infection, resulting from swimming or diving, dental abscesses or extractions, nasal allergies, nasal trauma, or colds. It also occurs as result of an exacerbation of chronic sinus infection. The etiology of chronic sinusitis is mostly related to physical conditions; however, it usually is a complication of an attack of acute sinusitis. Sometimes infections of bacteria or viruses from a neoplasm or dental disease lead to this condition.

Symptoms

Acute paranasal sinusitis. The symptoms resemble those of acute rhinitis but are more severe. Headache, facial pain, sore throat, cough, tenderness and swelling with nasal obstruction, and a purulent nasal and postnasal discharge are among the systemic symptoms. Occasionally there are toothaches, tenderness in the roof of the mouth, and fever.

Chronic paranasal sinusitis. Sometimes there may be no symptoms but postnasal discharge or a nonproductive cough with intermittent nasal obstruction.

Treatment

Acute. Oral nasal decongestants like 15-50mg phenylpropanolamine given three times daily or systemic antibiotics are used the most frequently to relieve the infection.

Chronic. For cases of infection by organisms, an antibiotic is given. Usually surgical correction is helpful in these types of cases.

Chinese Herb Formulas

1. Ko-ken-tang   葛根湯
(Pueraria Combination)

In the initial stage of acute cases, the symptoms of fever, sensation of heaviness in the head, stuffy nose, nasal drainage, and stiff shoulders can be cured by this combination.

2. Ko-ken-tang-chia-wei-fang   葛根湯加味方
(Pueraria Combination with additional herbs)

This combination is applied when the disease has progressed to a chronic stage. The formula is *Ko-ken-tang* with 2.0g each of cnidium, scute, platycodon, magnolia flower; 5.0g of gypsum and 0.5-1.0g of rhubarb should be added in cases of interior fever and a tendency toward constipation. This combination also relieves hypertrophic rhinitis or swollen mucous membranes, after an operation. Magnolia flower is often found in formulas for nasal diseases.

3. Ching-chieh-lien-chiao-tang-chia-hsin-i
                                                         荊芥連翹湯加辛夷
(Schizonepeta and Forsythia Combination with Magnolia Flower)

Patients most prone to paranasal sinusitis apparently are those whose body build is bony and skin color slightly dark. They exhibit abdominal muscle tension, a nervous temperament, and frequently perspiration in the limb areas. This formulas is given to this type of patient. It is also used when *Ko-ken-tang* fails to take effect.

4. Hsiao-chai-hu-tang   小柴胡湯
(Minor Bupleurum Combination)

This combination may be given to moderately strong patients with an inclination to slight weakness. 3.0g each of platycodon and gypsum may be added to this formula; *Ling-kuei-chu-kan-tang* may be taken along with this formula.

5. Ta-chai-hu-tang   大柴胡湯
(Major Bupleurum Combination)

To patients of a bony but firm physique with symptoms of hardness and tension below the heart, thoraco-costal distress, stiff shoulders and constipation, this formula with 3.0g of platycodon and 5.0g of gypsum may be given.

6. **Fang-feng-tung-sheng-san** 防風通聖散
   (Siler and Platycodon Formula)
   Gourmands with an obese build, a firm pulse and abdomen, and a tendency toward constipation should take this formula for a long time. Patients with a similar physique with acne-like rosacea or rhinophyma (nose tissue enlargement) also respond to this formula.

7. **Szu-ni-san** 四逆散
   (Bupleurum and Chih-shih Formula)
   Those with an abdominal conformation similar to that of *Ta-chai-hu-tang* and a slightly firm hardness with tension below the heart may be given this formula with hoelen, cnidium and coix added.

8. **Hsin-i-ching-fei-tang** 辛夷清肺湯
   (Magnolia Flower and Gypsum Combination)
   This formula will cure paranasal sinusitis, hypertrophic rhinitis, rhinophyma, anosmia, and severe stuffy nose when the preceding formulas fail to take effect. Also in the presence of heat toxin and pain, this combination may be tried.

9. **Li-tse-tung-chi-tang** 麗澤通氣湯
   (Angelica and Siler Combination)
   This combination is for the loss of the sense of smell.

10. **Ling-kuei-chu-kan-tang** 苓桂朮甘湯
    (Atractylodes and Hoelen Combination)
    Patients with a chronic condition, a tendency toward flaccid abdomens, the presence of intragastric water stagnation, dizziness, and positional vertigo may be given this formula or the combination of *Ko-ken-tang* and *Hsiao-chai-hu-tang*. For patients with intragastric water stagnation, *Fu-ling-yin* or *Hsiao-pan-hsia-chia-fu-ling-tang* has always been effective.

11. **Pan-hsia-pai-chu-tien-ma-tang** 半夏白朮天麻湯
    (Pinellia and Gastrodia Combination)
    This formula is generally effective for chronically ill patients

who have flaccid abdomens, gastroptosis, frequent gastric discomfort, and paroxysmal headaches and dizziness that lead to vomiting as a consequence of intragastric water stagnation. In these cases, this formula generally takes effect.

12. Pu-chung-i-chi-tang   補中益氣湯
(Ginseng and Astragalus Combination)
For those who easily tire and are anemic with a tendency to become chronically ill, this formula is given for a long period of time with 2.0g each of agastache and magnolia flower.

13. Shih-chuan-ta-pu-tang   十全大補湯
(Ginseng and Tang-kuei Ten Combination)
This formula is used for patients who have become more debilitated than those above; they tire more easily and are more anemic.

14. Kuei-chiang-tsao-tsao-huang-hsin-fu-tang
桂薑棗草黃辛附湯
(Cinnamon and Six Herb Combination)
This formula has the effect of bringing about an upturn of the great *ch'i* in those who have a weak constitution and a chill conformation and are becoming chronically ill. It is used when all other attempts have failed.

Sinusitis

Stagnant mucopurulent discharge in the paranasal cavity is called sinusitis. Acute sinusitis may be the result of acute rhinitis, influenza, measles, pneumonia, a deviated septum, or dental caries. Most cases of chronic sinusitis follow acute rhinitis or acute sinusitis.

Symptoms
The symptoms are excessive nasal drainage, a feeling of stuffiness in the nose, headache, and emotional instability. In acute sinusitis, the above symptoms will last for an extended period of time. The symptoms of chronic sinusitis are not as severe as those of the acute condition, but the patient still ex-

periences a feeling of persistent heaviness in the head, anxiety, nasal stuffiness, and occasionally amnesia and diminished olfaction.

Treatment

Patients with both acute and chronic sinusitis should conscientiously follow the doctor's orders. For acute nasal suppuration, surgery is not necessary. Antibiotics by mouth or injected into the paranasal cavity are effective. The patient should remain quiet. Cold cloths on the forehead are also soothing. Sinusitis is resistant to treatment. Under the doctor's guidance the patient should be instructed in how to properly wash the nasal cavity at home, and this should be done several times a day. Acupuncture, moxibustion, and acupressure are also effective but should only be done by experts.

Chinese Herb Formulas

1. **Ko-ken-tang** 葛根湯
    (Pueraria Combination)

This formula is to be taken during the primary stage of acute sinusitis. It is effective for stuffy nose, fever, headache, nasal drainage, and stiffness in the shoulders. Those having gastrointestinal weakness should avoid taking this formula.

2. **Hsin-i-ching-fei-tang** 辛夷清肺湯
    (Magnolia Flower and Gypsum Combination)

This formula is to be taken for sinusitis with nasal drainage and stuffiness.

3. **Pan-hsia-pai-chu-tien-ma-tang** 半夏白尤天麻湯
    (Pinellia and Gastrodia Combination)

This formula is effective for those with sinusitis who have gastrointestinal weakness.

4. **Ching-chieh-lien-chiao-tang-chia-hsin-i** 荊芥連翹湯加辛夷
    (Schizonepeta and Forsytnia Combination with Magnolia Flower)

This formula is to be taken by those with sinusitis who have a darkening of the skin and tense abdominal tendons.

5. **Hsiao-chai-hu-tang** 小柴胡湯
   (Minor Bupleurum Combination)
   This formula is to be taken for sinusitis by those who have a delicate constitution.

6. **Ta-chai-hu-tang** 大柴胡湯
   (Major Bupleurum Combination)
   This formula is to be taken for nose suppuration by those with a strong constitution, hardness beneath the heart, chest distention, shoulder stiffness, and constipation. 3.0g platycodon and 5.0g gypsum should be added to this formula.

7. **Fang-feng-tung-sheng-san** 防風通聖散
   (Siler and Platycodon Formula)
   This formula is to be taken by those with sinusitis who are obese and have a strong pulse, no gastrointestinal weakness, and a tendency towards constipation.

8. **Szu-ni-san** 四逆散
   (Bupleurum and Chih-shih Formula)
   This formula is to be taken for sinusitis by those with tenseness and a feeling of pressure beneath the heart.

9. **Pu-chung-i-chi-tang** 補中益氣湯
   (Ginseng and Astragalus Combination)
   This formula is to be taken for chronic sinusitis by those with a delicate constitution who have anemia or a tendency towards fatigue.

10. **Shih-chuan-ta-pu-tang** 十全大補湯
    (Ginseng and Tang-kuei Ten Combination)
    This formula is to be taken for sinusitis by those with a delicate constitution and a tendency towards fatigue or anemia.

11. **Kuei-chiang-tsao-tsao-huang-hsin-fu-tang** 桂薑棗草黃辛附湯
    (Cinnamon and Six Herbs Combination)
    This formula is to be taken for chronic sinusitis by those with a delicate constitution who have chills.

Epistaxis

A nosebleed may be caused by a blow to the nose or by congestion which results in breakage of the nasoseptal blood vessels. Epistaxis may also be caused by swollen nasal ulcers, hypertension, hemophilia, purpura, leukemia, scurvy, cirrhosis, spleen disease, arteriosclerosis, heart disease, anemia, and vibriss a hemorrhage. A nosebleed can also be a premonitory symptom of uremia. In some instances, women have nosebleeds during menses. Severe epistaxis will cause anemia and forgetfulness. The patient should be given a complete physical examination in order to determine the exact cause of the nosebleed.

Treatment

Temporary epistaxis requires no treatment. During the nosebleed, the patient should lie down and elevate his head higher than his feet. This will stop the blood flow naturally. When it is a symptom of another disease, the original condition must be treated and cured. However, when epistaxis occurs as a result of hypertension or menstruation, it may be considered a natural function of the body.

Chinese Herb Formulas

1. Huang-lien-chieh-tu-tang 黃連解毒湯
    (Coptis and Scute Combination)
This formula is to be taken by those who are excitable and flush readily, and who have anxiety and internal heat. This formula should be mixed with cold beverages.

2. Hisao-chien-chung-tang 小建中湯
    (Minor Cinnamon and Paeonia Combination)
This formula is effective for those having a delicate constitution with tendency towards fatigue, mild anemia, and nosebleed.

3. Kuei-chih-fu-ling-wan 桂枝茯苓丸
    (Cinnamon and Hoelen Formula)
This formula is to be taken for nosebleeds due to menstruation.

4. Kuei-pi-tang 歸脾湯
   (Ginseng and Longan Combination)
This formula is effective for nosebleeds due to leukemia, pernicious anemia, and purpura.

5. Ma-huang-tang 麻黃湯
   (Ma-huang Combination)
This formula is to be taken for nosebleeds due to influenza or febrile diseases with perspiration.

6. Chiung-kuei-chiao-ai-tang 芎歸膠艾湯
   (Tang-kuei and Gelatin Combination)
This formula is to be taken for nosebleeds due to menstruation. It is effective for those of weak conformation who have chills and anemia due to habitual nosebleeds.

7. Ching-chieh-lien-chiao-tang 荊芥連翹湯
   (Schizonepeta and Forsythia Combination)
This formula is to be taken for nosebleeds due to chronic rhinitis or sinusitis.

Adenoid Conditions and Hypertrophy of Tonsils

Adenoid hyperplasia refers to the glandular growth or enlargement of the tissues of the pharynx palate, tonsils, palatine tonsils and to various growths on the pharynx walls. Its occurrence is infrequent in infants and adults but common in children, especially those of school age. Its etiology is yet unknown, but it is frequently seen in children with weak physiques who have had scarlet fever and recurrent inflammations in the nasal, paranasal, and pharynx regions. Also, it can be congenital in nature or due to unhygienic habits and living conditions.

Symptoms

Nasal obstruction is the main symptom. Breathing through the mouth, snoring, and difficulty in swallowing and sleeping are frequently found with this condition. Besides, retardation of mental development, teeth derangement, memory loss, decrease in the ability to concentrate, and, at times, otitis media may result through inflammation of the Eustachian tube. Usually enlarged tonsils are coarse and undulating with trenches and furrows dissecting their surface. They are red in appearance and tender to touch.

Treatment

An adenoidectomy is usually performed, but on certain occasions it does more harm than good.

Chinese Herb Formulas

1. Ko-ken-tang   葛根湯
   (Pueraria Combination)
With stuffy nose as the major indication and heaviness of the head and headache as the accompanying symptoms, this formula can be used for long periods of time. It is most suitable for those who do not have a weak physique. 2.0g each of cnidium and platycodon, and 5.0g of gypsum are added to the formula.

2. Hsiao-chai-hu-tang   小柴胡湯
   (Minor Bupleurum Combination)
Adenoidal problems with thoraco-costal distress, swelling in the lymphatic gland of the neck, and an inclination toward nervousness are the indications for this combination. Most often 2.0g of platycodon and 5.0g of gypsum are added.

3. Hsiao-chien-chung-tang   小建中湯
   (Minor Cinnamon and Paeonia Combination)
Patients with a thin and weak physique who catch cold easily, tire rapidly, and who have a thin abdominal wall plus frequent nocturia and tension should take this combination for a long time.

4. Ching-chieh-lien-chiao-tang   荊芥連翹湯
   (Schizonepeta and Forsythia Combination)
Retarded children with a normal physique who look healthy but have suffered from chronic rhinitis or chronic otitis media and have a pale, dark skin may be given this formula to improve their physique. The foregoing formulas are also effective for treatment of tonsil hypertrophy or enlargement.

5. Huang-po-chien   黃柏煎
   (Phellodendron Decoction)

Patients suffering from a cold, enlarged tonsils, a high fever, and chronic tonsilitis may be cured by gargling a decoction of this formula each morning. It is best to continue administration for at least six months. It is more efficacious if the patient also takes *Hsiao-chai-hu-tang* in addition to gargling.

Sore Throat

Sore throat may be caused by acute laryngitis, pharyngitis, tonsillitis, peritonsillitis, and peritonsillar abscess. Laryngophthisis, diphtheria, and esophageal cancer may also cause this condition.

Treatment

The underlying cause must be treated first in order to cure the sore throat, which is a secondary symptom. Antitubercular agents with serum therapy are effective for sore throat caused by laryngophthisis or diphtheria. Esophageal cancer requires surgery.

Pharyngitis

Pharyngitis is an inflammation of the pharynx, whereas laryngitis is an inflammation of the larynx. The majority of those afflicted with this condition are suffering from a common cold. Air pollution may be a possible cause, since recently, sore throats have come to be a chronic condition. Smokers, drinkers, and people who work in an unsanitary environment often suffer from pharyngitis or laryngitis.

Symptoms

The symptoms of this condition are pain in the pharynx, swelling of the mucous membrane, copious sputum, and a febrile sensation. If the condition becomes chronic, there is a constant dry or itching sensation in the pharynx, causing a hacking cough. The patient with laryngitis will have swollen vocal cords and hoarseness.

Treatment
It is very important for the patient to take proper care of himself and keep warm. He should gargle and eat warm but bland foods, and he should abstain from smoking and speaking loudly. Sometimes, patent medicines are effective.

Chinese Herb Formulas
1. **Ko-ken-tang** 葛根湯
    (Pueraria Combination)
This formula is effective for the initial stages of a sore throat.

2. **Hsiao-chai-hu-tang** 小柴胡湯
    (Minor Bupleurum Combination)
This formula is to be taken for sore throat.

3. **Pan-hsia-hou-pu-tang** 半夏厚朴湯
    (Pinellia and Magnolia Combination)
This formula is to be taken for pharyngitis accompanied with hoarseness.

Tonsillitis

Tonsillitis is an acute inflammation of the palatine tonsils. It may be caused by streptococcus, staphylococcus, tubercular bacilli, or, less commonly, one of several viruses, such as those responsible for influenza, measles, or whooping cough. Chronic tonsillitis may develop when acute tonsillitis recurs frequently. Young children and teen-agers are more susceptible to this disease, but sometimes adults also suffer from it.

Tonsillitis often manifests itself in combination with peritonsillitis, peripyema, acute otitis media, palsy of the lips and mouth, edema, lymphadenitis of the neck, and acute multiple articular rheumatism.

Symptoms
This disease is divided into three categories.
1. Catarrhal tonsillitis: swelling in the epiglottis and tonsils.

2. Lacunar tonsillitis: suppuration in the fossula tonsillaris, severe chills, ague, high fever (39-40°C), pain during swallowing, arthralgia, and aching in the limbs.
3. Follicular tonsillitis: swelling of the follicles of the tonsils which become yellowish white spots, pain during swallowing, earache, high fever, loss of appetite, and indigestion. The primary symptoms in children will be vomiting and stomach cramps.

Treatment

Antibiotics cure this disease. Tonsillitis is frequently found in people who are prone to allergies. It is very important to improve the general health of the patient, making him more resistant to infection. The tonsils are an important indicator of other diseases. Surgery is only necessary when there is persistent pain.

Chinese Herb Formulas

1. **Ko-ken-tang** 葛根湯
   (Pueraria Combination)

This formula is to be taken in the first stage of tonsillitis when there is fever and a sore throat.

2. **Hsiao-chai-hu-tang** 小柴胡湯
   (Minor Bupleurum Combination)

This formula is to be taken when there is a fever that lingers for several days and a sore throat.

3. **Ching-liang-yin** 清涼飲
   (Gardenia and Mentha Combination)

This formula is to be taken for the pain and inflammatory congestion of a swollen throat.

4. **Ching-yin-li-ke-tang** 清咽利膈湯
   (Arctium Combination)

This formula is to be taken for lacunar tonsillitis.

5. **Chu-feng-chieh-tu-tang** 驅風解毒湯
   (Siler and Forsythia Combination)

This formula is to be taken for lacunar tonsillitis.

6. **Pai-nung-san** 排膿散
   (Platycodon and Chih-shih Formula)
   This formula is to be taken for tonsillitis accompanied with suppuration.

Throat Obstruction

Blockage in the throat is sometimes caused by esophagostenosis or esophageal cancer. However, the major causes of this condition are autonomic nervous system disorders, overwork, insufficient sleep, and stress. The patient who suffers from tonsillitis or peritonsillitis may also have this condition, along with a painfully swollen throat.

Although this condition is caused mainly by autonomic disorders, esophageal disorders should not be overlooked during diagnosis.

Chinese Herb Formula
Pan-hsia-hou-pu-tang 半夏厚朴湯
(Pinellia and Magnolia Combination)
This formula is to be taken for esophageal constriction and for those who experience the sensation of having foreign matter blocking the throat. This is especially effective for pharyngitis for esophageal inflammation.

Hoarseness

Hoarseness is caused by an abnormal condition of the vocal cords. Laryngitis, polyps and bleeding in the throat, laryngophthisis, syphilis, esophageal cancer, external injuries, and palsy of the vocal cords are the causes of this condition. In severe cases, dysphonia is present.

Treatment
Various treatments are available according to the needs of the individual case. Hoarseness caused by excessive talking can be cured easily. Hoarseness due to laryngophthisis, syphilis, or esophageal cancer is very difficult to cure, as it depends on the

prognosis of the originating disease.

Chinese Herb Formulas
1. **Pan-hsia-hou-pu-tang** 半夏厚朴湯
   (Pinellia and Magnolia Combination)
   This formula is effective for hoarseness due to bronchitis with a chronic cough. It is also good for neurotic hysteria.

2. **Mai-men-tung-tang** 麥門冬湯
   (Ophiopogon Combination)
   This formula is to be taken for hoarseness accompanied by a severe cough, copious sputum, and a dry or febrile sensation in the throat.

3. **Hsiang-sheng-po-ti-wan** 響聲破笛丸
   (Gasping Formula)
   This formula is to be taken for hoarseness due to overuse of the vocal chords.

4. **Kan-tsao-hsieh-hsin-tang** 甘草瀉心湯
   (Pinellia and Licorice Combination)
   This formula is to be taken for hoarseness due to nervous exhaustion or hysteria by those patients who have gastrointestinal weakness, a feeling of pressure beneath the heart, and emotional instability.

5. **Pai-ho-ku-chin-tang** 百合固金湯
   (Lily Combination)
   This formula is to be taken for hoarseness and sore throat due to tuberculosis.

6. **Tzu-yin-chiang-huo-tang** 滋陰降火湯
   (Phellodendron Combination)
   This formula is to be taken for hoarseness accompanied by sore throat, severe cough, and a darkening of the skin. It is recommended for those who have a tendency towards constipation.

Snoring

Snoring, which was not treated as a disease in ancient times, is a term referring to an abnormal sound from the upper respiratory organ during respiration. The snorer opens his mouth and breathes through his mouth and nose at the same time. Snoring most often occurs while asleep because as the snorer falls asleep, his masticatory muscle and other facial muscles tend to become lax, the mandible hangs down, the mouth opens, the tongue retreats to the inferior-posterior position thus narrowing the air passage. When air passes through it, the soft palate vibrates. Snoring is also liable to occur after drinking alcoholic beverages because the soft palate becomes slightly paralyzed.

Snoring also can be caused by nasal polyps, distortion in the nasal septum, glandular neoplasm (tumors), diseases of the nasal cavity, tonsilar hypertrophy (enlargement), and cerebral hemorrhage.

Treatment

Treatment depends on the individual cause, some of which are difficult to treat. The following formulas may be used depending upon the cause.

Chinese Herb Formulas
1. Ko-ken-tang   葛根湯
    (Pueraria Combination)
Snoring resulting from rhinitis and rhinophyma can be cured by this combination. Those with paranasal sinusitis should be treated by adding 2.0g each of cnidium, scute, platycodon, and magnolia to the formula.

2. Hsiao-chai-hu-tang   小柴胡湯
    (Minor Bupleurum Combination)
Patients with adenoidal tonsilar hypertrophy, thoraco-costal distress, and snoring resulting from scrofulosis should be given this combination with 3.0g platycodon and 5.0g of gypsum added.

3. Acupuncture
Obese and hypertensive patients who snore and have severe stiff-

ness in the shoulders and neck can be cured by acupuncture on the loci in the scapulas and simultaneously administering *Fang-feng-tung-sheng-san* or *Ta-chai-hu-tang*. The pasting of *Niu-huang-ching-hsin-wan* (Bos and Musk Formula) to the loci of *tien chu* and *chien ching* instead of acupuncture can also alleviate the condition.

OBSTETRIC DISEASES

Hyperemesis Gravidarum
(Vomiting During Pregnancy)

Women often vomit in the first, second, or third month of pregnancy. Most pregnant women experience this problem, some severely, others mildly. In Latin the condition is called *vomitus matutinus* or morning sickness because the vomiting and nausea usually occur in the morning when the stomach is empty. Other manifestations are a loss of appetite and an abnormal craving for sour-tasting food, both of which generally disappear spontaneously within the first five months of pregnancy. Additionally, there is often a hypersecretion of saliva (ptyalismus). Occasionally a pregnant woman will have such severe metabolic disturbances that she becomes so debilitated that she dies. Poisons generated by the pregnancy sometimes spread through the body causing toxemia. Other accompanying symptoms are anemia, gastric disturbances, uterine retroflexation, hysteria, neurosis, and pyelitis. The presence of these symptoms may aggravate the condition. The woman will have a lower pulse rate than normal but no fever. The prognosis depends on her general condition. If the pulse is over 110, the body temperature exceeds 38°C, the urine volume is decreased, and a large quantity of protein and round casts appear in the urine, then it is necessary to consider aborting the pregnancy.

Treatment
The patient must fast for one or two days. Up to 2.0 liters of glucose and insulin may be administered intravenously as needed. Drugs such as chlorpromazine or vitamins such as methionine, pantothenic acid, thioctan, and pyridoxin may be taken alone or in combination with fasting. Adrenocortical hormone may be helpful also. In very severe cases, abortion should be considered.

Chinese Herb Formulas
1. Hsiao-pan-hsia-chia-fu-ling-tang　　小半夏加茯苓湯
   (Minor Pinellia and Hoelen Combination)

This formula appears frequently in modern gynecological and obstetric journals. It is very effective and is usually used at the beginning for mild cases. The indications are discomfort beneath the heart, cardiac palpitations, and slight vertigo. Nausea and vomiting generally occur irregularly and in most cases there is gastric water stagnancy. This formula should be cool when taken.

2. Pan-hsia-hou-pu-tang　　半夏厚朴湯
   (Pinellia and Magnolia Combination)

This formula is extremely effective for women who have suffered from morning sickness for a lengthy period of time and who also have neurotic symptoms or nervousness and hysteria. She may feel as though there is something clinging to her throat, have frequent sweating and urination, an irritative cough, and dropsy.

3. Erh-chen-tang-chia-chien-fang　　二陳湯加減方
   (Citrus and Pinellia Combination Modified)

This combination is used for conditions similar to those in which the first formula is used except that the patient has a little fever and expectorates a thick sputum. This formula is composed of *Erh-chen-tang* plus 1.0g each of coptis, cardamon, and forsythia.

4. Szu-ling-tang　　四苓湯
   (Hoelen and Polyporus Combination)

This combination is for women suffering from thirst, slight fever, reduced urine, and vomiting whenever they drink any water. This formula tastes bland, but if the patient feels sick after taking the decocted form, she may take it in powder form.

5. Fu-lung-kan-chien   伏龍肝煎
   (Fu-lung-kan Decoction)

If the above formulas fail to take effect and the patient's condition is very severe, 4.0g of *fu-lung-kan* (the aged earth at the bottom of a Chinese family's old kitchen stove) is placed in a vessel to which is then added 600ml of water. It is stirred thoroughly, allowed to stand and settle, and then 500ml is taken from the top clear water. This same procedure is used to decoct the first formula, *Hsiao-pan-hsia-chia-fu-ling-tang*. Therefore, for the sake of convenience, 4.0g of *fu-lung-kan* may be added to *Hsiao-pan-hsia-chia-fu-ling-tang* and the two decocted together. The foregoing formulas are given to women with a tendency to have a firm fever in the initial stage of pregnancy who still have stamina. All of these formulas should be cool when taken.

6. Jen-sheng-tang   人參湯
   (Ginseng and Ginger Combination)

This formula is indicated for a weak conformation: a weak and debilitated physique with a sensitive stomach and intestines. It is for women who do not violently vomit but constantly secrete sour saliva, spit frequently, have a slow and weak pulse, a weak and soft abdomen, and a tendency to have diarrhea with stomachaches. This and the following formula are better when taken warm.

7. Kan-chiang-jen-sheng-pan-hsia-wan   乾薑人參半夏丸
   (Ginger, Pinellia, and Ginseng Gormula)

This formula is for women who have been suffering from the vomiting for quite a long period of time and are gradually beginning to have severer symptoms: constant nausea and vomiting, signs of somatic debility, a soft and weak abdomen, a weak and thin pulse, and an inability to take any nourishment due to the constant vomiting.

8. Wu-mei-wan   烏梅丸
   (Mume Formula)

This formula is for women whose condition has become quite dangerous. Such patients are suffering from malnutrition as a result of their inability to ingest food without vomiting. They may experience the uncomfortable sensation of worms crawling up the chest and throat.

9. Wu-chu-yu-tang 吳茱萸湯
(Evodia Combination)

This formula is for dangerous cases where the patient vomits food immediately after it is eaten. In addition, she will have headaches, giddiness, insomnia, and irritability. The formula is most suitable for patients having a submerged and slow pulse, distension and obstruction beneath the heart, and a chilly feeling in the limbs.

10. Hsuan-fu-hua-tai-che-shih-tang 旋覆花代赭石湯
(Inula and Hematite Combination)

When the Patient's condition has become a weak conformation and she has a bloated feeling beneath her heart at the stomach, a slight stomachache, vomiting of ingested foods, hyperacidity, heartburn, and a tendency toward constipation, this formula is good.

11. Baked Rice Decoction 炒米煎

When the symptoms have become extremely severe and the foregoing formulas have failed to take effect, the patient should gradually be given this decoction. It sometimes has a marvelous effect. Note that in this stage of the illness the patient is extremely frail and may become sick at the odor of other decoctions.

Toxemia of Pregnancy

Toxemia of pregnancy is mainly a condition occurring in the early or in the latter stage of pregnancy. When it occurs in the early stage, it is usually after about ten weeks; latter stage toxemia occurs after six months. It is thought that this condition is caused by the endotoxins of pregnancy, mainly by toxins from the placenta. However, strenuous work and careless diet are also primary causes.

Symptoms

The symptoms of pregnancy sickness are flushing or nausea in the early morning or a feeling of emptiness in the abdomen. The patient will vomit food, gastric juice, and, in severe cases, gall juice. There is also headache, dizziness, general tiredness, and occasional fever. Edema precedes the other symptoms in the latter stage toxemia. The edema appears first in the legs, then extends up to the hands and face.

In latter stage toxemia, the patient will also have albuminuria and hypertension. Severe édema is called "edema in pregnancy". In addition to the above symptoms, there will also be headache, dizziness, loss of consciousness, and convulsions.

If the patient has a decrease in urinary output, mental confusion, and loss of vision, then retinitis albuminuria, death of the fetus, eclampsia, or premature separation of the placenta may follow.

Treatment

In order to prevent toxemia of pregnancy, the patient should have regular examinations during the first five months of pregnancy; these should be done monthly during the sixth, seventh, and eighth month and weekly during the ninth month. Any disorder of pregnancy will become worse if there is constipation. The patient should have a bowel movement early every morning and eat generous amounts of vegetables. If she does become constipated, she should not take enemas or cathartics as they may induce abortion. She must avoid strenuous exercises and excessive mental work. She should eat small amounts of food at each meal, but may increase the number of meals in order not to feel hungry. The patient who suffers from latter stage toxemia must have physical and mental quiet and ample sleep, decrease salt intake, and eat sufficient, complete, low-calorie protein such as cheese, meat, eggs, and bean curd.

Chinese Herb Formulas
1. **Hsiao-pan-hsia-chia-fu-ling-tang**　　　　　　小半夏加茯苓湯
    (Minor Pinellia and Hoelen Combination)
A common formula for sickness of pregnancy; to be taken for vomiting and stomach discomfort.

2. **Szu-ling-tang**　　　　　　四苓湯
    (Hoelen and Polyporus Combination)
To be taken for thirst, fever, or decreased urinary output.

3. **Wu-ling-san** 五苓散
   (Hoelen Five Herb Formula)
To be taken for dry throat, oliguria, edema, hypertension, severe albuminuria, headache, and nausea.

4. **Chai-ling-tang** 柴苓湯
   (Bupleurum and Hoelen Combination)
It is effective for the conformation which is similar to that of *Wu-ling-san* (Hoelen Five Herb Formula), but with the symptoms of distension at the chest and heart, mild fever, headache, and nausea with anorexia.

5. **Yin-chen-hao-tang** 茵陳蒿湯
   (Capillaris Combination)
To be taken for fullness at the upper abdomen, distension at the chest and heart, thirst, constipation, dysuria, and edema. Sometimes, a combination with *Wu-ling-san* (Hoelen Five Herb Formula) may produce good results.

6. **Mu-fang-chi-tang** 木防己湯
   (Stephania and Ginseng Combination)
To be taken for distension at the heart, facial darkness, abdominal fullness, gasping, palpitation, difficult breathing, distension at the chest, edema, oliguria, thirst, and sunken pulse.

7. **Pa-wei-ti-huang-wan** 八味地黃丸
   (Rehmannia Eight Formula)
It is effective for edema with marked hypertension and albuminuria, thirst, dysuria, flushing, and pain at the waist and feet.

8. **Fen-hsiao-tang** 分消湯
   (Hoelen and Alisma Combination)
To be taken for mild edema at the limbs or face with obvious water stagnancy in the abdomen, hardened swelling at the abdomen (especially after a meal), and sunken, tense pulse.

9. **Tang-kuei-shao-yao-san** 當歸芍藥散
   (Tang-kuei and Paeonia Formula)
To be taken as a preventive and as treatment of toxemia of pregnancy.

Hydatidiform Mole

Hydatidiform mole is a degenerative disorder of the chorion (placenta) which occurs as a complication in about one in 1,500 pregnancies in the United States, usually during the first eighteen weeks. Although it is assumed to be of placental (fetal) origin, the precise cause is not known. Hydatidiform mole is more common among women over forty, and over five times more prevalent in the Orient than in the West. Malignant change (chorioepithelioma), which occurs in about 4 percent of cases in the United States, is often fatal.

Symptoms

Excessive nausea and vomiting occur in over one-third of patients having hydatidiform mole. Uterine bleeding beginning at six to eight weeks is observed in virtually all instances and is indicative of threatened or incomplete abortion. In about one-fifth of the cases the uterus is larger than would be expected in a normal pregnancy of the same duration. Intact or collapsed grape-like molar tissue may be passed through the vagina.

Eclamptogenic toxemia, frequently of the fulminating type, may develop during the second trimester of pregnancy.

A malignant tumor may be suspected if there is continued or recurrent uterine bleeding after evacuation of a mole, or the presence of an ulcerative vaginal tumor, pelvic mass, or evidence of distant metastatic tumor. The diagnosis is established by pathologic examination of curettings or by biopsy.

Amniography after the third month, either by transcervical or transcutaneous route, using intravenous urographic media may demonstrate a honeycomb appearance of the uterine contents.

Treatment

Emergency Measures. Hemorrhage indicative of abortion requires immediate hospitalization. The type and cross-match of the patient's blood must be done and at least two units of blood available for transfusion. Free bleeding will cease as soon as the uterine contents are evacuated and firm uterine contraction with oxytocin is established. Curettage will probably be required for removal of adherent tissue.

Specific Measures. The uterus must be evacuated as soon as

possible after the diagnosis of hydatidiform mole. If the uterus is larger than a five month pregnancy and the cervix is resistant to wide dilation, a hysterotomy (Cesarean section) may be indicated. Hysterotomy is rarely curative.

Antitumor Chemotherapy. Methotrexate, 3mg/kg IM, in divided doses over a five day period is a method of treatment.

Chinese Herb Formulas

1. **Tao-ho-cheng-chi-tang** 桃核承氣湯
   (Persica and Rhubarb Combination)

This prescription may dispel the hydatidiform mole in a patient with a forceful abdomen and pulse, pain when pressed at the lower abdomen, no anemia, and repeated, irregular hemorrhage.

2. **Kuei-chih-fu-ling-wan-liao** 桂枝茯苓丸料
   (Cinnamon and Hoelen Formula)

This formula should be taken for a lengthy time after an abortion to eliminate occlusion of blood, prevent the occurrence of pernicious chorioepithelioma, and improve the constitution.

3. **Tang-kuei-shao-yao-san** 當歸芍藥散
   (Tang-kuei and Paeonia Formula)

This formula restores body strength and thus cures anemia. It is for women of a cold conformation after having an abortion who have anemia, general weakness, and lethargy.

4. **Chiung-kuei-chiao-ai-tang** 芎歸膠艾湯
   (Tang-kuei and Gelatin Combination)

This combination is used for intermittent hemorrhaging and the resulting anemia. In most cases the patient will have poor muscle tone, a soft abdomen, anemophobia, and a minute and weak pulse.

5. **Shih-chuan-ta-pu-tang** 十全大補湯
   (Ginseng and Tang-kuei Ten Combination)

This formula is suitable for a weak conformation: general weakness, extremely severe anemia, deteriorated appetite, and extreme fatigue.

6. **Kuei-pi-tang** 歸脾湯
   (Ginseng and Longan Combination)

This formula is prescribed for severely anemic patients who have pain and hardness beneath the heart and aggravated neurotic symptoms such as insomnia and amnesia. It is taken after having taken the preceding formula.

Weak Pains
(Insufficient Contractions at Birth)

Uterine contractions at the time of delivery that are short and weak with long and irregular intervals between often delay delivery. In such cases the pains are referred to as weak pains.

Uterine contractions that are weak from the beginning of delivery are called primitive pains. If the contractions become weak during the course of delivery because of fatigue and exhaustion of uterine muscle, they are called secondary pains.

Primitive pains frequently occur in women giving birth to their first child. The causes are abnormal development of the uterus, inflammation, a tumor, excessive dilation, somatic disease, abnormality in the endocrinological system, an abnormal fetal position, or fetal teratogenecity (malformation).

Secondary pains are caused by a narrow pelvis, premature rupture of the amnion, an intrapelvic tumor, incomplete extension of the vagina, and abnormality in the fetus. They can result in fetal compression in the vagina and produce a comatose state. At times they cause uterine rupture. Although weak pains before amnionic rupture do not worry us much, if they occur after amnionic rupture appropriate emergency action must be taken to calm the woman and to increase her vitality.

Chinese Herb Formulas
1. **Ma-huang-tang** 麻黃湯
   (Ma-huang Combination)

This formula opens up the surface, so to speak; it is a sweating agent. The principle is: if we want the south wind to come in, we have to open the north window. Likewise opening up the surface opens up the interior so as to facilitate the delivery. Asada Dohaku said, "For premature rupture of the amnion and the resulting weak pains in the parturient woman who is experiencing anemophobia, lower back pain, and distress, *Ma-huang-tang* plus aconite should be used to hasten delivery."

2. Wu-chi-san 五積散
(Tang-kuei and Magnolia Formula)
For the parturient woman who has weak pains, delayed delivery, and pain and distress beneath the heart, this formula in thick decocted form in combination with one-half of a small winecup full of vinegar will relieve the thoracic distress and ease delivery. In ancient times people used *Ping-wei-san* to save parturient women from dangerous deliveries.

3. Chiung-kuei-tang 芎歸湯
(Cnidium and Tang-kuei Combination)
Also named *Fo-shou-san*, this very famous formula is prescribed for various complications before and after delivery. For those who have had weak pains during previous deliveries, the taking of this formula for one or two months before delivery may strengthen the uterine contractions and make delivery more easy.

4. Tu-sheng-tang 獨參湯
(Ginseng Combination)
A parturient woman with secondary pains and diminished body strength who has lost the amniotic fluid but the head of the fetus is in sight is given this formula to increase vitality.

5. Tang-kuei-shao-yao-san-liao 當歸芍藥散料
(Tang-kuei and Paeonia Formula)
This formula is for women who have habitual weak pains during delivery. It augments uterine contraction if it is taken continuously from the beginning of pregnancy. It can even prevent a difficult delivery.

6. Moxibustion 灸法
Moxibustion on the *san-yin-chiao* locus from the beginning of the pregnancy continuously to the end has a prophylactic effect.

7. I-kan-san-chia-shao-yao 抑肝散加芍藥
(Bupleurum Formula with Paeonia)
This formula is effective for the adverse ascending of pneuma (hyperventilation) that causes terror and worry during delivery.

Atonic Uterine Bleeding

Uterine contractions weaken just after delivery, but sometimes blood continues to come from the myometrial surface where the placenta separated from the uterus. This bleeding is mostly due to the secondary pains and a flaccid or atonic uterus but continuous bleeding leads to a dangerous loss of blood. Sometimes the blood flows out in large quantities and remains in the uterus. Occasionally this heavy bleeding causes acute anemia, pallor, cold sweats, and even death from exhaustion. In these cases emergency treatment is necessary.

A flaccid uterus can be caused by many things: multiple births, miscarriages, artificially induced abortions, abuse of oxytocics, twins, hyperamnion, incomplete separation or partial remnant of placenta, myometrial swelling and pain, underdevelopment, ovarian tumor, or fatigue.

Treatment
An ice bag at the lower end of the uterus with massage to promote contraction plus specialized obstetric therapy helps. Although these are necessary measures, the taking of the following Chinese herb formulas may also be helpful.

Chinese Herb Formulas
1. Tu-sheng-tang   獨參湯
   (Ginseng Combination)

In cases of extremely severe anemia leading to weakening of the heart, this formula can be administered in large quantities.

2. Jen-sheng-tang   人參湯
   (Ginseng and Ginger Combination)

For patients having pallor, cold sweats, and cardiac weakening, this formula is recommended following the administration of *Tu-sheng-tang*.

3. Fu-ling-szu-ni-tang   茯苓四逆湯
   (Hoelen, G.L. and Aconite Combination)

This formula is for severe anemia leading to shock, a collapsed state, cardiac weakening, minute and weak pulse, cold limbs, and cold sweats.

4. **Kuei-pi-tang** 歸脾湯
   (Ginseng and Longan Combination)
   This formula is used when the most severe phase of bleeding has passed but the patient remains severely anemic and has not yet recovered her bodily strength. The prescription must be continued for a long amount of time.

5. **Chiung-kuei-chiao-ai-tang** 芎歸膠艾湯
   (Tang-kuei and Gelatin Combination)
   This formula is prescribed for patients having only slight weakening in bodily strength, slight hemorrhage, and mild anemia.

6. **Shih-chuan-ta-pu-tang** 十全大補湯
   (Ginseng and Tang-kuei Ten Combination)
   This formula is for patients with a non-energetic G I function, dry skin, and no fever who have just passed the dangerous phase but still are somatically debilitated and anemic.

7. **Tang-kuei-shao-yao-san** 當歸芍藥散
   (Tang-kuei and Paeonia Formula)
   Women having a history of atonic uterine bleeding should be given this formula from the beginning of pregnancy. This formula is an excellent prophylactic.

Retention of the Placenta

In ancient times "still placenta" meant a placenta which had not been expelled. There are two conditions under which the placenta is retained. In the first instance the placenta fails to separate from the uterine wall. In the second instance the placenta separates from the uterine wall but cannot be expelled because of constriction of the uterus at its lower part or neck section. The former condition is caused by atonia of the uterus, chronic metritis, syphilis, or uterine myoma. The latter condition is caused by excessive uterine friction or abuse of oxytocics.

Occasionally a woman may have partial retention of the placenta or ovarian membrane which results in incomplete abortion. If the retention of the placenta causes abnormal bleeding, or bacterial infection leading to endometritis, a gynecological disposal is called for and may be done in conjunction with Chinese herbal medication.

Chinese Herb Formulas
1. **Kuei-chih-fu-ling-wan-liao** 桂枝茯苓丸料
   (Cinnamon and Hoelen Formula)
   When placental retention causes resistant pressing pain at the abdomen and uterine bleeding, administration of this formula can expel the retained placenta. If there is constipation, rhubarb may be added to the formula.

2. **Tao-ho-cheng-chi-tang** 桃核承氣湯
   (Persica and Rhubarb Combination)
   This formula is suitable for a tense abdominal wall, eminent resistance and pressing pain at the lower abdomen, general symptoms indicating inflammatory hyperemia, and a tendency toward constipation.

3. **Huo-hsieh-san-yu-tang** 活血散瘀湯
   (Cnidium and Persica Combination)
   This formula is to be used when the symptoms are milder than in the preceding conformation when the condition has lasted for several days.

4. **Chiung-kuei-tiao-hsieh-yin** 芎歸調血飲
   (Cnidium and Rehmannia Combination)
   When a portion of the retained placenta remains unexpelled, the taking of this formula will expel it. Continued administration will bring about the patient's recovery from her postpartum anemia by strengthening her vitality.

Eclampsia

The ancient name for this disease in Chinese is the same as the present day one. It occurs in paroxysmic form during pregnancy, delivery, or the puerperal period and is characterized by intermittent convulsions of the muscles all over the body. Additionally the patient experiences absent-mindedness. The occurring rates are: delivery, 60%; pregnancy, 22%; puerperium,

18%. It is the most serious complication caused by toxemia of pregnancy.

The symptoms of this disease can be divided into prodromal, paroxysmal, and post-episodic symptoms. The prodromal symptoms commonly are present several days or even weeks before the episode and include lower limb or somatic edema, reduced urine, proteinuria, headache, vertigo, lassitude, nausea, vomiting, occasional violent stomachache, hypertension, psychic instability, and blurring. Right before the incidence there will be scintillating scotoma, visual disturbance, and auditory deterioration.

The episodic state is exactly the same as in epilepsy or toxemia. It lasts about one to two minutes at the frequency of eight to ten convulsions or even as many as fifty to one hundred during the episode. The episode causes sudden visual disturbance or even blindness. The body temperature may rise to 38-40°C.

Mostly the symptoms disappear after delivery and the patient returns to normality. At times the disease may recur on and off after delivery. If the fetus dies, the convulsions cease and the fetus is expelled a few days later.

It is necessary to distinguish this disease from epilepsy, hysteria, toxemia, and meningitis.

The disease is treated with *Tang-kuei-san* or *Tang-kuei-shao-yao-san* from *Chin kuei yao lueh* from the initial stage of pregnancy in order to eliminate abdominal water stagnancy (ascites), activate occluded blood, cleanse blood fever, and, in doing so, bring about a prophylactic effect. If the disease occurs during the final term or delivery, prompt gynecological measures must be taken.

Symptoms

Symptoms are generalized tonic-clonic convulsions, coma followed by amnesia and confusion, 3-4+ proteinuria, marked hypertension preceding a convulsion and hypotension afterwards (also during coma or vascular collapse), stertorous breathing, rhonchi, frothing at the mouth, twitching of muscle groups (in the face and arms), nystagmus, and diminished or complete absence of urination.

Treatment

Emergency Care. If the patient is convulsing, she must be

turned on her side to prevent aspiration of vomit and mucus and to prevent the caval syndrome. A padded tongue blade or plastic tongue depressor inserted between the teeth prevents biting the tongue and maintains respiratory exchange. Fluid and food should be aspirated from the glottis or trachea, and oxygen given by face cone or tent. Magnesium sulfate, 10ml of 25% aqueous solution, given intravenously or by injection repeated in half doses four times daily prevents and controls convulsions, lowers blood pressure, and encourages urination. In cases of overdosage 20ml of a 10% aqeous solution of calcium gluconate given intravenously, slowly, and repeated every hour clears urinary, respiratory, and neurologic depression.

General Care. The patient should be kept in a single, darkened, quiet room to allow absolute bed rest with no visitors allowed. She should lie on her side with side rails for protection during convulsions. Unnecessary procedures (baths, enemas, or douches) should be delayed and the blood pressure cuff left on her arm. Typed and cross-matched whole blood must be available for immediate use because patients in eclampsia often develop premature separation of the placenta resulting in a hemorrhage. Also, they are susceptible to shock.

A convulsing patient must take nothing by mouth and fluid intake and output for each 24-hour period should be recorded. When she can eat and drink, she should be on a salt-free (less than 1.0g salt per day), high carbohydrate, moderate protein, low fat diet. Potassium chloride is a good salt substitute. Hydrochlorothiazide, 25-50mg orally or intravenously, may be given to promote urination in patients who are not anuric or severely oliguric. Phenobarbital should be given on admission and sedation maintained until improvement is established. Perenteral magnesium sulfate is given as necessary.

Because severe hypotensive disease, renal disease, and toxemia of pregnancy are usually aggravated by continuing pregnancy, the most direct method of treatment of any of these disorders is termination of the pregnancy. However, the eclampsia must be under control before attempting induction of labor or delivery. Labor is induced preferably by amniotomy alone when the patient's condition permits. Oxytocins to stimulate labor are used only if necessary. Regional anesthesia is the preferred method. Vaginal delivery is preferred if the patient is not at term or if labor is not inducible and if she is bleeding, but if there is a question of disproportion, cesarean section may be necessary. If so, procaine is used for local infiltration of the abdominal wall. After the baby is delivered, thiopental anesthesia is used for abdominal closure.

Chinese Herb Formulas
1. Emergency Care.

In ancient books this remedy is called "eclampsia aid". A patient with eclampsia feels as if something is moving in her abdomen and rushing toward her chest. Once this uprushing substance enters the chest cavity, the eclampsia also reaches its fulmination. Therefore, at the time of the incident, the patient must lie on her back while the doctor sits on the patient's left side facing toward the patient's feet. The doctor then clenches his right fist with the thumb bent inward, places his fist at the lower edge of the ribs immediately under the patient's breast, which is the location corresponding to the *pu zon* locus, and thrusts his fist inward with as strong a force as possible. In most cases the left side of the *pu zon* locus is compressed. However, if the patient feels distress at the right side, the right side *pu zon* locus must be compressed. During the attack the patient's tongue is slack and her tightly locked jaws could result in biting off her tongue. Hence it is necessary to insert a wooden plate or mouth opener between the teeth. In ancient times they used a wad of cotton or a handkerchief.

2. Ursi Fel 熊膽
(Bear's Gall)

As the seizure is ending, the patient should take 0.2-0.5g of bear's gall all at once. This drug has spasmolytic and sedative actions.

3. Sheng-lien-tang 參連湯
(Ginseng and Coptis Combination)

If there is no bear's gall at hand or immediately after the patient has taken bear's gall, she should take *Sheng-lien-tang* plus evodia.

4. Hsieh-hsin-tang-chia-chen-sha 瀉心湯加辰砂
(Coptis and Rhubarb Combination with Cinnabar)

If the patient is flushed and in an excited state implying mental instability, this formula works as a sedative.

5. Tao-ho-cheng-chi-tang 桃核承氣湯
    (Persica and Rhubarb Combination)
This formula is used for patients having more drastic symptoms than those of the preceding formula. These patients become severely flushed and display manic behavior. 2.0g of schizonepeta is added to the formula.

6. Ling-yang-chiao-tang 羚羊角湯
    (Antelope Horn Combination)
This remedy is indicated for the postpartum woman who is consistently lethargic and has repeated episodes of mild to severe physical exhaustion.

7. Wu-chu-yu-tang 吳茱萸湯
    (Evodia Combination)
This formula is used for postpartum women whose symptoms include vomiting, headache, vexation, irritation, and cold limbs. This conformation is not specific to postpartum women, it may also occur before delivery.

8. Leech Therapy 水蛭療法
Yamada Ko's report says, "For eclamptic women, the ancient people put thirty to fifty leeches on top of the sick woman. The leeches would suck out blood from the woman. It was definitely effective."

Puerperal Fever

Puerperal fever refers to a fever derived from the infection of genital wounds caused by intra-genital invasion of various bacteria during childbirth. Essentially it is the proliferation of putrefactive bacteria in necrotic tissues or body secretions. The metabolite and poisonous substances excreted by bacteria are absorbed into the body, which results in the so-called puerperal intoxication. The causative bacteria are chiefly septisemic streptococci (70-80%), and rarely, staphylococci pneumococci, *E. coli*, or enterocogen (15%). These, after entry into the tissues or bloodstream at the time of labor and postpartum manipulations, cause puerperal infections. Malnutrition and anemia augment these infections. In addition, there is another kind of infection, a combination of the two: the combined infection of putrefactive and streptococcus bacteria.

Puerperal fever is the collective term for the following diseases.

1. Sapraemia or toxemia is puerperal intoxication in which the pathogens have not yet entered the bloodstream so that no proliferation has occurred. In other words the disease is localized and generally mild in severity. Representative of this disease are putrid endometritis, uterine putrescentia, and lochia retention (absorption fever, putrefaction fever, or alternate fever).

2. Puerperal infection (such as bacteriaemia) is mostly caused by virulently toxic bacteria which enter the tissues and proliferate producing somatic and very serious symptoms which can be differentiated from mildly toxic and localized infections. Mild and localized infections are represented by puerperal ulcer and puerperal septic metro-endometritis. Somatic infections that disseminate via lymphatic vessels all over the body often advance slowly. Representative of this type of infection are puerperal parametritis, puerperal perimetritis, puerperal pelveoperitonitis, and puerperal septic peritonitis. In contrast, infections that disseminate via blood vessels often proceed rapidly. Representative diseases of the blood vessel type of infection are septic phlebitis, puerperal pyaemia, puerperal septicemia, and puerperal ulcerous endocarditis.

Chinese Herb Formulas
1. San-wu-huang-chin-tang 三物黃芩湯
   (Scute Three Herb Combination)

The intolerable heat in the limbs caused by blood fever is the target of treatment with this formula. This symptom appears in the initial stage: the puerperal woman has a vexatious sensation of fever in the palms of her hands and the soles of her feet, and her tongue and mouth become so dry that she wants to moisten them with water but yet doesn't drink much water. Her body strength at this point has not yet been exhausted to any extent.

2. **Hsiao-chai-hu-tang-chia-ti-huang** 小柴胡湯加地黃
   (Minor Bupleurum Combination with Rehmannia)
   This formula can be taken in the initial as well as the middle stage of infection when the patient has vexatious fever in the limbs, headache, alternate chills and fever, thirst, and loss of appetite. Occasionally, *Hsiao-chai-hu-tang* combined with *Szu-wu-tang* is given.

3. **Chih-kan-tsao-tang** 炙甘草湯
   (Baked Licorice Combination)
   This formula is suitable for patients whose symptoms have lasted for a couple of days. The symptoms it treats are a tendency toward weakness, cardiac hyperfunction, short breathing, knotty and irregular pulse, vexatious fever, pharyngeal dryness and thirst, constipation, and adverse flushing.

4. **Pa-wei-wan-liao** 八味丸料
   (Rehmannia Eight Formula)
   If fatigue and exhaustion are exacerbated leading to anuria and vexatious fever in the limbs or septicemic phlebitis, this formula is given.

5. **Kuei-chih-fu-ling-wan-liao** 桂枝茯苓丸料
   (Cinnamon and Hoelen Formula)
   This formula is used for puerperal infection when thrombosis occurs in the pelvis or clogging occurs in the chief veins of the legs and feet leading to thrombotic phlebitis and resultant circulation disturbance, severe edema and pyrexia, and pain.

6. **Tao-ho-cheng-chi-tang** 桃核承氣湯
   (Persica and Rhubarb Combination)
   This combination is used for more serious cases than the preceding one when the symptoms are accompanied by constipation.

Puerperal Lower Limb Thrombosis

Sometimes blood coagulates within the uterine wall (especially the part from which the placenta was separated) or within the pelvic connective tissues. If not yet infected by bacteria, it forms a thrombosis or clot within the pelvis or the veins of the thighs. Commonly, it occurs in one lower limb only. The resultant hyperemia and edema resemble those in septicemic phlebitis but are less feverish and painful than the latter.

Thrombosis occurs between the end of the first week after delivery and the beginning of the second week, or between the third and the fourth week, or suddenly when the puerperal woman begins walking. It aches at the site of the thrombosis and the hyperemic edema spreads from the calf upward to the thigh. She will have a fever in addition.

This illness is more often found in women having varicose veins or cardiac diseases. The prognosis is good; the coagulated blood can be absorbed spontaneously. The patient must keep quiet for four to five weeks and take the following formulas to shorten the duration.

Chinese Herb Formulas
1. **Kuei-chih-fu-ling-wan-liao** 桂枝茯苓丸料
   (Cinnamon and Hoelen Formula)

This combination is the most frequently employed formula for this disease. It is for those having blood occlusion and stagnation and resistant pain when pressed on the lower abdomen. If the patient has constipation, 1.0-2.0g of rhubarb is added to this formula.

2. **Tao-ho-cheng-chi-tang** 桃核承氣湯
   (Persica and Rhubarb Combination)

This formula is used for women who have more violent symptoms than in the preceding formula and have strong resistant pain in the abdomen and constipation.

3. **Ti-tang-tang** 抵當湯
   (Rhubarb and Leech Combination)

If the condition persists for some period of time and the preceding formula has failed to eliminate the blood clot and edema, this formula may then be worth trying.

4. **Tang-kuei-tiao-hsieh-yin** 當歸調血飲
   (Cnidium and Rehmannia Combination)

This formula is for patients with lingering pain, a lack of stamina, a deteriorated appetite, a proneness to anemia, and edema. It also can eliminate lochia and clogged blood and replenish the blood.

5. Tang-kuei-shao-yao-san-liao　　　　　　　　　當歸芍藥散料
   (Tang-kuei and Paeonia Formula)
This formula can be used for debilitated women who have anemia, fatigue, weakness, and chills that have persisted for a long time.

6. Chih-kan-tsao-tang　　　　　　　　　　　　　　炙甘草湯
   (Baked Licorice Combination)
This formula is for a weak conformation and is suitable for women with dry skin, cardiac hyperfunction, knotty and impeded pulse, vexatious fever, adverse flushing, dry throat, and a tendency toward constipation.

Milk Deficiency

In ancient times *zu nan* originally meant "difficult labor," but its meaning was later changed to "milk deficiency." Insufficient secretion of milk in a lactating woman renders her unable to breast feed the infant. It causes are an endocrine disturbance, underdevelopment of the mammae or various diseases of the mammae, atrophic yellowing disease, and such things as anemia, abnormality in sympathetic nerves, or extreme mental distress.

This condition can be effectively cured by treating the various causative diseases, enriching nutrition, taking sedatives, and eliminating frightening and anxiety producing factors. The following are effective formulas for these problems.

Chinese Herb Formulas
1. Ko-ken-tang　　　　　　　　　　　　　　　　　葛根湯
   (Pueraria Combination)
This formula is effective for women with normally developed mammae with sufficient milk but who are unable to breast feed because of obstruction and stagnation, and who feel pain in their shoulders or back. Pueraria has the effect of stimulating the secretion of milk and was used as a lactagogue in cake form in ancient times.

2. **Chiung-kuei-tiao-hsieh-yin** 芎歸調血飲
    (Cnidium and Tang-kuei Combination)

This combination is used as a postpartum healing agent to eliminate lochia, to activate blood circulation, to increase body strength, and to render luxuriant milk secretion.

3. **Shih-chuan-ta-pu-tang** 十全大補湯
    (Ginseng and Tang-kuei Ten Combination)

This combination increases the stamina in people with anemia, weak vitality, and excessive fatigue.

4. **Pu-kung-ying-tang** 蒲公英湯
    (Dandelion Combination)

Those who have underdeveloped mammae had best take this formula as soon as possible. To be effective the root of dandelion must be fresh and big. In ancient books it is recorded that a male's mammae swelled after taking this formula. However, we have never observed such an effect.

5. **Zu-chuan-san** 乳泉散
    (Trichosanthes Root Formula)

When a postpartum woman has obstructed milk, she may take the best quality trichosanthes root prepared in the form of pueraria cake and dipped in honey or sugar before taking. Pueraria cake alone may also be used and taken by first dipping in honey.

6. **Tsuei-zu-fang** 催乳方
    (Rehmannia and Honeycomb Formula)

Equal portions of *Vespae Nidus* (bee's nest) and cured rehmannia are roasted until charred and then made into pills the size of a sterculia seed with a gluing agent. The dosage is fifty pills each time taken along with a barley decoction. *Tsuei-zu-fang* is taken for about two weeks during which period no fish or meat is allowed. Recently fashion has changed the nutritive diet. The immediate ingestion of animal protein and fat were prohibited in ancient times. According to ancient bromatotherapy, the lactating woman was allowed only congee, salted prunes, or dried fish and she still had copious milk secretion.

7. Otsuka's Familial Prescription 大塚家方

White Bombyx batryticatus is pulverized and made into pills with *Han-mei-fen* (cold prune powder). *Han-mei-fen* is a substance produced by first freezing *Oryza glutinosa* during extremely cold winter days and then pulverizing it into powder. This drug is administered in dosages of 3.7g each time, twice each day, once in the morning and again in the evening. It should be taken along with wine within one hundred days after delivery. It should take effect in ten days. If after ten days the milk secretion is not increased, it is useless to continue taking it. However, its effectiveness rates 70 percent.

8. Folk Medicine 民間方
The following recipe is said to take effect after seven days of ingestion: 40g of tangerine leaves that have been dried in the shade, 40g of *Oryza glutinosa* and 8g of licorice. Pulverize the three substances into a powder and blend. Before using, stir the mixture into boiling water.

Puerperal Mastitis

Postpartum inflammation of the breast occurs most often after several weeks or more of nursing. Infection invades via the ducts following contamination of the nipple and is often caused by fissures in the nipple or obstructed milk flow. Hemolytic *Staphylococcus aureus* is the causative agent in most cases. Inflammation is unilateral in three fourths of patients. Most often affected are women giving birth to their first child (primiparas).

This disease is classified into (1) parenchymatous mastitis, (2) interstitial mastitis, (3) subareolar abscess, and (4) retromammary abscess. The first type is due to stagnation or obstruction of milk. The second type is due to bacterial infection through fissures in the nipple causing cellulitis. In the third type the abscess is located superficially, and in the fourth type the abscess is located deep inside the breast.

Symptoms

At the onset of this illness there are chills, fever, malaise, regional pain, tenderness, and induration. Localization, mass formation, fluctuation, and glandular disease in the armpit occur later. Fever and swelling in the breasts, as well as pain and swelling in armpit lymph nodes, occur. In most cases once infection is well established an abscess formation is unavoidable.

Treatment

Treatment consists of suspending nursing, supporting the breasts, prescribing antipyretics and analgesics, and giving intensive broad-spectrum antibiotic therapy. Incision and drainage are required if abscess formation occurs.

Prevention consists of proper initial nursing procedure and breast hygiene.

Chinese Herb Formulas
1. **Ko-ken-tang** 葛根湯
   (Pueraria Combination)
No matter if it is obstructed or purulent mastitis this formula plus 5.0g of gypsum can be used for the initial chills, fever, swelling, pain, and stiff shoulders.

2. **Szu-ni-tang-chia-mai-ya** 四逆湯加麥芽
   (Aconite and G.L. Combination with Malt)
For obstructed mastitis with stiff and aching breasts, 8.0g of malt is baked, crushed, and added to this formula. This is taken alternately with a decoction of malt alone. The decoction may suspend lactation but render dissipation of the swelling.

3. **Hsiao-chai-hu-tang** 小柴胡湯
   (Minor Bupleurum Combination)
After administration of *Ko-ken-tang*, the fever may drop temporarily, but the symptoms of tongue fur, thirst, and loss of appetite may persist. If such is the condition of the patient, this formula is indicated. This formula alone cures stagnant mastitis.

4. **Shih-wei-pai-tu-tang-chia-lien-chiao** 十味敗毒湯加連翹
   (Bupleurum and Schizonepeta Combination with Forsythia)
If the body temperature remains high and the reddening and aching continues after taking the preceding two formulas, no doubt pustulation has occurred and this formula plus 3.0g of

forsythia is indicated.

5. **Tuo-li-hsiao-tu-yin** 托裏消毒飲
   (Gleditsia Combination)

This combination is used for abscesses that are unlikely to rupture and for breasts that are stiff and swollen. For this purpose this formula has to be taken in large amounts.

6. **Chien-chin-nei-tuo-san** 千金內托散
   (Astragalus and Platycodon Formula)

After a period of time has elapsed, the body strength deteriorates. If the pus is not expelled, then this formula should be used. Externally *Chung-huang-kao* (Phellodendron and Curcuma Ointment) is applied to speed up the rupturing and discharging of pus. The formula must be taken continuously after rupture of abscesses to promote granulation.

7. **Pai-nung-san** 排膿散
   (Platycodon and Chih-shih Formula)

When suppuration is underway and abscesses are formed but the pus is not discharged and no other formulas can bring about rupture in the abscesses, then this formula may be given.

8. **Chung-huang-kao** 中黃膏
   (Curcurma and Phellodendron Ointment)

At the beginning of this illness the application of *Chung-huang-kao* plaster sometimes disperses the obstruction or stagnation or accelerates the opening of abscesses when there is suppuration.

9. **Folk Medicine** 民間方

For obstructed mastitis, the corm of water lily is ground into a paste, mixed with a little vinegar and flour, and applied to the lesion. It accelerates dissipation. However, the effect is less likely if suppuration is already underway.

Postpartum Clonus

Occasionally a few days after delivery there will be some kind of abdominal ache resembling the uterine contraction; this is commonly called postpartum abdominal ache. The Chinese term for it is *er-chen-tong* (infantile clonus) or *nung-tong* (stroking ache). *Er-chen-tong* is a natural physiological phenomenon caused by uterine contraction and generally disappears within a few days. However, the clonus may be extremely violent and persistent in multiparous or nervous women, or can occur if there is a remnant of the placenta or lochia and a blood clot.

Symptoms
Chinese medicine divides the symptoms into two categories: firm and weak conformations. The former has little bleeding, much lochia, and fullness of the abdomen which upon pressing will have an aching and unpleasant sensation. The latter has much bleeding, a proneness to anemia, and a soft abdomen which the patient herself likes to press.

Treatment
Western medical treatments are palliative, but the following Chinese formulas are quite effective.

Chinese Herb Formulas
1. **Kuei-chih-fu-ling-wan-liao** 桂枝茯苓丸料
   (Cinnamon and Hoelen Formula)

This formula is effective for a conformation exhibiting a firm and fully distended abdomen and resistance against pressure at the lower abdomen. It also treats placental remnants and excessive lochia, and alleviates patient discomfort. If the patient has constipation, 1.0-2.0g of rhubarb are added.

2. **Chiung-kuei-tiao-hsieh-yin** 芎歸調血飲
   (Cnidium and Tang-kuei Combination)

This formula is suitable for women having a not so firm conformation, a soft abdomen, pain when pressed in the lower abdomen, and obstructive stagnancy of lochia. As the lochia is purged the patient will feel much better.

3. **Tang-kuei-shao-yao-san-liao** 當歸芍藥散料
   (Tang-kuei and Paeonia Formula)

This formula is useful for women who have slight tension in the abdomen which is not full and firm and who have a proneness to anemia, love to press on their abdomens, and cannot take a purgative.

4. Hsiao-chien-chung-tang 小建中湯
   (Minor Cinnamon and Paeonia Combiantion)
   When the patient has copious bleeding, a feeble physique, proneness to anemia, weakened stamina, weak pulse, and a thin and tight yet feeble abdomen, this combination is used.

5. Tang-kuei-chien-chung-tang 當歸建中湯
   (Tang-kuei, Cinnamon, and Paeonia Combination)
   This combination is used for those parturient women who have prominent anemia, fatigue, and abdominal pain following delivery.

6. Kan-tsao-kan-chiang-tang 甘草乾薑湯
   (Licorice and Ginger Combination)
   This formula usually takes effect in those having a weak and chill conformation with severe, impetuous pain.

Postpartum Beriberi

Postpartum beriberi is commonly called *hsieh chiao chi* (blood beriberi), a condition which manifests itself conspicuously in women who have a proneness to beriberi, are fatigued, and suffer from poor nutrition after delivery. The mother's beriberi may cause the same in the infant.

Symptoms
The symptoms are the same as for ordinary beriberi. The patient experiences numb sensations, cardiac palpitation, edema, and loss of reflexes and coordination.

Treatment
Postpartum beriberi is generally treated with a prescription such as *Szu-wu-tang*.

Chinese Herb Formulas
1. Szu-wu-tang-chia-wei-fang 四物湯加味方
   (Tang-kuei Four Combination Supplemented)

This formula is commonly used for the so-called *hsieh chiao chi* (blood beriberi). The infant should be given *Hsia-pin-tang* (Pinellia and Areca Seed Combination) as a preventive. The formula is made by adding 3.0g each of chaenomeles and atractylodes and 6.0g of coix to *Szu-wu-tang*. If the numbness in the lower extremities is very strong and the woman has feeble legs, 3.0g each of turtle shell and haliotis are added to the formula which is then taken for a long period of time. However, caution must be used in giving this formula to patients having prominent anemia and a tendency to have diarrhea.

2. **Chiung-kuei-tiao-hsieh-yin** 芎歸調血飲
   (Cnidium and Tang-kuei Combination)

In milder cases this formula may be used to restore one's vitality and to diminish fatigue, to produce new blood, and to promote the appetite. Afterwards the beriberi symptoms will disappear and the patient will recover quickly.

3. **Pa-wei-ti-huang-wan-liao** 八味地黃丸料
   (Rehmannia Eight Formula)

This formula is suitable for patients whose lower abdomen is especially weak and feeble; who have a numb sensation in the mouth, lips, lower abdomen, and limbs; a hot feeling at the center of the soul; thirst; vexation; and difficulty in urinating. Preparations containing rehmannia may be administered whenever there is the symptom of weak legs and numbness.

4. **Shih-chuan-ta-pu-tang** 十全大補湯
   (Ginseng and Tang-kuei Ten Combination)

This combination is effective for patients with seriously deteriorated nutrition who exhibit anemia and dry skin.

5. **Wei-cheng-fang** 痿證方
   (Eucommia and Achyranthes Formula)

This formula is effective for patients who have a feeble lumbar making it impossible for them to stand up. These patients may also be paralyzed in their legs as a result of beriberi.

6. **Ta-fang-feng-tang** 大防風湯
   (Major Siler Combination)

This combination is used for the conformation much like that of *Shih-chuan-ta-pu-tang:* weakness in both *ch'i* and blood, and debilitated legs and knees which make walking almost impossible.

7. Hsia-pin-tang　　　　　　　　　　　　　　　夏檳湯
   (Pinellia and Areca Seed Combination)
This combination is often used for beriberi occurring in breast-fed infants. It also can be administered prophylactically to normal infants if their mothers have postpartum beriberi.

Habitual Abortion

Abortion occurring at a certain stage of each pregnancy is called "habitual abortion". About 30 percent of these are due to syphilis; others are caused by diabetes, kidney disease, and tuberculosis. Most, however, are the result of gynecological causes such as imbalance of hormones, abnormal oosperm, cervical weakness, improperly developed uterus, or incompatible blood types of husband and wife. Habitual abortion usually recurs for the same reason. Therefore, the sufferer must have a medical examination to learn the cause and the appropriate precautions.

Symptoms

The abortion often occurs about three months after conception. The preceeding symptoms are a weighty sensation in the legs, severe vaginal hemorrhage, and lumbago. Abortion follows in a few days. If the embryo has descended completely, bleeding will cease in a few days. Otherwise, the bleeding will continue and there is a danger of bacterial infection in the placenta. The embryo is well-developed after five months; abortion occurring after this point in the pregnancy will usually be complete and without residual bleeding. As in childbirth, abortion begins with grinding pain.

Treatment

Habitual abortion may often be prevented if the pregnant woman takes good care of herself. She should observe the following health practices: (1) Avoid hard work or excessive exercise. (2) Maintain even body temperature. (3) Avoid constipation and diarrhea. (4) Avoid influenza and infectious diseases. (5) Practice moderation in her sexual life. In Chinese medicine, women having weak and chilling physique accompanied by abnormal location of the uterus due to stagnant blood are prone to abortion. Ingestion of proper formulas can prevent habitual abortion.

Chinese Herb Formulas

1. Tang-kuei-shao-yao-san 當歸芍藥散
(Tang-kuei and Paeonia Formula)
To be taken for limbs chill, headache, and abdominal pain.

2. Wen-ching-tang 溫經湯
(Tang-kuei and Evodia Combination)
To be taken for weakness, fever, and thirst.

3. Fasting
Fasting for one or two weeks can improve the physical constitution and decrease the possibility of abortion. This should always be done under a physician's supervision.

GYNECOLOGICAL DISEASES

Leucorrhea

The vagina always has secretions to maintain moisture. Even the healthiest woman has a certain amount of these secretions. For some reason, however, they will sometimes increase or become mucopurulent, causing heavy vaginal drainage. At one time or another, almost all women suffer from this condition which is called "leucorrhea".

The healthy woman with leucorrhea two or three days before or after her menstrual cycle is of normal physiology and should not be concerned. Neither should the pregnant woman having colorless or white leucorrhea. But in a woman after menopause, leucorrhea should be suspected as a symptom of uterine carcinoma. If caused by other disease, the leucorrhea is usually milky or yellow with pus and sometimes mixed with blood. If caused by cancer or abortion, it will have an abnormal odor.

The genital tract of the woman is easily affected by outside causes and is prone to vaginitis, endometritis, ovaritis, and pelvic peritonitis. The causes of leucorrhea are mostly gynecological. Therefore, it is important not to neglect or feel shame about the symptom of leucorrhea. Always accept a medical doctor's examination so that the cause can be found and treated.

Treatment

If the leucorrhea is caused by a disease, cure the disease first. The best therapy for leucorrhea is douching.

Chinese Herb Formulas

1. **Lung-tan-hsieh-kan-tang**   龍膽瀉肝湯
   (Gentiana Combination)

It is effective for those having bladder inflammation, urethritis, and uteritis with severe heat of the strong type. To be taken also for leucorrhea with a yellow or red color due to endometritis, vaginitis, and vaginal trichomoniasis.

2. **Pa-wei-tai-hsia-fang**   八味帶下方
   (Tang-kuei and Eight Herb Formula)

To be taken for chronic leucorrhea with a white or yellow color and accompanied by moderate anemia and abdominal looseness. It is also effective for leucorrhea caused by gonococci or vaginal trichomoniasis.

3. **Kuei-chih-fu-ling-wan**   桂枝茯苓丸
   (Cinnamon and Hoelen Formula)

To be taken for acute or chronic leucorrhea with stagnant blood and pressure at the lower abdomen.

4. **Tang-kuei-shao-yao-san**   當歸芍藥散
   (Tang-kuei and Paeonia Formula)

To be taken by those of the weak conformation with leucorrhea of a white color and a tendency towards anemia.

5. **Ching-hsin-lien-tzu-yin**   清心蓮子飲
   (Lotus Seed Combination)

It is effective for those having chronic leucorrhea with gastrointestinal weakness, physical chills and weakness, and leucorrhea consisting of a large amount of watery discharge.

6. **Wu-chi-san**   五積散
   (Tang-kuei and Magnolia Formula)

To be taken for dilute leucorrhea due to cold. It is also effective for leucorrhea due to chilling resulting from an air-conditioned room or exercises.

7. **Chieh-keng-tang** 桔梗湯
   (Platycodon Combination)
   A common formula for lung pus, it is effective for leucorrhea with yellow color.

8. **Chia-wei-hsiao-yao-san** 加味逍遙散
   (Bupleurum and Paeonia Formula)
   Effective for those who have taken *Tang-kuei-shao-yao-san* in vain.

9. **Chang-yung-tang** 腸癰湯
   (Coix and Persica Combination)
   Effective for leucorrhea accompanied by resistant pressure or swelling in the lower abdomen, but without constipation. In severe cases with constipation, take rhubarb or *Ta-huang-mu-tan-pi-tang* with coix (Rhubarb and Moutan Combination with Coix).

10. **I-yi-fu-tzu-pai-chiang-tang** 薏苡附子敗醬湯
    (Coix, Aconite, and Thlaspi Combination)
    To be taken for chronic dilute leucorrhea, abdominal weakness, chilling at the waist and feet, and tense and sunken pulse.

11. **Chai-hu-chia-lung-ku-mu-li-tang** 柴胡加龍骨牡蠣湯
    (Bupleurum and Dragon Bone Combination)
    Kuei-chih-chia-lung-ku-mu-li-tang 桂枝加龍骨牡蠣湯
    (Cinnamon and Dragon Bone Combination)
    Chai-hu-kuei-chih-kan-chiang-tang 柴胡桂枝乾薑湯
    (Bupleurum, Cinnamon, and Ginger Combination)
    All are effective for leucorrhea.

12. **Pa-wei-wan** 八味丸
    (Rehmannia Eight Formula)
    To be taken by women with dark skin, abdominal weakness and swelling, and leucorrhea.

13. **Shih-chuan-ta-pu-tang** 十全大補湯
    (Ginseng and Tang-kuei Ten Combination)
    It is effective for those suffering from physical weakness, lack of vigor, anemia, tendency towards fatigue, weak pulse, and

continuous leucorrhea after childbirth or abortion.

14. Jen-sheng-tang 人參湯
(Ginseng and Ginger Combination)
To be taken for leucorrhea with chilling. If the patient has gastrointestinal weakness, *Liu-chun-tzu-tang* (六君子湯 , Major Six Herb Combination) may also be used.

15. Wen-ching-tang 溫經湯
(Tang-kuei and Evodia Combination)
To be taken for watery leucorrhea with chill at the waist.

16. Yu-che-san 羽澤散
(Alum and Apricot Seed Formula)
This is a suppository effective for a great amount of leucorrhea and for chilling and itching at the vagina.

Climacteric Disorder

When a woman is past forty years of age, her ovarian function decreases gradually. After the ovary has completely stopped functioning, ovulation and the menstrual cycle cease. The period of time between normal menstrual function and menopause is called "climacteric". It usually lasts for one to three years and occurs between forty and fifty years of age.

During menopause, the ovarian function ceases and loses chime with other endocrine organs, especially the thyroid gland, hypothalamus, and kidneys. As a result, there will be changes in the blood vessels, nerves, and emotional states, resulting in generalized pains. These are called the "symptoms of climacteric disorder". In addition to chilling, fever, headache, aching shoulders, sweats, palpitation, and painful menstruation, there may be irritability, depression, and insomnia. Occasionally, the abdomen, hips, and legs will become somewhat obese. The above symptoms vary with the individual. If a woman in menopause has several of the symptoms at the same time, it is not necessarily a disease.

Treatment
Administration of sedatives or analgesics may produce

good results, but this should be done under a doctor's guidance.

Chinese Herb Formulas
1. Kuei-chih-fu-ling-wan　　　　　　　　　桂枝茯苓丸
(Cinnamon and Hoelen Formula)

To be taken for resistant, pressing pain in the lower abdomen around the umbilicus, symptoms of stagnant blood, pelvic congestion, headache, abdominal pain, and menstrual difficulties. It is a strong conformation. Most of the patients are vigorous and have a ruddy face. Those having constipation should add rhubarb (0.5-2.0 g.) to this formula. In severe cases, take *Tao-ho-cheng-chi-tang* (Persica and Rhubarb Combination) instead.

2. Tang-kuei-shao-yao-san　　　　　　　　當歸芍藥散
(Tang-kuei and Paeonia Formula)

To be taken by women of the weak type with a tendency towards anemia and fatigue, chilling at the waist and feet, heaviness of head, vertigo, tinnitus, palpitation, and aching in the lower abdomen.

3. Chia-wei-hsiao-yao-san　　　　　　　　加味逍遙散
(Bupleurum and Paeonia Formula)

To be taken blood diseases, such as fever and chilling, and for fever in the lims, heaviness of head vertigo, ruddy face, night sweats, insomnia, generalized tiredness, and loss of appetite. This is a drug for the semi-strong and semi-weak type.

4. Nu-shen-san　　　　　　　　　　　　　女神散
(Tang-kuei and Cyperus Formula)

To be taken for congestion and vertigo. It is a remedy for climacteric disorder and blood diseases.

5. Szu-wu-tang　　　　　　　　　　　　　四物湯
(Tang-kuei Four Combination)

This is an excellent formula for gynecological disease, to be taken for anemia and nervousness. The patient with diarrhea should not take it.

6. **Chiung-kuei-tiao-hsieh-yin** 芎歸調血飲
   (Cnidium and Tang-kuei Combination)

To be taken for the postpartum diseases. It is especially effective for nervous ailments of blood diseases.

7. **Chai-hu-chia-lung-ku-mu-li-tang** 柴胡加龍骨牡蠣湯
   (Bupleurum and Dragon Bone Combination)

This is a sedative, to be taken for pressure at the chest, uncomfortable feeling at the umbilicus, palpitation, congestion, headache, vertigo, insomnia, and fatigue of the blood diseases.

8. **I-kan-san-chia-chen-pi-pan-hsia** 抑肝散加陳皮半夏
   (Bupleurum Formula with Citrus and Pinellia)

To be taken for nervousness with epilepsy, anxiety with proneness to anger, and insomnia.

9. **Pan-hsia-hou-pu-tang** 半夏厚朴湯
   (Pinellia and Magnolia Combination)

To be taken by patients of the weak type with a sensation of something blocking or itching and stimulating in the throat, a hoarse voice, a weak and sunken pulse, and a patting sound at the lower part of the heart.

10. **Kuei-chih-chia-lung-ku-mu-li-tang** 桂枝加龍骨牡蠣湯
    (Cinnamon and Dragon Bone Combination)

To be taken for a tendency towards physical weakness, nervousness, congestion, headache, insomnia, palpitation, fearfulness, sweating, and night sweats.

11. **Kan-mai-ta-tsao-tang** 甘麥大棗湯
    (Licorice and Jujube Combination)

To be taken for hysteria, nervousness, spasm, insomnia, tendency towards yawning, and, in severe cases, coma or mania.

12. **Ling-kuei-kan-tsao-tang** 苓桂甘棗湯
    (Hoelen, Licorice, and Jujube Combination)

To be taken for palpitation at the lower umbilicus, congestions, vomiting, headache, and decrease of urine.

13. Huang-lien-chieh-tu-tang　　　　　　　黃連解毒湯
    (Coptis and Scute Combination)
It is effective for ruddy face, congestion, insomnia, stress, palpitation, and stagnation of blood.

14. Chen-wu-tang　　　　　　　　　　　　眞武湯
    (Vitality Combination)
It is effective for weak conformation, easy fatigability, chilling, weak pulse and abdomen, stagnancy in the gastrointestinal tract, decrease in urine, abdominal pain and diarrhea, vertigo, and palpitation.

Uterine Carcinoma

Among cancers occurring in women, the number of uterine carcinomas is about equal to that of gastric carcinomas. Uterine carcinoma occurs in two areas, the endometrium and the cervix. Younger women are most likely to contract cervical carcinoma and older women, carcinoma of the endometrium. Generally, the older patients are between forty and sixty years of age.

Symptoms
In the initial stages, the cancer is nearly painless. When the malignant tissue begins to grow, hemorrhage and leucorrhea (usually after intercourse) occur. The amount of leucorrhea is small in the beginning, but it increases gradually, becoming malodorous, mixed with blood or pus, and causing itching at the vagina. When there is bleeding after intercourse, the patient should not ignore it; she should consider surgery. When the malignancy has become advanced, there is pain in the lower abdomen.

If the carcinoma has metastasized to other organs, it will cause pain in those areas. If it extends to the bladder or the large intestine, the patient will have fast urination and painful defecation. When it invades the peritoneum or pelvis, there will be pain in the lower limbs. The patient suffering from endometrial carcinoma will have recurrent pains and paleness, facial edema, and weakness.

Treatment

Presently, there is no cure other than surgery. The uterus is an independent organ, and once it has been removed, there is no possibility of recurrence of the cancer unless metastasis has already occurred.

It is important to detect the early symptoms of cancer and begin treatment immediately. Symptoms of hemorrhage or leucorrhea should be diagnosed and treated by a gynecologist. When there is frank hemorrhage, the condition is advanced. If the patient will not accept surgery, or as additional therapy after surgery, use the following Chinese herbal formulas.

Chinese Herb Formulas

Without surgery, the Chinese herbal formulas may not cure uterine carcinoma.

1. Kuei-chih-fu-ling-wan-chia-i-yi-jen 桂枝茯苓丸加薏苡仁
(Cinnamon and Hoelen Formula with Coix)
To be taken in the primary stage by the patient who has vigor and a sensation of weight in the lower abdomen.

2. Chiung-kuei-chiao-ai-tang 芎歸膠艾湯
(Tang-kuei and Gelatin Combination)
To be taken for bleeding, anemia, a sensation of pressure in the lower abdomen, pain during intercourse, and hemorrhage.

3. Shih-chuan-ta-pu-tang 十全大補湯
(Ginseng and Tang-kuei Ten Combination)
It is helpful to the patient who will not accept surgery but has severe anemia, physical weakness, and malodorous leucorrhea.

4. Kuei-pi-tang 歸脾湯
(Ginseng and Longan Combination)
It is effective for continuous bleeding, severe anemia, gastrointestinal weakness, and stagnancy at the chest after taking *Shih-chuan-ta-pu-tang*. (Ginseng and *Tang-kuei* Ten Combination)

Ovaritis and Oviduct Inflammation

Ovaritis, oviduct inflammation, pelviperitonitis, and periovaritis often occur together. These are called the "inflammation of uterine parts". The main causes of this disease are gonococci, staphylococci, tubercle bacilli, and other pathogenic bacteria.

The patient suffering from acute ovaritis will have severe pain and fever in the lower abdomen, occasional yellow pus, and continuous fever. In the chronic state, there will be ovarian swelling and pressing pain, continuous pain in the lower abdomen, lumbago, and pain on excretion and during intercourse. The patient will also experience severe discomfort before the menstrual cycle. When there is pus, it becomes ovary pustulation. The patient suffering from oviduct inflammation will have severe pain in the lower abdomen, spasm in the feet, difficulty in walking, high fever, and leucorrhea with pus. In severe case, it will lead to peritonitis and become recalcitrant. At this stage, there is continuous fever and a predisposition to tubercular oviduct inflammation and ovarian tumor.

In Chinese medicine, the similar formulas may be used in conjunction with antibiotics. For chronic cases, Chinese formulas alone are effective.

Chinese Herb Formulas

1. **Ta-huang-mu-tan-pi-tang** 　　　　　大黃牡丹皮湯
  (Rhubarb and Moutan Combination)
  To be taken for acute ovaritis and oviduct inflammation, obvious, resistant pressing pain in the lower abdomen, polyleucorrhea, and severe inflammation.

2. **Tao-ho-cheng-chi-tang** 　　　　　　桃核承氣湯
  (Persica and Rhubarb Combination)
  It is effective for acute and subacute resistant pressing pain in the lower abdomen, abdominal pain of the strong conformation, severe nervousness, leucorrhea, and constipation.

3. **Kuei-chih-fu-ling-wan** 　　　　　　桂枝茯苓丸
  (Cinnamon and Hoelen Formula)
  To be taken for chronic symptoms due to moderate inflammation with resistant pressing pain in the lower abdomen.

4. **Lung-tan-hsieh-kan-tang** 龍膽瀉肝湯
    (Gentiana Combination)

It is effective for chronic symptoms, prolonged leucorrhea, and tense *kan* (liver) meridian at both sides of the umbilicus.

5. **Che-chung-yin** 折衝飲
    (Cinnamon and Persica Combination)

It is effective for subacute or chronic symptoms, resistant pressing pain in the lower abdomen, leucorrhea, and prolonged ovaritis and oviduct inflammation.

6. **Huo-hsieh-san-yu-tang** 活血散瘀湯
    (Cnidium and Persica Combination)

To be taken after *Ta-huang-mu-tan-pi-tang* (Rhubarb and Moutan Combination) and *Tao-ho-cheng-chi-tang* (Persica and Rhubarb Combination). It is effective for subacute ovaritis and oviduct inflammation, severe stagnant blood, and constipation.

Abnormal Menstruations

(Amenstruation, vicarious menstruation, scanty menstruation, and excessive menstruation)

Abnormal menstruation include amenstruation and vicarious, precocious, scarce, scanty, frequent, excessive, and difficult menstruation.

Amenstruation (amenorrhea) is partly caused by growth defects and by secretion disorder of the ovary. The basic causes are nutritional deficiencies; the functional causes are emotional upsets and excitment.

Vicarious menstruation is a periodic bleeding from the nose, stomach, intestine, or lung instead of the uterus.

Precocious menstruation is due to premature development of ovarian function and swelling of the internal organs.

Scarce menstruation is due to defects in ovarian function or uterine development.

Frequent menstruation is due to abnormal function of an ovary, uterine myoma, Basdow's disease, or heart disease.

Chinese Herb Formulas

1. **Szu-wu-tang**　　　　　　　　　　　四物湯
   (Tang-kuei Four Combination)

   To be taken for amenstruation or at menopause by those who have a defect of uterine development, malfunction of the ovary, or atrophy of the endometrium.

2. **Chia-wei-hsiao-yao-san**　　　　　　加味逍遙散
   (Bupleurum and Paeonia Formula)

   To be taken for menopause, physical weakness, or a long-standing tendency towards anemia or tuberculosis. It is also taken for developmental uterine defects. Addition of 3.0g. each of rehmannia and cyperus will produce better results.

3. **Shih-chuan-ta-pu-tang**　　　　　　十全大補湯
   (Ginseng and Tang-kuei Ten Combination)

   It is effective for amenstruation and anemia caused by generalized fatigue, prolonged lactation, or massive hemorrhage during childbirth. If there is anorexia after taking this formula, the patient should take *Kuei-pi-tang* (Ginseng and Longan Combination) or *Pu-chung-i-chi-tang* (Ginseng and Astragalus Combination).

4. **Kuei-chih-fu-ling-wan**　　　　　　桂枝茯苓丸
   (Cinnamon and Hoelen Formula)
   Tao-ho-cheng-chi-tang　　　　　　桃核承氣湯
   (Persica and Rhubarb Combination)

   It is effective for uteritis or endometritis, resistant pressing pain in the lower abdomen, and stagnant blood. For constipation, add rhubarb (0.5-2.0 gm.). In severe cases with congestion, headache, and ruddy face, the patient should take *Tao-ho-cheng-chi-tang*. This formula is usually used for excessive and vicarious menstruation.

5. **Ta-huang-mu-tan-pi-tang**　　　　　大黃牡丹皮湯
   (Rhubarb and Moutan Combination)

   It is a formula to disperse stagnant blood, and for distention of the abdomen due to amenstruation.

6. **Ta-cheng-chi-tang** 大承氣湯
    (Major Rhubarb Combination)
To be taken for distension of the abdomen and for constipation with a strong conformation.

7. **Chai-hu-kuei-chih-tang** 柴胡桂枝湯
    (Bupleurum and Cinnamon Combination)
For distension at the chest and amenstruation due to tension in the lower abdomen; add rhubarb (0.5-2.0 gm.) to this formula to relieve chest distension and restore menstruation. In severe cases of the strong types, use *Ta-chai-hu-tang* (Major Bupleurum Combination).

8. **Tang-kuei-szu-ni-chia-wu-chu-yu-sheng-chiang-tang**
    當歸四逆加吳茱萸生薑湯
    (Tang-kuei, Evodia, and Ginger Combination)
It is effective for lumbago, abdominal pain, and menopause due to chilling.

9. **Pan-hsia-hou-pu-tang** 半夏厚朴湯
    (Pinellia and Magnolia Combination)
   Hsiang-su-san 香蘇散
    (Cyperus and Perilla Formula)
To be taken at menopause for anxiety, fear, sorrow, or other strong emotions. *Hsiang-su-san* is occasionally effective.

10. **Ti-tang-wan** 抵當丸
    (Rhubarb and Leech Formula)
It is effective for amenstruation due to resistance at the lower abdomen, stagnant blood, amnesia, and polyuria.

11. **Hsieh-hsin-tang** 瀉心湯
    (Coptis and Rhubarb Combination)
To be taken for vicarious menstruation with nosebleed, hemoptysis, ruddy face, congestion, headache, and stress. It is also effective for excessive menstruation.

12. **Huang-lien-chieh-tu-tang** 黃連解毒湯
    (Coptis and Scute Combination)
It is effective for moderate symptoms of *Hsieh-hsin-tang*.

13. Chiung-kuei-chiao-ai-tang   芎歸膠艾湯
(Tang-kuei and Gelatin Combination)
To be taken for vicarious menstruation, tendency towards anemia, and physical weakness due to chills. It is also effective for excessive menstruation.

14. Fu-tzu-li-chung-tang   附子理中湯
(Ginseng, Ginger, and Aconite Combination)
To be taken at menopause for physical weakness and chilling, and in order to recover vigor.

15. Fang-chi-huang-chi-tang   防己黃耆湯
(Stephania and Astragalus Combination)
It is effective for the obese woman with a tendency towards fatigue and scanty menstruation every two or three months.

Menstrual Aberration

The menstrual cycle recurs about every thirty days. However, a cycle that recurs between twenty-eight and thirty-six days is still considered normal. Menstrual aberration means a menstrual cycle too short (two to three weeks) or too long (over forty days). Short menstrual cycles are called "frequent menstruations," and long menstrual cycles are called "scarce menstruations". If the short and long menstrual cycles are not accompanied by illness and recur at regular intervals, they are regarded as normal. Usually there is a range of difference of not more than three or four days. Irregular phenomena often occur during menarche, menopause, and lactation.

The causes of frequent menstruations may be inflammation of uterine muscle, retroversion of the uterus, swelling of the uterus, or abnormal ovarian function with possible complications of heart disease, nephralgia, hypertension, and constipation. Most women having frequent menstruations also have excessive amounts of menstrual blood during periods which last from one week to ten days. This may result in anemia and general weakness. Some patients become more or less hysterical due to emotional instability. Scarce menstruations may be caused by uterine disorder, such as tuberculosis of the endometrium or excessive scraping during artificial abortion. It may also be caused by degeneration of the ovary due to tuberculosis, pneumonia, diabetes, malnutrition, and overwork.

Treatment

The patient should be treated with hormone therapy by a qualified physician. Meanwhile, it is important for her to control her own emotions.

Chinese Herb Formulas
1. **Kuei-chih-fu-ling-wan** 　　　　　　　桂枝茯苓丸
   (Cinnamon and Hoelen Formula)
   Effective for scarce menstruations.

2. **Tang-kuei-shao-yao-san** 　　　　　　當歸芍藥散
   (Tang-kuei and Paeonia Formula)
   Effective for both frequent and scarce menstruations.

Difficult Menstruation

Severely painful menstruation (lower abdominal pain or lumbago) that interferes with normal life is called "difficult menstruation." It is divided into three categories — premenstrual, mid-menstrual, and post-menstrual pain. There are various causes of difficult menstruation, and they are generally divided into the following three categories:

1) Organic: : Narrow cervical opening, ill-developed uterus, anteflexion of the uterus, uterine myoma.
2) Inflammatory: Endometritis, pelviperitonitis, oviduct inflammation.
3) Emotional: Nervousness, nervous exhaustion, hysteria, neurasthenia, anxiety, chlorosis.

Of all the causes, uterine abnormality results in the most severe pain.

Treatment

For emotional causes, administration of tranquilizers one week before menstruation will produce good results. But for other causes, a medical doctor should be consulted for proper therapy or surgery. Chinese herbal formulas are prepared for use where there is anemia, congestion, lack of vitality, and air stagnancy.

Chinese Herb Formulas

1. **Tang-kuei-shao-yao-san** 當歸芍藥散
   (Tang-kuei and Paeonia Formula)

   To be taken for difficult menstruation due to ill-developed uterus or narrow cervical opening, anemia, and chilling.

2. **Kuei-chih-fu-ling-wan** 桂枝茯苓丸
   (Cinnamon and Hoelen Formula)

   It is effective for anteflexion or retroflexion of the uterus, uterine myoma, resistant pressing pain in the lower abdomen, and pelvic congestion.

3. **Tao-ho-cheng-chi-tang** 桃核承氣湯
   (Persica and Rhubarb Combination)

   To be taken for difficult menstruation due to inflammation, post-menstrual pain, and hemorrhage. It is effective for cramping and pressing pain in the lower abdomen and for congestion. In severe cases, purge after taking this formula for two or three days, and then take *Che-chung-yin* (Cinnamon and Persica Combination). The condition will be relieved by using this therapy for several months.

4. **Che-chung-yin** 折衝飲
   (Cinnamon and Persica Combination)

   It is effective for subacute or chronic difficult menstruation due to endometritis, pelviperitonitis, and oviduct inflammation.

5. **Niu-hsi-san** 牛膝散
   (Achyranthes Formula)

   It is effective for scanty menstruation, stagnant blood in the lower abdomen, severe pain at the umbilicus or at the lower abdomen and waist, clonus, and aching at the chest.

6. **Hsiao-chien-chung-tang** 小建中湯
   (Minor Cinnamon and Paeonia Combination)

To be taken for lack of vitality, anemia, physical weakness, and difficult menstruation due to ill-developed uterus. The patient who has a tendency towards fatigue, chilling, and spasm around abnormal muscle should add *tang-kuei* (4.0 g.) to this formula.

7. Ta-chien-chung-tang   大建中湯
(Major Zanthoxylum Combination)
It is effective for weak abdomen, severe pain, chilling of the hands and feet, and weak pulse.

8. Cheng-chi-tien-hsiang-tang   正氣天香湯
(Lindera and Cyperus Combination)
It is effective for difficult menstruation due to nervousness, hysteria, or air stagnancy.

9. Tang-kuei-chien-chung-tang   當歸建中湯
(Tang-kuei, Cinnamon, and Paeonia Combination)
To be taken for severe abdominal pain, lumbago, and pain at the end of, or after menstruation.

Mastitis

Mastitis, or inflammation of the breast, is divided into two categories. One is acute suppurative mastitis caused by staphylococci at a nipple damaged during the mother's breast feeding. The other is stagnant mastitis which is caused by milk deficiency or stagnation. Basically, the two diseases have the same symptoms of endocrine or autonomic nerve disorder. This means that a nervous disorder can easily cause an inflammative constitution and predispose towards bacterial infection.

Around the time of menopause, the palpable masses of various sizes in one or both breasts should be diagnosed according to the patient's history. To be considered are whether or not she has borne children and how many, if she has had abortions or problems with breast feeding, and if she has had hormone injections.

Symptoms

Suppurative mastitis: A part of the breast hardens and swells, becoming very painful. The inflamed area is feverish and red.

In severe cases, there is pus, general tiredness, loss of appetite, and headache.

Stagnant mastitis: The breast becomes swollen and red. There is hardening of the mammary glands accompanied by pain and occasional fever (about 38°C), but no pus.

Soft tumors with painful symptoms can be cured easily in women in their thirties.

Treatment

This disease may be cured by cold therapy or taking antiphlogistics. The patient with suppurative mastitis must disinfect the nipples before breast feeding. The patient having stagnant mastitis should breast feed at regular intervals. If any milk remains after nursing the baby, it may be squeezed out manually or suctioned with a breast pump. Sedatives may be used with good results. But when the tumor hardens and there is swelling of the mammary duct and nipple, special treatment is necessary.

Chinese Herb Formulas

1. **Ko-ken-tang-chia-shih-kao** 葛根湯加石膏
   (Pueruria Combination with Gypsum)

For the patient in the primary stage with chills, fever, swelling, and pain.

2. **Hsiao-chai-hu-tang** 小柴胡湯
   (Minor Bupleurum Combination)

For the patient who has a fever after taking the first formula, but has no appetite.

3. **Shih-wei-pai-tu-san-chia-lien-chiao** 十味敗毒散加連翹
   (Bupleurum and Schizonepeta Formula with Forsythia)

For the patient who has taken the first formula but still has fever and pus.

4. **Tuo-li-hsiao-tu-yin** 托裏消毒飲
   (Gleditsia Combination)
   Chien-chin-nei-tuo-san 千金內托散
   (Astragalus and Platycodon Formula)

To be taken for suppurative swelling.

5. pai-nung-san 排膿散
    (Platycodon and Chih-shih Formula)
To be taken to help discharge pus.

6. Kuei-chih-fu-ling-wan 桂枝茯苓丸
    (Cinnamon and Hoelen Formula)
To be taken by the obese woman of middle age with stagnant blood at the lower abdomen. For constipation, add rhubarb (0.5-2.0 gm.).

7. Tao-ho-cheng-chi-tang 桃核承氣湯
    (Persica and Rhubarb Combination)
It is effective for aggravated stagnant blood at the lower abdomen, ruddy face, flushing up, headache, and severe constipation.

8. Tzu-ken-mu-li-tang 紫根牡蠣湯
    (Lithospermum and Oyster Shell Combination)
To be taken for prolonged mastitis when breast cancer is not suspecte

9. Shih-liu-wei-liu-chi-yin 十六味流氣飲
    (Tang-kuei Sixteen Herb Combination)
To be taken for swelling due to air stagnancy and undiagnosed tumors.

Breast Cancer

Breast cancer is a very common disease. The majority of patients are women between forty and fifty years of age who have had few or no childbirths. Others are those who have had several abortions or who have not breast-fed their infants.

Symptoms

There is a hard, painless lump in the breast which can be felt on palpation. When the lesion has grown to a certain size, the epidermis will sink and sometimes the nipple will bleed or become ulcerated. The cancer is usually located in the upper outer quadrant of the breast. Since carcinoma of the breast is a type of external cancer, it may be discovered easily by daily

observation. After each menstrual cycle, or on a fixed date every month for those past menopause, conduct the following self-examination to promote early discovery of any lesions:
1) In a well-lighted place, observe the nude upper body and compare the left with the right breast to see if they have the same shape.
2) Lift both hands above the head and see if there is puckering or dimpling of the skin of the breast.
3) Lay down, insert a sponge or folded towel under the left shoulder, raise the left arm above the head, and feel the left breast with the flat of the fingers of the right hand to check for any lumps.
4) Reverse step 3 to check the right breast.

Treatment

Like other cancers, it is important to discover breast cancer in the early stages and to treat is immediately. Whenever there is a hard lump, the patient must seek a doctor's diagnosis as soon as possible. Since not all lumps are cancerous, the patient should not worry when her doctor orders a biopsy.

Chinese Herb Formulas

The Chinese herbal formulas should be used in conjunction with surgery.

Kuei-chih-fu-ling-wan 桂枝茯苓丸
(Cinnamon and Hoelen Formula)
Shih-liu-wei-liu-chi-yin 十六味流氣飲
(Tang-kuei Sixteen Herb Combination)
To be taken for edema of the legs, fever, constipation, and related symptoms.

Retroflexion of the Uterus

Occasionally there are no obvious symptoms of this condition, but it usually causes menstrual aberration, excessive menstruation (menorrhagia), painful menstruation (dysmenorrhea), pressure on the bladder and rectum, pain in the lower abdomen, and lumbago. Sometimes it will cause infertility. In addition, it may predispose to the complications of endometritis, oviduct inflammation, and especially ovarian ptosis.

Disorder of the blood circulation at the pelvis is due to stagnant blood. In severe cases, intercourse is unpleasant and painful. Chinese herbal formulas can relieve these symptoms.

Chinese Herb Formulas

1. **Tang-kuei-shao-yao-san** 當歸芍藥散
    (Tang-kuei and Paeonia Formula)

To be taken by those having physical weakness, mild anemia, chilling, and a tendency towards fatigue, pain in the lower abdomen, and lumbago due to retroversion or retroflexion of the uterus.

2. **Kuei-chih-fu-ling-wan** 桂枝茯苓丸
    (Cinnamon and Hoelen Formula)

To be taken for retroflexion of the uterus due to endometritis or oviduct inflammation, and for resistant pressing pain in the lower abdomen. When there is constipation, add rhubarb (0.5-2.0 gm.).

3. **Tao-ho-cheng-chi-tang** 桃核承氣湯
    (Persica and Rhubarb Combination)

It is effective in severe cases for inflammation, ruddy face, congestion, and headache.

4. **Che-chung-yin** 折衝飲
    (Cinnamon and Persica Combination)

To be taken for chronic retroflexion of the uterus and swelling pain in the lower abdomen.

5. **Wen-ching-tang** 溫經湯
    (Tang-kuei and Evodia Combination)

To be taken for chilling, infertility due to retroflexion of the uterus, difficult menstruation, pain in the lower abdomen, hot palms, and dry lips.

6. **Chia-wei-hsiao-yao-san** 加味逍遙散
    (Bupleurum and Paeonia Formula)

To be taken for abdominal swelling, anemia, and nervousness.

Addition of 3.0 g. each of rehmannia and cyperus will produce better results.

Uterine Ptosis and Prolapse

Uterine ptosis is the state in which the uterus has dropped to the opening of the vagina, even the uterine neck. It is divided into complete and incomplete prolapse of the uterus.

Causes of this condition are relaxation of uterine ligaments, perineal wound, damage to the perineal tendon, functional disorder, abdominal fluid, and tumors of the uterus or ovary. Chinese herbal formulas are to be taken for improving body constitution or dispelling the pressure of the stagnant blood.

Chinese Herb Formulas

1. **Tang-kuei-shao-yao-san** 當歸芍藥散
   (Tang-kuei and Paeonia Formula)
   To be taken by the woman with chills, mild anemia, and physical weakness.

2. **Kuei-chih-fu-ling-wan** 桂枝茯苓丸
   (Cinnamon and Hoelen Formula)
   It is effective for the rather strong conformation of the woman with stagnant blood in the lower abdomen and pressure of a tumor. If there is constipation and severe stagnant blood, take *Tao-ho-cheng-chi-tang* (Persica and Rhubarb Combination).

3. **Pu-chung-i-chi-tang** 補中益氣湯
   (Ginseng and Astragalus Combination)
   It is effective for physical weakness and anemia. The formula is often combined with kaolin (3.0 gm.).

4. **Wen-ching-tang** 溫經湯
   (Tang-kuei and Evodia Combination)
   It is effective for uterine ptosis of the weak woman, menstrual aberration, waist chills and abdominal pain, congestion, chilling, dry lips, and hot palms.

5. Tang-kuei-szu-ni-chia-wu-chu-yu-sheng-chiang-tang
當歸四逆加吳茱萸生薑湯
(Tang-kuei, Evodia, and Ginger Combination)
It is effective for severe chills, a tendency towards anemia, abdominal pain when the patient feels cold, and severe ptosis.

Endometritis

(A Common Gynecological Disease)

Endometrium is most important as the base of the developing oosperm. Endometritis is an inflammation of the uterine neck and endometrium, and it can be classified as an acute or chronic inflammation. It is caused by the growth of suppurative bacteria resulting from unsanitary hygeine during or after intercourse, childbirth, abortion, or menstruation. Infection may also occur during uterine curettage, probe insertion, and careless forceps insertion. The bacteria most frequently involved are gonococcus, tubercle bacillus, escherichia coli, staphylococci, and streptococci.

Other causes of this disease are general blood disorder, irregular diet and life, malposition of the uterus, retained placenta, uterine myoma, and lead poisoning. Three interchangeable terms are applied to this condition — endometritis, substantial inflammation, and peripheral inflammation. In severe cases, infection will spread to the uterine wall itself. Since endometritis easily becomes chronic, it must be cured as soon as possible. Those who wish to have children should be aware of this disease, since it can cause sterility or habitual abortion.

Symptoms consist of discomfort or pain at the lower abdomen and malodorous leucorrhea consisting of a mixture of pus and mucus which is milky or yellow in color. Sometimes the discharge contains blood. There is also itching at the outside of the vagina, painful menstruation, bleeding during intercourse, vaginal infection, chilling, fever, irritability, and loss of appetite.

Treatment

The patient should obtain diagnosis and proper therapy as soon as possible, since household remedies do not cure endometritis. It will become chronic and leave many complications if not immediately and completely eradicated. Those who are past menopause are particularly susceptible to chronic infection since they have no menstrual cycle for replacement of the endometrium. When the primary symptoms of leucorrhea and discomfort appear, the patient must seek examination immediately. Antibiotics should be prescribed for acute inflammations. For chronic inflammations, Chinese herb formulas will be effective.

Chinese Herb Formulas

1. Lung-tan-hsieh-kan-tang   龍膽瀉肝湯
   (Gentiana Combination)
   To be taken by those of the strong conformation for moisture heat of the *kan* (liver) meridian, and for acute or chronic endometritis due to bacterial infection. It is also effective for leucorrhea as a complication of urethritis and cystitis. In addition, it is suitable for tense abdominal tendon, resistant pressing pain at the lower abdomen along the *kan* (liver) meridian, and strong pulse. Generally, smilax (3 g.) and coix (5 g.) should be added.

2. Kuei-chih-fu-ling-wan   桂枝茯苓丸
   (Cinnamon and Hoelen Formula)
   To be taken by those of strong conformation with endometritis due to retained placenta, myoma of the uterus with leucorrhea, abdominal pain, a sensation of heavy pressure at the lower abdomen, and excessive or difficult menstruation. If constipation occurs, add rhubarb (0.5-2.0 g.).

3. Tao-ho-cheng-chi-tang   桃核承氣湯
   (Persica and Rhubarb Combination)
   To be taken for more serious endometritis.

4. Ta-huang-mu-tan-pi-tang   大黃牡丹皮湯
   (Rhubarb and Moutan Combination)
   To be taken for the most serious endometritis, great amounts of leucorrhea with pus and odor, pain and fullness at the lower abdomen, urethritis, cystitis, severe pain during urination, and pelvic congestion.

5. Pa-wei-tai-hsia-fang　　　　　　　　　　八味帶下方
    (Tang-kuei and Eight Herb Formua)
    To be taken for subacute or chronic endometritis with yellow or white leucorrhea. If there is no constipation, rhubarb may be omitted.

6. Tang-kuei-shao-yao-san　　　　　　　　當歸芍藥散
    (Tang-kuei and Paeonia Formula)
    To be taken by the woman of weak conformation without inflammation, but with congestion, mild anemia, chills, and a tendency towards fatigue, leucorrhea due to chronic endometritis, frequent urination, and abdominal pus and lumbago.

7. Chia-wei-hsiao-yao-san　　　　　　　　加味逍遙散
    (Bupleurum and Paeonia Formula)
    It is effective for the patient with chronic and weak conformation, disorder of the autonomic nervous system, menstrual aberration, abdominal pain, leucorrhea, and stagnant blood.

8. Chiung-kuei-chiao-ai-tang　　　　　　　芎歸膠艾湯
    (Tang-kuei and Gelatin Combination)
    It is effective for chronic conformation, leucorrhea, tendency toward anemia, frequent bleeding of the uterus, hot sensation in the limbs, spasm at the left side of the abdomen, weakness at the abdomen, and abdominal pain.

9. Kuei-pi-tang　　　　　　　　　　　　　歸脾湯
    (Ginseng and Longan Combination)
    To be taken for the symptoms of loss of appetite, nervousness, insomnia, and amnesia.

10. I-yi-fu-tzu-pai-chiang-tang　　　　　　薏苡附子敗醬湯
    (Coix, Aconite, and Thlaspi Combination)
    It is effective for chronic and weak conformation, a tendency toward weakness, water leucorrhea, fatigue and weakness, dry skin, and weak and sunken pulse.

Uterine Myoma

Tumors (sarcomas) of the myometrium (uterine wall) are not malignant. They are the most easily grown of myomas, so patients with this disease are rather common. After middle age, about 40 percent of women develop myomas. The basic cause has not yet been found, and the only fact known is that the growth of uterine myomas is related to the function of ovarian hormones. Sizes of myomas range from that of a finger to that of a child's head.

The patient with this disease has delayed, painful, and excessive menstruation. When the myoma occurs beneath mucous membrane, it will cause endometritis and abnormal menstruation. At the cervix uteri, it will put pressure on the bladder and rectum. The uterine myoma occurring beneath mucous membrane will become degenerative muscle, and the patient's parturition will be called "parturition from myoma".

Symptoms

The tiny myoma is without symptoms that are apparent to the patient. When it reaches a certain size, it sometimes causes irregular bleeding or excessive menstruation. When even larger, it will put pressure on the rectum and bladder, causing constipation or blockage. Some patients will have symptoms of waist chilling, lumbago, or painful menstruation. Massive hemorrhage will induce anemia and even palpitation, gasping, and rapid pulse rate of the heart. Young patients become aware of myomas only after abortion.

Treatment

The Chinese herb formulas are not absolutely effective for myoma of the uterus. A small myoma should be observed for a time before surgery. If it does not show signs of growth, treatment is unnecessary. However, the patient should receive regular physical examinations. Occasionally, the deextravasated blood agents can dispel an egg-size tumor or promote myoma parturition. But in severe cases which have been treated for a month or two without improvement, the patient should undergo surgery immediately. Some patients worry that a myoma is a latent cancer. They can be reassured that uterine myomas are completely different from, and do not become cancer.

Chinese Herb Formulas
Although Chinese herbal formulas cannot completely cure, they can decrease the uncomfortable symptoms of uterine myomas that have grown to a moderate size before menopause.

1. **Kuei-chih-fu-ling-wan-chia-pieh-chia-ta-huang** 桂枝茯苓丸加鱉甲大黃
   (Cinnamon and Hoelen Formula with Tortoise Shell and Rhubarb)
   A common formula for uterine myoma, it can decrease excessive menstruation and pain in the lower abdomen.

2. **Chiung-kuei-chiao-ai-tang** 芎歸膠艾湯
   (Tang-kuei and Gelatin Combination)
   To be taken for severe, irregular hemorrhage, lumbago, and painful menstruation.

3. **Tao-ho-cheng-chi-tang** 桃核承氣湯
   (Persica and Rhubarb Combination)
   It is effective for obvious, resistant, pressing pain in the lower abdomen.

4. **Che-chung-yin** 折衝飲
   (Cinnamon and Persica Combination)
   To be taken for painful menstruation, menstrual aberrations, and lower abdominal pain due to uterine myoma.

5. **Ti-tang-wan** 抵當丸
   (Rhubarb and Leech Formula)
   It is effective for uterine myoma, a sensation of fullness in the lower abdomen, frequent urination, and amnesia. If the patient has taken this formula for two or three months and the tumor has not shrunk, she should discontinue it.

6. **Chiung-kuei-tiao-hsieh-yin** 芎歸調血飲
   (Cindium and Rehmannia Combination)
   To be taken for uterine myoma after childbirth or abortion.

7. Fasting

One week of fasting can decrease the size of a small myoma. However, this must be done under the supervision of an experienced instructor, and the patient must maintain her strength during this time.

Ovarian Tumor

Eighty percent of ovarian tumors are benign. The part of the ovary in which they grow contains ovarian secretions and forms a sac shape which is called "sac tumor". The size of this tumor may vary from that of a first to that of an adult's head. The basic cause of this disease is still not clear. It occurs most frequently in women between thirty and forty years of age.

Symptoms

The tumor will not cause pain until it reaches a certain size. So in the early stages, patients are not aware of it. By the time the tumor reaches the size of a child's head, it can be felt on palpation like a hard muscle at the left or right side of the abdomen. At this stage, the tumor will put pressure on the rectum and the bladder, which are located beside the ovary. Symptoms include a weighty sensation in the lower abdomen, pain, and constipation. When the tumor is still small, there is occasionally a severe pain at the ovary. This occurs because the tumor has stagnant blood or is bleeding. If the patient ignores it, the benign tumor will grow, putting pressure on the lungs and heart, thereby causing symptoms of palpitation and dyspnea. There is also a general malnutrition.

Treatment

When it is discovered, the tumor should be removed surgically as soon as possible.

Chinese Herb Formulas

1. Tao-ho-cheng-chi-tang   桃核承氣湯
 (Persica and Rhubarb Combination)
 To be taken for severe symptoms due to the tumor's size, for constipation, and for pain in the abdomen.

2. **Kuei-chih-fu-ling-wan** 桂枝茯苓丸
   (Cinnamon and Hoelen Formula)
   For relatively moderate symptoms.

3. **Fasting**
   This can increase the health of the whole body by decreasing some of the symptoms. But patients with progressing tuberculosis, gastric hemorrhage, duodenal ulcer, and extreme emaciation should not fast.

Infertility

When no pregnancy occurs for three years after marriage, the condition is called "infertility". Those who have never conceived are said to have "congenital infertility"; those who have had one pregnancy but none following are said to have "acquired infertility". The problem may originate with either the husband or the wife or both.

Male infertility may be the result of many factors: i.e., spermacrasia, impotence, deformed penis, incomplete physical development, endocrine imbalance due to diabetes, and sexual weaknesses.

Female infertility may also be due to many factors: i.e., abnormal or malfunctioning genital organs, absense of menses,, nonovulational menses, oviduct blockage, retroflexion or myoma of the uterus, endometritis, vaginal spasm, narrow opening of the uterus and cervix uteri, vaginitis, cystitis, dislocation of the uterus, uterine ulcer, edema of the oviduct, chronic ovaritis, morphine intoxication, obesity, hysteria, frigidity, and defects of uterine development.

Treatment

Both the husband and wife should seek a physician's examination. If the results are found to be aspermia in the husband or oviduct blockage in the wife, it is useless to expect a pregnancy. In all other cases, pregnancy may be possible after proper treatment. Those having endometritis, dislocation of the uterus, pelviperitonitis, defects of uterine development, chilling, or frigidity may hope for pregnancy after taking Chinese herb formulas.

Chinese Herb Formulas
1. **Tang-kuei-shao-yao-san** 當歸芍藥散
   (Tang-kuei and Paeonia Formula)
   To be taken for infertility due to defects of uterine development, chilling, anemia, and physical weakness.

2. **Hsiao-chien-chung-tang** 小建中湯
   (Minor Cinnamon and Paeonia Combination)
   It is effective for the woman with physical weakness, gastrointestinal weakness, a tendency towards fatigue. If there is a tense abdominal tendon, *tang-kuei* (3.0 g.) should be added.

3. **Kuei-chih-fu-ling-wan** 桂枝茯苓丸
   (Cinnamon and Hoelen Formula)
   It is effective for infertility due to endometritis, ovaritis, pelviperitonitis, malposition of the uterus, and stagnant blood with resistant pressing pain at the lower abdomen.

4. **Tao-ho-cheng-chi-tang** 桃核承氣湯
   (Persica and Rhubarb Combination)
   To be taken for severe inflammation and congestion, and by the strong type with constipation.

5. **Ta-huang-mu-tan-pi-tang** 大黃牡丹皮湯
   (Rhubarb and Moutan Combination)
   It is effective for pelviperitonitis, cystitis, severe, resistant pressing pain in the lower abdomen of the strong conformation, and malodorous leucorrhea.

6. **Lung-tan-hsieh-kan-tang** 龍膽瀉肝湯
   (Gentiana Combination)
   To be taken for infertility due to chronic endometritis, vaginitis, pain in urination, and chronic gonorrhea of the strong conformation.

7. **Wen-ching-tang** 溫經湯
   (Tang-kuei and Evodia Combination)
   To be taken by the woman with physical weakness, chilling at

the waist and feet, hot palms, dry lips, menstrual aberration, leucorrhea, occasional hemorrhage, lumbago, diarrhea during menstruation, and a swollen sensation in the lower abdomen.

8. Chia-wei-hsiao-yao-san 加味逍遙散
(Bupleurum and Paeonia Formula)
To be taken for infertility due to defects of uterine development, functional disorder of the ovary, hysteria, chlorosis with physical weakness, and a tendency towards long-standing anemia.

9. Shih-chuan-ta-pu-tang 十全大補湯
(Ginseng and Tang-kuei Ten Combination)
It is effective for severe symptoms of paragraph 8, anemia, and severe fatigue and weakness.

Chill

The patient with this condition will feel chilled, especially at the hands, feet, and waist. When she goes to bed each night, she will still feel chilled at the waist for a long time after retiring, even though the other parts of her body are warm. The basic causes are still not clear. Perhaps the finest part of the nerve fiber has undergone a change and the blood circulation has been disturbed.

The causes of chilling are anemia and disorders of the blood circulation such as stagnant blood. Local chills may be due to an imbalance in body fluids, gastrointestinal weakness, gastroptosis, lack of vigor, functional disorder of metabolism, or disorder of the autonomic nervous system. Depending of the area of the body affected and the severity of chilling, we may presume to designate the basic causes of this condition. For example:

    Women who feel chilled at the legs and waist . . . . disorder of menopause, difficult menstruation, endometritis, myoma of the uterus

    Those with a low temperature in one part of the body . . . . anemia, hypotension, heart disease, disorder of the autonomic nervous system

    Those with normal body temperature who feel chilled . . . . nervousness, hysteria, other emotional states

There are various types of chills. Some patients feel general chilling, and some feel chilled only at the feet. The latter will wear cloth stockings in summer and cannot stand on the floor comfortably for even five minutes without foot covering. Some feel chilled at the head; others feel ice-cold at the back, stomach, and waist; still others feel chilled at the back of the knees, but have a hot face. Chill patients are mostly women, especially those under twenty years of age and those who are past menopause. The symptoms are rather common in winter, but some patients still feel chilled in summer.

Treatment
It is relatively simple to cure this condition. First, keep the body warm, then take more Vitamin B (good for the nerves) and Vitamin E (good for dilatation of the blood vessels). Sedatives may help to improve blood circulation and relax the nerves. Of course, if other disease are causing the condition, cure them first.

Chinese Herb Formulas
1. Tang-kuei-shao-yao-san　　　　　　　當歸芍藥散
   (Tang-kuei and Paeonia Formula)
To be taken for waist chills, leg chills, sensation of tiredness, and a tendency towards anemia. It is also effective for headache, dizziness, and shoulder aching.

2. Tang-kuei-szu-ni-chia-wu-chu-yu-sheng-chiang-tang
   　　　　　　　　　　當歸四逆加吳茱萸生薑湯
   (Tang-kuei, Evodia, and Ginger Combination)
For chills in women past middle age. It is especially effective for chilling of the hands and feet and for stagnant blood at the limbs with chilblain. To be taken by those having a weak and sunken pulse, fullness at the abdomen, and abdominal pain and hernia.

3. Ling-chiang-chu-kan-tang　　　　　　苓薑朮甘湯
   (Hoelen and Ginger Combination)
It is effective for severe chilling from waist to feet and for polyuria. It may be used by those having normal upper body temperature but severe chilling of the lower body.

4. **Kuei-chih-chia-fu-tzu-tang** 桂枝加附子湯
   (Cinnamon and Aconite Combination)
   To be taken by those having chills who must wear cloth stockings in summer to put their feet on the floor and who also have abdominal pain when it is cold.

5. **Chen-wu-tang** 眞武湯
   (Vitality Combination)
   Fu-tzu-tang 附子湯
   (Aconite Combination)
   It is effective for metabolic disorder, lack of vigor, tendency towards fatigue, chilling at the hands and feet, water stagnancy at the abdomen, and pain and diarrhea when it is cold. When chilling is associated with neuralgia and rheumatism, the patient should take *Fu-tzu-tang*.

6. **Fu-tzu-li-chung-tang** 附子理中湯
   (Ginseng, Ginger, and Aconite Combination)
   Li-chung-tang 理中湯
   (Ginseng and Ginger Combination)
   Li-chung-tang may be taken for gastrointestinal weakness, gastroptosis, emaciation, lack of vigor, mild anemia, and general chilling. For severe chills, take *Fu-tzu-li-chung-tang*.

7. **Szu-ni-tang** 四逆湯
   (Aconite and G. L. Combination)
   To be taken for severe chilling of the hands and feet and after diarrhea when the patient has severe chills, weak and sunken pulse, pale face, and fatigue.

8. **Ching-shih-hua-tan-tang** 清濕化痰湯
   (Pinellia and Arisaema Combination)
   To be taken for chilling, great amounts of phlegm, or neuralgia at the ribs.

9. **Pai-hu-tang** 白虎湯
   (Gypsum Combination)
   To be taken for surface chilling.

Blood Disease

The blood disease is an abnormal state of women. The mental and emotional disorders due to menstruation, pregnancy, childbirth, puerperal fever, menopause, abortion, and contraception are its characteristics.

The blood disease often causes autonomic nervous system symptoms such as ruddy face, congestion, limb fever, chills after sweating, palpitation, pressure at the heart, vertigo, tinnitus, and unstable blood pressure. There are also the emotional symptoms of nervousness, easy excitability, hysteria, melancholy, amnesia, confusion, tendency towards fatigue, headache, and shoulder stiffness. The main disease of the young woman is chilling and of the middle aged, disorder of menopause.

Treatment

Since it is a type of emotional disease, a life without stress can bring about very good results. Sometimes, administration of tranquilizers can also be helpful. Chinese herbal formulas are used according to air, blood, and water stagnancy.

Chinese Herb Formulas
1. Kuei-chih-fu-ling-wan　　　　　　　　　　桂枝茯苓丸
   (Cinnamon and Hoelen Formula)

To be taken for resistant, pressing pain in the lower abdomen around the umbilicus, symptoms of stagnant blood, pelvic congestion, headache, abdominal pain, and menstrual difficulties. It is a strong conformation. Most of the patients are vigorous with a ruddy face. Those having constipation should add rhubarb (0.5-2.0 gm.) to this formula. In severe cases, take *Tao-ho-cheng-chi-tang* (Persica and Rhubarb Combination) instead.

2. Tang-kuei-shao-yao-san　　　　　　　　　當歸芍藥散
   (Tang-kuei and Paeonia Formula)

To be taken by women of the weak type with a tendency towards anemia and fatigue, chilling at the waist and feet, heaviness of the head, vertigo, tinnitus, palpitation, and aching in the lower abdomen.

3. **Chia-wei-hsiao-yao-san** 加味逍遙散
   (Bupleurum and Paeonia Formula)

To be taken for the obvious neuroses of the blood disease, such as fever and chills. It is also for fever in the limbs, heaviness of the head, vertigo, ruddy face, night sweats, insomnia, generalized tiredness, and loss of appetite. This is a medication for the semi-strong and semi-weak type.

4. **Nu-shen-san** 女神散
   (Tang-kuei and Cyperus Formula)

To be taken for flushing up and vertigo. It is a remedy for climacteric disorder and blood diseases.

5. **Szu-wu-tang** 四物湯
   (Tang-kuei Four Combination)

This is a perfect formula for gynecological diseases, to be taken for anemia and nervousness. The patient with diarrhea should not take it.

6. **Chiung-kuei-tiao-hsieh-yin** 芎歸調血飲
   (Cinidium and Rehmannia Combination)

To be taken for postpartum diseases. It is especially effective for nervous ailments due to blood diseases.

7. **Chai-hu-chia-lung-ku-mu-li-tang** 柴胡加龍骨牡蠣湯
   (Bupleurum and Dragon Bone Combination)

This is a sedative to be taken for pressure at the chest, uncomfortable feeling at the umbilicus, palpitation, flushing up, headache, vertigo, insomnia, and fatigue due to the blood diseases.

8. **I-kan-san-chia-chen-pi-pan-hsia** 抑肝散加陳皮半夏
   (Bupleurum Formula with Citrus and Pinellia)

To be taken for nervousness with epilepsy, anxiety accompanied by proneness to anger, and insomnia.

9. **Pan-hsia-hou-pu-tang** 半夏厚朴湯
   (Pinellia and Magnollia Combination)

To be taken by patients of the weak type who have a sensation of something blocking or itching and stimulating in the throat, a hoarse voice, weak and sunken pulse, and a patting sound at the lower part of the heart.

10. Kuei-chih-chia-lung-ku-mu-li-tang   桂枝加龍骨牡蠣湯
    (Cinnamon and Dragon Bone Combination)
To be taken for a tendency towards physical weakness, nervousness, congestion, headache, insomnia, palpitation, fearfulness, sweating, and night sweats.

11. Kan-mai-ta-tsao-tang   甘麥大棗湯
    (Licorice and Jujube Combination)
To be taken for hysteria, nervousness, spasm, insomnia, tendency towards yawning, and, in severe cases, coma or mania.

12. Ling-kuei-kan-tsao-tang
    (Hoelen, Licorice, and Jujube Combination)
To be taken for palpitation at the lower umbilicus, congestion, vomiting, headache, and decrease in urinary output.

13. Huang-lien-chieh-tu-tang   黃連解毒湯
    (Coptis and Scute Combination)
It is effective for ruddy face, congestion, insomnia, stress, palpitation, and stagnation of blood.

14. Chen-wu-tang   眞武湯
    (Vitality Combination)
It is effective for weak conformation, proneness to becoming tired, chilling, weak pulse and abdomen, stagnancy in the gastrointestinal tract, decrease in urinary output, abdominal pain and diarrhea, and vertigo or palpitation.

Vaginal Trichomoniasis

    This disease is usually caused by parasitic vaginal trichomonas of the digestive system, which have invaded and remained in the vaginal cavity. Children and elderly, as well as adult women suffer from this disease. The mode of infection is still not clear, but it is commonly believed that the protozoa is spread during intercourse or bathing.

Symptoms

There is massive leucorrhea of milky or yellow color, and the mouth of the vagina becomes fiery red. Pain and itching are severe. The vaginal wall will also become fiery red and will hemorrhage. Trichomonas vaginalis is a rather large protozoa that can be seen with an ordinary microscope. Any questions concerning this disease should be referred to a gynecologist.

Treatment

Irrigation of the vaginal cavity alone may bring about fairly good results. After several days therapy, the painful symptoms should decrease. If this disease cannot be completely cured, it will cause inflammation again immediately. Therapy must be maintained for at least three weeks, after which symptoms should be minimal.

Chinese Herb Formulas

1. **Glyrrhizae Radix** 甘草一味
   (Licorice Root)

When the outside or external orifice of the vagina has been broken down, application of a dressing of licorice extract on the wound will check the pain.

2. **Lung-tan-hsieh-kan-tang** 龍膽瀉肝湯
   (Gentiana Combination)

To be taken for leucorrhea or itching at the outside of the vagina.

Frigidity

Frigidity usually means the lack of a pleasant feeling during sexual intercourse. It also includes women past a certain age who have no sexual desire.

The reasons for frigidity include underdevelopment of the female genital organs and of the endocrine and nervous systems, immaturity of the male genital organs, lack of sex knowledge, imcompatible personalities of the couple, fear of pregnancy, diabetes, and other general diseases. However, high expectation of prompt satisfaction during intercourse is another reason.

Frigidity in the woman has nothing to do with the act of

insemination or an ensuing pregnancy. Impotence of the male, however, would prevent conception.

Treatment
The physical causes of frigidity require a physician's help, but the mental causes can be eliminated by cooperation between husband and wife. For the wife, a little wine or a sedative can decrease her emotional tension and accomplish very good results.

Chinese Herb Formulas
1. Chai-hu-chia-lung-ku-mu-li-tang　　　柴胡加龍骨牡蠣湯
   (Bupleurum and Dragon Bone Combination)
   Chia-wei-hsiao-yao-san　　　加味逍遙散
   (Bupleurum and Paeonia Formula)
   I-kan-san　　　抑肝散
   (Bupleurum Formula)

Effective for frigidity due to emotional causes such as nervousness and anxiety.

Postoperative Symptoms

There are symptoms which occur after surgical removal of the uterus due to uterine myoma, of an ovary due to abnormal pregnancy or sac-tumor, or of the breast due to breast cancer. Physically, most of these patients are slender and have cold hands and feet.

Symptoms
The patient will have facial or upper-body fever, chills, dizziness, palpitation, aching shoulders, headache, and other symptoms. Those who have undergone abdominal surgery will have abdominal pain, constipation, and the sensation of abdominal distention.

Treatment
Because the endocrine system has been greatly affected by the surgery, administration of sedatives and stimulants may bring about good results.

Chinese Herb Formulas
1. **Kuei-chih-chia-shao-yao-tang**　　　桂枝加芍藥湯
   (Cinnamon and Paeonia Combination)
   To be taken for hardening of the abdominal muscles and abdominal pain.

2. **Tang-kuei-szu-ni-chia-wu-chu-yu-sheng-chiang-tang**
   　　　　　　　　　　當歸四逆加吳茱萸生薑湯
   (Tang-kuei, Evodia, and Ginger Combination)
   To be taken for abdominal distension, abdominal pain, chilling, and a tendency towards tiredness.

SKIN DISEASES

Hyperhidrosis

Hyperhidrosis is excessive sweating when no inducing environmental factors such as humidity, body exercise, or heat are present. There are two types: generalized and localized. Generalized hyperhidrosis occurs in people who are nervous and mentally excitable or who are suffering from Basedow's disease, anemia, apoplexy, tabes (emaciation) or an endocrine disturbance. On the other hand, in localized hyperhidrosis the sweating occurs in isolated areas of the body such as the hands and feet or where the sweat glands are located. Sometimes the sweating occurs on one side of the face only or on the lower torso below the waist but not on the upper torso. It is thought to be caused by a disturbance of the sympathetic nervous system.

Symptoms

In localized hyperhidrosis excessive perspiration occurs in the armpits, on the face, palms of the hands and soles of the feet, and on the external genitalia. Excessive sweating in the armpits leads to offensive odor, the formation of carbuncles, and fungus infections like ringworm in adults. In children it leads to prickly heat. Hyperhidrosis soaks the skin of the palms and feet making them pale, soft, and cold to the touch.

Treatment
Dust the affected areas with talc powder or urotropine powder. Surgical removal of the sweat glands may be necessary for local hyperhidrosis in extreme cases.

Chinese Herb Formulas
1. **Kuei-chih-chia-huang-chi-tang**　　　　　桂枝加黃耆湯
    (Cinnamon and Astragalus Combination)
This combination is usually taken by patients with weak physiques or by those who look strong but easily catch cold because of the hyperhidrosis.

2. **Fang-chi-huang-chi-tang**　　　　　　　　防己黃耆湯
    (Stephania and Astragalus Combination)
Pale-skinned women with a dropsical, obese constitution are most likely to have hyperhidrosis along with fatigability and frequent urination. They will also have anemophobia and painful urination after having a cold. These women respond well to this combination. It is also good for armpit odor and underarm perspiration of obese patients.

3. **Chai-hu-chiang-kuei-tang**　　　　　　　　柴胡薑桂湯
    (Bupleurum, Cinnamon, and Ginger Combination)
Physical debility, excessive perspiration above the neck, *ch'i* tending to flush-up, and persistent low-grade fever are the targets of this combination. Tubercular nightly sweating can also be treated with this formula.

4. **Tang-kuei-liu-huang-tang**　　　　　　　　當歸六黃湯
    (Tang-kuei and Six Herb Combination)
This combination is for a weak-fever conformation of night sweats and for tubercular night sweats. It also may alleviate protracted night sweats of unknown causes.

5. **Pu-chung-i-chi-tang**　　　　　　　　　　補中益氣湯
    (Ginseng and Astragalus Combination)
For people who sweat too easily after illness or become easily fatigued this combination strengthens dermal functions and

restores vigor.

6. **Shih-chuan-ta-pu-tang** 十全大補湯
 (Ginseng and Tang-kuei Ten Combination)
This formula is for anemia and severe fatigue accompanied by spontaneous night sweats following a serious disease.

7. **Pu-yin-tang** 補陰湯
 (Tang-kuei and Rehmannia Combination)
This combination cures patients who perspire even on cold days, tire easily, and ache around the waist.

8. **Mu-li-san** 牡蠣散
 (Oyster Shell Formula)
This formula is for spontaneous sweating, especially while asleep, in people who have been debilitated by a serious illness. It is taken if the above mentioned formulas have been ineffective.

Trichophytia Pompholyciformis
(Ringworm)

Ringworm is a genus of Trichophyton that attacks the outer skin causing small white vesicles that eventually burst and itch intensely. Sometimes a severe infection of pyogenic bacteria such as Trichophyton precipitates an inflammation of the lymph nodes. Both of these infections are subject to relapse.

Symptoms
On the palms and soles small white vesicles appear which turn purulent (with pus) in most cases. At times the skin peels and cracks causing itching

Treatment
0.25-0.5g of microcrystalline griseofulvin taken orally once or twice daily for two weeks is effective. Two percent miconazole cream of one percent clotrimazole cream may be applied twice daily also.

Chinese Herb Formulas

1. Ma-hsing-i-kan-tang　　　　麻杏薏甘湯
(Ma-huang and Coix Combination)

This formula works for thin patients afflicted with dandruff.

2. Lien-chiao-tang　　　　連翹湯
(Forsythia Combination)

For a dry lesion that has become more serious in nature than the preceding conformation, this combination can be effective.

3. Shih-wei-pai-tu-tang　　　　十味敗毒湯
(Bupleurum and Schizonepeta Combination)

This combination is taken to cure suppurative Trichophyton with itching and pus effusions. 3.0g forsythia and 5.0g coix are added.

4. Kuei-chih-fu-ling-wan-liao　　　　桂枝茯苓丸料
(Cinnamon and Hoelen Formula)

This formula is for people with "stagnant blood" who have a pimply Trichophyton infection with red, cloud-like margins and a burning, itching sensation. 5.0g of coix should be added.

5. Tao-ho-cheng-chi-tang　　　　桃核承氣湯
(Persica and Rhubarb Combination)

People with symptoms similar to those in the preceding instance with more severe inflammation, as well as constipation, should take this combination.

6. Fang-feng-tung-sheng-san　　　　防風通聖散
(Siler and Platycodon Formula)

This formula is for people with obese physiques—gourmands with food and water toxicity and a tendency to be constipated.

7. Tang-kuei-shao-yao-san　　　　當歸芍藥散
(Tang-kuei and Paeonia Formula)

Women with debilitated physiques, chills, and poor complexions may take this formula with coix added.

8. I-yi-fu-tzu-pai-chiang-san　　　　薏苡附子敗醬散
(Coxi, Aconite, and Thlaspi Formula)

Weak conformations with chronic, unhealed, dry, scaly ringworm may take this formula.

9. San-wu-huang-chin-tang　　　　　三物黃芩湯
   (Scute Three Herb Combination)

People with dry, itching, sore, and cracked skin experiencing thirst and feverish limbs should take this combination.

10. Tzu-yun-kao　　　　　紫雲膏
    (Lithospermum Ointment)

This ointment is particularly effective in treating dry ringworm and is sometimes efficacious for moist or suppurative ringworm.

Keratoderma Tylosis Palmaris Progressiva

Keratosis is one of several types of inflammatory skin diseases. It is usually found in young girls, especially after the first or second year of menstruation. It begins on the lower side of the final segments of the right hand fingers in a righthanded person or the left hand figners in a lefthanded person. The skin turns dry, cracked,and coarse and peels. Gradually the condition spreads and extends to the front half of the palm. Microscopically epithelial proliferation is found. This is followed by a thickening and hardening of the skin: the stratum corneum of the skin of the palms thickens, sometimes with painful lesions resulting from the formation of fissures. Keratosis is often found with other abnormalities, including baldness and vitiligo, the spotty lack of skin pigmentation. The disease usually worsens in winter. Now it is generally believed that the condition is caused by the external stimuli associated with heavy housework. This etiology has replaced the old explanation that it was caused by the presence of abnormal female hormones.

Symptoms

Lesions usually appear on the lower side of the fingers. The skin turns arid and coarse and begins to peel. The prints of the fingers diminish and small fissures appear. If untreated the epidermal cells eventually enlarge.

Treatment

External exacerbating stimuli such as heavy work or excessive contact with cold water, dirt, and hay must be avoided, X-ray therapy, chemical pastes, and injections of female hormones may prove to be helpful. The wearing of cotton or rubber gloves while working will prevent further progression.

Chinese Herb Formulas

1. Ma-hsing-i-kan-tang 麻杏薏甘湯
(Ma-huang and Coix Combination)

Pathologically this disease is believed to be due to poor surfacial blood circulation. Thus this combination is for the disturbance of blood circulation and dry skin caused by dampness and cold. It is especially effective against dandruff.

2. Chia-wei-hsiao-yao-san 加味逍遙散
(Bupleurum and Paeonia Formula)

Weak women with minor anemia who have menstrual problems and neurosis can take this formula with 3.0g of lycium and 2.0g of schizonepeta added.

3. Kuei-chih-fu-ling-wan-liao 桂枝茯苓丸料
(Cinnamon and Hoelen Formula)

Women with firm physiques and blood diseases, such as stagnant blood beneath the abdomen indicated by resistant pain when palpated and menstrual problems, can take this formula with 6.0g of coix added.

4. I-yi-fu-tzu-pai-chiang-tang 薏苡附子敗醬湯
(Coix, Aconite, and Thlaspi Combination)

Slack abdominal muscles, weak pulse, and a tendency toward anemia are the indications for this combination. Chronic diseases such as scleroderma (hardening and thickening of the skin), verruca (warts), and lichen (skin lesions) can also be treated with this combination.

5. San-wu-huang-chin-tang 三物黃芩湯
(Scute Three Herb Combination)

Dry, itching, and cracked skin; thirst; and feverish limbs are the symptoms treated with this combination.

6. Tzu-yun-kao 紫雲膏
   (Lithospermum Ointment)
   This ointment lubricates and moistens dry skin. Hence it is the most popular remedy for this disease. It also is used to treat cheiropompholyx (itching skin disease), callouses, keloids, and warts.

7. Wen-ching-tang 溫經湯
   (Tang-kuei and Evodia Combination)
   People with yin-weak physiques, blood and *ch'i* weakness, chills, warm palms, dry mouth, and menstrual problems, or ascending chills can taken this combination.

8. Tang-kuei-szu-ni-chia-wu-chu-yu-sheng-chiang-tang
   當歸四逆加吳茱萸生薑湯
   (Tang-kuei, Evodia, and Ginger Combination)
   This combination cured a woman of 32 who had chills, frostbite evey winter, and cracked and dry palms which itched during the night.

Urticaria

Like eczema, urticaria is caused by a particular irritation in an urticaria-prone physique. The irritation is usually caused by a food to which the person is allergic. Raw mackerel, bonito, egg, and unfresh fish are common allergens. Direct sunshine and cold air may also bring on urticaria. Those having constipation, gastrointestinal disorders, hepatitis, and nephritis are very susceptible to this disease.

Symptoms
Urticaria forms a map-like erythema on the skin and is accompanied by severe itching. It will subside after several hours, and the patient will recover completely in one to seven days.

Treatment
Prophylaxis is better than treatment. Those who are susceptible to this condition should avoid all known allergens. If it is caused by another disease, that disease should be cured first

in order to prevent a relapse of the urticaria.

Chinese Herb Formulas

1. Yin-chen-hao-tang　　　　　　　　　　　茵陳蒿湯
    (Capillaris Combination)
This is effective for acute urticaria. To be taken for discomfort in the area between the heart and armpits, loss of appetite, constipation, and itching.

2. Hsiao-chai-hu-tang　　　　　　　　　　　小柴胡湯
    (Minor Bupleurum Combination)
This is effective for those of average structure with discomfort in the area between the heart and armpits, resistance when pressure is applied to the abdomen, and food allergy. It is good for urticaria in women and children.

3. Shih-wei-pai-tu-san　　　　　　　　　　　十味敗毒散
    (Bupleurum and Schizonepeta Formula)
This is effective for repetitive urticaria.

4. Kuei-chih-ma-huang-ko-pan-tang　　　　桂枝麻黃各半湯
    (Cinnamon and Ma-huang Combination)
To be taken for primary urticaria with severe itching and mild fever.

5. Ko-ken-tang　　　　　　　　　　　　　　葛根湯
    (Pueraria Combination)
This is a common formula for primary urticaria. It is effective for severe chills, fever, swelling, and severe itching. In cases with high fever, add gypsum 5.0 g. In cases with a tendency towards constipation, add rhubarb 1.0 g.

6. Hsiang-su-san　　　　　　　　　　　　　香蘇散
    (Cyperus and Perilla Formula)
This is effective for urticaria initiated by eating fish.

7. Tiao-wei-cheng-chi-tang　　　　　　　　調胃承氣湯
    (Rhubarb and Mirabilitum Combination)
This is effective for urticaria due to food poison. In severe cases with abdominal swelling, *Ta-cheng-chi-tang* (大承氣湯, Major

Rhubarb Combination) should be used.

8. **Tao-ho-cheng-chi-tang** 桃核承氣湯
    (Persica and Rhubarb Combination)
To be taken by the woman of hearty constitution with facial redness, stagnant blood, and a tendency towards constipation. Mild cases should be treated with *Kuei-chih-fu-ling-wan* (桂枝茯苓丸, Cinnamon and Hoelen Formula)

9. **Ta-chai-hu-tang** 大柴胡湯
    (Major Bupleurum Combination)
To be taken by those of hearty constitution with chest fullness and recalcitrant symptoms.

10. **Fang-feng-tung-sheng-san** 防風通聖散
    (Siler and Platycodon Formula)
To be taken by those of obese constitution with chronic urticaria and constipation.

11. **Pai-hu-tang** 白虎湯
    (Gypsum Combination)
This is effective for severe itching, a sensation of fever, thirst, and insomnia.

12. **Pa-wei-wan** 八味丸
    (Rehmannia Eight Formula)
To be taken by the elderly for urticaria accompanied by thirst and dysuria.

13. **Hsiao-feng-san** 消風散
    (Tang-kuei and Arctium Formula)
This is effective for inflammation, secretion, and severe itching.

Eczema

Eczema is the most common skin disease, comprising thirty to fifty percent of all skin diseases. It is said that almost every person suffers from this condition at least once or twice in his lifetime.

In the past, this disease was thought to be an effusive symptom; now it is considered to be an allergy revealed on the skin. Nephritis, gastrointestinal disorders, obesity, and gynecopathy are some of the causes of this disease; most of the cases, however, are thought to be the result of external irritation of the eczema-prone skin. Some cases are also due to the application of cosmetics, the wearing of nylon underwear, and exposure to the sun. The causes vary from individual to individual. The most susceptible areas of the body are the head, face, and genitalia.

Symptoms

The first symptom of acute eczema is a red swelling on the skin. Gradually, the affected area becomes covered with pimples which turn into itching blisters. After a short time, the blisters break, suppurate, and secrete viscous fluid. The secretion dries and forms a yellow crust which drops off and is replaced by new tissue. In chronic eczema, the yellow crust drops off and the skin becomes red with pimples repeatedly. There is no known cure for this. The skin of the affected area becomes thick, itchy, and dark brown in color.

Treatment

Apply steroid and antihistamine ointments on the affected area. For chronic eczema, a disease related to the condition of the whole body, it is very important to improve the constitution of the patient by diet therapy. He should avoid fat and protein of animal origin and eat foods containing high amounts of calcium, Vitamin B, and iodine. Herb baths are occasionally effective for this disease.

According to Chinese medicine, eczema is not only a skin disease but also an internal disease resulting from stagnant blood, accumulated sputum, food poisons, and venereal disease. The patient should accept treatment of the whole body.

Chinese Herb Formulas

1. **Shih-wei-pai-tu-san** 十味敗毒散
   (Bupleurum and Schizonepeta Formula)

This is a common formula for eczema. It is effective for small, red pimples with little secretion but severe itching.

2. **Hsiao-feng-san** 消風散
   (Tang-kuei and Arctium Formula)
   To be taken for encrustation formed by continuous secretion. This type of eczema becomes more severe in summer.

3. **Tang-kuei-yin-tzu** 當歸飲子
   (Tang-kuei and Tribulus Combination)
   To be taken for eczema characterized by dry skin, little secretion, and itching. It may become worse in winter.

4. **Ko-ken-tang** 葛根湯
   (Pueraria Combination)
   To be taken for the initial stage of acute eczema with symptoms of inflammation, itching, and a hot sensation. It is also effective for chronic eczema with little secretion. In severe cases with itching and a burning feeling, add gypsum 8.0g.; in cases with constipation, add rhubarb 1.0g.

5. **Yueh-pi-chia-chu-tang** 越婢加尤湯
   (Atractylodes Combination)
   To be taken for secretion, swelling, difficult urination, and thirst.

6. **Tiao-wei-cheng-chi-tang** 調胃承氣湯
   (Rhubarb and Mirabilitum Combination)
   To be taken for constipation with abdominal swelling. In severe cases *Ta-cheng-chi-tang* (大承氣湯, Major Rhubarb Combination) should be used.

7. **Tao-ho-cheng-chi-tang** 桃核承氣湯
   (Persica and Rhubarb Combination)
   To be taken for a tendency towards chronic eczema, stagnant blood in the infected area, severe itching, lower abdominal pain, and stagnation.

8. **Ta-huang-mu-tan-pi-tang** 大黃牡丹皮湯
   (Rhubarb and Moutan Combination)
   To be taken for abdominal swelling and pressing pain.

9. **Ta-chai-hu-tang** 大柴胡湯
   (Major Bupleurum Combination)

To be taken by those of hearty constitution with lower heart distention.

10. Fang-feng-tung-sheng-san 防風通聖散
   (Siler and Platycodon Formula)
This is effective for those of obese constitution with constipation and abdominal fullness.

11. Pai-hu-tang 白虎湯
   (Gypsum Combination)
This is effective for the patient with severe itching, a sensation of having a fever, and dry throat.

12. Ching-shang-fang-feng-tang 清上防風湯
   (Siler Combination)
This is effective for eczema of the head or face with facial redness and congestion. If there is constipation, add rhubarb 1.0g.

13. Chia-wei-hsiao-yao-san with Szu-wu-tang
加味逍遙散加四物湯
   (Bupleurum and Paeonia Formula with Tang-kuei Four Combination)
This is effective for the woman of delicate constitution with mild anemia and a tendency towards chronic, dry, itching eczema with little secretion.

14. Wen-ching-yin 溫清飲
   (Tang-kuei and Gardenia Combination)
This is effective for eczema.

15. Chen-wu-tang 眞武湯
   (Vitality Combination)
To be taken for chilling constitution with moist eczema, fatigue, mild anemia, and itching.

Facial Boils

Staphylococci, the most resistant pyogenic cocci, may invade the deep layers of the skin from the sebaceous or sweat glands and cause inflammation or boils. When this occurs on the face, it is called "facial boils".

Because of their proximity to the brain, severe facial boils may occasionally invave the cerebral tissue and cause meningitis. People fear this disease because of the possibility of such a severe complication.

Symptoms

There is a particle at the center of the pore which becomes red and begins to swell, causing pain. It will then enlarge and discharge pus. Severe cases are accompanied by chills, fever, and loss of appetite.

Treatment

The patient should remain completely quiet, apply intermittent, moist heat to the lesions, and take antibiotics. For severe swelling, surgery should be performed at the proper time. Cleanliness is very improtant so that the bacteria are not spread to other broken areas of the skin.

Chinese Herb Formulas

1. Shih-wei-pai-tu-san　　　　　　　　　　十味敗毒散
   (Bupleurum and Schizonepeta Formula)
This is effective during the initial stage and for mild facial boils.

2. Nei-tuo-san　　　　　　　　　　　　　　內托散
   (Astragalus and Platycodon Formula)

Rosacea

Rosacea—a chronic disease affecting the skin of the nose, forehead, and cheeks—exhibits a red flushing of the face due to dilation of the capillaries and pimples or acne-like pustules. It occurs most commonly in adults, being most obvious during temperature changes or the imbibing of spirits. Etiological factors include congestion of face and head, a disturbed digestive system, consumption of alcohol, anemia, and gynecological problems.

Symptoms

Rosacea is divided into three stages. During the initial stage both bright and dark red coloration spreads over the face due to dilation of the capillaries and activation of the sebaceous glands. The second stage is characterized by the development of pimples or acne resulting from the swelling of hair folicles due to the glandular secretions. The third stage exhibits rhinophyma (marked enlargement of the blood vessels, sebaceous glands, and connective tissue of the nose). The redness and swollen tissues may extend from the tip of the nose across both cheeks to the forehead.

Treatment

The first and second stages can be treated by mercury, quartz lamp or by applying ointments. The third stage can be treated by surgery and/or X-ray therapy.

Chinese Herb Formulas

1. **Ko-ken-hung-hua-tang** 葛根紅花湯
   (Pueraria and Carthamus Combination)

Usually this combination is prescribed for the congested blood in the head and on the surface of the face. Since the disease cannot be cured rapidly, the formula is taken as a long-time medication.

2. **Huang-lien-chieh-tu-tang** 黃連解毒湯
   (Coptis and Scute Combination)

A minor case with only the symptoms of flushing and congestion of blood can be cured by this combination.

3. **Ko-ken-huang-lien-huang-chin-tang** 葛根黃連黃芩湯
   (Pueraria, Coptis, and Scute Combination)

A combined prescription of the above two formulas, this remedy is for patients who drink too much alcohol and who have frequent congestion of blood in the face or head.

4. **Fang-feng-tung-sheng-san** 防風通聖散
   (Siler and Paltycodon Formula)

This combination is taken by obese people over a long period of time for conditions caused by congestion of blood in the head. It is also given to those people who eat a lot of meat and drink alcohol.

External Treatment

1.0g of *liu-huang* (sulphur), 1.0g of *hsing-jen* (apricot seed) and 0.5g of *ching-fen* (calomel). A mixture made of the above components compounded with honey is applied topically on the infected parts and washed off the next morning. It is said to be effective if continued for several months.

Melanosis

Melanomas, or lentigo, are oval, flat, brown, pigmented spots on the skin caused by an increased deposit of melanin and an increased number of melanocytes on the epidermal junction. They result from sunlight stimulating the clusters of melanocytes to a higher than normal tyrosinase activity. The spots are mainly located on the face and at times symmetrically on the dorsal sides of both hands. The coloration tends to be darker in the summer than winter. Mainly found in females, the condition begins at the age of five or six years and becomes increasingly manifest towards puberty.

The direct cause is the ultra violet rays of the sun, but other factors include pregnancy, ovary and uterus disturbances, and mental and physical fatigue.

Treatment

In general the avoidance of direct sunlight arrests the condition. Specifically, dosages of vitamin C and the application of topical chemotherapy may prove helpful.

Chinese Herb Formulas

1. Tang-kuei-shao-yao-san-liao　　　　　當歸芍藥散料
    (Tang-kuei and Paeonia Formula)

Emaciated, anemic and chill-prone women who have acquired the freckles during their pregnancies take this combination. Most of them are unlikely to be cured within a short period. This formula is prescribed with the addition of 6.0g of coix.

2. **Kuei-chih-fu-ling-wan-liao** 桂枝茯苓丸料
   (Cinnamon and Hoelen Formula)

This combination is effective for slightly overweight people with resistance and pain when palpated in the lower abdomen that comes from stagnated blood. Add 6.0g of coix to the combination for use. If there have been no bowel movements, add 1.0g of rhubarb.

3. **Tao-ho-cheng-chi-tang** 桃核承氣湯
   (Persica and Rhubarb Combination)

The conformation for this combination is stronger resistance and pain in the lower abdomen than in the above case. It is also for those whose faces are red with flushing and fever who have severe extravasated blood, and who are constipated.

4. **Chia-wei-hsiao-yao-san-ho-szu-wu-tang**
   加味逍遙散合四物湯
   (Bupleurum and Paeonia Formula with Tang-kuei Four Combination)

For emaciated, anemic women who have not yet entered menopause, this combination is effective.

Riehl's Melanosis

Riehl's melanosis is a rare pigmentatory affliction of the skin of the face. The affected skin turns red initially and eventually brown. Occasionally the skin becomes arid and peels. It is seen more frequently in females than in males and is known by the term *melanosis faciei feminis*. The major causes of this condition are the overuse of low-grade, harmful cosmetics and nutritional deficiencies. Other physical reasons may also contribute to this malady.

Symptoms

Spotty redness followed by a brown pigmentation is the most evident symptom, but small pimples with peeling and occasionally an arid surface are also evident.

Treatment

There is no specific remedy for this disease; however, any direct exposure to causative agents such as sunlight and cosmetics should be avoided. Water-soluble ointments to treat the hyperpigmentation may be used.

Chinese Herb Formulas

1. Huang-lien-chieh-tu-tang 黃連解毒湯
   (Coptis and Scute Combination)

This combination is effective for initial flushing which gradually darkens.

2. Wen-ching-yin 溫清飲
   (Tang-kuei and Gardenia Combination)

This combination is effective for melanosis when the surface of the skin is as arid as the bark of a pine tree.

3. Chia-wei-hsiao-yao-san or Chia-wei-hsiao-yao-san-ho-szu-wu-tang 加味逍遙散或加味逍遙散和四物湯

(Bupleurum and Paeonia Formula or Bupleurum and Paeonia Formula with Tang-kuei Four Combination)

Menopausal women with a tendency toward emaciation and anemia should take these combinations for improvement of skin coloration.

Psoriasis Vulgaris

This disease occurs after puberty and is of long duration. Its development advances and regresses with a relapse rate of 70 percent.

At the beginning it assumes the form of red, flat spots ranging from as small as a point to as large as a bean in size. The papules are definitely formed with distinctive boundaries. Most often they occur symmetrically on the elbows, knees or over the whole body. Soon a layer of glossy, silver-white, dry, thick scales form which then gradually enlarge. The scales are difficult to peel off. If one willfully peels them off, the peeled surface bleeds. Itching is rare though it can occur.

The cause of this dermatosis is unknown. Some doctors believe its origin is genetic, while others believe psoriasis is caused by infection or by a disturbance in adipose metabolism. Because limitation in the intake of animal fats may have a beneficial effect, it is also believed to be related to the endocrine system and to metabolic functions.

Treatment

Limitation of the intake of animal fats, application of coaltar ointment, and irradiation with a sunlamp are the general treatments.

Chinese Herb Formulas

1. Kuei-chih-chia-huang-chi-tang   桂枝加黃耆湯
(Cinnamon and Astragalus Combination)
This preparation for patients who are not physically strong is mostly used during the early stage when the disease has not progressed too far.

2. Huang-lien-ah-chiao-tang   黃連阿膠湯
(Coptis and Gelatin Combination)
Generally this combination is prescribed for people with weak conformations. The symptoms relieved are inside fever and aridity of body fluids. Usually it is used to moisten the red and arid infected parts.

3. Fang-feng-tung-sheng-san   防風通聖散
(Siler and Platycodon Formula)
With the addition of 3.0g rehmannia, this formula is usually prescribed for patients with a strong, burly physique who love to eat fats and protein, both of which abound in food poisons. Consequently, they are apt to have frequent constipation as well as a solid abdomen.

4. Hsiao-feng-san   消風散
(Tang-kuei and Arctium Formula)
This combination is mainly used to remedy the "heat of the blood" and moisten "dry blood." Its targets are inside fever, secretions that form scabs, thirst, the redness of infected skin, and severe itching.

5. Wen-ching-yin   溫清飲
   (Tang-kuei and Gardenia Combination)
This combination is well suited for patients with chronic symptoms of brownish skin which is as dry and coarse as sand paper, has very little natural oil, and itches severely in infected areas that bleed when scratched. A patient with this conformation exhibits a more obstinate inside fever and aridity than patients of the previous conformation. It is very difficult to differentiate between the two conformations, and at times the two formulas may be alternately prescribed.

6. Ta-huang-mu-tan-pi-tang   大黃牡丹皮湯
   (Rhubarb and Moutan Combination)
   Kuei-chih-fu-ling-wan   桂枝茯苓丸
   (Cinnamon and Hoelen Formula)
For patients with an abdominal conformation of extravasated blood, this formula may be effective according to their evacuation condition and the severity of the psoriasis.

Neurodermatitis

Neurodermatitis, or allergic dermatitis, is a general term for skin ailments presumed to be caused by itching due to external stimuli or emotional upsets. It manifests itself in atopic dermatitis (chronic, itching, superficial inflammation of the skin), *lichen simplex chronicus* (thickening of the skin), and other skin problems. Atopic dermatitis occurs in persons with a genetic predisposition. Individuals often react to allergens, notably wool and animal fur. The disease usually occurs in infancy, disappears at the age of two or three years, recurs in early youth, and thereafter tends to be chronic. *Lichen simplex chronicus* is a persistent, well localized plaque commonly found on the neck, wrists, or ankles. A "scratch-itch" cycle is its prominent feature. It is more common in women over forty years of age, especially in persons of Oriental extraction living in the USA.

Symptoms

Atopic dermatitis. Itching, exudative, or thickened eurptions occur on the face, neck, upper trunk, wrists and hands, and in the folds of the knees and elbows. The itching may be extremely severe and long-lasting, leading to emotional disturbance.

Lichen simplex chronicus. Dry, leathery, enlarged, thick plaques appear on the neck, wrists, perineum, thighs, and other parts of the body. The patches are localized, rectangular, thickened, pigmented, well-defined, and circumscribed by exaggerated skin lines.

Treatment

Topical corticosteroids, lotions, ointments, pastes, or creams may bring relief. All lesions should be bandaged or covered and all possible allergens avoided.

Chinese Herb Formulas

1. Chih-tou-chuang-i-fang 治頭瘡一方
   (Lonicera and Forsythia Formula)

This formula (from the Fukuis' family Imperial prescription) is widely known as a drug for curing head sores. It is generally believed that head sores come from embryo toxemia, possibly related to genetic factors which determine an individual's hypersensitivity. The formula is used for skin diseases that affect the head, face, neck, armpits, genitalia, and other parts of the body. The afflicted part first has red papules followed by blisters which eventually ulcerate and form into scabs. If there is a discharge, then the component of rhubarb should be excluded. It is usually taken continuously for one or two months.

2. Ma-ming-tang 馬明湯
   (Silkworm Molt Combination)

This combination is applicable to head eczema of patients who have greater thirst, more ugly pimples, and more secretion and scabbing than in the previous formula.

3. Hsiao-feng-san 消風散
   (Tang-kuei and Arctium Fromula)

This combination is recommended if the above two prescriptions fail.

Infantile Lichen

A disease often found in children from a few months old up to around six years old, it appears most frequently on the arms and legs in the form of bean-sized spots. It recurs repetitively from early summer to autumn. It is an outgrowth of gastrointestinal disturbances, dyspepsia, constipation, and food-related allergies. Occasionally it is caused by insect bites, especially lice. The disease is not serious in itself, but the lesions itch so intensely that the sleep is disturbed causing neurotic symptoms. Hence it requires immediate treatment to avoid the accompanying irritability and emotional problems.

Symptoms
From spring to autumn, the red bean-sized macules or spots appear on the arms and legs, especially on the outer sides, and occasionally on the shoulders and buttocks. When scratched, the spots redden and swell like hives and gradually develop an induration; sometimes a vesicle will be formed at the center of the hardness. Such a skin eruption can appear anywhere on the body. At times it appears like hives in clusters admixed with various kinds of eruptions. It itches so violently that the infant cannot sleep. It will disappear only to return the next season. However, after the age of six the disease spontaneously heals.

Treatment
If the infant has an upset stomach and constipation, these symptoms must be cured first of all. Protein foods such as processed pork, dairy products, and fish may induce this disease and should be avoided whenever the condition is aggravated. Drugs used include internal medicines such as antihistamines, sedatives, and digestants; antihistaminic ointment may also be applied externally. If the condition is very severe a steroid preparation is used in combination with the above drugs. Sometimes an injection of a vaccine which will change the infant's constitution is also very effective. Scratching can cause bacterial infection with complicating boils, impetigo, lymphadenitis, etc. Bacterial infections may also induce nephritis. They should be treated as soon as possible. Environmental sanitation is important to drive off mosquitoes, flies, and especially lice. Care

should be taken to prevent emotional and behavior problems in the child. The child or infant needs a thorough daily bath with ordinary soap so as to keep the skin clean. Parents should keep some antihistamines and antipruritic ointment for use when the condition calls for it.

Chinese Herb Formulas
1. **Wu-ling-san** 　　　　　　　　　　　　　　　　　五苓散
   (Hoelen Five Herb Formula)

This combination has been widely used since Kairotsuka published an account of its applicability to summer diseases which are characterized by blisters and miliaries appearing on the skin. For infantile lichen, this formula is usually tried first, other formulas being considered only if this formula fails.

2. **Kuei-chih-chia-huang-chi-tang** 　　　　　　桂枝加黃耆湯
   (Cinnamon and Astragalus Combination)

This combination is often used for people who are prone to overly perspire and easily tire.

3. **Shih-wei-pai-tu-tang** 　　　　　　　　　　　十味敗毒湯
   (Bupleurum and Schizonepeta Combination)

This Combination is prescribed as a long-term regimen to improve the physical condition of the patient.

Scleroderma

Scleroderma is a chronic disease of undetermined cause characterized by the insidious proliferation of connective tissue in the dermis and in multiple internal organs. Unlike fibrosis, there is early and progressive small arterial involvement. The disease occurs most frequently in middle-aged women.

Localized forms of scleroderma are usually benign; 50 percent of the nodular localized forms, however, become systemic. The overlapping syndromes of scleroderma are distinguished by definite skin changes and definite myositis that is usually responsive to small doses of corticosteroids. Moreover, there is a high incidence of positive findings of antinuclear antibodies. The systemic syndromes (progressive systemic sclerosis) are of two types: the rare diffuse progressive form (5 percent of cases) that shows rapid systemic progression with little or no incidence of Raynaud's phenomenon; and the common form of progressive systemic sclerosis (95 percent of cases) which is dominated in the early stages by Raynaud's phenomenon and acrosclerosis. (Raynaud's phenomenon presents bluish-colored or pale fingers with a tingling sensation caused by spasms of the capillaries.)

Symptoms

Stiffness of the hands, sweating of the hands and feet, and Raynaud's phenomenon may at times be present for years before the condition becomes apparent. The skin eventually becomes hard, thick, parchment-like, and glossy with no pitting edema, and the fingers and toes become fixed in position. Gradually the entire integument becomes involved; and telangiectasia, pigmentation and depigmentation, widespread or local calcification of the skin especially around the joints, and abnormal nail growth and ulceration of the fingers and toes occur. Esophageal involvement presenting inability or difficulty in swallowing may occur early. Disturbance of gastrointestinal motility may also occur. Resulting constriction of the thorax, pulmonary fibrosis, and recurrent bronchial pneumonia may lead to decreased vital capacity, decreased compliance, and a low diffusing capacity even in patients whose chest X-rays show no abnormality. Pericardial disease is usually subtle. Myocardial disease may result in an irregular heartbeat or congestive heart failure; the latter has a poor prognosis. Arthritis sometimes results, but the findings are not conspicuous. Neurologic manifestations may show but are uncommon. Laboratory findings are helpful but not diagnostic. The erythrocyte sedimentation rate and serum globulin may elevate. The number of antinuclear antibodies rises in 50 percent of cases. Concomitant autoimmune hematologic disorders (thrombocytopenia and hemolytic anemia) are rare. Proteinuria and casts are found frequently, however. In rare cases, renal involvement is extensive ending in death within months. X-rays show subcutaneous calcification, osteoporosis of bone, and destruction of the fingers and toes. Gastrointestinal X-rays may show loss of normal peristalsis. Scleroderma-like lesions have been found in patients with carcinoid syndrome.

Treatment

Treatment is symptomatic and supportive. Orally administered doses of reserpine may improve the capillary blood flow in patients with Raynaud's phenomenon. Corticosteroids should be used only if definite polymyositis is a component.

The condition usually progresses slowly. The prognosis for long survival is best in young white women. Only about a third of all patients with scleroderma survive beyond seven years. Death is usually due to renal or cardiac failure or to toxicity.

Although Chinese herbal treatment is also not completely healing, if the formula complies with the conformation, the symptoms will be alleviated.

Chinese Herb Formulas

1. **Chia-wei-hsiao-yao-san-ho-szu-wu-tang** 加味逍遙散合四物湯
   (Bupleurum and Paeonia Formula with Tang-kuei Four Combination)

   Shih-chuan-ta-pu-tang 十全大補湯
   (Ginseng and Tang-kuei Ten Combination)

   These formulas will take effect after prolonged intake in women with a weak conformation, endocrinological disturbances, and emotional instability.

2. **Kuei-chih-fu-ling-wan-liao** 桂枝茯苓丸料
   (Cinnamon and Hoelen Formula)

   For those patients who still have some stamina this formula combined with 10.0g of coix is for blood blockage in the lower abdomen with resultant pain from the pressure.

3. **Tang-kuei-szu-ni-chia-wu-chu-yu-sheng-chiang-tang** 當歸四逆加吳茱萸生薑湯
   (Tang-kuei, Evodia, and Ginger Combination)

   This formula cured a forty-five year-old male who got scleroderma after being frostbitten; his skin became soft again after lengthy intake.

4. **Yi-i-fu-tzu-pai-chiang-tang** 薏苡附子敗醬湯
   (Coix, Aconite, and Thlaspi Combination)

   This formula is for patients whose condition has progressed to a chronic and weak conformation. Originally this was a remedy for warts, matacarpal keratodermia, and other dermatoses, but it also is effective for localized scleroderma.

Pruritus

Pruritus is the disagreeable sensation of itching. It is the most common symptom in dermatological maladies and includes localized or generalized itching, stinging, crawling, and burning sensations. Pruritus, a modified form of pain, is far less tolerable than pain.

Transient, mild pruritus is a natural, normal phenomenon. It may also be a symptom of a specific dermatologic disorder of spontaneous, unknown origin. It may foreshadow or accompany a serious disease of internal origin, such as lymphomas and other neoplasma—especially Hodgkin's disease—hepatic or biliary disease, diabetes mellitus, nephritis, or drug intoxication or habituation. Perhaps the most common causes of generalized pruritus are excessive dryness of the skin resulting from overbathing, especially in the elderly; borderline forms of ichthyosis; and senile degeneration complicated by irritation from soaps and the low humidity caused by artificial heating and cold weather. Other causes are constant pressure and chafing; irritation from chemicals, including drugs; and allergies, as well as emotional factors.

Treatment

General measures. Relief centers on the avoidance of rich and spicy foods. Test diets of elimination diets may expose suspected food allergies. If pruritus is believed to be primarily a manifestation of an emotional disorder, psychotherapy is in order. External irritants, such as rough clothing or occupational hazards, should be avoided. People with dry, irritated skin should not bathe with soap or put their hands in detergent water while washing clothes or dishes. Baths with a small amount of bath oil soothe dry skin. Scratching should be avoided or controlled, and to this end the nails should be kept trimmed and clean. All unnecessary medication should be discontinued since some medicines themselves often produce pruritus.

Specific measures. The removal or treatment of the specific causes whenever possible is, of course, the most desirable of cures.

Local measures. Lotions, emulsions, and ointments incorporating volatile analgesics and antipruritics may relieve itching. If the skin is too dry, an excellent procedure is to wet it as in a bath to hydrate the keratin and then apply petroleum jelly to the wet skin to trap the moisture. If the skin is too oily, drying agents may afford relief; wet dressings, soaks, lotions, and powders, especially if the condition is acute, are efficaceous. Lukewarm baths of 15 minutes two or three times daily may often effectively control generalized pruritus. However, elderly patients with dry skin should bathe as infrequently as possible. After bathing, the skin should be blotted, not rubbed, dry. Caution: Overbathing, prolonged bathing periods, and exposure to drafts after bathing cause excessive drying of the skin.

Use of topical corticosteroid creams. Covering selected lesions of psoriasis, lichen, and localized eczemas each night with the corticosteroid wrapped with a thin plastic pliable film, such as Saran wrap, enables between 1-2 percent of the ointment to be absorbed. Complications from these creams include miliaria, cracking, pus-producing lesions, adrenal cortical suppression, localized skin atrophy, bad odors, fungal infections, and red hives. Thus the cure can be worse than the disease.

Systemic antipruritic drugs. Antihistamines and antiserotonins may be tried for certain cases of pruritus of allergic or undetermined cause. There is no preferred antihistamine, although 4mg of chlorpheniramine two to four times daily is inexpensive and less likely to cause drowsiness than the other antihistamines. Epinephrine injection 0.25-1.0ml of 1:1000 solution every four hours may be palliative with acute hives or nettle rash. Phenobarbital in 15-30mg doses two to four times daily may sedate agitated or distracted patients. Barbituates in themselves rarely produce dermatitis. Cortisotropin or the corticosteroids may also provide relief.

Prognosis

Elimination of external instigators and irritating agents is most successful in giving complete relief from itching. Pruritus that accompanies a specific skin disease subsides when the disease is brought under control. Spontaneous pruritus or that accompanying serious internal diseases may not respond to any type of therapy.

Chinese Herb Formulas
1. **Kuei-chih-ma-huang-ko-pan-tang** 桂枝麻黃各半湯
   (Cinnamon and Ma-huang Combination)
   This formula is for the initial stage of pruritus with feverishness when the external, visible symptoms are mild.

2. **Kuei-chih-huang-chi-wu-wu-tang** 桂枝黃耆五物湯
   (Astragalus Five Combination)
   This formula is for the initial stage when patients have dry skin, a lessening of skin fat, and pain.

3. **Ta-ching-lung-tang**
   (Major Blue Dragon Combination)
   This combination is for young men who have generalized pruritus especially at night, a buoyant pulse, and listlessness. The symptoms lessen in the daytime.

4. **Tang-kuei-yin-tzu** 當歸飲子
   (Tang-kuei and Tribulus Combination)
   Generally this formula is for older people with "senile pruritus," a condition which does not show any abnormal manifestations on the skin surface. However, old and young men who have insufficient skin fat or dry skin may also take this formula.

5. **Szu-wu-tang-chia-ching-chieh-fu-ping** 四物湯加荊芥浮萍
   (Tang-kuei Four Combination with Schizonepeta and Lemna)
   If the preceding formula fails to take effect, this one may be taken.

6. **Wen-ching-yin** 溫清飲
   (Tang-kuei and Gardenia Combination)
   This formula is for patients with a firm physique who have a sanguine temperament, up-flushing, and itchy skin that is as dry and harsh as sand paper with a brownish tinge.

7. **Pai-hu-chia-kuei-chih-tang** 白虎加桂枝湯
   (Cinnamon and Gypsum Combination)
   This formula is for severe pruritus with feverishness and intoler-

able thirst.

8. **Lung-tan-hsieh-kan-tang** 龍膽瀉肝湯
   (Gentiana Combination)

This formula for women with vulval pruritus is taken orally. In addition, on those occasions when the itching becomes violent, a compress of *Ku-sheng-tang* (Sophora Combination) applied to the affected area is helpful.

9. **Pa-wei-wan-liao** 八味丸料
   (Rehmannia Eight Formula)

This formula is for diabetics with vulval pruritus. It is also suitable for senile pruritus when accompanied by fatigue, thirst, and skin aridity.

10. **Chen-wu-tang** 眞武湯
    (Vitality Combination)

This formula is effective for senile or debilitated people with itching during the winter. As long as there is no abnormal skin condition, this remedy may be used.

11. **Ku-sheng-tang** 苦參湯
    (Sophora Combination)

This formula may be applied externally in the form of a wash or a compress for a severe pruritic condition.

Trichophyton Eczema (Fungus Infection)

Trichophyton, the principal genus of fungus, can cause an infection of or near the groin. Usually the infection causes complicated eczema which results in a severe itching sensation. Often the genitalia or the groin is involved and the itching extends to the lower abdomen or hips and even up to below the breasts or armpits. Profuse sweating aggravates the condition which is recurrent. The affected area appears brown at the center, mixed with papules, vesicles, crust, and scales while the peripheral area is red and swollen.

Chinese Herb Formulas

1. Shih-wei-pai-tu-tang　　　　　　　　十味敗毒湯
　　(Bupleurum and Schizonepeta Combination)
If the infection is complicated with eczema, this formula plus 6.0g of coix is commonly used.

2. Yueh-pi-chia-chu-tang　　　　　　　越婢加朮湯
　　(Atractylodes Combination)
This formula is suitable for a moist and dirty lesion that is secreting and has a strong stench.

3. Ta-huang-mu-tan-pi-tang　　　　　　大黃牡丹皮湯
　　(Rhubarb and Moutan Combination)
This formula is for people with a firm conformation and habitual constipation who are suffering from a persistent case of trichophyton infection that manifests dark brown scabes, fetid secretions, and extremely severe itching.

4. Tao-ho-cheng-chi-tang　　　　　　　桃核承氣湯
　　(Persica and Rhubarb Combination)
This combination is used when the patient has blood stagnation, resistant pain or pressure at the lower abdomen, and constipation.

5. Lung-tan-hsieh-kan-tang　　　　　　龍膽瀉肝湯
　　(Gentiana Combination)
This formula is for women who have extremely severe itching and pain in the genitalia.

6. Chai-hu-sheng-shih-tang　　　　　　柴胡勝濕湯
　　(Bupleurum and Cimicifuga Combination)
Recorded in *Lan shih mi tsang* (A Private Collection of the Orchid Room), this formula treats eczema (stubborn tinea or Trichophyton eczema) in both the groin and the scrotum, and severe pruritus that occurs repeatedly on the inside of the thighs, hips, and the genitalia during the summer or in humid climates. When other formulas have failed to cure, this one may be tried.

Recalcitrant Tinea

Adolescent males are most susceptible to this disease which is caused by a white fungus. It often occurs together with eczema. Recalcitrant tinea grows mainly in the moist skin folds of the groin, hips, armpits, or other areas having heavy secretion. This disease is aggravated by hot temperatures and humid weather; so people are most susceptible to it during the summer. The reason for this is that the fungi multiply rapidly during this season when sweat accumulates in skin folds and the genital area. Swimming pools and sea-bathing are the most common places to contract this infection. Fresh water should always be used to clean the body after swimming. Tinea is very difficult to cure, and relapses are frequent. Radical treatment should be used.

Symptoms

During the initial stages, the tinea are contained in small papules. Later the surrounding skin begins to swell and the central site of infection becomes red and itchy. When scratched, the infection will spread to the surrounding skin.

Treatment

It is important to keep the infected areas clean. The patient should wear loosen, cotton underwear. After bathing, the area should be dried completely and talcum powder applied to the infected parts. When there is itching, apply steroid ointment or antihistamine and then talcum powder. Addition of a sulphur agent to the bath water is also effective in treating this disease.

Chinese Herb Formulas

1. Chai-hu-sheng-shih-tang　　　　　　　　柴胡勝濕湯
   (Bupleurum and Cimicifuga Combination)

This is an effective formula for recalcitrant tinea. To be taken for repeated relapses and itching.

2. Lung-tan-hsieh-kan-tang　　　　　　　　龍膽瀉肝湯
   (Gentiana Combination)

To be taken by women with itching and severe pain in the genital area.

3. **Shih-wei-pai-tu-san** 十味敗毒散
   (Bupleurum and Schizonepeta Formula)
   This is effective for recalcitrant tinea.

4. **Yueh-pi-chia-chu-tang** 越婢加朮湯
   (Atractylodes Combination)
   This is effective for secretions and an unpleasant odor at the infected area.

5. **Tao-ho-cheng-chi-tang** 桃核承氣湯
   (Persica and Rhubarb Combination)
   This is effective for stagnant blood, resistant pressing pain, and constipation.

6. **Ta-huang-mu-tan-pi-tang** 大黃牡丹皮湯
   (Rhubarb and Moutan Combination)
   This is effective for the strong conformation of lingering recalcitrant tinea, constipation, secretion with unpleasant odor, and severe itching.

Alopecia

Alopecia is partial or complete loss of hair on the head. Although aging may be responsible, there are other causes also. These are listed as follows:

1) *Alopecia in maturity* – The causes of this form of male alopecia is unknown. It begins around thirty years of age, and it is said that a heredity factor is involved.

2) *Mechanical alopecia* – Those who often wear wigs or use hair dye (actors and actresses) will develop thinning of their hair. After a period of time, the hair begins to fall out. This occurs in both men and women.

3) *Alopecia furfuracea* – The patient has many bran-like skin chips on the scalp, and the hair from the forehead to the top of the head begins to fall out. Before long, all the hair falls out except a certain amount around the ears and on the back of the head. In addition to heredity factors, the causes may be gastrointestinal disturbances, anemia, excessive mental strain, and female disorders.

4) *Round alopecia* — The patient will unexpectedly suffer from one or several dime-size patches of alopecia. The skin of the affected area is normal, but the outlines of the hair loss are very clear. In some cases, the areas will increase in size or number. It is not contagious and has no particular symptoms other than hair loss. Its causes are still not clear. With proper therapy, normal hair growth will resume after two or three months. The spontaneous cure rate of this condition is 20%, and the rate of relapse is 30 to 50%. Severe cases are sometimes difficult to cure.
5) *Atrophic alopecia* — The skin on the top of the head or at the hair root becomes atrophic. This is followed by hair loss which does not extend over the whole scalp. The cause of the atrophy is unknown. Treatment can only stop the progress of the hair loss; growth of new hair cannot be expected.
6) *Symptomatic alopecia* — This type of alopecia is caused by a serious systemic disease, especially one with high fever or severe stress. The hair will grow again after recovery from the disease.
7) *Others* — Scar-like alopecia due to injury, alopecia syphilitica, and leprous alopecia.

Treatment

Therapies are described according to the above alopecia categories. They are as follows:
1) Oral intake of arsenic agents, ferralium, and pilocarpin is effective.
2) Prophylaxis is better than therapy. Do not cut or dye the hair too often.
3) Cure the known causes first. Apply tincture of dilute phenol and rub olive oil on the skin. Tranquilizers have sometimes resulted in a cure.
4) Injections of Vitamins B_1 and B_2 at the affected areas and oral intake of pituitary hormone, arsenic agents, and tranquilizers are effective. Infrared and light therapy are also effective.
5) Use of sulfur ointment on the affected areas and diathermy can prevent its spread. The patient should seek a doctor's diagnosis.

Chinese Herb Formulas

1. **Chai-hu-chia-lung-ku-mu-li-tang** 柴胡加龍骨牡蠣湯
(Bupleurum and Dragon Bone Combination)
This is effective for round alopecia. To be taken by those of hearty constitution with resistance or pressing pain from the chest cavity to the armpits, palpitation at the umbilicus, and nervousness.

2. **Kuei-chih-chia-lung-ku-mu-li-tang** 桂枝加龍骨牡蠣湯
(Cinnamon and Dragon Bone Combination)
This is also effective for round alopecia. To be taken by those of delicate constitution with vertigo, chilling of the feet, and palpitation at the umbilicus.

3. **Ta-chai-hu-tang** 大柴胡湯
(Major Bupleurum Combination)
To be taken by those of hearty constitution with heart distention and a tendency towards constipation.

4. **Hsiao-chai-hu-tang** 小柴胡湯
(Minor Bupleurum Combination)
To be taken for alopecia in young children and adolescents, or those of delicate constitution with symptoms of chest distention.

5. **Fang-feng-tung-sheng-san** 防風通聖散
(Siler and Platycodon Formula)
To be taken by those of delicate constitution with the symptoms of chest congestion, food poisoning, alcoholism, and constipation.

Leukoderma

Leukoderma is a deficiency of skin pigment which causes white patches. The majority of patients are middle-aged. This disease is thought to be caused by malnutrition and a disorder of the autonomic nervous system. The true causes, however, have not yet been clearly established. The white patches will gradually extend to other areas. When they reach an area of hair growth, the hair will turn white without itching or any other symptom of which the patient is aware. Intestinal diseases with fever, scarlet fever, neurosis, sensitivity to external medications, injury, and continuous pressure are other factors thought to cause this disease.

Treatment

Leucoderma is very difficult to cure, and at present there is no effective medication available.

Chinese Herb Formulas

1. **Kuei-chih-chia-huang-chi-tang** 桂枝加黃耆湯
   (Cinnamon and Astragalus Combination)

To be taken by the patient with delicate skin and a tendency towards perspiration. Use of this formula in the initial stage will cure this disease.

2. **Kuei-chih-fu-ling-wan** 桂枝茯苓丸
   (Cinnamon and Hoelen Formula)

To be taken by the patient having a resistant sensation in the lower abdomen.

Herpes Zoster (Shingles)

In ancient times this disease was called "fire band sores." A viral infection, it occurs most often in spring and autumn. Generally there is no warning symptom. Occasionally there will be neuralgia, fever, lassitude, and a loss of appetite followed by the skin reddening a few days after being infected. This syndrome, caused by the same virus as varicella (chickenpox), usually involves a single, unilateral dermatome. Pain, sometimes very severe, may precede the appearance of the skin lesions. The lesions follow the distribution of a nerve root, usually thoracic and lumbar roots but cervical roots and the trigeminal nerve may be involved. The skin lesions are similar to those of chickenpox and develop in the same way from maculopapules to vesicles to pustules, and finally to dark brown scabs. The disease lasts two to three weeks. In severe cases, it may last for more than one month and the vesicles may enlarge and become either hemorrhagic or gangrenous.

Such complications as lingering neuralgia, impairment of the sense of touch, lack of coordination, as well as local lymphatic swelling, may develop. Secondary bacterial infection of the lesions is common and may produce a pitted scar. Cellulitis, erysipelas, and surgical scarlet fever may occur. In patients whose immune system has been suppressed due to chemotherapy, *herpes zoster* may spread producing skin lesions beyond the affected area, visceral lesions, and encephalitis. This is a serious, sometimes fetal, complication.

Treatment

General measures. The skin must be kept clean by means of frequent tub baths or showers when no fever is present. Calamine lotion applied locally and antihistamines taken orally may relieve the itching.

Treatment of complications. Secondary bacterial infection of local lesions may be treated with bacitracin-neomycin ointment; if extensive, an injection of penicillin may be needed. Cystarabine has not been shown to be effective in the control of *herpes zoster* in an immunosuppressed host. Tests with adenine arabinoside are being made presently. While zoster immune globulin is not helpful for clinical therapy, it has proved useful as a prophylactic.

Prognosis

The total duration from onset of symptoms to the disappearance of crusts rarely exceeds two weeks. Fatalities are rare except in immunosuppressed patients.

Chinese Herb Formulas
1. **Ko-ken-tang** 葛根湯
   (Pueraria Combination)

This formula can be prescribed for the prodromal stage when there are feverish symptoms and for the initial stage of vesicle eruption.

2. **Hsiao-chai-hu-tang** 小柴胡湯
   (Minor Bupleurum Combination)

Within one to two weeks of onset the vesicles erupt and the

patient has a fever with thoracic pain. This formula is then a suitable therapy.

3. **Ta-chai-hu-tang** 大柴胡湯
   (Major Bupleurum Combination)

This formula is suitable for people with strong physiques, pain and hardness beneath the heart, thoraco-costal distress, and violent abdominal pain.

4. **Shih-wei-pai-tu-tang** 十味敗毒湯
   (Bupleurum and Schizonepeta Combination)

This formula can be taken after adding 3.0g of forsythia to alleviate vesicle eruption and lingering pain, and to prevent the development of gangrene.

5. **Chen-wu-tang** 眞武湯
   (Vitality Combination)

This formula is given to patients whose illness and pain have persisted so long that fatigue is setting in.

6. **Acupuncture and Moxibustion Therapy**

Acupuncture or moxibustion, when applied to the nerve roots affected, is an efficacious form of therapy.

Underarm Odor

This is an unpleasant odor originating in the armpits. It is due to oversecretion of the sweat glands in both sexes. Since these glands become active during adolescence, underarm odor also begins at this time. Sweat gland activity is minimal in old age, so there is no problem with odor during this time.

Treatment

The best way to avoid excessive underarm odor is to have the specific sweat glands surgically removed. However, keeping the armpits clean and sprinkling talcum powder on them is more or less effective as a method of control. Deodorants are available that are temporarily effective.

Chinese Herb Formulas
1. **Fang-chi-huang-chi-tang** 防己黃耆湯
   (Stephania and Astragalus Combination)
This is effective for those having white and tender skin, a tendency toward fatigue, and ephidrosis.

2. **Lung-tan-hsieh-kan-tang** 龍膽瀉肝湯
   (Gentiana Combination)
This is effective for those having liver disturbances, tea-brown skin color, tense abdomen, venereal disease, and moist toxin. This is effective for a certain degree of suppuration in facial boils.

3. **Po-chou-san** 伯州散
   (Eriocheir and Viper Formula)
To be taken at the onset of suppuration. It is also effective for pus drainage. Do not put this powder on the infected area.

Systemic Lupus Erythematosus (SLE)

In the past this disease was regarded as one of the collagenous diseases. However, today it has been excluded from them and is regarded as an allergy due to a tubercular lesion.

Lupus erythematosus is divided into the chronic and the acute or metastasis types. The former has no somatic symptoms and a good prognosis; the latter has strong somatic symptoms and a poor prognosis.

The chronic type shows red, asymptomatic, localized plaques usually on the face, often in butterfly distribution on both sides of the nose and across the bridge, with greyish white scales. The patient experiences a sensation of scorching heat when exposed to sunshine.

Systemic lupus erythematosus (SLE), an inflammatory syndrome of unknown cause, primarily involves the vascular and connective tissues of many organs with a resultant multiplicity of local and systemic manifestations. The disease (or at least an SLE-like syndrome) may be initiated by the use of certain drugs: diphenylhydantoin and other anticonvulsants, hydralazine, isoniazid, phenothiazines, procainamide, quinidine, sulfonamides, and thiouracils. Heredity probably plays a role in SLE; an increased frequency of antinuclear antibodies are found in families of patients. SLE has also been reported to have occurred in several sets of identical twins.

Although the pathogenesis of SLE has been studies extensively, the underlying mechanisms remain vague. The pathologic changes in SLE apparently involve an alteration of the immunogenic mechanism. An antibody to DNA is found in most people with severe, active SLE antinuclear antibodies, although a frequent serologic finding of SLE can also be demonstrated in normal older individuals, particularly women, as well as in clinical disorders other than SLE. The absence of antinuclear antibodies in active untreated SLE is unusual. Free DNA is a frequent finding in the serum of patients with SLE. It is felt that the anticomplementary activity of SLE serum is due to the complement consumption by circulating DNA antigen-antibody complexes. Fluorescent antibody studies of the renal glomeruli of SLE patients showed antigens, antibodies, and complements, pointing to an immune complex deposition in the pathogenesis or renal lesions. Serum complement is normal in drug-induced SLE, which may account for the decrease in renal involvement in the drug-induced disease. It has been reported that serious renal disease is less frequent in patients with precipitating antibodies to DNA-protein antigen than in those who have complement fixation antibodies to double-stranded DNA.

The type, severity, time of onset, and duration of the pathologic involvement gives a highly variable clinical pattern and prognosis. Pathologic changes are nonspecific but include widespread fibrinoid vascular changes and widespread inflammation of the arteries.

Pathologic alterations, as demonstrated by ordinary postmortem and light microscope studies, do not necessarily reflect the clinical severity of the condition. Patients who have died of the fulminant disease may show subtle nonspecific changes, whereas biopsies of living patients with moderate clinical disease may show necrotizing vasculitis.

Symptoms

Systemic reaction: weakness, fatigue, malaise, fever, sweating, and weight loss may occur.

Skin: discoid lupus erythematosus may occasionally precede the systemic disease. Conversely, disk-like lesions may develop during the course of the systemic disease. A redness of skin of exposed surfaces due to sensitivity to sunlight—especially the classical symmetric malar erythema, the so-called butterfly rash—and erythematosus rashes of the neck, elbows, and hands are the most common dermatologic manifestations. Purpura, angioneurotic edema, baldness, vitiligo (patchy lack of pigmentation), mucosal ulceration, or hyperpigmentation occurs less frequently.

Lymph nodes and spleen: half of the patients have generalized lymphadenopathy; one-fourth have splenomegaly.

Eyes: corneal and retinal involvement, including cotton wool retinal exudates, have been reported in about 20-25 percent of patients.

Hematopoietic system: hematologic involvement occurs in all patients. There may be severe hemolytic anemia or thrombocytopenic purpura. Hypersplenism has been described. Splenomegaly (enlargement of the spleen) occurs in about 20-25 percent of cases.

Lungs: pulmonary dysfunction with basilar atelectatic pneumonitis and pleurisy, with or without effusion, are common.

Cardiovascular system: pericariditis, with or without effusion, occurs in about half of the cases. Myocarditis with excessivly fast heartbeat, a galloping rhythm, and disturbances of rhythm may result in heart failure. Verucous endocariditis may also occur. Coronary arteritis is a rare but serious complication. Arterial hypertension may be a manifestation of renal disease. Raynaud's phenomenon is common and vasculitis of nearly any blood vessel may occur.

Gastrointestinal system: ulcerative lesions of the mucous membranes, especially the mouth, are very common. There may be loss of appetite, nausea and vomiting, difficulty in swallowing, diarrhea, abdominal pains, ileus, peritonitis, and bloody stools. The intestinal involvement may be the result of extensive vasculitis, of ulceration or perforation, or of coexisting ulcerative colitis or ileocolitis.

Liver-hepatomegaly (enlargement of the liver): often accompanies SLE with evidence of hepatic dysfunction occurring in about one-third of the cases. Chronic, active hepatitis with LE cells, hyperglobulinemia, and other immunologic phenomena has been mistakenly termed "lupoid hepatitis"; however, it is not true SLE.

Kidney: complications are a serious feature of SLE. Three different types of lupus nephritis have been described. Focal proliferative lupus nephritis is characterized by proteinuria and microscopic hematuria, but the nephrotic syndrome and kidney failure are rare. Response to corticosteroids is favorable. Diffuse proliferative lupus nephritis and membranous lupus nephritis are usually characterized by the nephrotic syndrome and renal insufficiency. Although remissions can be induced in some cases, the prognosis is generally unfavorable, and most patients die of the complications of renal failure within three years.

Musculoskeletal system: myalgia (muscular pain) and arthralgia (joint pain) occur in over 90 percent of patients. Myositis (inflammation of muscles) with elevation of muscle enzymes is common. About a third of the patients develop polyarthritis which is difficult to distinguish from rheumatoid arthritis. However, advanced destruction of articular cartilage, ankylosis, contractures, spinal involvement, and pannus formation are uncommon. "Rheumatoid" nodules and cysts of synovial surfaces may cause pain and deformity of the involved joints.

Nervous system: involvement of the central nervous system (CNS) is common and may vary from mild neurotic traits to psychosis, mild to severe convulsions, hemiplegia (paralysis of one side of the body), and coma. Peripheral neuritis is not uncommon.

In October 1967 at the twenty-third session of the Japanese Oriental Medical Association, the Kanto Branch, Aimi Saburo delivered a report on the treatment of SLE with Chinese herb medicine. In the report blood stagnancy was found to be a common phenomenon; hence he concluded that extravasation and the consequent tissue disturbances were a result of the denaturization of fibrinoid which in turn caused the denaturization of blood vessels and the final microscopic changes. Thus the Chinese herbal remedies for stagnant blood—*Kuei-chih-fu-ling-wan* for internal use and *Tzu-yun-kao* for external use—are used to treat SLE.

Treatment

It is extremely difficult to evaluate the results of present-day treatment in a disease with such variable dominant features, severity, and course as SLE. Patients with CNS involvement or diffuse proliferative or membranous nephritis generally do not respond to treatment as well as those without involvement of these systems; they have a poorer prognosis. Treatment may be followed by subjective improvement, reduction in anti-DNA attackers, an increase in complement, and a decrease in proteinuria. Controlled studies now in progress have not been continued long enough to determine the effect on longevity or the course of the disease. Use of cytotoxic immunosuppressive agents should be reserved for symptomatic patients or those with a life-threatening disease which fails to respond to more conservative therapy.

Corticosteroids and corticotropin may exert a favorable effect in some patients, but the results are variable. Treatment with 7-15mg of prednisone daily given orally is usually more effective in the early phases of the illness. Many patients obtain marked temporary benefit during acute episodes or when there is involvement of vital organs. Large doses may be necessary for patients with hemolytic anemia, thrombocytopenia, pericarditis, diffuse renal disease, or CNS involvement.

Chinese Herb Formulas

1. **Hsiao-chai-hu-tang** 　　　　　　　　　　　小柴胡湯
   (Minor Bupleurum Combination)

This formula is indicated for patients with a tubercular physique who have thoraco-costal distress. If blood stagnation is a further complication, this formula is used in combination with *Kuei-chih-fu-ling-wan* or with *Wu-ling-tang*.

2. **Shih-wei-pai-tu-tang** 　　　　　　　　　　十味敗毒湯
   (Bupleurum and Schizonepeta Combination)

This formula is for patients who have a physique that is more likely indicative of *Hsiao-chai-hu-tang* conformation with the manifestation of thoraco-costal distress; it is generally used for patients with boils and allergic eczema.

3. **Kuei-chih-fu-ling-wan-liao** 桂枝茯苓丸料
   (Cinnamon and Hoelen Formula)

This formula is usually effective for nodal erythematosus. The administration of this formula must be guided by the abdominal symptoms or other symptoms that are indicative of blood-stagnation conformation.

Yueh-pi-chia-chu-tang or *Fang-chi-huang-chi-tang* plus *ma-huang* always works for nodal erythematosus.

4. **Kuei-chih-fu-ling-wan-liao-chia-chien-fang**
   桂枝茯苓丸料加減方
   (Cinnamon and Hoelen Formula Modified)

The effectiveness of this formula for nodal erythematosus has been reported by Aimi Saburo.

Trichophytia Superficialis Facialis
(T. S. Facialis)

In ancient times this type of dermatosis was called *tinea capitis* (tinea on the head). In the vernacular, it is called ringworm. It is mostly found in children of seven or eight, especially boys. It appears on the head or face in the form of a round macula like a pityriasis with a clear border and slight depigmentation exhibiting a whitish color. The macula gradually enlarges and develops a bran-like substance that clings to the surface. Affected hair easily falls out. Sometimes it becomes vesicular and forms abscesses and scabs. This dermatosis, though fungal in origin, cannot be proved to have any association with athlete's foot. It is now regarded to be a simple pityriasis instead of trichophytosis, meaning caused by a trichophyton fungi.

Treatment

Treatment is as for pityriasis: local application of boric acid and zinc oxide ointment, and systemic steroidal therapy.

Chinese Herb Formulas
1. **Ching-shang-fang-feng-tang** 清上防風湯
   (Siler Combination)

When the head and face of the patient have become reddish and there is fever and itching, this formula is indicated.

2. **Shih-wei-pai-tu-tang** 十味敗毒湯
   (Bupleurum and Schizonepeta Combination)
This formula is indicated when vesicles or abscesses have developed and there is itching.

3. **Ma-hsing-i-kan-tang** 麻杏薏甘湯
   (Ma-huang and Coix Combination)
This formula is for trichophytia that is uperficial and dry with copious exfoliation of the head.

4. **Tzu-yun-kao** 紫雲膏
   (Lithospermum Ointment)
This ointment is suitable for external application on the affected lesions.

5. **Gypsum** 石膏
Only the single ingredient gypsum is used. 10g of gypsum are soaked in 50ml of vinegar solution diluted to half concentration. Then it is stirred well and allowed to stand overnight. The supernatent layer is skimmed and applied to the lesion. It can have a marvelous effect. This therapy was recorded in Katakura Tsururei's *Ching nagn suo tan*. The author has also tried this method and obtained good results.

Scabies

Scabies is a skin disease caused by the itch mite (very small, length about 0.6 mm) which is parasitic and multiplies in burrows in the skin. The lesions occur between the fingers, at the bends of the wrists and arms, in the armpits, and on the lower abdomen and genital areas.

One way of contracting this disease is to shake hands with someone who has it. Another way is to sit on a seat recently used by an infected person. When there is scabies patient in the family, the clothes of the whole family should be disinfected in boiling water.

Symptoms
There are small mites on the skin which secrete a viscous

fluid and cause itching. They will burrow beneath the skin in a fine, wavy, dark line with a tiny papule at the end. This is rapidly covered by secondary lesions. The infected area itches intensely, becoming worse when it is warm and at night.

Treatment

The entire family as well as the patient should be treated. Treatment consists of a long bath in a mineral hot-spring or in water containing a sulfur agent. After the skin is dried, the whole body should be dusted with a sulfur agent, paying particular attention to the infected area. This procedure should be repeated on three consecutive nights.

Athlete's Foot
(Hongkong Foot)

This is a recalcitrant skin disease caused by *tinea alba*. It annoys many in the summer. Those having ephidrosis or who often wear closed shoes or nylon socks will be most susceptible to this disease. Its symptoms seem to disappear in winter but will recur during the summer.

Symptoms

At first there are a number of blisters on the skin between the fingers and toes. They will soon become dry, break open, and itch. When scratched, a fluid will flow out and the area will become moist. This is followed by suppuration.

Treatment

The areas most susceptible to athlete's foot (between the toes and fingers) should be kept clean, dry, and well-protected. Shoes and socks should be made of material that provides good ventilation. Nylon socks, shoes made of snythetic material, and shoes with latex soles are not ventilating at all and should be avoided. Those having ephidrosis at the toes should always wear wool or cotton socks. These should be changed twice a day, and the same pair of shoes should not be worn for two consecutive days during the summer. Use of infrared light and fomentations of carbolic acid solution are also effective treatments.

Chinese Herb Formulas
1. Ma-hsing-i-kan-tang 麻杏薏甘湯
 (Ma-huang and Coix Combination)
This is effective for dry athlete's foot that is not suppurative.

2. San-wu-huang-chin-tang 三物黃芩湯
 (Scute Three Herb Combination)
This is effective for those having hot feet, thirst, a sensation of fever, and dry, chapped skin in the area affected.

3. Tzu-yun-kao 紫雲膏
 (Lithospermum Ointment)
This ointment is for external use on the affected areas.

Cracks on the Hands and Feet

The skin, especially that of the hands and feet, may become red, cracked, and rough due to cold air or a diet that is deficient in fat. A severe case is known as chilblains.

Treatment
The skin should be protected from chilling and filthy substances, and the fat content in the patient's diet should be increased. The hands and feet should be washed with warm water and then some cream should be applied. Intake of larger amounts of Vitamins A and E is also effective.

Chinese Herb Formulas
1. Tzu-yun-kao 紫雲膏
 (Lithospermum Ointment)
This is effective for cracks on the hands and feet.

Prickly Heat

Sweat is secreted from the openings of the sweat gland ducts. When the openings are blocked or there is a disorder due to high fever, the sweat cannot be secreted completely and it will stay beneath the skin surface causing inflammation. The resultant swelling and rash is called "prickly heat". Those having delicate skin are most susceptible to this condition. Children suffer from it more often than adults.

Symptoms

There are a number of small, red lesions on the skin and pain when the sweat invades the outer portion of the skin. The lesions will quickly become itchy, transparent blisters. If the patient scratches the blisters with dirty hands, suppuration leading to eczema will follow. To soothe the itching, a hot towel can be placed over the affected area or a soft brush used to scrape it gently.

Treatment

Make sure the skin is clean at all times and keep sweat or dirt from blocking the openings of the sweat gland ducts. After bathing, apply talcum powder. If the patient suffers from unbearable itching, spread a hot towel over the powder. When the sweat or dirt has been removed and the pores are open, apply steroid ointment or antihistamine, then talcum powder.

Chinese Herb Formula

1. **Kuei-chih-chia-huang-chi-tang** 桂枝加黃耆湯
   (Cinnamon and Astragalus Combination)
   This is effective for prickly heat resulting from ephidrosis.

Psoriasis and Tinea Alba

Psoriasis is a chronic, relapsing skin disease, the cause of which is unknown. It first appears on the scalp and often spreads to other parts of the body. *Tinea alba* is a superficial infection of the skin caused by a white fungus. It is often found on the scalp, but in certain susceptible people, it may appear on other parts of the body as well.

Symptoms

In the initial stage, psoriasis appears in gray-white patches; gradually these patches enlarge, causing the skin to dry out. The affected area is neither itchy nor painful; when scratched, particles will fall off in bran-like flakes.

Tinea alba causes a patchy loss of hair after which the skin itches and becomes coarse with a white scale-like substance. When scraped too hard, it will become inflamed and suppurate. This should be cured immediately; otherwise, the infected areas will become larger and the hair will fall out.

Treatment

There is no specific sure for psoriasis. Good care of the skin may eventually bring about improvement and remission of the disease. The patient who suffers from *tinea alba* may buy an over-the-counter preparation and apply it to the infected parts.

Chinese Herb Formulas
1. Shih-wei-pai-tu-san 十味敗毒湯
   (Bupleurum and Schizonepeta Formula)
To be taken for blisters with suppuration and itching.

2. Ma-hsing-i-kan-tang 麻杏薏甘湯
   (Ma-huang and Coix Combination)
To be taken by those with dry, infected areas and scaling of the skin.

Acne

Acne in young people is due to excessive sebum that has blocked the pores of the skin or to a suppuration caused by the invasion of a pyogenic cocci. In Western medical science, the coccus is known as "acne vulgaris."

During adolescence, the sexual or paracortiadrenal gland secretes an excessive amount of hormones causing those with sebaceous skin to be susceptible to acne. Gastrointestinal disturbances, liver disorder, disorder of hormone secretion, and constipation are secondary causes.

Symptoms

Acne occurs on the face, the chest, and the back. At first, the pore is blocked by the sebum cutaneum and keratin. These substances then harden and become yellow. The skin swells around them and suppurates. When the suppuration subsides, the skin returns to normal unless the lesion was also infected by bacteria. If it was, scarring could result.

Treatment

Acne is a symbol of adolescence. If the patient worries about it, the result will be an imbalance of the internal secretions, unstable emotions, insufficient sleep, constipation, and an aggravation of the condition. In therapy, keep the skin clean by washing the face carefully with lukewarm water, making sure to rinse off all the fat and soap elements. Sulfur-containing cleansers are more effective than regular soap for this disease. During inflammation, gently squeeze out the pus and fat and then apply penicillin ointment.

Chinese Herb Formulas

1. Tang-kuei-shao-yao-san-chia-i-yi-jen　當歸芍藥散加薏苡仁
   (Tang-kuei and Paeonia Formula with Coix)

To be taken for a tendency towards anemia, pallor, and small whiteheads.

2. Ching-shang-fang-feng-tang　清上防風湯
   (Siler Combination)

To be taken for red acne.

Dark Spots

Dark spots are tea-brown in color and range in size from that of a soybean to that of the palm of the hand. Some spots may be easily distinguished from the skin, while others may not. Women past middle age are susceptible to this condition which appears on the face, forehead, and below the eyes.

The spots may be a side effect of pregnancy, female disorders, liver disease, or excessive sunshine. They may be related to the action of paracorticoadrenal hormone. The real causes, however, are not yet clear.

Symptoms

In some cases, the patient feels neither pain nor itching,

but when the affected area is scraped, the skin will detach in small scales. The spots are not always apparent, but will appear when the patient feels tired or nervous. Some young women suffer from this condition before or during menstruation.

Treatment

Cure the known causes of this disease and the dark spots will disappear. Principally, one should eat a well-balanced diet and avoid excessive work, exposure to sun or wind, the use of too much soap, and unnecessary stimulation of the skin. Adequate daily intake of Vitamins C and E and use of soap containing sulfur may also cure this disease. Eating an orange a day for a month has cured this condition in some people.

Chinese Herb Formulas
1. Chia-wei-hsiao-yao-san-chia-ti-huang-chuan-chiung

加味逍遙散加地黃川芎

(Bupleurum and Paeonia Formula with Rehmannia and Cnidium)
This is effective for nervous female patients with climacteric disorder, mild anemia, and spots on the face.

2. Kuei-chih-fu-ling-wan-chia-i-yi-jen   桂枝茯苓丸加薏苡仁
(Cinnamon and Hoelen Formula with Coix)
This is effective for female patients having an average structure, resistant pressure at the lower abdomen, and spots on the face.

3. Tang-kuei-shao-yao-san   當歸芍藥散
(Tang-kuei and Paeonia Formula)
To be taken by the woman of delicate constitution with dark spots, anemia, and chilling during pregnancy.

4. Tao-ho-cheng-chi-tang   桃核承氣湯
(Persica and Rhubarb Combination)
To be taken for severe resistant pressing pain in the lower abdomen, facial flushing with fever, severe stagnant blood, and constipation.

Blisters

A blister is an inflammation which may occur on the hands or feet due to rough manual labor or friction of shoes against the feet.

Treatment

An ancient method of treatment is to penetrate the blister with a needle to dispel the fluid inside. The needle should first be dipped in mercurochrome, and the blister should be covered with a Band-aid. After two or three days, healing will occur.

Chinese Herb Formula
Tzu-yun-kao 紫雲膏
(*Lithospermum Ointment*)
Spread *Tzu-yun-kao* on the blisters.

Warts

The real cause of warts is unknown. It is presumed to be a type of virus infection. Some people will contract warts, while others will not. There are ordinary warts, flat warts of youth, condyloma, and senile warts.

Symptoms

Warts are usually found on the hands and the feet. They have a rough surface and will gradually increase in number. They are neither painful nor itchy. If neglected, they will sometimes disappear spontaneously. Warts of youth usually grow on the face of a young person. A number of small warts may appear in one spot, and all are small and soft. If scratched, they will soon reappear; the majority will disappear spontaneously. A condyloma has a long stem and is like a mushroom. People over 40 years of age may have black-brown senile warts that are not hard. These will appear on the hands and feet.

Skin Diseases

Treatment

Ordinary warts and warts of youth may disappear spontaneously. But it is better to remove a condyloma. At present, there is no effective therapy for senile warts.

Chinese Herb Formulas
1. I-yi-jen-chien   薏苡仁煎
   (Coix Decoction)
This is effective for ordinary warts and warts of youth.

2. Pan-hsia-hsieh-hsin-tang-chia-i-yin-jen   半夏瀉心湯加薏苡仁
   (Pinellia Combination with Coix)
This is effective for chest cavity blocking with borborygmus, and for gastritis and warts.

UROLOGICAL DISEASES

Orchitis (Epididymitis)

Orchitis, an inflammation of the testicles, can be caused by an accidental blow, a gonococcal infection, syphilis, tuberculosis, mumps, or a viral invasion. About 25 percent of the cases are a complication of mumps contracted after puberty.

Symptoms
Orchitis caused by gonococcus results in swelling of the testes and scrotum, intense pain, chills and persistent high fever, hiccups, and vomiting. With mumps orchitis often the salivary glands swell but the other symptoms are comparatively slight.

Treatment
The routine treatment for orchitis is bed rest, use of scrotum supporters, ice-bags, and analgesics. If the cause is not mumps, antibiotics are used.

Chinese Herb Formulas
1. Lung-tan-hsieh-kan-tang　　　　　　　　　龍膽瀉肝湯
   (Gentiana Combination)
This combination is for inflammation, congestion, swelling, pain in

the lower abdomen or the genitalia, and specifically, gonococcal orchitis. In Chinese medicine "moist-fever" of the liver meridian corresponds to gonococcal urethritis, cystitis, and orchitis.

2. **Kuei-chih-fu-ling-wan-liao** 桂枝茯苓丸料
   (Cinnamon and Hoelen Formula)

This formula with 6.0g of coix is for extravasated blood in the lower abdomen; resistance and pain in the abdomen; and prolonged swelling of the testicles.

3. **Teng-lung-tang** 騰龍湯
   (Moutan and Persica Combination)

Stronger than the two preceding formulas, this formula is for patients with a stronger physique who have severe inflammation, congestion, swelling, and pain. If there is no constipation, the rhubarb and mirabilitum may be left out.

4. **Ta-huang-mu-tan-pi-tang** 大黃牡丹皮湯
   (Rhubarb and Moutan Combination)

This combination is for conformations similar to *Teng-lung-tang* except that the symptoms are more severe and urgent.

5. **Hsiao-chai-hu-tang** 小柴胡湯
   (Minor Bupleurum Combination)

This remedy is most frequently for orchitis caused by mumps or tuberculosis. If treatment has been delayed for a long time, this formula along with *Kuei-chih-fu-ling-wan-liao* is recommended.

Urethritis

The symptoms of acute urethral inflammation are not the same for men and women. In the male the external sphincter is the focal point for diagnosis. Urethritis occurring in the area in front of the sphincter is called anterior urethritis, and that behind it posterior urethritis. Inflammation involving the whole part, including the front and rear, is called total urethritis. With anterior urethritis the first cup in the Thompson twin cup test is turbid, the external urethra becomes reddened, and pus is discharged. In addition, the man complains of urethral pruritus itching, a burning sensation on urination, lack of control of urination, and dysuria. With posterior urethritis, both cups in the Thompson twin cup test are turbid, and the patient complains of frequent and painful urination, bleeding, and a feeling of residual urine even though there is no discharge to be seen at the opening of the urethra. With total urethritis all the above symptoms are present.

In the female there is reddening of the external urethra and a discharge of pus. The subjective symptoms are milder than those in the male, and include a burning sensation during urination, mild pain, and frequent urination. In chronic cases there are practically no subjective symptoms at all; there is a filiform substance floating in the first urine after awakening and the external urethral opening is obstructed. So far as we know, the cause for these problems is primarily from bacterial infection of gonococcus. Urethritis from other bacterial infections is quite rare. Known pathogens involved in urethritis are streptococcus, *E. coli*, pneumococcus, and influenza bacteria, all of which often cause acute inflammation. Tubercular urethritis is an extension of tuberculosis to the upper part of the urethral tract and is always accompanied by urethral constricture and peri-urethritis (inflammation of connective tissue).

The external causes of this disease include the following: mechanical, thermal, or chemical stimulation which causes artificial urethritis; foreign bodies which cause foreign body urethritis; catheterization which causes catheterization urethritis; trauma which causes traumatic urethritis; and the continuous excretion of solid components in the urine, such as oxalate, phosphorous, and urate. Another kind of chronic urethritis whose cause is unknown is called Waelsch chronic nongonorrheal urethritis.

Chinese Herb Formulas
1. **Chu-ling-tang** 猪苓湯
    (Polyporus Combination)

This formula is mostly used to alleviate painful, frequent, and bloody urination.

2. **Lung-tan-hsieh-kan-tang** 龍膽瀉肝湯
    (Gentiana Combination)

This formula is for women with severe inflammation that impedes urination causing pain and discomfort. Leukorrhea, a vaginal discharge of mucous and pus, is also present.

3. Wu-lin-san 五淋散
   (Gardenia and Hoelen Formula)
When the disease is chronic and the preceding formulas fail to take effect, this formula is suitable.

Urethral Stenosis

In its broadest sense stenosis refers to urethral conditions that are caused by congenital deformity, spasms, inflammations, tumid ulcers, and obstruction or compression due to the presence of foreign substances.

Symptoms
During urination the urine changes from a thread-like form and becomes separated or spiral; the stream becomes weak and discontinuous. Ultimately urination stops completely, the retention causing uremia. This condition is most frequently found in those who have or have had gonorrhea.

Chinese Herb Formulas
1. Teng-lung-tang 騰龍湯
   (Moutan and Persica Combination)
This combination is for urethral stenosis in those with a firm conformation. It is used for symptoms that are not very serious. If there is no constipation, the rhubarb and mirabilitum may be deleted.

2. Ta-huang-mu-tan-pi-tang 大黃牡丹皮湯
   (Rhubarb and Moutan Combination)
This remedy is for inflammation, dysuria, and unendurable disstress. Large quantities (6-10g) of rhubarb and mirabilitum may be added.

3. Lung-tan-hsieh-kan-tang 龍膽瀉肝湯
   (Gentiana Combination)
This combination is for patients with gonorrhea who have slight

inflammation, and frequent and painful urination.

4. **Pa-wei-wan or liao** 八味丸或料
   (Rehmannia Eight Formula)

This formula is for chronic cases without inflammation but with dysuria, a sensation of residual urine, nocturia, and fatigue. Persons who tend to have a firm conformation take this formula along with *Teng-lung-tang* without the rhubarb and mirabilitum.

Hydrocele

A hydrocele is a cystic collection of fluid in the scrotum near the testes. It usually disappears in childhood. However, if the hydrocele sac becomes acutely infected or enlarged, it should be removed surgically.

Symptoms
The scrotum is swollen but without pain. In infants it can be as large as an egg; in adults it may grown to be as large as an adult's head. Sometimes it heals spontaneously in boys. In adults surgery may become necessary.

Treatment
The palliative treatment uses the puncture drainage method. The eradicative treatment calls for Winkelmann's operation. However, before undergoing surgery it is best to first try the following formulas.

Chinese Herb Formulas
1. **Wu-ling-san-chia-che-chien-tzu-mu-tung** 五苓散加車前子木通
   (Hoelen Five Herb Formula with Plantago and Akebia)

This formula is effective in children as well as adults. Children should take it for at least one month.

2. **Pan-hsia-hou-pu-tang** 半夏厚朴湯
   (Pinellia and Magnolia Combination)

This formula is effective for symptoms of "stagnant water" (edema) in the arms, legs, and facial area, and for gastric water stagnation, a condition in which the water migrates downward to the lower torso causing hydrocele. This formula may work if the preceding one fails.

3. **Lung-tan-hsieh-kan-tang** 龍膽瀉肝湯
   (Gentiana Combination)
This combination is effective for orchitis accompanied by edema.

4. **Fang-chi-huang-chi-tang** 防己黃耆湯
   (Stephania and Astragalus Combination)
This remedy is for white-skinned, flabby people with hydrocele, dysuria, excessive perspiration, and "stagnant water" in the lower torso.

Cystic Kidney

Cystic kidney is a congenital (inherited) condition in which numerous cysts are present in the parenchyma of both kidneys. Simultaneously the same cysts appear in the liver, spleen, and pancreas. Infants usually die. In adults the cysts appear between the ages of thirty and forty. Because of the cystic suppression, the renal parenchyma atrophies and kidney function declines.

Symptoms
First an abdominal tumor in the muscle walls, pain, and blood in the urine appear; then kidney function degrades. There is a resultant increase in residual blood nitrogen and the presence of protein in the urine. The blood pressure also increases. If the disease lasts, in about ten years the patient dies of uremia, cerebral hemorrhage, or heart failure.

Treatment
This disease is bilaterally progressive and there is no specific method to prevent its development. In Chinese medicine there are several formulas prescribed according to the different conformations. These remedies are designed to slow the development of the disease and restore the patient's vitality.

Chinese Herb Formulas
1. **Kuei-pi-tang** 歸脾湯
   (Ginseng and Longan Combination)
   This formula is for hematuria which in time causes anemia, pallor, a weak pulse, and softness of the whole abdomen except in the area of the tumor.

2. **Hsiao-chien-chung-tang** 小建中湯
   (Minor Cinnamon and Paeonia Combination)
   This combination is effective for the patient suffering from cystic kidney with a weak constitution. It treats the abdominal pain especially.

VENEREAL DISEASES

Condyloma Latum

The Chinese term for condyloma latum is "plum hemorrhoid." This is an apt term to describe the dull pink or gray mucous patches that occur in secondary syphilis. They appear in the corner of the mouth, around the eye, in the anal canal and rectum, and on the vulva, the breast, and the scrotum. Papules also develop at mucocutaneous junctions causing the skin to erode and become dirty gray in appearance.

Symptoms
These lesions are caused by the spirochete *Treponema pallidum* and are extremely infectious. The syphilitic condyloma latum begins to bulge on the surface of the skin. It becomes moist and red and begins excreting fluid. The skin becomes milky white as it absorbs the exudate, and gradually the latum coalesces to become as big as a child's palm.

Treatment
A 25% podophyllin in benzene tincture is applied to the lesion. For an intra-anal condyloma latum, a proctoscope may be used to confine the medication to the lesion. If it does not cause

any discomfort, powder may be dusted onto the lesion, or electric cautery treatment used under anesthesia, a method which is most effective in polyplasmic cases. Local cleansing and dusting are necessary as condyloma lata recurs quite readily. Other effective forms of treatment include intramuscular injections of 1.2 million units of benzathine penicillin G for a total of 2.4 million units; intramuscular injection of 2.4 million units of procaine penicillin G along with aluminum stearate, then 1.2 million units every three days until the total dose reaches 4.8 million units; and daily intramuscular injections of procaine penicillin G 600,000 units for eight to ten days in succession.

Chinese Herb Formulas
1. **Hsiang-chuan-chieh-tu-chi** 香川解毒劑
   (Smilax and Akebia Combination)
   Huang-lien-chieh-tu-san-chia-ching-fen 黃連解毒散加輕粉
   (Coptis and Scute Formula plus Calomel)

These are the formulas frequently given to syphilitic patients who are not very strong. The two formulas are used simultaneously for five to seven days followed by suspension of the medication for five to seven days. Since calomel is poisonous, this formula must be used with caution. If general antisyphilis therapy has already been employed, the calomel may be eliminated. Presently, calomel is hard to acquire; therefore, *Shih-wei-pai-tu-tang* plus forsythia and coix may be pulverized and used in its place.

2. **Fang-feng-tung-sheng-san** 防風通聖散
   (Siler and Platycodon Formula)
   I-yi-jen-san 薏苡仁散
   (Coix Formula)

Patients with a stalwart and obese physique and an inclination to constipation may be given *Fang-feng-tung-sheng-san* for a prolonged time. It is often administered with *I-yi-jen-san* which has been pulverized into a powder.

Men's Gonorrhea

In ancient times there were records on the five urine-stuttering and turbid conformations, which are the equivalent of gonorrhea.

The incubation period is two to three days following exposure. It begins with urethritis which is characterized by an itching and burning pain present during urination in conjunction with a serous discharge from the urethra followed by a purulent discharge.

Medical treatment for gonorrhea in males differs from treatment of the disease in women. According to the phase of infection men's gonorrhea may be divided into (1) acute anterior urethral gonorrhea; (2) acute posterior urethral gonorrhea; and (3) chronic urethral gonorrhea. As the inflammation reaches the posterior part, there will be polyuria, post-urination pain, dripping of blood, and hematuria. Regardless of whether it is first or second stage gonorrhea, the urine is turbid. When it progresses toward chronicity, the subjective symptoms disappear. Each morning at the urethral opening a serous substance appears. During the second stage some filiform or floating substance will appear.

Symptoms

Initially there is burning on urination and a serous or milky discharge. One to three days later the urethral pain is more pronounced and the discharge becomes yellow, creamy and profuse, sometimes blood-tinged. Without treatment the disorder may regress and become chronic or progress to involve the prostate, epididymis, and periurethral glands with acute, painful inflammation. This in turn becomes chronic with prostatitis and urethral strictures. Rectal infection is common in homosexual males, systemic involvement is listed below. Asymptomatic infection is common.

Complications

The forms of local extension of the initial infection have been described. However, unusual sites of primary infection (e.g. the pharynx) must always be considered. Systemic complications follow the dissemination of gonococci from the primary site, the genital tract, via the blood stream. Gonococcal bacteremia is associated with intermittent fever, arthralgia, and skin lesions ranging from maculopapular to pustular or hemorrhagic. Rarely, gonococcal endocarditis or meningitis develops. Arthritis and tenosynovitis are common complications, particularly involving the knees, ankles, and wrists. Several joints are commonly involved. Gonococci can be isolated from only a third of arthritides, and cell wall deficiency forms in a few cases. In the remainder it is possible that some immune complex disease or hypersensitivity reaction is responsible. Gonococcal arthritis may be accompanied by iritis or conjunctivitis with negative cultures. The commonest form of eye involvement is the direct inoculation of gonococci in the conjunctival sac. This may occur as ophthalmia neonatorum (in the newborn), or by auto-inoculation of a person with genital infection. The purulent conjunctivitis may rapidly progress to panophthalmitis and loss of the eye unless treated promptly.

Treatment

Uncomplicated gonorrhea. The usual treatment in this instance is 4.8 million units IM of aqueous procaine penicillin G injected into two or more sites at the same time together with 1.0g probenecid given orally prior to the injections. This treatment can also be effective in aborting syphilis within two weeks after infection.

Alternatively, give ampicillin, 3.5g orally, together with probenecid, 1.0g orally, given at one time. Never treat gonorrhea with benzathine penicillin G. When a penicillin is not indicated or is ineffective, give tetracycline, 1.5g orally stat, then 0.5g orally four times daily for four days (total 9.0g); or spectinomycin, 4.0g IM in two injection sites at the same time.

Follow-up Treatment. Urethral or rectal specimens must be obtained from men seven days after completion of treatment. Serologic tests for syphilis are required two weeks and two months later.

Treatment of Complications. In general, prostatitis, epididymitis, bacteremia, arthritis, eye infections, and other complications are best treated with penicillin G, 10-20 million units IV daily for one to two weeks or longer. Full doses of tetracyclines are probably also effective. Postgonococcal urethritis and chlamydial urethritis can be treated with tetracycline, 0.5g orally four times daily for seven to ten days. In post-gonococcal urethritis, signs and symptoms persist after adequate drug regimen and no further evidence of gonococci. Gonococcal ophthalmia requires topical as well as systemic penicillin treatment.

Additional supportive treatment is needed for most complications. Prostatitis may be relieved by hot sitz baths or diathermy; acute epididymitis requires bed rest, cold compresses and support to the scrotum, and analgesics. Acute salpingitis requires bed rest during the acute stage and surgical evaluation if chronic pain and signs of inflammation continue. Aspiration of joints may be necessary to relieve severe pressure followed by physical therapy as inflammation subsides.

Chinese Herb Formulas
1. **Ma-huang-tang** 麻黃湯
   (Ma-huang Combination)
Symptoms at the beginning of infection are anemophobia, low back pain, and a buoyant pulse in strong patients. This formula may be administered in one dose for the alleviation of acute symptoms.

2. **Tzu-yuan** 紫圓
   (Croton and Hematite Formula)
One dose of this formula may alleviate acute symptoms at the initial stage in strong patients.

3. **Chu-ling-tang** 豬苓湯
   (Polyporus Combination)
This combination is suitable for the initial symptoms of painful sensation on urination, polyuria, and hemorrhage.

4. **Huang-lien-chieh-tu-tang** 黃連解毒湯
   (Coptis and Scute Combination)
At the acute phase of the disease, when the hematuria is very serious, this formula is generally indicated along with the formula of *Chu-ling-tang*.

5. **Ta-huang-mu-tan-pi-tang** 大黃牡丹皮湯
   (Rhubarb and Moutan Combination)
This formula is indicated for severe symptoms in the initial stage when painful urination and dysuria, and even mucous discharge, is present. For a purulent, bloody discharge and a tendency to be constipated, the portions of rhubarb and mirabilitum may be increased up to 6.0g each to purge the discharges and alleviate the symptoms.

6. **Lung-tan-hsieh-kan-tang** 龍膽瀉肝湯
   (Gentiana Combination)

No matter whether it is acute, subacute, or chronic gonorrhea, this formula is used for slight inflammation.

7. **Fang-feng-tung-sheng-san** 防風通聖散
   (Siler and Platycodon Formula)

This formula is suitable for prolonged administration to those who have an obese physique and a tendency to be constipated and whose illness is advancing toward chronicity; there are no excessive subjective symptoms, except the feeling of fatigue or an increase in "gonorrheal threads" (turbidity) because of poor nutrition.

8. **Tuo-li-hsiao-tu-yin** 托裏消毒飲
   (Gleditsia Combination)

Patients having a tendency toward fatigue and debility in whom the gonorrhea has become chronic and the discharge of pus lengthy use this formula.

9. **Ching-hsin-lien-tzu-yin** 清心蓮子飲
   (Lotus Seed Combination)

This formula is suitable for persons who are weak in the stomach and intestines, anemic, and inclined to neurasthenia. Often the patient is run down from working too hard. The patient will have difficulty urinating, and the urine will be turbid and characterized as "gonorrheal threads."

10. **Pa-wei-ti-huang-wan** 八味地黃丸
    (Rehmannia Eight Formula)

This formula is suitable for patients with chronic gonorrhea who have dysuria, urine retention, thirst, low back pains, numbness beneath the navel, and heat at the centers of the soles of the feet. It is, however, unsuitable for urethral constriction and prostatomegaly. This formula is most effective in persons who have a healthy stomach and intestines. The patient's appetite will not decrease after using this remedy. If the patient has a weak stomach and intestines, distention and obstruction beneath the heart, anorexia, and diarrhea after taking this formula, the drug should be suspended at once.

Women's Gonorrhea

Gonorrhea in women is almost exclusively contracted through coitus. Occasionally women become infected in a bathing area or may have been infected in childhood due to a babysitter's carelessness.

With acute gonorrhea the external genitalia become reddened and moist, and a purulent substance is discharged from the vagina and urethra. Inflammation may invade from the cervix into the uterus, then via the fallopian tubes to the peritoneal membrane and result in peritonitis. It may also attack the kidney by way of the ureters.

If the condition is accompanied by urethritis, there will be burning and severe pain on urination and polyuria will occur as a consequence. This is commonly called *"hsiao ker"* (exhaustion and thirst) in Chinese.

Endometritis generally alters from an acute to a chronic problem. Salpingitis commonly progresses slowly. Aching during coitus and menstruation signals developing ovaritis and peritonitis.

The chief difference between men's and women's gonorrhea is the wide variety of inflammations which develop in women's organs; therefore, prescriptions indicated differ.

Symptoms

Pain, frequency and urgency in urination may occur with a purulent urethral discharge. Vaginitis and cervicitis with inflammation of Skene's and Bartholin's glands are common. Usually, however, the infection is asymptomatic showing only slightly increased vaginal discharge and moderate cervicitis on examination. Infection may remain as a chronic cervicitis, the cervix being the largest reservoir of gonococci in the human body. The infection may progress to involve the uterus and tubes causing acute and chronic salpingitis with ultimate scarring of the tubes and sterility. Rectal infection is common both from the organism spreading from the genital tract and from infection by anal coitus. Systemic involvement is the same as listed under men's gonorrhea.

Treatment

Treatment is the same for both men and women. So the

treatment for men can also be applied to women.

Chinese Herb Formulas

1. Chu-ling-tang   豬苓湯
(Polyporus Combination)

This combination is used for urethritis that has affected the bladder causing polyuria, dysuria, and hematuria.

2. Lung-tan-hsieh-kan-tang   龍膽瀉肝湯
(Gentiana Combination)

This formula is used commonly for men as well as women. In women it is used for vulvitis, major vestibulitis, urethritis, cystitis, vaginitis, endometritis, polyuria, discomfort on urination, and leukorrhea. It is used for either acute or chronic cases.

3. Ta-huang-mu-tan-pi-tang   大黃牡丹皮湯
(Rhubarb and Moutan Combination)

This combination is used for the acute or subacute stage if the symptoms are very evident; the inflammation has spread from the accessory organs to peritoneal membrane; and there are resisting pain in the lower abdomen, constipation, a purulent discharge, pain on urination, polyuria, dysuria, and intolerability. 6.0g of coix and 3.0g of paeonia are added to this formula before use.

4. Kuei-chih-fu-ling-wan   桂枝茯苓丸
(Cinnamon and Hoelen Formula)

This formula is for milder conditions than those above: there is no constipation and the resisting pain in the lower abdomen is slight.

5. Che-tsung-yin   折衝飲
(Cinnamon and Persica Combination)

This combination is used when endometritis has spread to the ovaries and the fallopian tubes, although the condition is not very severe.

6. Tang-kuei-shao-yao-san   當歸芍藥散
(Tang-kuei and Paeonia Formula)

This formula is used for chronic cases in which the patient has a weak physique, slight inflammation, anemia, inflammation of the uterus and its accessory organs, leukorrhea, and climacteric nervous symptoms.

7. Tang-kuei-chien-chung-tang 當歸建中湯
(Tang-kuei, Cinnamon, and Paeonia Combination)
This combination is used for patients when the symptoms are becoming chronic and the inflammation is not serious. However, the patient's vitality has deteriorated, and she has severe abdominal pain because of inflammation of the uterus and its accessory organs.

8. Pa-wei-tai-hsia-fang 八味帶下方
(Tang-kuei and Eight Herb Formula)
This formula has xanthorrhea and leukorrhea as its targets. It is given when other symptoms are slight and the patient has a rather weak conformation.

9. Pa-wei-shan-chi-fang 八味疝氣方
(Cinnamon and Akebia Formula)
This combination is for subacute and chronic cases when the patient has lower abdominal pain, low back pain on encountering coldness, and leukorrhea.

10. Pa-wei-wan 八味丸
(Rehmannia Eight Formula)
This formula is used for patients who have dysuria due to chronic urethritis, cystitis, and a feeling of retaining urine, or leukorrhea that exudes without any sign of cessation. Such patients may also experience low back pain, thirst, and fatigue.

Syphilis

In ancient times syphilis had many names to describe the various symptoms and stages. For example, in the initial stage when the lesions are still hard, the disease was called "chancre"; inguinal bubo, which is an inflammatory enlargement of lymph nodes, was called "urine toxin"; skin eruptions caused by syphilitic infection were referred to as "plum abscesses"; and syphilis in its latent stage as a "festering plum." (This latter term apparently indicating that the disease has reached a stage without any surface manifestations.)

Today it is known that syphilis is caused by the organism *Spirochaeta pallida* and that the disease progresses through three definable stages. Within two to three weeks following infection, a local hard node, the chancre, is formed. Skin eruptions in the form of pityriasis rosea, impetigo, and papules follow. Several months later syphilitic alopecia (patches of baldness) appears. Rheumatic pain may be felt in both the arms and legs, along with serpenginous syphilid, tinea siccus, and condyloma latum.

In the third stage there are rubber-like swellings, syphilitic leukoderma, rubroderma, and ulcers.

Symptoms

Primary Syphilis. This is the stage of infection that may pass unrecognized. The typical lesion is the chancre at the site or sites of inoculation, most frequently the penis, labia, or anorectal region. Occasionally the primary lesion occurs in the oropharynx (lip, tongue, or tonsils) and, rarely, on the breast or finger. The chancre starts as a small erosion ten to ninety days (average three to four weeks) after infection. It rapidly develops into a painless superficial ulcer with firm indurated margins, and the enlarged regional lymph nodes become rubbery, discrete, and insensitive. Secondary infection of the chancre, which can be painful, is not uncommon. Healing occurs without treatment, but a scar usually remains, especially in cases with secondary infection.

Treatment

Benzathine penicillin G, 1.2 million units in each buttock for a total dosage of 2.4 million units; or procaine penicillin G with aluminum monostearate in oil (PAM), 2.4 million units IM initially and then 1.2 million units IM every third day until a total of 3.8 million units is reached; or procaine penicillin G, 600,000 units daily IM for eight to ten consecutive days.

Symptoms

Secondary Syphilis. This stage of syphilis usually develops in a few weeks (but may appear up to six months) after the chancre. The most common manifestations are skin and mucosal papular, pustular, or follicular (or combinations of any of these types) rashes with manulopapular rash being the most common. The skin lesions are usually generalized; involvement of the palm and soles in especially suspicious. Annual lesions simulating ringworm are observed in blacks. Mucous membrane lesions range from ulcers and papules of the lips, mouth, throat, genitalia, and anus ("mucous patches") to a diffuse redness of the pharynx. Both skin and mucous membrane lesions are highly infectious at this stage.

Meningeal, hepatic, renal, bone, and joint invasion with resulting cranial nerve palsies, jaundice, nephrotic syndrome, and periositis may occur. Alopecia, iritis, and iridocyclitis may also occur. A transient myocarditis manifested by temporary ECG changes has been noted.

Treatment

Treatment is as for primary syphilis unless CNS disease is present, in which case treatment is as for neurosyphilis. Isolation of the patient is important.

Symptoms

Tertiary Syphilis. This stage may occur any time after secondary syphilis, even after years of latency. Late lesions probably represent, at least in part, a delayed hypersensitive reaction of the tissue to the organism and are usually divided into two types: (1) a localized gummatous reaction with a relatively rapid onset and generally prompt response to therapy ("benign late syphilis") and (2) diffuse inflammation of a more insidious onset which characteristically involves the CNS and large arteries, is often fatal if untreated, and is at best arrested by treatment. Gummas (small tumors) may appear in any area or organ of the body, but most often involve the skin or long bones. Cardiovascular disease is usually manifested by aortic aneurysm, aortic insufficiency, or aortitis. Various forms of diffuse or localized CNS involvement may occur.

Treatment

Treatment is as for latent syphilis, i.e. with benzathine penicillin G, three doses of 3 million units at seven day intervals;

procaine penicillin G with aluminum monostearate suspension, six doses of procaine penicillin G, twelve doses of 600,000 units daily. There is no known method for reliable eradication of the Treponema from man in the late stages of syphilis.

Chinese Herb Formulas

1. Ta-chai-hu-tang   大柴胡湯
(Major Bupleurum Combination)

For distention and hardness beneath the heart, this formula or *Szu-ni-san* is first administered followed by antitoxins (mercurials).

2. Hsiang-chuan-chieh-tu-chi   香川解毒劑
(Smilax and Akebia Combination)

This formula is an antisyphilitic agent that has been widely used for initial necrosis, inguinal bubo, and syphilis. For this purpose 2.0g of schizonepta and 3.0g each of siler and forsythia are added. For syphilitic neuralgia 3.0g of cinnamon, 2.0g of pharbitidis, 0.5g of aconite are added. For syphilitic keratitis, 1.5g of chrysanthemum, 3.0g each of plantago, platycodon, and siler, and 4.0g of talc are added.

3. Huang-lien-chieh-tu-tang   黃連解毒湯
(Scute and Coptis Combination)

This combination is used for latent syphilis with flush-up, mental instability, tinnitus, vertigo, insomnia, and similar nervous symptoms.

4. Chieh-keng-chieh-tu-tang   桔梗解毒湯
(Platycodon and Hoelen Combination)

This combination is for patients with syphilis that has attacked the throat causing hoarseness and ulceration.

5. Lung-tan-hsieh-kan-tang   龍膽瀉肝湯
(Gentiana Combination)

This combination is suitable for chancre, inguinal bubo (enlarged lymph nodes of the groin), and especially for excessive leukorrhea, vulval itch, and pain. For women with musty leukorrhea, 4.0g of smilax is added.

6. Shih-wei-pai-tu-tang　　　　　　　十味敗毒湯
   (Bupleurum and Schizonepeta Combination)
   This combination is suitable for various skin eruptions and lymphatic swelling. 3.0g of forsythia is added to this formula.

7. Fang-feng-tung-sheng-san　　　　　防風通聖散
   (Siler and Platycodon Formula)
   Patients who are stalwart and muscular and in the latent stage of syphilis are given this formula for the purgation of pus.

8. Tzu-ken-mu-li-tang　　　　　　　紫根牡蠣湯
   (Lithospermum and Oyster Shell Combination)
   This combination is suitable for rubbery swelling or for superficial infections.

9. Ta-pai-chung-yin　　　　　　　　大百中飲
   (Achyranthes and Smilax Combination)
   This formula is indicated for syphilis that has been lingering for a very long time.

10. Hua-tu-wan　　　　　　　　　　化毒丸
    (Mastic and Realgar Formula)
    This formula is prepared by replacing the calomel with raw milk. It can be used in combination with the above formula but not for initial latent syphilis nor in weak patients.

Congenital Syphilis

This illness is also called hereditary syphilis because it is transmitted from the parents, especially from the mother through the placenta. In most instances of infection, the fetus dies as a consequence of spontaneous abortion, premature delivery, or stillbirth. Infants who are born will exhibit various syphilitic symptoms.

Children with congenital syphilis will have acute or chronic dermatitis (pemphigus) on the palms and soles, skin syphilis, rhagades on the lips and eyelids, lymphatic swelling, rubbery swelling at various parts of the body, and encephalohydrocele (enlargement of the head). Their mental development is poor and their condition may lead to epilepsy, meningitis, or idiocy. The so-called syphilis *congenita tarda* (retarded congenital syphilis) is syphilis that appears after school age. It is characterized by a rubbery swelling in the bones or visceral organs, the appearance of Hutchinson symptoms (an anomaly of teeth in crescent form along the external margin of the frontal teeth), keratitis, and inner ear diseases that often lead to deafness.

Symptoms

The clinical manifestations of congenital syphilis are quite similar to those of the secondary stage of the acquired form. Skin and mucous membrane lesions, generally highly infectious, are often present at birth or in early infancy. Signs of the disease, however, may be minimal and may be ascribed to minor infections or allergies unless adequate diagnostic measures are taken. Characteristic later stigmas of congenital syphilis include interstitial keratitis (clouding of the cornea), Hutchinson's teeth, 8th nerve deafness (Hutchinson's triad), saddle nose, rhagades, saber shins and other bone changes, hepar lobatum (syphilitic cirrhosis), pneumonia alba, and mental retardation. Any of the tertiary sequelae of the adult disease (CNS, visceral, or cardiovascular) may occur. The newborn is infectious, and suitable precautions must be taken to prevent contagion of others.

Treatment

Early congenital syphilis (less than two years of age) is treated with 50,000 units/kg of benzathine penicillin G as a single injection or with a total of 100,000 units/kg PAM IM given at two to three day intervals in divided doses. The treatment of late congenital syphilis is the same as for latent syphilis. Neurosyphilis of congenital origin should be treated the same as acquired syphilis.

Chinese Herb Formulas
1. Tzu-yuan   紫圓
   (Croton and Hematite Formula)

Infants having head abscesses and skin symptoms may be purged with *Tzu-yuan* along with other decoctions.

2. **Wu-wu-chieh-tu-tang** 五物解毒湯
   (Cnidium and Lonicera Combination)
   This formula is used as a general antitoxin agent for congenital syphilis.

3. **Shih-wei-pai-tu-tang** 十味敗毒湯
   (Bupleurum and Schizonepeta Combination)
   This formula is suitable for children over five or six years of age who have various symptoms of congenital syphilis, especially the skin symptoms that are quite severe.

4. **Hsiao-chai-hu-tang** 小柴胡湯
   (Minor Bupleurum Combination)
   This formula is used for congenital syphilis with complications of hepatomegaly and splenomegaly. It may be used continuously for a long time.

5. **Hsiao-kan-yin** 消疳飲
   (Cinnamon and Apricot Seed Combination)
   This combination is used for patients with the foregoing symptoms who are in a weak physical state.

6. **Chai-hu-ching-kan-tang** 柴胡清肝湯
   (Bupleurum and Rehmannia Combination)
   This formula, when used in combination with *Tzu-yuan*, may act as an antitoxicating agent and will improve the physique of patients having pale dark skin and tensive abdominal muscles.

Chancroid

Chancroid is an acute, localized venereal disease caused by the short gram-negative bacillus *Haemophilus ducreyi*. Infection occurs by contact during intercourse, although nonvenereal inoculation has occurred in medical personnel through contact with chancroid patients. The incubation period is three to five days.

Symptoms

The initial lesion at the site of inoculation is a macule or vesicopustule which soon breaks down to form a painful, soft ulcer with a necrotic base, surrounding erythema, and undermined edges. Multiple lesions — started by autoinoculation — and inguinal adenitis often develop. The adenitis is usually unilateral and consists of tender, matted nodes of moderate size with overlying erythema. The nodal mass softens, becomes fluctuant, and may rupture spontaneously. With lymph node involvement, fever, chills and malaise may occur.

The chancroid skin test may become positive and remain positive for life. Mixed venereal infection is very common.

Balanitis (inflammation of the glans penis or glans clitoris) and phimosis are frequent complications. Infection of the ulcer with fusiforms, spirochetes, and other organisms is common.

Treatment

Give either sulfisoxazole, 1.0g orally four times daily, or tetracycline, 0.5g orally four times daily for one to two weeks. The drugs are equally effective. Cleansing of ulcerations with soap and water twice daily promotes healing. Fluctuant buboes may be aspirated by needle. Chancroid usually responds well to treatment. Even without treatment it usually is self-limited.

Chinese Herb Formulas
1. **Hsiang-chuan-chieh-tu-chi** 香川解毒劑
   (Smilax and Akebia Combination)
This formula is used for patients in whom the symptoms have become chronic and stabilized.

2. **Lung-tan-hsieh-kan-tang** 龍膽瀉肝湯
   (Gentiana Combination)
This remedy is suitable for patients having symptoms appearing on the clitoris, labia, glans penis, prepuce or with inguinal bubo and adenitis (inflammation of a gland or lymph node).

3. **Ah-chiao-fu-tzu-tang** 阿膠附子湯
   (Gelatin and Aconite Combination)
Administration of this formula may alleviate the symptoms and accelerate healing of the so-called "candle chancroid" that has very severe gangrenous erosion and is quite painful. The dose of aconite must be considered with caution.

4. Sophora Wash, Coptis Powder
苦參湯之洗用，黃連末之散佈

The sophora decoction should be used to wash the ulcers. It is very effective. If there is bleeding, dust the area with coptis powder.

Inguinal Bubo

Generally, bubo means the swelling of the inguinal (groin) lymph glands due to inflammation; sometimes inflammatory swelling in the superficial or axilla lymph glands is also called bubo. However, inguinal bubo refers exclusively to the inguinal lymph gland. Bubo is caused by various conditions: external wounds, glandular pests, syphilis, chancroid, gonorrhea. The fourth venereal disease, it results in bubo simplex, bubo pestilentis, bubo indolens, bubo dolens, tripperbubo, or climactic bubo.

Symptoms

Pain is felt in the groin area because the inguinal lymph glands become swollen and red. These symptoms are accompanied by a high fever and increasing pain, and finally the formation of a pustule. However, bubo of gonococcal origin generally has little pustulation and is painless. When the lymph nodes harden they become isolated from each other. On the other hand the bubo from chancroid has very serious swelling, severe inflammation, and pustulation.

Treatment

Treatment is generally the same as for syphilis.

Chinese Herb Formulas

1. **Teng-lung-tang** 騰龍湯
   (Moutan and Persica Combination)

During the initial period when the lymph nodes are swollen and aching, this formula is indicated. If constipation is not severe, the doses of rhubarb and mirabilitum may be reduced.

2. **Ta-huang-mu-tan-pi-tang** 大黃牡丹皮湯
   (Rhubarb and Moutan Combination)

This formula is used at the stage when the symptoms are very severe, the swelling and aching are very evident, and suppuration is taking place.

3. Tuo-li-hsiao-tu-yin 托裏消毒飲
   (Gleditsia Combination)

If suppuration has been prolonged and pus drainage persists without signs of cessation, this formula may be administered in combination with *Po-chou-san* (伯州散 Eriocheir and Viper Formula).

4. Hsiang-chuan-chieh-tu-chi 香川解毒劑
   (Smilax and Akebia Formula)

This formula is used to disperse the toxin when the violent symptoms are over and no surface symptoms are present. It is best to continue administration of this formula for two or three months.

5. Lung-tan-hsieh-kan-tang 龍膽瀉肝湯
   (Gentiana Combination)

This combination is used for slight symptoms.

Gonococcal Prostatitis

This disease occurs as a continuation of urethral gonococcal infection. Only in very rare cases is it caused by bacterial invasion from the rectum through masturbation and copulation.

Along with a high fever, the genitalia ache drastically, especially following urination. There is often dysuria that usually leads to urine retention, and in very severe cases it may proceed toward prostatic ulceration. Occasionally a fistula may develop between the prostate and the urethra or rectum from which pus is discharged. The symptoms may be eased temporarily.

Bacteria may reach the prostate via the blood stream or tuberculosis or the urethra. Prostatitis is thus commonly associated with urethritis (gonococcal, chlamydial, mycoplasmal) or with an active infection of the lower urinary tract. Perineal pain, lumbosacral backache, fever, and dysuria and frequent urination may be symptoms of prostatic bacterial infection (prostatosis).

Prostatitis may be acute or chronic. However, acute prostatitis commonly evolves into a chronic state, and overmanipulation of chronic prostatitis gives rise to acute symptoms.

Symptoms

Symptoms of acute prostatitis usually are perineal pain, fever, dysuria, frequent urination, and urethral discharge. To the palpating finger the prostate feels enlarged, boggy, and very tender; fluctuation occurs only if an abscess has formed. Even gentle palpation of the prostate results in a copious purulent discharge.

Symptoms of chronic prostatitis may include lumbosacral backache, perineal pain, mild dysuria and frequency, and scanty urethral discharge. Palpation reveals an irregularly enlarged, firm, and slightly tender prostate.

Epididymitis and cystitis, as well as urethritis, commonly accompany acute prostatitis. Chronic prostatitis commonly predisposes to recurrent urinary tract infection and occasionally to urethral obstruction and acute urinary retention.

Treatment

Specific treatment. For acute prostatitis the initial treatment may consist of co-trimoxazole (sulfamethoxazole, 400mg plus trimethorprim 80mg), six to eight tablets daily; or tetracycline, 2g daily by mouth until the culture of prostatic fluid and susceptibility tests indicate the drug of choice. Treatment for two weeks usually results in subsidence of the acute inflammation but chronic prostatitis may continue.

Eradication of bacteria in chronically infected prostatic tissue is exceedingly difficult. Antimicrobial drugs diffusing best into prostatic acini must be lipid-soluble and basic (e.g. trimethorprim sulfamethoxazole—co-trimoxazole). Erythromycins are quite effective in the prostate but mainly against gram-positive organisms, which are rare in urinary tract infections and prostatitis. Conversely, most drugs which are active against gram-negative coliform bacteria (the commonest cause of prostatitis) fail to reach the prostatic acini.

General Measures. During the acute phase the patient must have bed rest, adequate hydration, analgesics, stool softeners, and sitz baths. Urethral instrumentation and prostatic massage must be avoided.

Chronic prostatitis should be treated by prolonged antimicrobial therapy accompanied by vigorous prostatic massage once weekly to promote drainage. Total prostatectomy is a possible treatment but has a high morbidity and a significant mortality rate. Transurethral prostatectomy offers only uncertain benefits.

Chinese Herb Formulas
1. Ta-huang-mu-tan-pi-tang 大黃牡丹皮湯
(Rhubarb and Moutan Combination)
In acute cases with severe symptoms, such as dysuria that lead to urine retention or obstruction, or pustulation that has yet to happen, this formula may be administered to purge the pus and ease the symptoms. Doses of rhubarb and mirabilitum may be increased to 5.0g and over.

2. Teng-lung-tang 騰龍湯
(Moutan and Persica Combination)
This formula is used for acute or subacute conditions not as severe as the one above. Doses of rhubarb and mirabilitum may be modified according to the severity.

3. Chu-ling-tang 豬苓湯
(Polyporus Combination)
This combination is suitable for frequent urination, dysuria, pain on urination, and hematuria. At times it is used in combination with the preceding formula.

4. Ching-hsin-lien-tzu-yin 清心蓮子飲
(Lotus Seed Combination)
This combination is indicated for patients having a chronic disease, debilitated stamina, a weak stomach and intestines, slight anemia, easy fatigability, nervous hypersensitivity, and an uncomfortable, heavy pressure sensation when urinating.

5. Pa-wei-ti-huang-wan 八味地黃丸
(Rehmannia Eight Formula)
This formula is often used for chronic cases in which the symptoms after urination are easy fatigability, thirst, low back pain, and feverish feet. It is used jointly with *Teng-lung-tang* in many cases.

ORAL DISEASES

Halitosis

Halitosis is offensive or foul-smelling breath. The primary causes are stomatitis and gastritis. Other causes are:
1. Tooth decay, pulpitis, pyorrhea, stomatitis, dental plaque, and dental tophus.
2. Chronic pharynitis, inflammation of the upper palate, and chronic rhinitis.
3. Tracheitis and pulmonary diseases.
4. Sour stomach, esophageal cancer, gastric cancer, gastric ulcer, and chronic gastritis.
5. Diabetes, habitual constipation, and febrile diseases.
6. Leukemia and agranulocytosis.
7. Foods such as cheese, onions, garlic, scallions, and wine, as well as smoking.
8. Nervous disorders.

Individual treatment is very important. The patient should choose the Chinese formula according to his conformation.

Chinese Herb Formulas
1. **Pan-hsia-hsieh-hsin-tang**
   (Pinellia Combination)

This formula is recommended for patients with chronic gastritis, subcardiac distention, nausea, white tongue coating, bitter taste, and halitosis.

2. Kan-tsao-hsieh-hsin-tang 甘草瀉心湯
   (Pinellia and Licorice Combination)

This formula is appropriate for patients with gastrointestinal disorders with borborygmus, diarrhea, stress, nervousness, stomatitis, ulcers in the mouth, and halitosis.

3. Szu-chun-tzu-tang 四君子湯
   (Major Four Herb Combination)
   Liu-chun-tzu-tang 六君子湯
   (Major Six Herb Combination)

These formulas may be taken by patients of delicate constitution with gastrointestinal weakness, gastroptosis, abdominal distention, anemia, sweet taste, and halitosis.

4. Kuei-chih-wu-wu-tang 桂枝五物湯
   (Cinnamon Five Herb Combination)

This formula is to be taken for stomatitis and pyorrhea with halitosis.

Stomatitis

Stomatitis is an inflammative and suppurative condition of the mucous membrane in the mouth. The mucous membrane of the mouth may be locally irritated by artificial teeth, by the build-up of tartar, bacteria or capsicum on the teeth, or by fish bones or pepper. General causes of stomatitis may be gastrointestinal disorders, acute febrile diseases, menstrual disorders, pregnancy, blood disease, drug toxication, vitamin deficiency, and malnutrition.

When a patient suffers from the common cold, his gums, lips, and tongue become red and painful; this condition is called simple stomatitis. Aphthous stomatitis, or canker sores, is characterized by elliptical grainlike swelling with white centers. When there are yellowish-white, severely painful ulcers on the gums or mucous membrane of the upper palate, the condition is called ulcerative stomatitis. In addition, other forms of the disease are traumatic stomatitis, herpetic stomatitis, and gangrenous stomatitis.

Symptoms
The patient with this condition has symptoms of aphthous ulcers in the mouth with roughness, suppuration, severe pain, halitosis, abundant salivation, thirst, and dysphagia.

Treatment
Vitamins B_2, B_6, and B_{12} are effective for this condition. Tranquilizers with steroids may produce better results, but the patient should use them only under doctor's guidance. Baking soda is also effective. In severe cases, silver nitrate, steroid ointment, or gentian violet solution are also effective.

Chinese Herb Formulas
1. San-huang-hsieh-hsin-tang　　　　　　　三黃瀉心湯
    (Coptis and Rhubarb Combination)
This formula may be taken during the primary stage of stomatitis by patients with a febrile feeling in the mouth and a tendency toward constipation.

2. Kan-tsao-hsieh-hsin-tang　　　　　　　甘草瀉心湯
    (Pinellia and Licorice Combination)
This formula is to be taken for stomatitis with gastric discomfort and distention below the chest.

3. Chia-chien-liang-ke-san　　　　　　　加減涼膈散
    (Forsythia and Paeonia Formula)
This formula is to be taken for stomatitis with swelling of the mucous membrane.

4. Ching-je-pu-hsieh-tang　　　　　　　清熱補血湯
    (Cnidium and Moutan Combination)
This formula is to be taken for aphthous stomatitis.

5. Wen-ching-yin-chia-lien-chiao　　　　　温清飲加連翹
    (Tang-kuei and Gardenia Combination with Forsythia)
This formula should be taken frequently for persistent stomatitis and a tendency towards recurrent stomatitis.

6. **Ching-je-pu-chi-tang** 清熱補氣湯
   (Tang-kuei and Cimicifuga Combination)
   This formula is appropriate for patients of the weak conformation with persistent stomatitis and a tendency toward fatigue.

7. **Chih-tzu-kan-tsao-shih-tang** 梔子甘草豉湯
   (Gardenia, Licorice, and Soja Combination)
   This formula is used to treat stomatitis with a febrile feeling in the mouth and lips.

8. **Ko-ken-tang** 葛根湯
   (Pueraria Combination)
   This formula is to be taken for stomatitis.

Salivary Calculus

Salivary calculus are stones in the salivary duct formed by the precipitation of calcium salts from the saliva as a result of chronic inflammation in the salivary gland. There are several theories concerning the etiology. One hypothesis is that occlusion of the blood causes the formation of solid concretions of mineral substances. A second theory suggests that the condition results from a foreign body invading the excretion duct of the salivary gland. A factor of great importance is the constitution of the patient. The calculus is formed in the tissues of the salivary gland and migrates toward the excretion ducts. This condition is mainly found in middle-aged men.

Diagnosis is based on the appearance of oval shaped calculi at the floor of the oral cavity or on the submaxilla (the lower jawbone). Another symptom assisting the diagnosis is increased saliva secretion that occurs while eating. This condition also manifests itself clearly by means of X-rays.

Treatment

Surgical operation is necessary to open up the obstructed duct. This treatment is done by inserting a catheter into the duct. If the calculus recurs, total removal of the gland is necessary.

Chinese Herb Formulas

1. **Chih-tzu-kan-tsao-tang**　　　　　　　　梔子甘草湯
   (Gardenia and Licorice Combination)

   A woman who was suffering from a severe pain caused by a polyp under her tongue previously had undergone successful treatment for an esophageal polyp. Therefore, she was again given the same formula, *Chih-tzu-kan-tsao-tang.* On the second day a bean-sized, brownish calculus appeared and was removed with pincers.

2. **Chih-tzu-kan-tsao-chih-shih-shao-yao-tang**
   　　　　　　　　梔子甘草枳實芍藥湯
   (Gardenia, Licorice, Chih-shih, and Paeonia Combination)

   Another woman had a small bulge under her tongue. In a few days the bulge suddenly enlarged and hurt so much that she could not close her mouth. She was diagnosed as having salivary calculus and given *Chih-tzu-kan-tsao-chih-shih-shao-yao-tang.* On the second day, a bean-sized calculus was excreted spontaneously and she was cured.

Periodontitis

Periodontitis is the inflammation of periodontal tissues surrounding a tooth. Accumulations of microorganisms and substrate (plaque) on tooth surfaces calcify and form calculi. Food, bacteria, and calculi in the dental pockets cause an inflammation and the formation of pus (pyorrhea) with or without discomfort or other symptoms. If the disease proceeds without treatment, the involved teeth are eventually lost because of reabsorption of supporting alveolar bone.

Symptoms

At onset the accumulation of pus leads to acute swelling and pain. Eventually the patient may experience fever, insomnia, anorexia, and sometimes anemophobia, trembling, and other manifestations.

Pathologic changes in the tissue through chronic swelling and inflammation eventually lead to the formation of fistulas.

Treatment

Antibiotics may be prescribed for an abscess. Local drainage and oxygenating mouth rinses can be applied. Curetage, gingivectomy and even extraction are other methods of treatment. Selection of treatment is based on the condition and degree of damage.

Chinese Herb Formulas

1. **Ko-ken-tang**   葛根湯
    (Pueraria Combination)

This combination is generally used at the early onset of the disease. Often it is used with the addition of 3.0g each of cnidium and astragalus.

2. **Kuei-chih-wu-wu-tang**   桂枝五物湯
    (Cinnamon Five Herb Combination)

This combination is widely applicable to diseases of the mouth. It is also recommended for toothache. This preparation was Yoshimasu Todo's favorite formula which he employed for periodontitis, pyorrhea, and other periodontal problems.

3. **Wu-wu-ta-huang-tang**   五物大黃湯
    (Rhubarb Five Herb Combination)

This combination is effective for pyogenic symptoms when inflammation occurs.

4. **Liang-ke-san**   涼膈散
    (Forsythia and Rhubarb Formula)
   Chia-chien-liang-ke-san   加減涼膈散
    (Forsythia and Paeonia Formula)

This formula is employed for swelling and pain in dental roots accompanied by fever and constipation. It is also recommended for acute inflammation, pyorrhea, and a tendency to constipation. For more severe inflammation *San-huang-hsieh-hsin-tang-chia-mang-hsiao* (三黃瀉心湯加芒硝) Coptis and Rhubarb Combination with Mirabilitum) is recommended.

5. **Li-hsiao-san**   立效散
    (Asarum and Cimicifuga Formula)

A superior remedy for toothache, this prescription of Tung-heng

Lee's is found in the book *Chung fang kuei chu* (Directions to All Prescriptions).

Dental Caries

Dental caries and pyorrhea are the two main diseases of the mouth. Their causes are very complicated and still not clear yet. The bacteria that cause tooth decay attach to remnant food. The fermenting bacteria produces lactic acid, which dissolves the protein, and invades the tooth enamel. In addition to the above direct cause, there are indirect causes of tooth decay such as insufficient calcium and vitamins, systemic diseases, and impaction of the teeth. People especially fond of eating sweet foods and pregnant women usually suffer from this condition.

Symptoms

There is no pain when the surface of the enamel is invaded by bacteria. But when bacteria penetrate the dentin and stimulate the nerves, the patient will feel pain when drinking water.

Treatment

Early treatment is very effective for dental caries and can bring about a complete cure. The patient should brush his teeth after eating or before sleeping, and see a dentist twice a year.

Chinese Herb Formulas
1. Ko-ken-tang-chia-chuan-chiung-huang-chin

葛根湯加川芎黃芩

   (Pueraria Combination with Cnidium and Scute)
This formula may be taken for toothache. It is contraindicated for elderly patients and those having gastrointestinal weakness or a delicate constitution.

2. Kuei-chih-wu-wu-tang   桂枝五物湯
   (Cinnamon Five Herb Combiantion)
This formula is effective for toothache in those of delicate constitution and the elderly.

3. **Ching-wei-hsieh-huo-tang** 清胃瀉火湯
   (Scute and Mentha Combination)

This formula is recommended for patients of strong conformation with "internal heat" in the stomach and mouth, halitosis, and a coating on the tongue.

4. **Pai-hu-tang** 白虎湯
   (Gypsum Combination)

This formula may be taken for tooth decay with gingivitis, severe swelling, fever, and thirst.

5. **Tao-ho-cheng-chi-tang** 桃核承氣湯
   (Persica and Rhubarb Combiantion)

This formula is used to treat patients of strong conformation with flushing up, shoulder stiffness, a tendency toward constipation, toothache, and gingivitis.

Pyorrhea

Pyorrhea or peridontitis is a continuous discharge of pus in the gum tissues. The gum tissues of the teeth become purplish and swollen, and there is inflammation and bleeding. The build-up of tartar on the teeth, an overabundance of animal fat in the diet, general disease (gout, rheumatism, diabetes, kidney disease, liver disease, syphilis, and tuberculosis) will also cause this condition.

Symptoms

The symptoms of this condition are halitosis, swollen gum tissue, a loosening of the teeth, and pus. Patients of tubercular constitution have symptoms of anemia, dry gums, and little pus. Patients who consume an overabundance of animal fat in their diet show copious salivation and pus, moisture in the gum tissues, and redness. Those with nephritis or diabetes show bleeding and little pus in the gum tissues. During times of excessive work or stress, the patient will suffer from severe pain and bleeding in the gums.

Treatment

The tartar is removed from the teeth, and iodine tincture or glycerine is spread on the gum tissues; in severe cases, peridontal surgery is necessary. When bleeding of the gum tissues occurs, the patient should take sufficient vitamins C and E, perhaps by eating an orange every day or a lemon every other day. For prophlactic treatment at home, the patient with pyorrhea should massage his gums regularly and brush his teeth with toothpaste and a special brush. Rinsing the mouth is also important for good oral hygiene. Above all, the known causes of this condition should be treated and cured.

Chinese Herb Formulas

1. **Kuei-chih-wu-wu-tang** 桂枝五物湯
    (Cinnamon Five Herb Combination)
    This formula is to be taken for pyorrhea. The main herbs of this formula are hoelen, cinnamon, and scute.

2. **Tao-ho-cheng-chi-tang** 桃核承氣湯
    (Persica and Rhubarb Combination)
    This formula is effective for those of strong constitution with flushing up, aching shoulders, constipation, headache, purplish gums, and bleeding.

3. **Pu-chung-i-chi-tang-chia-ti-huang-mu-tan-pi-fu-ling-shao-yao**
    補中益氣湯加地黃牡丹皮茯苓芍藥
    (Ginseng and Astragalus Combination with Rehmannia, Moutan, Hoelen, and Paeonia)
    This formula may be used to treat patients of delicate constitution with anemia, a tendency toward fatigue, and pyorrhea.

4. **Ko-ken-tang-chia-chuan-chiung-huang-chin**
    葛根湯加川芎黃芩
    (Pueraria Combination with Cnidium and Scute)
    This formula is effective for primary pyorrhea.

5. **Pai-hu-chia-jen-sheng-tang** 白虎加人參湯
    (Ginseng and Gypsum Combination)
    This formula is recommended for pyorrhea with a febrile sensation and thirst.

6. **Fang-feng-tung-sheng-san** 防風通聖散
    (Siler and Platycodon Formula)

This formula is used to treat obese patients with constipation, abundant salivation, marked inflammation, and pyorrhea.

7. **Su-tzu-chiang-chi-tang** 蘇子降氣湯
   (Perilla Fruit Combination)

This formula is effective for those of delicate constitution with flushing up, cold feet, heart disease, and pyorrhea.

8. **Pai-nung-san** 排膿散
   (Platycodon and Chih-shih Formula)

This formula is effective for pyorrhea with painful swelling, pus in the gums, and purplish gum tissue.

9. **Kan-lu-yin** 甘露飲
   (Sweet Combination)

This formula is recommended for persistent pyorrhea.

10. **Shih-chuan-ta-pu-tang** 十全大補湯
    (Ginseng and Tang-kuei Ten Combination)

This formula is used to treat pyorrhea in patients with marked anemia and a delicate constitution.

11. **Pa-wei-ti-huang-wan** 八味地黃丸
    (Rehmannia Eight Formula)

This formula may be taken for pyorrhea by patients with diabetes and fatigue.

Pulpitis

When tooth decay becomes serious and extends to the dental pulp, it will cause pulpitis. At this stage, if the condition of the tooth is irreversible—the pulp is abscessed and dying—there is no other treatment except extracting or dentizing the tooth. In addition, bacteria that attack the dental pulp can invade the root of the tooth, as well as the blood and lymph, and may cause the inflammation of the circulatory organs, nerves, blood, and skin. The patient should be aware of the complications caused by this condition.

Symptoms
There is pricking pain in the dental pulp that becomes intense when the patient is sleeping at night; in severe cases, the patient will feel pain during the day.

Treatment
The abscess that occurs in the pulp should be completely disinfected. In severe cases, the tooth should be extracted and an artificial tooth put in its place. When the patient is suffering from toothache, baking soda may be used to rinse the mouth; aspirin and sedatives are also effective for this condition.

Chinese Herb Formulas
Ko-ken-tang-chia-chuan-chiung-huang-chin 葛根湯加川芎黃芩
(Pueraria Combination with Cnidium and Scute)
Kuei-chih-wu-wu-tang 桂枝五物湯
(Cinnamon Five Herb Combination)
Both of these formulas are effective for painful pulpitis.

EXPLANATION OF CHINESE HERBAL FORMULAS

EXPLANATION OF CHINESE HERBAL FORMULAS

An-chung-san
(Cardamon and Fennel Formula)

Main Herbs
- 4.0g cinnamon
- 1.0g cardamon
- 3.0g corydalis
- 0.5g galanga
- 3.0g oyster shell
- 1.0g licorice
- 1.5g fennel

Effects
Used to treat patients of a delicate constitution and slender physique with a weak pulse and flaccid muscles and skin, abdominal weakness, ascites, palpitations at the umbilicus, subcardiac pain, nausea, vomiting, and dragging pain in the lower abdomen and the lumbar region.

Uses
Neurotic gastralgia, gastric ulcers, duodenal ulcer, prolapsed stomach, chronic gastritis, gastric tumor, pyloric obstruction, painful menstruation, and "morning sickness".

Erh-chen-tang
(Citrus and Pinellia Combination)

Main Herbs
- 4.0g citrus
- 1.0g licorice
- 3.0g ginger
- 5.0g hoelen
- 5.0g pinellia

Effects

Given to patients with copious watery sputum; vertigo; palpitations; stomach discomfort; occasional fever; a submerged weak pulse; and vomiting and nausea due to stagnant water in the stomach.

Uses

Vomiting, nausea, vertigo, headaches, eclampsia, stagnant ch'i, hangover, apoplexy, prolapsed stomach, and emotional disorders.

Nu-sheng-san
(Tang-kuei and Cyperus Formula)

Main Herbs

3.0g tang-kuei	2.0g cinnamon
1.5g saussurea	1.5g coptis
1.5g licorice	2.0g areca seed
0.5-1.0g rhubarb	3.0g atractylodes
2.0g scute	2.0g ginseng
3.0g cyperus	1.0g clove
3.0g cnidium	

Effects

Used for treating neurotic symptoms, blood diseases, flushing up, vertigo, and menopausal problems.

Uses

Menopausal disturbance and prepartum and postpartum neuroses.

Chai-hu-chia-lung-ku-mu-li-tang
(Bupleurum and Dragon Bone Combination)

Main Herbs

5.0g bupleurum	2.5g dragon bone
4.0g pinellia	2.5g oyster shell
1.0g rhubarb	2.5g ginseng

    3.0g hoelen   2.5g ginger
    3.0g cinnamon   2.5g jujube
    2.5g scute

Effects

Used for harmonizing the "interior" and the "exterior" and sedating the mind. It is indicated for distention in the chest and beneath the heart, decreased urine and constipation, palpitations above the naval, insomnia, mental instability, irritability, melancholy, jumpiness, anxiety, and even the manifestations of hysteria and spasms, or exhaustion which cause the person to have a general feeling of heaviness making it difficult to move his body.

Uses

Neurosis, hysteria, epilepsy, nervous insomnia, climacteric disorders, neurotic cardiac palpitations, neurotic impotence, hypertension, apoplexy, valvular diseases, angina pectoris, chronic nephritis, renal atrophy, edema, uremia, beriberi, monoplegia, heatstroke, stiff shoulders, cirrhosis of the liver, and baldness.

Chai-hu-ching-kan-tang
(Bupleurum and Rehmannia Combination)

Main Herbs

2.0g bupleurum	1.5g coptis	1.5g platycodon
1.5g *tang-kuei*	1.5g scute	1.5g arctium
1.5g paeonia	1.5g phellodendron	1.5g trichosanthes
1.5g cnidium	1.5g gardenia	1.5g mentha
1.5g rehmannia	1.5g forsythia	1.5g licorice

Effects

Used for improving glandular problems in children who have a slightly dark or bluish white complexion, relieving tension in the straight abdominal muscles, and reducing inflammation in the liver, gallbladder, and triple warmer meridians.

Uses

Improvement of the glandular constitution in little children, lymphadenitis of the lungs, adenoidal problems, lymphadenectasis of the neck, chronic tonsillitis, skin diseases, disorders following measles, poor metabolism, and pleurisy.

Chai-hu-kuei-chih-kan-chiang-tang
(Bupleurum, Cinnamon, and Ginger Combination)

Main Herbs
- 6.0g bupleurum
- 3.0g cinnamon
- 3.0g trichosanthes
- 3.0g scute
- 3.0g oyster shell
- 2.0g ginger
- 2.0g licorice

Effects
Used for persons with a delicate constitution who have alternating chills and fever, chest distention, mild stagnancy and irritation, decreased urine, extreme thirst, sweating of the head, heart palpitations, cold hands and feet, and soft stool or diarrhea.

Uses
Common cold, pneumonia, bronchitis, tuberculosis, pleurisy, peritonitis, gastric atonia, hyperfunctional cardiac palpitations, insomnia, climacteric disorders, hepatitis, and gallstones.

Chai-hu-kuei-chih-tang
(Bupleurum and Cinnamon Combination)

Main Herbs
- 5.0g bupleurum
- 4.0g pinellia
- 1.5g licorice
- 2.0g jujube
- 2.5g cinnamon
- 2.0g scute
- 2.0g ginseng
- 2.5g paeonia
- 1.0g ginger

Effects
Effective for persons with a somewhat delicate constitution who have a tendency to become fatigued; also for gastrointestinal weakness, headaches, heaviness in the head, neuralgia, fever, mild chillphobia, floating pulse, distention and hardening beneath the heart, periumbilical or lower abdominal pain, and tenseness around the rectus abdominus muscle.

Uses
1. Common cold, influenza, pneumonia, pulmonary tuberculosis, and pleuritis.
2. Stomachache, gastrosia, gastric distress, gastric ulcer,

duodenal ulcer, acute colitis, ulcerative colitis, pancreatitis, gallstones, hepatitis, jaundice, and gallstones.
3. Chronic appendicitis, peritonitis, abdominal pain, abdominal distention, and constipation.
4. Intercostal neuralgia, headaches, arthralgia, nephritis, inflammation of the pelvis of the kidney, neurotic behavior, neurasthenia, irritability, insomnia, female problems, hysteria, epilepsy, and cerebral disorders.

Chai-ko-chieh-chi-tang
(Bupleurum and Pueraria Combination)

Main Herbs
- 4.0g bupleurum
- 4.0g pueraria
- 2.0g *chianghuo*
- 2.0g angelica
- 3.0g scute
- 3.0g paeonia
- 2.0g platycodon
- 5.0g gypsum
- 2.0g licorice
- 2.0g jujube
- 1.0g ginger

Effects
Given to patients with a common cold for whom both *Kuei-chih-tang* (Cinnamon Combination) and *Ma-huang-tang* (Ma-huang Combination) have been ineffective. Further symptoms are absence of perspiration, high fever, headaches, extreme thirst, generalized aching, and nosebleeds.

Uses
Pneumonia, cold, influenza, and febrile diseases.

Chai-shao-liu-chun-tzu-tang
(Bupleurum, Paeonia, and Six Major Herb Combination)

Main Herbs
- 4.0g ginseng
- 4.0g atractylodes
- 3.0g paeonia
- 2.0g citrus

>   4.0g hoelen   2.0g jujube
>   4.0g pinellia   2.0g ginger
>   3.0g bupleurum   1.0g licorice

Effects

Used for people who have a *Liu-chun-tzu-tang* (Six Major Herb Combination) conformation together with spasms of the rectus abdominus muscle, or abominal pain.

Uses

Gastrointestinal weakness, gastritis, gastroptosis, gastric ulcer, indigestion, chronic peritonitis, loss of appetite, and vomiting.

Chen-wu-tang
(Vitality Combination)

Main Herbs

>   5.0g hoelen   3.0g ginger
>   3.0g paeonia   0.5-1.0g aconite
>   3.0g atractylodes

Effects

Used for treating metabolic disorders, painful urination from stagnant fluids, abdominal pain, diarrhea, vertigo, cardiac palpitations, abdominal weakness, severe fatigue, cold hands and feet accompanied by pain.

Uses

Common cold of a yin-conformation, influenza, pneumonia, pleurisy, tuberculosis, neurasthenia, cerebral bleeding, hypertension, valvular diseases, gastrointestinal weakness, chronic enteritis, indigestion, intestinal tuberculosis, gastroptosis, peritonitis, ascites, cyclic vomiting, nephritis, kidney atrophy, partial paralysis, rheumatalgia, and senile itching.

Chi-pi-tang
(Lotus and Citrus Combination)

Main Herbs

>   4.0g atractylodes   3.0g lotus seed   2.0g citrus

4.0g hoelen   3.0g dioscorea   2.0g alisma
3.0g ginseng   2.0g crataegus   1.0g licorice
                     (hawthorn)

Effects
Used for treating watery diarrhea due to gastrosplenic weakness, indigestion in children, loss of appetite, persistent diarrhea, frequent abdominal pain, frequent vomiting, and jaundice.

Uses
Indigestion, chronic gastroenteritis, intestinal tuberculosis, watery diarrhea, chronic diarrhea, loss of appetite after sickness, digestive problems in infants.

Chia-wei-hsiao-yao-san
(Bupleurum and Paeonia Formula)

Main Herbs
3.0g *tang-kuei*   2.0g moutan
3.0g paeonia   2.0g gardenia
3.0g atractylodes   2.0g licorice
3.0g hoelen   1.0g ginger
3.0g bupleurum   1.0g mentha

Effects
Used for gynecological problems such as aching in the arms and legs, dizziness, mental instability, flushing, thirst, night sweats with fever, loss of appetite, narcolepsy or insomnia, cardiac and limb fever, earaches, abdominal distention near the umbilicus, turbid or residual urine, and menstrual irregularity.

Uses
Climacteric disturbances, blood vessel disorders, infertility, premenstrual tension, menstrual irregularity, stomatitis, leukorrhea, chronic endometritis, chronic hepatitis, cirrhosis, urethritis, cystitis, constipation, eczema, hyperkeratosis of the palms, lack of skin pigmentation, and hyperthyroidism.

Chieh-keng-pai-san
(Platycodon and Croton Formula)

Main Herbs
    1.0g platycodon   0.3g croton seed
    1.0g fritillaria

Effects
    A strong expectorant with pus-discharging effects and a purgative action. Contraindicated for people with a feeble physique.

Uses
    Pulmonary gangrene, acute pneumonia, the initial stage of diphtheria, apoplexy, paroxysms of asthma. To be taken in a single dose.

Chien-chin-nei-tuo-san
(Astragalus and Platycodon Formula)

Main Herbs
    2.5g ginseng   2.0g platycodon
    3.0g *tang-kuei*   2.0g magnolia
    2.0g astragalus   2.0g cinnamon
    2.0g cnidium   1.0g angelica
    2.0g siler   1.0g licorice

Effects
    Used for treating carbuncles, suppurating skin lesions, pain, and polyps in a delicate constitution.

Uses
    Carbuncles, hemorrhoids, periproctitis, suppurative mastitis, lymphadenitis, and suppurative otitis media.

Chih-kan-tsao-tang
(Baked Licorice Combination)

Main Herbs

3.0g licorice   3.0g linum   3.0g ginseng
3.0g ginger   3.0g jujube   2.0g gelatin
3.0g cinnamon   6.0g ophiopogon   6.0g rehmannia

Effects

Used for treating palpitations; increased respiratory rate; knotty, alternating, quick, or irregular pulse; dry and coarse skin; annoying fever in the hands and feet; a tendency to tire easily, and thirst.

Uses

Valvular disease, palpitations, anemia, endocarditis, hyperthyroidism, anxiety, hypertension, arteriosclerosis, tuberculosis, and puerperal fever.

Chih-shih-chih-tang
(Kaolin Combination)

Main Herbs

4.0g astragalus   3.0g *tang-kuei*
2.0g ginger   1.5g licorice
4.0g ginseng   2.0g citrus
2.0g jujube   1.0g cimicifuga
4.0g atractylodes   3.0g kaolin
2.0g bupleurum

Effects

Used for treating chronic prolapsis of the anus.

Chih-tou-chuang-i-fang
(Forsythia and Lonicera Formula)

Main Herbs

    3.0g forsythia   2.0g siler   1.0g carthamus
    3.0g cnidium   2.0g lonicera   1.0g licorice
    3.0g atractylodes   1.0g schizonepeta   0.5g rhubarb

Effects

Used for treating children with sores on their heads accompanied by itching and scabbing, and reddening papules, and vesicles; erosions with scabs on the face, neck, armpits, and pudenum.

Uses

Head eczema in children, fetal poisoning, and inflammatory dermatitis.

Chih-tzu-kan-tsao-shih-tang
(Gardenia, Licorice, and Soja Combination)

Main Herbs

    3.0g gardenia   2.0g licorice
    4.0g soja (soybean relish)

Effects

Used for the conformation *Chih-tzu-shih-tang* (Gardenia and Soja Combination) when there are acute symptoms such as superficial respiration or severe itching.

Uses

Esophageal constriction; insomnia; jaundice; inflammation of the tongue, larynx, or the pharynx; weakness and discomfort following sweating and vomiting; somatic fever, hypertension, neurasthenia, eczema, dry ringworm, herpes, and hives.

Chih-tzu-sheng-chiang-shih-tang
(Gardenia, Ginger, and Soja Combination)

Main Herbs
    3.0g gardenia   4.0g ginger
    4.0g soja (soybean relish)

Effects
    Used for treating a *Chih-tzu-shih-tang* conformation with the additional symptom of vomiting.

Uses
    Catarrhal jaundice, esophageal cancer, esophageal constriction, insomnia, inflammation of the mouth and pharynx, neurasthenia, hemoptysis, and fatigue after heavy sweating or vomiting.

Chih-tzu-shih-tang
(Gardenia and Soja Combination)

Main Herbs
    3.0g gardenia   4.0g soja (soybean relish)

Effects
    Used for treating fevers, irritability, insomnia, chest distention, loss of appetite, reddening of the tongue with yellowish fur.

Uses
    Catarrhal jaundice, esophageal cancer, esophageal constriction, insomnia, inflammation of the mouth, pharyngitis, neurasthenia, hemoptysis, and fatigue after heavy sweating or vomiting.

Ching-chieh-lien-chiao-tang
(Schizonepeta and Forsythia Combination)

Main Herbs
    2.0g schizonepeta   2.0g *chih-shih*

2.0g forsythia
2.0g siler
2.0g *tang-kuei*
2.0g cnidium
2.0g paeonia
2.0g bupleurum
2.0g scute
2.0g gardenia
2.0g angelica
2.0g platycodon
1.0g licorice

Effects

Used especially for diseases located in the upper warmer and adenoids of patients with dark skin and greasy sweat on their palms and soles, and a tense pulse and abdomen; also for inflammation and suppuration of the ears and nasal passages (otitis and rhinitis).

Uses

Inflammation of the middle ear, sinusitis maxillaris, hypertrophic rhinitis, tonsillitis, nosebleeds, hyperplastic pulmonary tuberculosis, acne, baldness, and inflamed adenoids in children.

Chin-chiu-pieh-chia-tang
(Chin-chiu and Tortoise Shell Combination)

Main Herbs

2.0g *chin-chiu*
2.0g *ching-hao*
2.0g *mume*
2.0g anemarrhena
3.0g *tang-kuei*
3.0g tortoise shell
3.0g bupleurum
3.0g lycium bark
1.5g ginger

Uses

Pneumonia, hyperplastic tuberculosis, and pleurisy.

Ching-fei-tang
(Platycodon and Fritillary Combination)

Main Herbs

2.0g scute
2.0g platycodon
2.0g morus
3.0g jujube
2.0g bamboo
3.0g hoelen

2.0g apricot seed
2.0g gardenia
3.0g ophiopoton
2.0g fritillary
2.0g citrus

3.0g *tang-kuei*
2.0g asparagus
0.5g schizandra
0.5g ginger
1.0g licorice

Effects

Treat chronic respiratory diseases with a fever in the chest and an incessant cough, difficult expectoration; and copious, thick sputum of a green, yellow, white, or other color.

Uses

Chronic bronchitis, chronic laryngitis, pneumonia, pulmonary tuberculosis, bronchodilation, bronchial asthma, and cardiac asthma.

Ching-hsin-lien-tzu-yin
(Lotus Seed Combination)

Main Herbs

4.0g lotus seed
3.0g plantago
2.0g astragalus

4.0g ophiopogon
3.0g scute
2.0g lycium bark

4.0g hoelen
3.0g ginseng
2.0g licorice

Effects

Used for treating spleen, lung, and kidney injuries due to excessive drinking and sexual indulgence; polyuria; turbid urine; spermatorrhea; bed wetting; a feeling of residual urine; abnormal leukorrhea; neurotic diabetes; loss of appetite; and generalized fatigue in a delicate constitution.

Uses

Kidney stones, renal tuberculosis, gonorrhea, cystitis, leukorrhea, prostatitis, impotence, urinary retention, diabetes, sexual impotence, and inflamed mouth.

Ching-je-pu-chi-tang
(Tang-kuei and Cimicifuga Combination)

Main Herbs

    3.0 ginseng   3.5g hoelen
    3.0g *tang-kuei*   2.0g scrophularia (figwort)
    3.0g paeonia   0.5g cimicifuga
    3.0g ophiopogon   1.0g schizandra
    3.5g atractylodes   1.0g licorice

Effects

    Given to persons with a weak conformation suffering from chronic gastritis, tongue ulceration, and a loss of tongue papilla caused by weakness and fever in the stomach.

Uses

    Inflammation of the mouth or mouth ulcers, reddened tongue after a fever, a postpartum or malignant tumor, ulceration of a red tongue caused by weak *ch'i*, and numbness and loss of the sense of taste due to chronic gastritis.

Ching-je-pu-hsieh-tang
(Cnidium and Moutan Combination)

Main Herbs

    3.0g *tang-kuei*   1.5g anemarrhena
    3.0g paeonia   1.5g phellodendron
    3.0g cnidium   1.5g moutan
    3.0g rehmannia   1.5g schizandra
    3.0g ophiopogon   1.5g bupleurum
    1.5g scrophularia (figwort)

Effects

    Used to replenish and nourish the blood, and to expel fever from it.

Uses

    Ulcerated mouth and tongue due to postpartum blood dryness and pyelitis; ulcerated and inflamed mouth due to Behcet's disease or syphilis.

Ching-shang-fang-feng-tang
(Siler Combination)

Main Herbs

1.5g schizonepeta	3.0g cnidium
1.5g coptis	3.0g scute
1.5g mentha	3.0g forsythia
1.5g *chih-shih*	3.0g angelica
1.5g licorice	3.0g platycodon
3.0g gardenia	3.0g siler

Effects

Used for purging anxiety and inner heat in the upper body and for curing facial boils and thriving fever.

Uses

Boils on the head and face, acne, head eczema, facial flushing, conjunctivitis, acne rosacea, inflammation of the middle ear, inflammation of the gums, and fungal infections caused by Trichophyton.

Chiu-wei-ping-lang-tang
(Areca Seed Nine Combination)

Main Herbs

4.0g areca seed	1.0g rhubarb
3.0g magnolia bark	1.0g ginger
3.0g cinnamon	1.0g saussurea
3.0g aurantium	1.0g evodia
1.5g perilla	3.0g hoelen
1.0g licorice	

Effects

Suitable for beriberi. It is used for edema of the feet and gasping.

Uses

Emotional distress, rapid heartbeat due to anxiety, hypertension, Basedow's disease, gastroenteritis, multiple neuritis (lesions of a nerve or nerves), herpes, rheumatism, fatigability, and climacteric disorders.

Chiung-kuei-chiao-ai-tang
(Tang-kuei and Gelatin Combination)

Main Herbs
- 3.0g cnidium
- 4.0g *tang-kuei*
- 3.0g gelatin
- 3.0g artemisia
- 5.0g rehmannia
- 4.0g paeonia
- 3.0g licorice

Effects

A tonic and hemostatic, the formula is used to treat bleeding, stagnant blood, and anemia.

Uses

Uterine bleeding, endometritis, uterine cancer, habitual spontaneous abortion, excessive uterine bleeding, rectal bleeding, hemorrhoidal bleeding, intestinal bleeding, blood in the urine or sputum, bleeding due to injuries, extravasated blood in the eye, purpura, and anemia.

Chu-ling-tang
(Polyporus Combination)

Main Herbs
- 3.0g polyporus
- 3.0g hoelen
- 3.0g alisma
- 3.0g talc
- 3.0g gelatin

Effects

Effective for urethral inflammation accompanied by extreme

thirst, fever, cough, vomiting, discomfort, insomnia, and pain in the lower abdomen.
Uses
Nephritis, pyelitis, renal cirrhosis, cystitis, urethritis, hematuria, uterine bleeding, intestinal bleeding, enteritis, gonorrhea, diarrhea, edema, and insomnia.

Chu-yeh-shih-kao-tang
(Bamboo Leaves and Gypsum Combination)

Main Herbs
    6.0g ophiopogon   2.0g bamboo leaves
    6.0g oryza   2.0g licorice
    4.0g pinellia   10.0g gypsum
    3.0g ginseng

Effects
Used for treating people with a delicate constitution, deficiency of saliva, coarse skin, thirst, dry tongue, pneumonia, measles, influenza, fever, cough, abnormal sweating, and night sweats.

Uses
Common cold, influenza, pneumonia, bronchitis, bronchial asthma, whooping cough (pertussis), pulmonary emphysema, pulmonary gangrene, tuberculosis, measles, scarlet fever, and diabetes.

Fang-chi-huang-chi-tang
(Stephania and Astragalus Combination)

Main Herbs
    5.0g stephania   1.5g licorice
    5.0g astragalus   3.0g jujube
    3.0g atractylodes   3.0g ginger

Effects

Used for stimulating spleen function, increasing vitality, increasing the flow of urine, and reducing swelling.

Uses

Rheumatism, arthritis, abnormal sweating, obesity, nephritis, hernia of the testis, edema of the legs, and menstrual irregularity.

Fang-feng-tung-sheng-san
(Siler and Platycodon Formula)

Main Herbs

1.2g *tang-kuei*	1.2g siler	1.2g mentha
1.2g paeonia	1.5g mirabilitum	2.0g platycodon
1.2g gardenia	1.2g *ma-huang*	2.0g scute
1.2g cnidium	1.2g ginger	2.0g licorice
1.2g forsythia	1.5g rhubarb	3.0g talc
1.2g schizonepeta	2.0g atractylodes	2.0g gypsum

Effects

Given to persons with an obese constitution and firm muscles, and a strong pulse and abdomen for cardiac disorders, habitual constipation, stiff shoulders, numb hands and feet, fatigue, headaches, and heavy head.

Uses

Obesity, hypertension, apoplexy, arteriosclerosis, diabetes, chronic nephritis, beriberi, asthma, habitual constipation, scabies, red nose, arthritis, and nasal suppuration.

Fen-hsiao-tang
(Hoelen and Alisma Combination)

Main Herbs

2.5g atractylodes	2.0g alisma
2.5g white atractylodes	1.0g *chih-shih*
2.5g hoelen	1.0g areca

2.0g citrus   1.0g cardamon
2.0g magnolia bark   1.0g saussurea
2.0g cyperus   1.0g juncus
2.0g polyporus   1.0g ginger

Effects

Used for treating stagnant *ch'i,* stagnant food, edema, the initial stage of ascites, distention beneath the heart, insufficient stools, severe constipation, gas in the intestines, sour stomach, and loss of appetite.

Uses

Peritonitis, nephritis, ascites, tympanites (gas in the intestines), and cirrhosis.

Fu-ling-szu-ni-tang
(Hoelen, G. L. and Aconite Combination)

Main Herbs

2.0g licorice   0.5-1.0g aconite
2.0g ginseng   2.0g ginger
4.0g hoelen

Effects

Used for treating chills, diarrhea, vomiting, abdominal distention, cold hands and feet, anemia, palpitations, anxiety, edema and decreased urine.

Uses

Influenza, typhoid fever, cholera, diarrhea, autointoxication, appendicitis, gastroenteritis, indigestion, jaundice, abnormal perspiration, hemorrhaging due to external injuries from surgery or childbirth.

Fu-ling-tse-hsieh-tang
(Alisma, Hoelen, and Ginger Combination)

Main Herbs

    4.0g hoelen   3.0g ginger
    2.0g cinnamon   3.0g atractylodes
    4.0g alisma   1.5g licorice

Effects

Used for treating gastric regurgitation and thirst, decreased urine, palpitations, flushing up, headaches, vertigo, abdominal distention, and abdominal pain.

Uses

Gastric atonia, gastroptosis, gastrectasis, gastric ulcers, gastric cancer, "morning sickness", spitting up of milk in little children, and pyloric obstruction.

Fu-ling-yin
(Hoelen Combination)

Main Herbs

    5.0g hoelen   3.0g citrus
    4.0g atractylodes   3.0g ginger
    3.0g ginseng   1.5g *chih-shih*

Effects

Used for treating stagnant fluid and *ch'i* in the stomach, nausea, heartburn, and mild resistance beneath the heart.

Uses

Gastritis, gastroptosis, enlargement of the stomach, excessive stomach acid, and gastrointestinal weakness.

Fu-tzu-keng-mi-tang
(Aconite and Oryza Combination)

Main Herbs
    0.5-1.0g aconite   3.0g jujube
    7.0g oryza   1.5g licorice
    5.0g pinellia

Effects
    Given to people with a delicate constitution who have metabolic disorders, a cold feeling in the abdomen, gas, violent paroxyms of pain, flushing up, chest distention, nausea, and vomiting.

Uses
    Intestinal colic, gastric spasms, gastric ulcers, peritonitis, gallstones, pancreatitis, pylorospasm.

Fu-tzu-tang
(Aconite Combination)

Main Herbs
    0.5-1.0g aconite   5.0g atractylodes
    4.0g hoelen   3.0g ginseng
    4.0g paeonia

Effects
    Used for treating generalized pain, arthralgia, severe cold in the back, cold hands and feet, white coating on the tongue, submerged and weak pulse, and generalized anemia.

Uses
    Common cold, influenza, neuralgia, rheumatism, arthritis, abdominal pain due to chills, peritonitis, edema, ascites, stomatitis, abdominal pain in pregnant women, apoplexy, facial paralysis, monoplegia (paralysis of a single limb or area), dermatitis, eczema, and hives.

Hsiang-sha-liu-chun-tzu-tang
(Cyperus and Cardamon Combination)

Main Herbs

6.0g ginseng	3.0g licorice
6.0g pinellia	3.0g citrus
6.0g atractylodes	1.5g saussurea
6.0g hoelen	1.5g cardamon

Effects

Used for treating patients with *Liu-chun-tzu-tang* conformation who have distention beneath the heart, stagnancy of *ch'i*, a loss of appetite, and stagnated food in the stomach.

Uses

Chronic gastroenteritis, gastroptosis, gastric atonia, gastric ulcer, gastric cancer, chronic peritonitis, loss of appetite during convalescence, a delicate constitution in the elderly, and apoplexy.

Hsiang-su-san
(Cyperus and Perilla Formula)

Main Herbs

3.5g cyperus	1.0g licorice
1.5g perilla	1.0g ginger
3.0g citrus	

Effects

Used for treating a common cold due to stagnated *ch'i* and stagnated food.

Uses

Common cold, neurasthenia, abdominal pain of emotional origin, climacteric neurosis, absence of menstruation, food poisoning caused by eating poisoned fish, loss of the sense of smell, nasal congestion, belching, and vomiting.

Hsiao-chai-hu-tang
(Minor Bupleurum Combination)

Main Herbs
- 7.0g bupleurum
- 3.0g scute
- 5.0g pinellia
- 3.0g ginseng
- 3.0g jujube
- 2.0g licorice
- 4.0g ginger

Effects
Mainly given to patients with thoraco-costal distress and abdominal distention. It generally improves the physical constitution.

Uses
Common cold, acute and chronic bronchitis, pleuritis, pneumonia, hepatitis, cholecystitis, gallstones, jaundice, gastritis, sour stomach and gastric disorders, lymphadenitis, tonsillitis, mumps, mastitis, pyelitis, puerperal fever, severe chills and fever due to uterine disease, stuttering, epilepsy, impotence in young men, neurosis, baldness, mental instability in children.

Hsiao-cheng-chi-tang
(Minor Rhubarb Combination)

Main Herbs
- 2.0g rhubarb
- 2.0g *chih-shih*
- 3.0g magnolia bark

Effects
Used for treating bloating, constipation, moist fever, and a sinking pulse.

Uses
Acute febrile diseases, habitual constipation, hypertension, obesity, food poisoning, epilepsy, emotional disorders, food stagnation, tetanus, dysentery, and difficult and painful urination (dysuria).

Hsiao-chien-chung-tang
(Minor Cinnamon and Paeonia Combination)

Main Herbs

4.0g cinnamon	4.0g jujube
4.0g ginger	2.0g licorice
6.0g paeonia	20.0g maltose

Effects

Given to persons having a delicate constitution with a tendency towards fatigue.

Uses

Children of a delicate constitution who wet the bed, urinate frequently, cry at night, and have gastritis, diarrhea or constipation, hernias or frequent headaches; necrosis; arthritis; rickets; neurosis; asthma; purpura; tonsillitis; and neurasthenia and neuropalpitations.

Hsiao-ching-lung-chia-shih-kao-tang
(Minor Blue Dragon Combination Incorporating Gypsum)

Main Herbs

6.0g pinellia	3.0g licorice	3.0g asarum
3.0g *ma-huang*	3.0g cinnamon	3.0g schizandra
3.0g paeonia	3.0g ginger	5.0g gypsum

Uses

For patients with a *Hsiao-ching-lung-tang* conformation plus irritability.

Hsiao-ching-lung-tang
(Minor Blue Dragon Combination)

Main Herbs

6.0g pinellia	3.0g cinnamon
3.0g *ma-huang*	3.0g ginger

3.0g paeonia (peony)   3.0g asarum
3.0g licorice   3.0g schizandra

Effects

Used to treat subcardiac edema, anhidrosis (absence of sweating), general aching, dry coughs, fever, asthmatic cough or labored breathing, frothy sputum, decreased urine, and occasional chills in the back.

Uses

1. Cough with fever, stridor, headaches, severe chills, flushing up, hiccups, and dizziness.
2. Bronchial stridor and watery sputum.
3. Allergic rhinitis.
4. Whooping cough, bronchial dilation, pulmonary asthma.
5. Renal cirrhosis, swelling due to primary nephritis, and colds accompanied by cough and swelling.
6. Conjunctivitis, inflammation of the tear ducts, periorbital edema and tearing.
7. Edematous arthritis.

Hsiao-hsien-hsiung-tang
(Minor Trichosanthes Combination)

Main Herbs

1.5g coptis   3.0g trichosanthes seed
6.0g pinellia

Effects

Used for treating subcardiac pressure and pain, chest pain on coughing or deep breathing, labored breathing, viscid sputum, and a floating pulse.

Uses

Pneumonia, bronchitis, pleurisy, gastritis, indigestion, intercostal neuralgia, and gallstones.

Hsiao-feng-san
(Tang-kuei and Arctium Formula)

Main Herbs

3.0g *tang-kuei*	1.5 anemarrhena
3.0g rehmannia	1.5g sesame
3.0g gypsum	1.0g cicada
2.0g siler	1.0g sophora
2.0g atractylodes	1.0g schizonepeta
2.0g akebia	1.0g licorice
2.0g arctium	

Effects

Used to treat skin diseases of "internal heat", copious discharges, and severe itching.

Uses

Recalcitrant eczema, chronic hives, itching, prickly heat, lichen, and skin diseases which aggravate in the summer.

Hsiao-kan-yin
(Cardamon and Shen-chu Combination)

Main Herbs

2.0g ginseng	2.0g atractylodes	1.0g cardamon
2.0g *shen-chu*	1.0g coptis	1.0g licorice
2.0g hoelen	1.0g blue citrus peel	0.5g picrorrhiza

Effects

Used for treating abdominal distention (like a frog's belly) resulting from tubercular peritonitis caused by mesenteric tuberculosis.

Uses

A weaker condition than that of *Tsing-fu-tang* (Bupleurum and Pinellia Combination) conformation in which there is no fever, and slight thirst.

Hsiao-pan-hsia-chia-fu-ling-tang
(Minor Pinellia and Hoelen Combination)

Main Herbs
    8.0g pinellia   5.0g ginger   5.0g hoelen

Effects
    Used for treating vomiting due to stagnant water in the stomach, eclampsia, flushing up, nausea, subcardiac distention, vertigo, and palpitations.

Uses
    Pernicious vomiting, acute gastroenteritis, gastroptosis, beriberi, and pleurisy.

Hsu-ming-tang
(Ma-huang and Ginseng Combination)

Main Herbs
    3.0g *ma-huang*   3.0g *tang-kuei*   2.0g licorice
    3.0g cinnamon   2.0g cnidium   4.0g apricot seed
    3.0g ginseng   2.0g ginger   6.0g gypsum

Effects
    Used for treating apoplexy, paralysis, sensory or speech disturbances, faintness, and strong fevers accompanied by headaches, stridor, generalized aching, and excessive thirst.

Uses
    Apoplexy, abnormal softening of the cerebrum, hypertension, neuralgia, partial paralysis, facial palsy, arthritis, edema, and bronchitis.

Hsuan-fu-hua-tai-che-shih-tang
(Inula and Hematite Combination)

Main Herbs

3.0g inula	5.0g pinellia
2.0g licorice	3.0g jujube
3.0g hematite	4.0g ginger
2.0g ginseng	

Effects

Treats gastrointestinal weakness and stagnant water that has brought about obstruction and hardening beneath the heart, together with flushing up, heartburn, vomiting, frequent belching, and a weak pulse, in addition to a weak conformation.

Uses

Stomach diseases: gastrectasia, gastric atonia, gastroptosis, gastritis, gastric ulcer, gastric cancer, constriction of the pyloric part of the stomach, severe vomiting during pregnancy, and vomiting in children.

Huang-chi-chien-chung-tang
(Astragalus Combination)

Main Herbs

6.0g paeonia	3.0g jujube	1.5g astragalus
3.0g cinnamon	3.0g licorice	20.0g maltose
3.0g ginger		

Effects

Used for a *Hsiao-chien-chung-tang* conformation: patients, especially children, with a delicate constitution who also have spontaneous sweating, night sweats, abdominal spasms, abdominal pain, cardiac palpitations, adynamia, fatigue, dry skin, and suppurative swelling.

Uses

Weakness during convalescence, night sweats, chronic middle ear inflammation, cervic glandular tuberculosis, abscesses, chronic ulceration, hemorrhoidal fistula, carbuncles, furuncles, and bone gangrene.

Huang-chi-pieh-chia-tang
(Astragalus and Tortoise Shell Combination)

Main Herbs

2.0g bupleurum
2.0g astragalus
2.0g tortoise shell
2.0g paeonia
2.0g rehmannia
3.0g asparagus
3.0g hoelen
1.0g ginseng
1.0g morus

1.0g pinellia
1.0g platycodon
1.0g cinnamon
1.5g lycium bark
1.5g anemarrhean
1.5g *chin-chiu*
1.5g aster
1.0g licorice

Effects

Used for treating a chronic cough; remittent, continuous, or wasting fever following a thoracic disease; aggravation of a common cold that causes weakness and fatiguing fever in tuberculosis patients; or a lingering mild fever after antibiotic treatment.

Uses

Pulmonary tuberculosis, chronic bronchitis, pneumonia, and chronic malaria.

Huang-chin-chia-pan-hsia-sheng-chiang-tang
(Scute, Pinellia, and Ginger Combination)

Main Herbs

4.0g scute
3.0g paeonia
3.0g licorice

4.0g jujube
5.0g pinellia
3.0g ginger

Effects

Used for treating patients with a *Huang-chin-tang* conformation accompanied by vomiting and nausea.

Uses

Acute gastroenteritis.

Huang-chin-tang
(Scute and Licorice Combination)

Main Herbs
    4.0g scute   3.0g licorice
    3.0g paeonia   4.0g jujube

Effects
Used for treating diarrhea, obstruction beneath the heart, abdominal spasms, fever, headaches, vomiting, dry heaves, and excessive thirst.

Uses
Acute enteritis, colitis, indigestion, acute appendicitis, abdominal pain due to inflammation of the ancillary organs of the uterus, and hemoptysis and nosebleeds due to vicarious menstruation.

Huang-lien-ah-chiao-tang
(Coptis and Gelatin Combination)

Main Herbs
    3.0g coptis   2.5g paeonia
    3.0g gelatin   one egg yolk
    2.0g scute

Effects
Good for treating weak conformations with cardiac palpitations, chest discomfort, and insomnia; it can also be used for geriatric insomnia, hemorrhaging from various conditions, diarrhea, and skin diseases.

Uses
Insomnia, neurosis, schizophrenia, hemorrhage, pneumonia, typhoid fever, scarlet fever, cerebral hemorrhage, and itching.

Huang-lien-chieh-tu-tang
(Coptis and Scute Combination)

Main Herbs

1.5g coptis	3.0g scute
1.5g phellodendron	2.0g gardenia

Effects

Used for treating congestion, emotional instability, inflammation, anxiety, hemorrhage, submerged and forceful pulse, subcardiac distention and resistance.

Uses

Febrile diseases, hemoptysis, nosebleeds, hematuria, melena, climacteric disorders, anxiety, cardiac palpitations, insomnia, neurasthenia, hysteria, hives, itching, apoplexy, and hypertension.

Huang-lien-tang
(Coptis Combination)

Main Herbs

3.0g coptis	3.0g cinnamon
3.0g licorice	3.0g jujube
3.0g ginger	6.0g pinellia
3.0g ginseng	

Effects

Used for treating obstruction and distention beneath the heart, a feeling of pressure, loss of appetite, nausea, vomiting, thoracic fever, gastric chills, abdominal pain, halitosis, and yellowish white fur on the tongue.

Uses

Acute gastroenteritis, gastrosia, hangover, inflammation of the mouth, cholera, diarrhea, abdominal pain, acute poisoning, and climacteric disorders.

Huang-tu-tang
(Fu-lung-kan Combination)

Main Herbs

7.0g *fu-lung-kan*	3.0g atractylodes
3.0g gelatin	2.0g licorice
3.0g rehmannia	0.5-1.0g aconite
3.0g scute	

Effects

Used for treating hemorrhaging, hemoptysis, and nosebleeds in patients with a delicate constitution and coarse skin, a weak abdomen, flushing up, restlessness, a sensation of heat in the palms, generalized fever, chillphobia, decreased urine, abdominal pain, and diarrhea.

Uses

Intestinal bleeding, anal bleeding, hemorrhoids, clear urine, rectal ulcer, rectal cancer, endometritis, uterine bleeding, nosebleeds, autonomic nervous disorders, amnesia, insomnia, and epilepsy.

Huo-hsiang-cheng-chi-san
(Agastache Formula)

Main Herbs

1.0g agastache	1.5g angelica
3.0g atractylodes	1.0g perilla
3.0g pinellia	1.0g areca
3.0g hoelen	1.0g jujube
2.0g magnolia bark	1.0g ginger
2.0g citrus	1.0g licorice
1.5g platycodon	

Effects

Used for treating internal injuries caused by eating or drinking raw, cold foods; and caused by external contraction of the wind, cold air "evils" that brings about gastrointestinal weakness,

headaches, stagnancy beneath the heart, vomiting, diarrhea, pain in the heart and abdomen, anhidrosis, forceful abdomen and pulse.
Uses
Common cold in the summer, acute gastroenteritis, diarrhea in the summer, heatstroke, vomiting, abdominal pain of emotional origin after childbirth, warts, children's coughs due to stagnant food, eye diseases, toothache, and sore throat.

I-kan-san
(Bupleurum Formula)

Main Herbs

4.0g atractylodes	3.0g gambir
4.0g hoelen	2.0g bupleurum
3.0g *tang-kuei*	1.5g licorice
3.0g cnidium	

Effects
Used for treating irascibility and irritability due to excessive liver *ch'i;* nervousness; excitability; insomnia due to hepatic hyperfunction; and epilepsy.
Uses
Neurosis, epilepsy, hysteria, insomnia, night crying of children, febrile disease, climacteric disorders, rickets, and spasms.

I-kan-san-chia-chen-pi-pan-hsia
(Bupleurum, Pinellia, and Citrus Formula)

Main Herbs

3.0g *tang-kuei*	4.0g atractylodes	1.5g licorice
3.0g gambir	4.0g hoelen	3.0g citrus
3.0g cnidium	2.0g bupleurum	5.0g pinellia

Effects
Indicated for adults with obvious pyschological problems, a weak pulse and abdomen, and strong palpitations from the left

side of the navel to beneath the heart, and for epileptic children.
Uses
Neurasthenia, hysteria, menopausal disorders, fear of the dark, insomnia, gout, atrophied limbs, "morning sickness".

I-tzu-tang
(Cimicifuga Combination)

Main Herbs
    1.5g cimicifuga   5.0g bupleurum
    6.0g *tang-kuei*   3.0g scute
    1.0g rhubarb   2.0g licorice

Effects
This formula is specifically for hemorrhoids. It is effective for constipation with bleeding and severe localized pain.

Uses
Hemorrhoidal pain, anal fissure, hemorrhoidal bleeding, prolapse of the rectum, and pudendal itching in women.

I-yi-fu-tzu-pai-chiang-tang
(Coix, Aconite, and Thlaspi Combination)

Main Herbs
    10.0g coix   0.5-1.0g aconite
    3.0g thlaspi

Effects
Used for treating tumors of the intestines, a condition equivalent to today's appendicitis, in weak-conformation patients with the symptoms of dry, scaly abdominal skin, spastic and lax abdominal wall, weak and quick pulse, no fever, pale facial complexion, and general weakness.

Uses
Appendicitis, local peritonitis, suppurative inflammation in accessory organs, hemorrhoidal fistula, eruptions on the palms, fungal diseases, warts, and leukorrhea.

I-yi-jen-tang
(Coix Combination)

Main Herbs

4.0g *ma-huang*   4.0g atractylodes
3.0g cinnamon   2.0g licorice
4.0g *tang-kuei*   8.0g coix
3.0g paeonia

Effects

Used for correcting disorders of blood circulation, dispelling fluids effused and accumulated in the joints and tissues, and relieving muscular tension.

Uses

Polyarthritic rheumatism, serious arthritis, tubercular arthritis, muscular rheumatism, beriberi, nephritis, pulmonary edema, and moist pleurisy.

Jen-sheng-tang
(Ginseng and Ginger Combination)

Main Herbs

3.0g ginseng   3.0g atractylodes
3.0g ginger   3.0g licorice

Effects

Used for gastrointestinal weakness, pallor, moist tongue without coating, polyuria, proneness toward fatigue and cold arms and legs, loose stools, frequent vomiting, headache with fever, body aches, edema, insomnia, spitting of blood, and intestinal bleeding. In addition, it is effective as a demulcent when treating excessive salivation and chills in the chest occurring during convalescence.

Uses
Acute and chronic gastroenteritis, gastric weakness, prolapsed stomach, dilatation of the stomach (gastrectasia), pernicious vomiting, excessive salivation, peptic ulcers, diarrhea, tapeworm, dyspepsia, mild labor pains, contraception, intoxication, diabetes, aching shoulders, cholera, hemorrhoidal bleeding, uterine bleeding, leukorrhea, and sneezing from a common cold.

Jun-chang-tang
(Linum and Rhubarb Combination)

Main Herbs

3.0g tang-kuei	2.0g chih-shih
3.0g rehmannia	2.0g scute
3.0g raw rehmannia	2.0g magnolia bark
2.0g linum	2.0g rhubarb
2.0g persica	1.5g licorice
2.0g apricot seed	

Effects
Used for treating habitual constipation due to lack of mucilage in the large intestine.

Uses
Habitual constipation, geriatric constipation, and constipation due to hypertension; arteriosclerosis; and chronic nephritis.

Kan-mai-ta-tsao-tang
(Licorice and Jujube Combination)

Main Herbs

5.0g licorice	6.0g jujube
20.0g wheat	

Effects
Good for treating overexcitement, spasms, hysteria, nervousness, insomnia, emotional instability, and frequent uncontrollable yawning.

Uses

Hysteria, nervous exhaustion, neurosis, insomnia, epilepsy, muscular twitching, sleep walking, gastrointestinal spasms, uterine cramping, spasmodic coughing, and night crying in children.

Kan-tsao-fu-tzu-tang
(Licorice and Aconite Combination)

Main Herbs
    2.0g licorice   4.0g white atractylodes
    0.5-1.0g aconite   3.5g cinnamon

Effects

Used for treating severe arthralgia, rheumatism, swelling in the joints, "water posioning", and difficult or painful urination.

Uses

Rheumatoid arthritis, neuralgia, arthritis, periostitis, influenza, lower back pain, and pain in a tendon.

Kan-tsao-hsieh-hsin-tang
(Licorice and Pinellia Combination)

Main Herbs
    3.5g licorice   2.5g ginger
    5.0g pinellia   2.5g jujube
    2.5g ginseng   1.0g coptis
    2.5g scute

Effects

Used for treating distention beneath the heart, gas, diarrhea, nausea, stress, and mental instability.

Uses

Gastroenteritis, hysteria, nervous exhaustion, insomnia, sleep walking, and inflammation of the mouth (stomatitis).

Kan-tsao-kan-chiang-tang
(Licorice and Ginger Combination)

Main Herbs
    4.0g licorice   2.0g ginger

Effects
    Good for treating cold arms and legs, irritability, dryness of the mouth, hiccups and vomiting; usually given to persons with cold conformation; frequent urination; copious, thin saliva; cold arms and legs; and vertigo or to a woman with uterine bleeding and weak postpartum pains.

Uses
    Frequent urination in the aged and debilitated, bed wetting, atrophy of the kidneys, urethritis, hypersalivation, infantile slobbering, atonic uterine bleeding, weak postpartum pains, vertigo, and hiccups.

Kan-tsao-tang
(Licorice Combination)

Main Herbs
    8.0g licorice

Effects
    Used for treating severe pain in the throat, abdominal pain, and coughs.

Uses
    Acute laryngitis, gastric spasms, spasmodic cough, hoarseness, recurrent abdominal pain, toothache, kidney failure, difficult urination, pain from carbuncles, and food poisoning.

Ko-ken-chia-pan-hsia-tang
(Pueraria and Pinellia Combination)

Main Herbs

4.0g pueraria	2.0g cinnamon
3.0g *ma-huang*	2.0g paeonia
3.0g ginger	2.0g licorice
3.0g jujube	8.0g pinellia

Effects

Used for patients with a *Ko-ken-tang* conformation accompanied by vomiting and nausea.

Ko-ken-huang-lien-huang-chin-tang
(Pueraria, Coptis, and Scute Combination)

Main Herbs

6.0g pueraria	3.0g scute
3.0g coptis	2.0g licorice

Effects

Used for treating generalized fever, diarrhea, annoying fever in the chest, excessive thirst, gasping, and excessive sweating.

Uses

Dysentery, infectious diarrhea, acute gastroenteritis, influenza of gastrointestinal type, asthma, hangover, fever after moxibustion or burns, erysipelas, measles, ophthalmic disorders, toothaches, inflammation of the mouth, and hypertension.

Ko-ken-tang
(Pueraria Combination)

Main Herbs

8.0g pueraria	4.0g jujube

4.0g *ma-huang* 2.0g licorice
3.0g cinnamon 1.0g ginger
3.0g paeonia

Effects

Used for treating colds with or without fever, chillphobia, floating and forceful pulse, tension in the neck and back, inflammation, congestion, diarrhea, and acute muscular spasms.

Uses

1. Common cold, influenza, pneumonia, bronchitis, and headaches.
2. Stiff shoulders, forty-years' wrist, fifty-years' shoulders, and neuralgia.
3. Skin diseases, eczema, hives, measles, furuncles, and boils.
4. Skin eruptions, styes, conjunctivitis, and trachoma.
5. Inflammation of the middle ear, runny nose, stuffy nose, and inflammation of the external ear.
6. Meningitis, lymphadenitis, mastitis, and scarlet fever.

Kou-teng-san
(Gambir Formula)

Main Herbs

3.0g gambir 2.0g siler
3.0g aurantium 2.0g chrysanthemum
3.0g pinellia 5.0g gypsum
3.0g ophiopogon 1.0g licorice
3.0g hoelen 1.0g ginger
2.0g ginseng

Effects

Used for treating emotionally disturbed middle-aged patients who have headaches, vertigo, irritability, ocular hyperemia, flushing up, insomnia, obstruction beneath the heart, stiff shoulders, and spasms in the shoulders and back.

Uses

Neurosis, headache, vertigo, pain in shoulders, climacteric disorders, arteriosclerosis, hypertension, chronic nephritis, and cerebral arteriosclerosis.

Kua-lu-chih-shih-tang
(Trichosanthes and Chih-shih Combination)

Main Herbs

3.0g *tang-kuei*	2.0g scute
3.0g hoelen	2.0g ginger
3.0g fritillary	1.0g cardamon
2.0g trichosanthes seed	1.0g *chih-shih*
2.0g platycodon	1.0g bamboo
2.0g citrus	1.0g saussurea
1.0g gardenia	1.0g licorice

Effects
Used for treating fever in stomach and dry and thick sputum.

Uses
Acute bronchitis, pneumonia, pleuritis, intercostal neuralgia, asthma, asthmatic bronchitis, pulmonary emphysema, pulmonary tuberculosis, apoplexy, cough due to smoking, dry thick sputum due to arteriosclerosis, angina pectoris, gastrosia, stiff shoulders, hypertension, and speech impairment due to brain lesion.

Kuei-chih-chia-fu-tzu-tang
(Cinnamon and Aconite Combination)

Main Herbs

4.0g cinnamon	4.0g ginger
4.0g paeonia	4.0g jujube
2.0g licorice	0.5-1.0g aconite

Effects
Used for treating incessant sweating, severe anemophobia, painful urination, muscular spasms of the arms and legs, neuralgia, and arthralgia.

Uses
Common cold, neuralgia, arthralgia, migraines, chilling abdominal pain, partial paralysis, rheumatism, purpura, spasms, poliomyelitis, impotence, postpartum hyperephidrosis (excessive sweating), cold arms and legs.

Kuei-chih-chia-huang-chi-tang
(Cinnamon and Astragalus Combination)

Main Herbs

    3.0g astragalus   4.0g ginger
    4.0g cinnamon   4.0g jujube
    4.0g paeonia   2.0g licorice

Effects

Used for treating sweating in the upper body but lack of sweating in the lower body, dragging pain in the waist and legs, nonspecific pain, anxiety, painful urination, jaundice, superficial moisture, flaccid skin, night sweats, and numbness.

Uses

The common cold in people with a delicate constitution; skin diseases; night sweats; inflammation of the middle ear; facial numbness; jaundice; and "yellow sweating".

Kuei-chih-chia-ko-ken-tang
(Cinnamon and Pueraria Combination)

Main Herbs

    4.0g cinnamon   4.0g ginger
    4.0g paeonia   2.0g licorice
    4.0g jujube   5.0g pueraria

Effects

Used when the patient has a *Kuei-chih-tang* conformation with tension in the neck and back.

Uses

Common cold, various fever diseases in the initial stage, neuralgia, rheumatism, conjunctivitis, stiff shoulders especially in the elderly.

Kuei-chih-chia-ling-chu-fu-tang
(Cinnamon and Atractylodes Combination)

Main Herbs

4.0g cinnamon	1.5g licorice
3.0g paeonia	0.5-1.0g aconite
3.0g ginger	5.0g hoelen
3.0g jujube	5.0g atractylodes

Effects

Used for treating headaches, chillphobia, spontaneous sweating, painful urination, mild spasms in the arms and legs, neuralgia, and arthralgia.

Uses

Paralysis following a stroke, arthritis, arthralgia, and neuralgia.

Kuei-chih-chia-lung-ku-mu-li-tang
(Cinnamon and Dragon Bone Combination)

Main Herbs

4.0g cinnamon	3.0g oyster shell
4.0g paeonia	2.0g licorice
4.0g ginger	4.0g jujube
3.0g dragon bone	

Effects

Used for treating persons whose physical strength is deteriorating and who have recurring fever, headaches, vertigo, spontaneous sweating, night sweats, insomnia, hyperfunctional cardiac palpitations, spasms in the lower abdomen, cold genitals, nocturnal emissions, excitability, and fatigability.

Uses

Genital neurasthenia, nervousness, palpitations, insomnia, incontinence, bed wetting, premature ejaculation.

Kuei-chih-chia-shao-yao-ta-huang-tang
(Cinnamon, Paeonia, and Rhubarb Combination)

Main Herbs
- 4.0g cinnamon
- 4.0g ginger
- 4.0g jujube
- 2.0g licorice
- 6.0g paeonia
- 1.0g rhubarb

Effects

Used for unresolved "superficial evil", fever with chillphobia, abdominal distention, constipation with severe pain, and straining due to diarrhea.

Uses

Colitis, chronic peritonitis, febrile dysentery, dysentery, intestinal colic, constipation, food poisoning, and indigestion.

Kuei-chih-chia-shao-yao-tang
(Cinnamon and Paeonia Combination)

Main Herbs
- 6.0g paeonia
- 4.0g cinnamon
- 4.0g ginger
- 4.0g jujube
- 2.0g licorice

Effects

Used for treating persons of a delicate constitution with abdominal pain, diarrhea, abdominal distention, and spasms in the abdominal straight muscles.

Uses

Abdominal pain, diarrhea, enteritis, appendicitis, food poisoning, abdominal pain from inflammation of the abdominal lining.

Kuei-chih-chu-shao-yao-chia-ma-huang-fu-tzu-hsi-hsin-tang
(Cinnamon, Ma-huang, Aconite, and Asarum Combination)

Main Herbs

4.0g cinnamon	4.0g *ma-huang*
4.0g jujube	3.0g asarum
4.0g ginger	0.5g aconite
2.0g licorice	

Effects
Used for hardening as large as a plate beneath the heart.

Uses
Various geriatric disorders, emaciation, and chronic diseases; bronchitis; asthma; common cold; neuralgia; rheumatism; lower back pain; breast cancer; spleen hemorrhage; sinusitis maxillaris; acute infectious disease; edema; and partial paralysis.

Kuei-chih-chu-shao-yao-chia-shu-chi-lung-ku-mu-li-chiu-ni-tang
(Cinnamon, Dichroa, Dragon Bone, and Oyster Shell Combination)

Main Herbs

4.0g cinnamon	5.0g dragon bone
4.0g ginger	4.0g jujube
4.0g dichroa	2.0g licorice
6.0g oyster shell	

Effects
Used for treating symptoms resulting from heat therapy (pyrotherapy) such as sweating or lack of sweating, mental instability, terror, psychotic behavior, absent-mindedness, coma, and delirium. Usually the patients have shallow respiration, decreased urine, and even bloody urine.

Uses
Burns, scalds, sunburns, neurotic disorders, and fevers due to moxibustion.

Kuei-chih-fu-ling-wan
(Cinnamon and Hoelen Formula)

Main Herbs

    4.0g cinnamon   4.0g persica
    4.0g hoelen   4.0g moutan
    4.0g paeonia

Effects

Given to those with a strong constitution and a flushed face; firm abdomen; pain when palpated at the umbilicus; tense and submerged, slow pulse; headaches; stiff shoulders, vertigo; and cold feet.

Uses

1. Gynecological diseases: endometritis, ovaritis, inflammation of the oviduct, uterine tumors, climacteric disorders, menstrual irregularity, abnormal leukorrhea, lower back pain, stiff shoulders and headaches.
2. Skin diseases: eczema, hives, dermatitis, black spots, pimples, and frigorism (condition caused by long exposure to cold).
3. Mental disorders: nervousness, neurosis, and hysteria.
4. Eye diseases: styes, effusion of blood into the eye (hemophthalmia), inflammation of the eyelids and the cornea.
5. Other ailments: enlarged prostate, hypertension, arthritis, neuralgia, and rheumatism.

Kuei-chih-jen-sheng-tang
(Cinnamon and Ginseng Combination)

Main Herbs

    4.0g cinnamon   2.0g ginger
    3.0g licorice   3.0g atractylodes
    3.0g ginseng

Effects

Used for warming the body and "resolving surface symptoms" and for headaches, fever, sweating, anemophobia, diarrhea, obstruction and hardening beneath the heart, pain in the heart and abdomen, palpitations beneath the heart, weak limbs, cold feet, and frequent urination.

Uses

Acute gastroenteritis, neurotic palpitations, heart disorders, habitual headaches, common colds, and influenza.

Kuei-chih-tang
(Cinnamon Combination)

Main Herbs

4.0g cinnamon	2.0g licorice
4.0g ginger	4.0g jujube
4.0g paeonia	

Effects

Used for stimulating blood circulation, warming the body, and strengthening the interior organs.

Uses

Common cold, neuralgia, headaches, abdominal pain due to chill, delicate constitution, "morning sickness", and neurasthenia.

Kuei-pi-tang
(Ginseng and Longan Combination)

Main Herbs

2.0g astragalus	2.0g *tang-kuei*
3.0g ginseng	1.0g ginger
3.0g atractylodes	1.0g jujube
3.0g hoelen	1.0g polygala
3.0g zizyphus	1.0g licorice
3.0g longan	1.0g saussurea

Effects

Used for treating patients with a weak conformation with

anemia, cardiac palpitations, amnesia, insomnia, hemorrhage, pallor, eroded vitality, fatigability, weak gastrointestinal, post-illness weakness, and frequent fever in whom other tonics cause stomach discomfort.

Uses

Anemia, hemorrhages, amnesia, insomnia, neurasthenia, neurotic palpitations, gastric ulcers, leukemia, menstrual irregularities, uterine cancer, endometritis, itching and burning in the vagina, involuntary emission, impotence, and chronic gonorrhea.

Li-ke-tang
(Pinellia and Gardenia Combination)

Main Herbs
    8.0g pinellia   0.5-1.0g aconite
    3.0g gardenia

Effects

Used for the treatment of stricture of the middle section of the esophagus which results in impairment of speech, vomiting, sticky sputum, and thirst.

Uses

Esophageal cancer, gastric cancer, esophageal stenosis, esophageal polyps, throat obstructions, and pain.

Liang-chih-tang
(Galanga and Chih-shih Combination)

Main Herbs
    6.0g hoelen   2.0g licorice
    6.0g pinellia   1.0g galanga
    4.0g cinnamon   2.0g *chih-shih*
    4.0g jujube

Effects

Used for subcardiac or abdominal convulsive pain accom-

panied by vomiting.
Uses
Gastrectasis, gastric ulcers, duodenal ulcers, gastric cancer, gastroptosis, gallstones, pancreatitis.

Lien-chu-yin
(Tang-kuei and Atractylodes Combination)

Main Herbs

    5.0g hoelen   3.0g paeonia
    4.0g cinnamon   3.0g rehmannia
    3.0g *tang-kuei*   3.0g atractylodes
    3.0g cnidium   2.0g licorice

Effects

Used for all the symptoms derived from anemia such as palpitations, vertigo, ringing in the ears, tinnitus, and facial edema. It may also be used for uterine bleeding, and hemorrhoidal bleeding in the male; it is contraindicated for serious anemia or gastrointestinal weakness that tends to cause diarrhea.

Uses

Anemia, palpitations and tinnitus, valvular diseases, chlorosis due to anemia, and anemia because of worms in the duodenum.

Ling-chiang-chu-kan-tang
(Ginger and Hoelen Combination)

Main Herbs

    6.0g hoelen   3.0g atractylodes
    3.0g ginger   2.0g licorice

Effects

Used for treating chilling in lower portion of the body—from the waist to the feet — clear urine, frequent urination and a feeling of extreme heaviness of the body, especially in the abdominal wall.

Uses
Lower back pain, sciatica, leukorrhea, and bed wetting.

Ling-kan-chiang-wei-hsin-hsia-jen-huang-tang
(Hoelen, Schizandra, and Rhubarb Combination)

Main Herbs
Ling-kan-chiang-wei-hsin-hsia-jen-tang with rhubarb
Effects
Used for treating patients with a *Ling-kan-chiang-wei-hsin-hsia-jen-tang* conformation who have constipation, flushing up, and a drunkard's face.

Ling-kan-chiang-wei-hsin-hsia-jen-tang
(Hoelen and Schizandra Combination)

Main Herbs
4.0g hoelen	2.0g ginger
4.0g pinellia	2.0g asarum
4.0g apricot seed	3.0g schizandra
2.0g licorice	

Effects
Used for treating stridor; cough; dropsy; a proneness to anemia; a submerged and weak pulse; cold hands and feet in the absence of such surface symptoms as fever, severe chills, headache and generalized pain; and the condition of chronic weakness.
Uses
Acute and chronic bronchitis, bronchial asthma, pulmonary emphysema, edema, ascites, chronic nephritis, atrophied kidney, effusive pleurisy, pulmonary edema, beriberi, and cardiac asthma.

Ling-kuei-chu-kan-tang
(Atractylodes and Hoelen Combination)

Main Herbs
    6.0g hoelen   3.0g atractylodes
    4.0g cinnamon   2.0g licorice

Effects
    Used for palpitations, increased respiratory rate, distention in the chest near the heart, vertigo upon standing, decreased urine, mild edema, headaches, cold feet, a submerged pulse, a weak abdomen, and flushing up due to water toxin.

Uses
1. Nervous disorders: neurasthenia, general nervousness, hysteria, cardiac palpitations, instability of the autonomic nervous system, and motion sickness.
2. Heart disease: valvular disease, cardiac asthma, neurogenic palpitations.
3. Eye ailments: conjunctivitis, chronic optic nerve disorders, optic nerve atrophy, and nebula.
4. Kidney disease: chronic nephritis, severe generalized edema, and renal atrophy.
5. Miscellaneous: hypertension, sinusitis, anemia, rhinitis, hyperthyroidism.

Ling-kuei-kan-tsao-tang
(Hoelen, Licorice, and Jujube Combination)

Main Herbs
    4.0g cinnamon   6.0g hoelen
    2.0g licorice   4.0g jujube

Effects
    Used for treating hysterical, rapid heart palpitations, hyperventilation, and severe abdominal pain.

Uses
    Cardiac disorders, neurotic palpitations, neurasthenia, hysteria, uterine spasms, gastric spasms, and epilepsy.

Ling-kuei-wei-kan-tang
(Hoelen, Licorice, and Schizandra Combination)

Main Herbs
- 6.0g hoelen
- 4.0g cinnamon
- 3.0g schizandra
- 2.0g licorice

Effects
Used for treating patients with cold arms and legs, flushing up, ruddy facial complexion, and dizziness together with cough and cardiac hyperfunction, a submerged and small pulse, and decreased urine.

Uses
Bronchitis, exudative inflammation of the middle ear, pulmonary emphysema, edema.

Liu-chun-tzu-tang
(Six Major Herb Combination)

Main Herbs
- 4.0g pinellia
- 4.0g ginseng
- 4.0g atractylodes
- 4.0g hoelen
- 1.0g licorice
- 2.0g citrus
- 2.0g ginger
- 2.0g jujube

Effects
This formula may treat gastrointestinal weakness: stagnant water in the stomach, indigestion, distention beneath the heart, loss of appetite, a tendency to be tired, loss of weight, anemia, a weak abdomen, a weak pulse, and cold hands and feet.

Uses
Chronic gastritis, gastroptosis, gastric distention, gastric ulcer, gastric cancer, chronic peritonitis, indigestion, loss of appetite, rickets, neurotic vomiting, vomiting, toxemia of pregnancy, and nervous exhaustion.

Lung-tan-hsieh-kan-tang
(Gentiana Combination)

Main Herbs

1.0g gentiana	3.0g alisma	1.0g gardenia
5.0g *tang-kuei*	5.0g rehmannia	3.0g plantago
1.0g licorice	5.0g akebia	3.0g scute

Effects

Effective for treating patients with a tense and sensitive zone along the outer sides of the rectus abdominis muscle and the symptoms of pain in the ribs; ocular, lingual and oral hyperemia; deafness; swollen ears; blood in the urine; gonorrhea; swelling and itching in the genital areas; abnormal leukorrhea; yellow-coated tongue, chordal and quick pulse; and redness on the edge of the tongue.

Uses

Urethritis, cystitis, endometritis, vaginitis, leukorrhea, pudendal itching and pain, chancre, bubo, inflammation of a testis, and pudendal eczema.

Ma-hsing-i-kan-tang
(Ma-huang and Coix Combination)

Main Herbs

4.0g *ma-huang*	2.0g licorice
3.0g apricot seed	10.0g coix

Effects

Used for treating rheumatics who suffer from generalized pain and a high fever in the evening.

Uses

Muscular rheumatism, arthritic rheumatism, neuralgia, warts, calluses and skin eruptions on the hands or feet, frostbite, eczema, dandruff, and asthma.

Ma-hsing-kan-shih-tang
(Ma-huang and Apricot Seed Combination)

Main Herbs
    4.0g *ma-huang*   2.0g licorice
    4.0g apricot seed   10.0g gypsum

Effects
    Used for treating fever due to stagnant heat in the lungs and thirst, or cough, and a floating, quick pulse in the presence or absence of sweating.

Uses
    Common cold, pneumonia, bronchitis, bronchial asthma, cardiac asthma, whooping cough, diphtheria, measles, and hemorrhoids.

Ma-huang-chia-chu-tang
(Ma-huang and Atractylodes Combination)

Main Herbs
    5.0g *ma-huang*   1.5g licorice
    5.0g apricot seed   4.0g cinnamon
    5.0g atractylodes

Effects
    Effective for patients with a *Ma-huang-tang* conformation accompanied by fever, chillphobia, anhidrosis, generalized aching, pain in muscles and joints, edema, and frequent urination.

Uses
    Rheumatic pain, arthralgia, acute nephritis, renal cirrhosis, edema, intoxication from carbonic oxide, habitual spontaneous abortions, nasal suppuration, and hypertrophic rhinitis.

Ma-huang-hsi-hsin-fu-tzu-tang
(Ma-huang, Aconite, and Asarum Combination)

Main Herbs
    4.0g *ma-huang*   0.5-1.0g aconite
    3.0g asarum

Effects
Used for the symptoms of chillphobia, mild fever, submerged and thin pulse, generalized lassitude, weakness, and somnolence.

Uses
Feeble and geriatric patients who have a common cold, influenza, bronchitis, bronchial asthma, pneumonia, rhinitis, sinusitis maxillaris, trigeminalgia, and headaches from the wind and cold.

Ma-huang-tang
(Ma-huang Combination)

Main Herbs
    5.0g *ma-huang*   5.0g apricot seed
    4.0g cinnamon   1.5g licorice

Effects
Used for external fevers and a firm conformation of greater yang disease exhibiting the symptoms of anhidrosis, floating and tense pulse, common cold, headaches, fever, anemophobia, generalized aching, chest distention, cough, and asthma.

Uses
Common cold, influenza, typhoid fever, pneumonia, bronchitis, bronchial asthma, measles, rhinitis, stuffy nose, neurosis, bed wetting, cystitis, arthritic rheumatism, and weak pain.

Ma-tzu-jen-wan
(Linum and Apricot Seed Formula)

Main Herbs
    5.0g linum   2.0g *chih-shih*
    4.0g rhubarb   2.0g magnolia bark
    2.0g paeonia   2.0g apricot seed

Effects
Effective for gastrointestinal heat, dry stools, frequent urination, floating and harsh pulse, hemorrhoids, and constipation.

Uses
Habitual constipation, geriatric constipation, bed wetting, frequent urination, constipation due to atrophic kidneys, and hemorrhoids.

Mai-men-tung-tang
(Ophiopogon Combination)

Main Herbs
    10.0g ophiopogon   2.0g ginseng
    3.0g jujube   5.0g pinellia
    5.0g oryza   2.0g licorice

Effects
Used for treating spasmodic coughing due to the flushing up of *ch'i*.

Uses
Bronchitis, bronchial asthma, pneumonia, laryngitis, whooping cough, tuberculosis of the pharynx, pulmonary tuberculosis, hoarseness, diabetes, hypertension and arteriosclerosis.

Mai-men-tung-yin-tzu
(Ophiopogon and Trichosanthes Combination)

Main Herbs

7.0g ophiopogon	2.0g trichosanthes root
3.0g pueraria	6.0g hoelen
1.0g licorice	1.0g bamboo leaves
2.0g ginseng	3.0g anemarrhena
4.0g rehmannia	1.0g schizandra

Effects

Used for nourishing "dry blood" and quenching thirst due to diabetes, and treating polyuria, emaciation, coarse skin, lack of energy in diabetics, coughing in those suffering from diabetes associated with tuberculosis, and night coughing in the elderly.

Uses

Coarse skin due to diabetes, chronic bronchitis, and pulmonary tuberculosis.

Mu-fang-chi-chu-shih-kao-chia-fu-ling-mang-hsiao-tang
(Stephania and Ginseng Combination without Gypsum and incorporating Hoelen and Mirabilitum)

Main Herbs

4.0g stephania	4.0g hoelen
3.0g cinnamon	5.0g mirabilitum
3.0g ginseng	

Effects

Used for patients with a *Mu-fang-chi-tang* conformation whose symptoms have returned after being ameliorated.

Mu-fang-chi-tang
(Stephania and Ginseng Combination)

Main Herbs
- 4.0g stephania
- 10.0g gypsum
- 3.0g cinnamon
- 3.0g ginseng

Effects
Used for treating heart trouble, stagnant water in the chest, rapid breathing, asthma, palpitations, distention beneath the heart, abdominal pain, painful urination, and a submerged and tight pulse.

Uses
Valvular diseases, heart trouble, cardiac asthma, nephritis, edema, beriberi, and bronchial asthma.

Pa-chen-tang
(Tang-kuei and Ginseng Eight Combination)

Main Herbs
- 3.0g *tang-kuei*
- 3.0g paeonia
- 3.0g cnidium
- 3.0g rehmannia
- 3.0g ginseng
- 3.0g atractylodes
- 3.0g hoelen
- 1.5g licorice
- 1.5g jujube
- 1.5g ginger

Effects
Used for treating weakness in both blood and *ch'i*, general weakness, emaciation, anemia, and weak stomach and intestines.

Uses
Weakness during convalescence, anemia, lower back pain in women, menstrual irregularity, and climacteric disorders.

Pa-wei-tai-hsia-fang
(Tang-kuei and Eight Herb Formula)

Main Herbs

5.0g *tang-kuei*	4.0g smilax
3.0g cnidium	2.0g citrus
3.0g hoelen	1.0g lonicera
3.0g akebia	1.0g rhubarb

Effects

Good for treating abnormal leukorrhea (discharge from the vagina) with "moist heat", mild anemia, subacute inflammation, and congestion.

Uses

Malodorous, purulent leukorrhea; and gonorrheal leukorrhea.

Pa-wei-wan
(Rehmannia Eight Formula)

Main Herbs

5.0g rehmannia	1.0g aconite
3.0g hoelen	3.0g moutan
1.0g cinnamon	3.0g dioscorea
3.0g alisma	3.0g cornus

Effects

This formula reactivates degenerated kidneys, adrenal glands, and reproductive organs, and acts as a preventative of and a remedy for senility. It is given to patients with severe fatigue and lassitude; sluggish gastrointestinal function; constipation; painful, frequent, or difficult urination; cold or feverish arms and legs; thirst accompanied by a dry tongue; lower back pain; weakness beneath the umbilicus; and hardness and tenseness in the pelvic area.

Uses

1. Nephritis: nephrosclerosis, nephrolithiasis, nephrotuberculosis, pyelitis (nephro-atrophy), albuminuria, and edema.

2. Cystitis, cystolithiases, cysto-tuberculosis, senile cysto-atrophy, enlarged prostrate, painful urination, urinary incontinence, and nocturia.
3. Diabetes and urinary incontinence.
4. Cerebral hemorrhage, arteriosclerosis, hypertension, and hypotension.
5. Psychological neurasthenia, anmnesia, nocturnal emissions, uncontrolled emissions, impotence, and involuntary erection.
6. Lower back pain, sciatica, deformed vertebra, numbness of the legs, and beriberi.
7. Cataracts, glaucoma, decreased vision, and keratitis.
8. Eczema, fungal disease (tinea), senile itching, vaginal itching, dry skin, and hives.

Pai-hu-chia-jen-sheng-tang
(Ginseng and Gypsum Combination)

Main Herbs
5.0g anemarrhena   10.0g oryza
15.0g gypsum   2.0g licorice
3.0g ginseng

Effects

Given to patients with a *Pai-hu-tang* conformation manifesting the symptom of excessive thirst due to dehydration as a result of high fever.

Uses

Influenza, pneumonia, inflammation of the brain, heatstroke with high fever and thirst, diabetes, cerebral bleeding, hyperthyroidism, dermatitis, hives, eczema, itching, congestion in an infected area, nephritis, uremia, inflammation of the gallbladder, and bed wetting.

Pai-hu-chia-kuei-chih-tang
(Gypsum and Cinnamon Combination)

Main Herbs
    5.0g anemarrhena   2.0g licorice
    8.0g oryza   4.0g cinnamon
    15.0g gypsum

Effects
    Used for patients with a *Pai-hu-tang* conformation who exhibit external symptoms and have a tendency to "flushing up".

Pai-hu-tang
(Gypsum Combination)

Main Herbs
    15.0g gypsum   2.0g licorice
    5.0g anemarrhena   8.0g oryza

Effects
    Treats high fevers and sweating with a flushed face, thirst due to stress, white coating on the tongue, and frequent urination.

Uses
    Common cold, influenza, measles, erysipelas, scarlet fever, typhoid fever and meningitis with high fever, thirst, anxiety, diabetes, emotional disorders, eczema, and itching.

Pai-nung-san
(Platycodon and Chih-shih Formula)

Main Herbs
    5.0g *chih-shih*   2.0g platycodon
    5.0g paeonia

Effects

Effective for treating suppurative swelling together with reddening and pain, tension around a lesion, severe inflammatory infiltration with delayed suppuration, and hardening in the epigastrium with spasm of rectus abdominis muscle.

Uses

Carbuncles, boils, lymphadenitis, felons, subcutaneous abscess, inflammation of a voluntary muscle (myositis), tonsillitis, sinusitis maxillaris, pyorrhea, inflammation of the external ear, hemorrhoids, inflammation of the tissues surrounding the rectum and anus, and mastitis.

Pai-nung-tang
(Platycodon and Jujube Combination)

Main Herbs

3.0g licorice	6.0g jujube
4.0g platycodon	3.0g ginger

Effects

Used for the treatment of all suppurations in patients with a weak conformation during the initial stages of infection (the swelling is not conspicuous), or when the fulmination is over and the condition has become chronic (tension and infiltration of the lesion are not severe and swelling and granules are not rigid, but there is slight suppuration).

Uses

Carbuncles, furuncles, abscesses, suppurative ulcers, inflammation of the middle ear, sinusitis maxillaris, pyorrhea, hemorrhoids, tonsillitis, lung abscess, and lung gangrene.

Pan-hsia-hou-pu-tang
(Pinellia and Magnolia Combination)

Main Herbs
    6.0g pinellia   4.0g ginger
    3.0g magnolia bark   2.0g perilla
    5.0g hoelen

Effects
    Treats neuroses, melancholia, esophageal constriction, intestinal weakness, flaccid muscles and skin, abdominal fullness, and ascites.

Uses
    Neurosis, pyschological neurasthenia, hysteria, nervousness, insomnia, fearfulness, neurotic esophageal constriction, recurrent palpitations, esophageal spasms, bronchitis, hoarseness due to a common cold, asthma, whooping cough, toxemia during pregnancy, blood vessel disorders, gastric laxity, and edema.

Pan-hsia-hsieh-hsin-tang
(Pinellia Combination)

Main Herbs
    6.0g pinellia   3.0g ginseng
    3.0g scute   3.0g licorice
    1.0g coptis   3.0g jujube
    3.0g ginger

Effects
    Treats obstruction and hardening beneath the heart, nausea, vomiting and loss of appetite.

Uses
    Gastritis, enteritis, indigestion, enlargement of the stomach, gastroptosis, gastric ulcer, duodenal ulcer, stomatitis, and motion sickness.

Pan-hsia-pai-chu-tien-ma-tang
(Pinellia and Gastrodia Combination)

Main Herbs

    3.0g pinellia   2.0g *shen-chu*
    3.0g white atractylodes   1.5g astragalus
    3.0g hoelen   1.5g ginseng
    3.0g citrus   1.5g alisma
    3.0g atractylodes   1.0g phellodendron
    3.0g malt   1.0g dried ginger
    2.0g gastrodia   2.0g ginger

Effects

Treats recurrent headaches, gastrointestinal weakness, stagnant gastric fluid, water poisoning, vomiting, vertigo, cold feet, and fatigue.

Uses

Recurrent headaches and vertigo, sleepiness after eating, weak hands and feet, hypertensive headache and vertigo in patients with weak stomachs and intestines, headaches and vertigo due to hypotension, gastric laxity, gastroptosis, and sinusitis maxillaris.

Pien-chih-hsin-chi-yin
(Areca and Evodia Combination)

Main Herbs

    5.0g hoelen   2.0g *chih-shih*
    5.0g pinellia   1.0g morus
    3.0g akebia   1.0g licorice
    2.5g cinnamon   1.0g evodia
    2.5g areca seed   2.0g tortoise shell
    2.0g perilla fruit

Effects

Used for treating cardiac asthma, hardening and water stagnancy or agitation beneath the heart, stiff shoulders and back,

labored breathing, and cardiac palpitations.
Uses
Cardiac asthma, chronic bronchitis, and angina pectoris.

Ping-wei-san
(Magnolia and Ginger Formula)

Main Herbs

4.0g atractylodes	2.0g jujube
3.0g magnolia bark	1.0g licorice
3.0g citrus	1.0g ginger

Effects

Increases digestive absorption and removes stagnant water in the stomach.

Pu-chi-chien-chung-tang
(Magnolia and Alisma Combination)

Main Herbs

4.0g hoelen	3.0g atractylodes	2.0g ophiopogon
4.0g white atractylodes	4.0g ginseng	2.0g scute
3.0g citrus	2.0g alisma	2.0g magnolia bark

Effects

Used for treating edema, ascites, and fullness of the intestines in patients with a weak conformation.

Uses

Edema, ascites, abdominal distention, cirrhosis of the liver, chronic peritonitis, chronic nephritis, and edema due to valvular disease.

Pu-chung-i-chi-tang
(Ginseng and Astragalus Combination)

Main Herbs

4.0g astragalus	2.0g bupleurum
2.0g ginger	3.0g *tang-kuei*
4.0g ginseng	1.5g licorice
2.0g jujube	2.0g citrus
4.0g atractylodes	1.0g cimicifuga

Effects

Used for treating weak pulse, lassitude, weak voice, weak eyesight, mild fever, loss of appetite, headaches, night sweats, decreased gastrointestinal function, and palpitations at the umbilicus.

Uses

Improvement of delicate constitutions, common cold in those with a delicate constitution, peritonitis, pulmonary tuberculosis, gastroptosis, loss of appetite, gastric atonia, emaciation in the summer, neurasthenia, impotence, uterine prolapse, hemorrhoids, rectal prolapse, partial paralysis, abnormal sweating, hernia, chronic gonorrhea, diarrhea, persistent malaria, sinusitis maxillaris, and hemorrhages.

Pu-huan-chin-cheng-chi-san
(Pinellia, Atractylodes, and Agastache Formula)

Main Herbs

4.0g atractylodes	1.0g licorice
3.0g citrus	3.0g ginger
6.0g pinellia	3.0g jujube
1.0g agastache	3.0g magnolia bark

Effects

Used for treating the common cold, "morbid" mountain air, alternating chills and fever, cholera, vomiting, diarrhea, dysentery, and epidemics.

Uses

Acute gastroenteritis, poisoning due to contaminated drinking water, cholera, and acclimation problems.

San-huang-hsieh-hsin-tang
(Coptis and Rhubarb Combination)

Main Herbs
  1.0g rhubarb   1.0g coptis
  1.0g scute

Effects

Good for symptoms of congestion, flushing up, irritability, stiff shoulders, and gastric stagnancy when accompanied by constipation and a forceful pulse.

Uses
1. Habitual constipation, diarrhea, skin disease, hives, contusions, and burns.
2. Vertigo, tinnitus, stiff shoulders, heavy head, headaches, impaired hearing, cardiac palpitations, mental instability, flushing up, and firm conformations.
3. Nervousness, neurosis, epilepsy, anxiety.
4. Hypertension, arteriosclerosis, liver disorders, and the prevention of and recuperation from apoplexy.
5. Hemorrhoids, hemorrhoidal bleeding, intestinal bleeding, blood in the urine or sputum, uterine hemorrhage, and flushing of the face.

San-wu-huang-chin-tang
(Scute Three Herb Combination)

Main Herbs
  3.0g scute   6.0g rehmannia
  3.0g sophora

Effects

Used for treating postpartum fever, stress fever, fatigue, dry tongue, and annoying heat in the palms and feet.

Uses

Postpartum fever, tuberculosis, insomnia, autonomic nerve disorders, stomatitis, hemorrhage during childbirth, hemoptysis, hemorrhage, chilblain, burns, hives, eczema, fungal infections, menopausal disorders, and annoying fever in the palms and feet in summer.

Shao-yao-kan-tsao-fu-tzu-tang
(Paeonia, Licorice, and Aconite Combination)

Main Herbs

3.0g paeonia   0.5-1.0g aconite
3.0g licorice

Effects

Used for patients with a *Shao-yao-kan-tsao-tang* conformation who have cold arms and legs and chillphobia.

Uses

Spasms in the back, knees and waist; spasms of the gastrocnemius (calf) muscle; sciatica; lower back pain; stiff shoulders; muscular rheumatism; intestinal hernia; biliary, renal, and hemorrhoidal colic; pain on urination; rigid tongue.

Shao-yao-kan-tsao-tang
(Paeonia and Licorice Combination)

Main Herbs

6.0g paeonia   6.0g licorice

Effects

Used for treating weakness in the legs and severe, painful muscle spasms in the stomach, intestines, bronchi, gallbladder, and ureters.

Uses
Muscle spasms around the waist and in the back and stomach, intestinal cramps, sciatica, fifty year's shoulder, muscular rheumatism, intestinal colic, pancreatitis, painful urination, bronchial asthma, spasmodic cough, hemorrhoidal pain, bladder pain, toothache, beriberi, palsy of the legs, weak legs, and noctiphobia (fear of the dark).

Shen-mi-tang
(Ma-huang and Magnolia Combination)

Main Herbs

5.0g ma-huang	3.0g magnolia back
2.0g licorice	2.0g bupleurum
4.0g apricot seed	2.5g citrus
1.5g perilla	

Effects
Used for treating a persistent cough, abdominal weakness, slight chest distress, deficient saliva, labored breathing, and neurosis.

Uses
Bronchial asthma, pediatric asthma, and pulmonary emphysema.

Sheng-chiang-hsieh-hsin-tang
(Pinellia and Ginger Combination)

Main Herbs

5.0g pinellia	2.5g licorice
2.0g ginger	2.5g jujube
2.5g ginseng	1.5g dried ginger
2.5g scute	1.0g coptis

Effects
Used for treating belching, gas, and diarrhea.

Uses

Inflammation of the stomach and intestinal track, excess of hydrochloric acid in the stomach, gastric distention, fermented diarrhea, and dilatation of the stomach.

Sheng-ling-pai-chu-san
(Ginseng and Atractylodes Formula)

Main Herbs

    3.0g ginseng   1.5g licorice
    1.5g dioscorea   3.0g atractylodes
    2.0g platycodon   5.0g coix
    4.0g dolichos   3.0g hoelen
    4.0g lotus seed   2.0g cardamon

Effects

Used to treat gastrointestinal weakness, loss of appetite, anemia, fatigue, chilling, watery diarrhea, weak pulse, weak abdomen, abdominal distention, gas, gas stagnancy, and the severe fatigue of convalescence.

Uses

Chronic gastroenteritis, chronic diarrhea, intestinal tuberculosis, indigestion, prolapsed stomach, loss of appetite after an illness, abnormal leukorrhea, and uterine bleeding.

Shih-chuan-ta-pu-tang
(Ginseng and Tang-kuei Ten Combination)

Main Herbs

    3.0g ginseng   3.0g hoelen
    3.0g astragalus   3.0g rehmannia
    3.0g atractylodes   3.0g cnidium
    3.0g *tang-kuei*   3.0g cinnamon
    3.0g paeonia   1.0g licorice

Effects

This formula treats men and women with debilities such as loss of appetite, decreased gastrointestinal function, loss of weight, loss of blood, and weakness due to prolonged disease. Indicative symptoms are remittent fever, muscle spasms, coarse skin, nocturnal emissions, pallor, weakness, and anxiety. It is also suitable for treating three types of ulcers: (1) with a small amount of pus; (2) without pus; (3) with pus but without tissue disintegration. However, it is not effective for severe, acute disorders with high fever.

Uses

Debility after illness, childbirth, and surgery; anemia, bloody dysentery, malaria, carbuncles, hemorrhoidal bleeding, caries, scrofula, leukemia, nocturnal emissions and hernia (rectocele); tuberculosis of the kidney, tuberculosis of the bone, decreased vision, chilblains, uterine carcinoma, menopausal disorders, postpartum beriberi, poliomyelitis, skin diseases, and ear ailments.

Shih-wei-pai-tu-tang
(Bupleurum and Schizonepeta Combination)

Main Herbs

3.0g bupleurum	3.0g platycodon
1.0g ginger	3.0g cnidium
2.0g *tuhuo*	1.0g schizonepeta
2.0g siler	3.0g cherry bark
3.0g hoelen	1.0g licorice

Effects

Especially effective for eczema, pimples, and hives. Better results are obtained in the treatment of suppuration and in skin nourishment when coix is added to the basic formula.

Uses

Carbuncles, furuncles, boils, lymphadenitis, mastitis, dermatitis, urticaria, eczema, acne, styes, allergic ophthalmia, nasal suppuration, inflammation of the middle and inner ear.

Shu-ching-huo-hsieh-tang
(Clematis and Stephania Combination)

Main Herbs

2.0g *tang-kuei*	1.5g siler
2.0g rehmannia	1.5g gentiana
2.0g atractylodes	1.5g ginger
2.0g cnidium	1.5g citrus
2.0g persica	1.0g angelica
2.0g hoelen	1.0g licorice
2.5g paeonia	1.5g stephania
1.5g achyranthes	1.5g *chianghuo*
1.5g clematis	

Effects

Used for increasing blood circulation, dispelling stagnant blood, and treating rheumatism.

Uses

Gout, serious arthritis, lower back pain, sciatica, numbness in the legs and feet, beriberi, edema, purpura, partial paralysis, hypertension, and postpartum thrombotic pain.

Su-tzu-chiang-chi-tang
(Perilla Fruit Combination)

Main Herbs

3.0g perilla fruit	2.5g cinnamon
4.0g pinellia	2.5g *tang-kuei*
2.5g citrus	1.5g jujube
2.5g magnolia	1.0g licorice
2.5g peucedanum	1.5g ginger

Effects

Used for treating cold legs and feet, labored breathing, weakness below the umbilicus, decreased urine, copious sputum, increased respiration, flushing up, chordal and tense pulse, and stagnancy beneath the heart.

Uses

Chronic bronchitis, asthmatic bronchitis, pulmonary emphysema, tinnitus, hemoptysis, nosebleeds, pyorrhea, putrid ulcer in the mouth, oral cancer, edema, and beriberi.

Suan-tsao-jen-tang
(Zizyphus Combination)

Main Herbs

10.0g zizyphus   5.0g hoelen
3.0g anemarrhena   1.0g licorice
3.0g cnidium

Effects

Used for treating patients with a delicate constitution and lack of energy, weak abdomen, weak pulse, and insomnia due to anxiety or somnolence due to fatigue.

Uses

Insomnia, somnolence, neurasthenia, night sweats, amnesia, nightmares, fright.

Szu-chun-tzu-tang
(Four Major Herb Combination)

Main Herbs

4.0g ginseng   4.0g hoelen
4.0g atractylodes 1.5g licorice

Effects

Good for treating gastrointestinal weakness, loss of appetite, vomiting, gas, diarrhea, weak abdomen, pallid complexion, and weakness of the arms and legs.

Uses

Gastrointestinal weakness, gastroptosis, gastric laxity, gastritis, anemia, vomiting, diarrhea, bleeding, weak conformation weak hands and feet, paralysis of a single limb, and bedwetting.

Szu-ni-chia-jen-sheng-tang
(G. L. and Aconite Combination with Ginseng)

Main Herbs

0.5-1.0g aconite	3.0g licorice
2.0g ginger	2.0g ginseng

Effects

Good for treating severe fatigue, severe anemia, cold hands and feet, absence of sweating, rapid respiration, and a weak and submerged pulse.

Uses

Febrile diseases, acute vomiting and diarrhea, dysentery.

Szu-ni-san
(Bupleurum and Chih-shih Formula)

Main Herbs

5.0g bupleurum	2.0g *chih-shih*
4.0g paeonia	1.5g licorice

Effects

Used for treating chest distention, abdominal spasms, cold hands and feet, and irritability caused by nervousness.

Uses

Inflammation of the gallbladder, gallstones, gastritis, gastric ulcer, pleurisy, rhinitis, neurosis, epilepsy, and tubercular peritonitis.

Szu-ni-tang
(Aconite and G. L. Combination)

Main Herbs
  0.5-1.0g aconite   3.0g licorice
  2.0g ginger

Effects
  Used for treating severe chills throughout the body, pallor, diarrhea, vomiting, abdominal pain, weak pulse, facial redness, and superficial fever.

Uses
  Influenza, intestinal fever, diarrhea, neurotic vomiting, indigestion, edema, jaundice, weak heart brought on by excessive bleeding, and cold hands and feet.

Szu-wu-tang
(Tang-kuei Four Combination)

Main Herbs
  4.0g *tang-kuei*   4.0g cnidium
  4.0g paeonia   4.0g rehmannia

Effects
  Menstrual irregularity, paroxysmal pain at the umbilicus and abdomen, uterine bleeding, abdominal pain during pregnancy, intestinal or anal bleeding, and postpartum blood clots or bleeding.

Uses
  Abnormal menstruation, abnormal leukorrhea, infertility, climacteric disorders, mastitis, anemia, ailments due to dry skin, paralysis of the legs and feet, hypertension, and apoplexy.

Ta-cheng-chi-tang
(Major Rhubarb Combination)

Main Herbs
 2.0g rhubarb 2.0g *chih-shih*
 2.0g mirabilitum 5.0g magnolia bark

Effects

Effective for treating patients with a strong abdomen, abdominal distention, a sensation of heaviness of the body, abnormal amount of sweating, a sinking-strong pulse, constipation, moist fever, and a dry tongue and mouth.

Uses

Acute pneumonia, typhoid, influenza, measles, meningitis, hypertension, tetanus, beriberi, habitual constipation, emotional distress, food poisoning, obesity, dysentery, and hemorrhoids.

Ta-chien-chung-tang
(Major Zanthoxylum Combination)

Main Herbs
 2.0g zanthoxylum 5.0g ginger
 3.0g ginseng 20.0g maltose

Effects

Suitable for treating internal chills, abdominal pain, weak abdomen, stagnant water, stagnant *ch'i*, vomiting, weak pulse, cold hands and feet, hacking cough, and edema.

Uses

Intestinal constriction, intestinal laxity, inflammation of the lining of the abdominal cavity (peritonitis), abdominal pain due to round worms, intestinal colic, acute appendicitis, and bladder and kidney stones.

Ta-ching-lung-tang
(Major Blue Dragon Combination)

Main Herbs
6.0g *ma-huang*   3.0g cinnamon
2.0g licorice   10.0g gypsum
5.0g apricot seed   3.0g zizyphus
3.0g ginger

Effects
Used for treating lack of perspiration, tight pulse, stress, fever, chillphobia, and body aches and pain.

Uses
Influenza, acute pneumonia, measles, febrile diseases, conjunctivitis, corneal ulcer, styes, acute nephritis, acute edema, acute arthritis, and erysipelas.

Ta-fang-feng-tang
(Major Siler Combination)

Main Herbs
3.0g *tang-kuei*   3.0g eucommia   1.5g achyranthes
3.0g paeonia   3.0g atractylodes   1.5g licorice
3.0g rehmannia   3.0g cnidium   1.5g zizyphus
3.0g astragalus   1.5g ginseng   1.5g ginger
3.0g siler   1.5g *chianghuo*   0.5-1.0g aconite

Effects
Used for nourishing the blood and *ch'i* and for alleviating paralysis, stiffness, swelling, pain in the knees and feet.

Uses
Arthritis, rheumatoid arthritis, atrophy of the spinal cord, inflammation of the spinal cord, partial paralysis, beriberi, paralysis of the legs and feet, and neuralgia.

Ta-huang-fu-tzu-tang
(Rhubarb and Aconite Combination)

Main Herbs
    1.0g rhubarb   0.5-1.0g aconite
    2.0g asarum

Effects
Used for treating pain in the armpits, waist, and legs; fever; a tight pulse; and mild abdominal tension.

Uses
Gastric spasms, intestinal spasms, inflammation of kidney and pelvis, kidney stones, gall stones, pancreatitis, intestinal colic, hernia pain, sciatica, intercostal neuralgia, migraine, and chronic appendicitis.

Ta-huang-mu-tan-pi-tang
(Rhubarb and Moutan Combination)

Main Herbs
    2.0g rhubarb   4.0g mirabilitum
    4.0g moutan   6.0g benincasa
    4.0g persica

Effects
This formula is for a patient with a strong conformation with a tendency to be constipated, fever and suppuration, and tumors in the lower abdomen.

Uses
Appendicitis; inflammation of areolar tissues in region of the rectum and anus; colitis; ulcerative enteritis; hemmorrhoids; rectal prolapse; inflammation of the peritoneal covering of the uterus; testitis; gonorrhea; abnormal leukorrhea; inflammation of lining of the abdominal cavity; inflammation of the pelvis of the kidney and its calices; cystitis; and stones in the ureter.

Tang-kuei-chien-chung-tang
(Tang-kuei, Cinnamon, and Paeonia Combination)

Main Herbs

    5.0g paeonia   4.0g ginger
    4.0g *tang-kuei*   4.0g jujube
    4.0g cinnamon   2.0g licorice

Effects

    Used for treating persons with a delicate constitution who have severe anemia, continuous abdominal pain radiating toward the waist and back, bleeding, abdominal weakness, hemorrhage on the lower body, and abdominal spasms.

Uses

    Abdominal pain in women, postpartum abdominal pain, pelvic peritonitis, abnormal uterine bleeding, sciatica, lower back pain, hernia, vertebral caries, kidney stones, renal tuberculosis, hemorrhoids, chronic peritonitis, prolapse of the anus, and chronic appendicitis.

Tang-kuei-shao-yao-san
(Tang-kuei and Paeonia Formula)

Main Herbs

    3.0g *tang-kuei*   3.0g cnidium
    4.0g paeonia   4.0g hoelen
    4.0g atractylodes   4.0g alisma

Effects

    Used to ease abdominal pain during pregnancy and various other abdominal aches in women. It cures men as well as women of weak conformation with anemia, pallor, general lassitude, and pain in the lower abdomen, waist, and heart.

Uses

    1. Pregnancy disorders: edema, habitual abortion, premature rupturing of the membrane, hemorrhoids, abdominal pain, cystitis, and lower back pain.

2. Postpartum weakness.
3. Menstrual irregularity, difficult menstruation, and female disorders.
4. Chronic nephritis, partial paralysis, vascular disease, and beriberi.

Tang-kuei-szu-ni-chia-wu-chu-yu-sheng-chiang-tang
(Tang-kuei, Evodia, and Ginger Combination)

Main Herbs

3.0g *tang-kuei*	2.0g licorice
3.0g cinnamon	5.0g jujube
3.0g paeonia	2.0g evodia
2.0g asarum	4.0g ginger
3.0g akebia	

Effects

Used for treating stagnancy of stale chilling humor, chest discomfort, vomiting, pain in the waist and abdomen, diarrhea, cold hands and feet, and thin pulse.

Uses

Weak pulse; cold hands and feet resulting from oversweating due to treatment of a febrile disease; chillblains; eruptions on the palms; sciatica; gangrene; intervertebral hernia; skin disease showing purpura due to blood stagnancy; uterine pain; chills; and diarrhea.

Tang-kuei-szu-ni-tang
(Tang-kuei and Jujube Combination)

Main Herbs

3.0g *tang-kuei*	5.0g jujube
3.0g cinnamon	2.0g asarum
3.0g paeonia	2.0g licorice
3.0g akebia	

Effects

Used for treating cold hands and feet, a minute and weak pulse, abnormal sweating in a febrile disease, abdominal distention, weak abdomen, and abdominal spasms.

Uses

Frostbite, eruptions of the palms, sciatica, intervertebral hernia, lower back pain, gangrene, stagnant blood in the skin showing purpura, intestinal colic, uterine pain, abdominal spasms in women, chills, and diarrhea.

Tang-kuei-yin-tzu
(Tang-kuei and Tribulus Combination)

Main Herbs

5.0g tang-kuei	1.5g schizonepeta
3.0g tribulus	3.0g cnidium
2.0g polygonum	4.0g rehmannia
3.0g paeonia	1.5g astragalus
3.0g siler	1.0g licorice

Effects

Used for treating itching due to "blood weakness", "blood dryness", and "wind heat", as manifested by the symptoms of anemia, dry skin, minimal secretions, dryness with mild reddening and itching of the skin.

Uses

Itching, scabies, chronic eczema, dry skin, abscesses and other conditions in which the chief complaints are dryness and itching.

Tao-ho-cheng-chi-tang
(Persica and Rhubarb Combination)

Main Herbs

5.0g persica   2.0g mirabilitum

4.0g cinnamon   1.5g licorice
3.0g rhubarb

Effects

Used for treating stagnant blood with marked flushing up, headaches, vertigo, ringing in the ears, insomnia, palpitations, constipation, frequent urination, mental instability, delirium, sensations of generalized fever, cold waist and feet, and palsy.

Uses

1. Gynecological: menstrual irregularity, dysmenorrhea, climacteric disorders, endometritis, ovaritis, spontaneous abortions, hemorrhage due to retained placenta, and stillbirths.
2. Internal problems: cystitis, gallstones, kidney stones, urethritis, prostatitis, enlarged prostate.
3. Skin diseases: dermatitis, eczema, hives, acne, athelete's foot, ringworm, frostbite, and warts.
4. Eye diseases: inflammation of the eyelid, eyebrow, cornea, retina, or conjunctiva; trachoma; blood in the eye, and glaucoma.
5. Internal bleeding: blood in the sputum or urine and bleeding of the gums, tongue, intestines, anus, and uterus.
6. Other ailments: chronic constipation, hypertension, arteriosclerosis, and discharges of purulent matter (pyorrhea).

Teng-lung-tang

(Moutan and Persica Combination)

Main Herbs

4.0g moutan   8.0g coix
4.0g persica   1.0g licorice
5.0g benincasa   1.5g rhubarb
4.0g atractylodes   5.0g mirabilitum

Effects

Used for treating inflammation and swelling pain in the lower abdomen.

Uses
Periproclitis, inflammation of the testes, appendicitis, prostatitis, pelvic peritonitis, endometritis, uterine tumors, and the initial stage of uterine cancer.

Ti-tang-tang
(Rhubarb and Leech Combination)

Main Herbs
  1.0g leech   1.0g gadfly
  3.0g rhubarb   1.0g persica

Effects
Used for treating stagnant blood, distention in the lower abdomen, resistance and pain in the abdomen when palpated, frequent urination, polyuria, dark stools, amnesia, and anxiety.

Uses
Absence of menstruation (amenorrhea), menstrual irregularity, uterine myoma (tumor), gangrene, amnesia, schizophrenia, and contusions from a fall or war wounds from battle.

Tiao-wei-cheng-chi-tang
(Rhubarb and Mirabilitum Combination)

Main Herbs
  2.5g rhubarb   1.0g licorice
  1.0g mirabilitum

Effects
Used for treating patients of a delicate constitution with a severe fever, submerged and firm pulse, elastic abdomen, vomiting, delirium, and a dry tongue and mouth.

Uses
Febrile diseases with constipation, habitual constipation, constipation in the elderly, food poisoning, acute gastroenteritis, and food stagnation.

Tuo-li-hsiao-tu-yin
(Gleditsia Combination)

Main Herbs

5.0g *tang-kuei*	3.0g paeonia
5.0g hoelen	2.0g gleditsia spine
3.0g ginseng	1.5g astragalus
3.0g cnidium	1.5g lonicera
3.0g platycodon	1.0g angelica
3.0g white atractylodes	1.0g licorice

Effects

Given to patients with a somewhat delicate constitution for treating suppuration with fever.

Uses

Carbuncles, suppurative lymphadenitis, inflammation of the voluntary muscles, bone gangrene, and discharges from the ear.

Tseng-sun-mu-fang-chi-tang
(Stephania and Perilla Fruit Combination)

Main Herbs

4.0g stephania	3.0g ginger
10.0g gypsum	5.0g perilla fruit
3.0g cinnamon	3.0g morus
3.0g ginseng	

Effects

Used to render diuresis and to treat stridor.

Tsing-fu-tang
(Bupleurum and Pinellia Combination)

Main Herbs

3.0g bupleurum	1.5g sparganium	1.0g ginger
2.0g pinellia	1.5g zedoaria	1.0g jujube
3.0g hoelen	1.5g crataegus	1.0g licorice
1.5g alisma	1.5g ginseng	1.5g polyporus
2.0g atractylodes	1.0g coptis	1.5g scute

Effects

Used for treating children with tension and a hard mass in the abdomen (mesenteric tubercular coalescence) or with glandular problems (adenopathic physique).

Uses

Tuberculous peritonitis, mesenteric tubercles of tuberculous origin, indigestion, indigestive stagnancy, epilepsy, physique, and high fever of unknown origin in children.

Tsou-ma-tang
(Croton and Apricot Seed Combination)

Main Herbs

1.0g croton   1.0g apricot seed

Effects

A cathartic, the formula is given in a single dose to stalwart individuals who suddenly contract an acute disease.

Uses

Apoplexy, uremia, convulsions caused by tetanus, contusions and wounds resulting from accidents, acute food poisoning, cerebral diseases, and other conditions in which the patient has thoracic distress or becomes unconscious.

Tung-mo-szu-ni-tang
(Licorice, Aconite, and Ginger Pulse Combination)

Main Herbs
    3.0g licorice   0.5-1.0g aconite
    4.0g ginger

Effects
Used for treating a *Szu-ni-tang* conformation accompanied by the symptoms of vomiting, diarrhea, severely cold hands and feet, and a seriously weak pulse.

Uses
Influenza, typhoid fever, diarrhea, autointoxication, appendicitis, gastroenteritis, indigestion, jaundice, excessive sweating, and edema in a weak conformation.

Tzu-ken-mu-li-tang
(Lithospermum and Oyster Shell Combination)

Main Herbs
    5.0g *tang-kuei*   4.0g oyster shell
    3.0g paeonia   2.0g astragalus
    3.0g cnidium   1.0g licorice
    1.5g rhubarb   1.5g lonicera
    2.0g cimicifuga   3.0g lithospermum

Effects
Used for treating recalcitrant carbuncles of unknown cause and malignant skin diseases.

Uses
Breast cancer, mastitis, lymphadenitis of the neck, gangrene of the lungs, syphilitic skin lesions.

Tzu-yin-chiang-huo-tang
(Phellodendron Combination)

Main Herbs

2.5g *tang-kuei*	2.5g rehmannia
2.5g paeonia	2.5g citrus
2.5g asparagus	1.5g phellodendron
2.5g ophiopogon	1.5g anemarrhena
3.0g atractylodes	1.5g licorice

Effects

Used for weakness and fire agitation, fever, coughing, sputum, gasping, night sweats, and dry mouth.

Uses

Hyperplastic pulmonary tuberculosis, acute and chronic bronchitis, acute and chronic pyelitis, tuberculosis of the kidneys, diabetes, dry pleurisy, and involuntary emissions.

Tzu-yuan
(Croton and Hematite Formula)

Main Herbs

4.0g croton	4.0g kaolin
4.0g hematite	8.0g apricot seed

Effects

Used for removing stagnant food in stomach and intestines and treating distention in the chest and abdomen.

Uses

Food poisoning, acute gastroenteritis, dysentery, uremia, infantile regurgitation of milk, cerebral diseases, paralysis of the intestines, fetal toxin, cerebral edema, night crying in children due to abdominal distention and constipation, beriberi, hyperlipemia, and contusions.

Tzu-yun-kao
(Lithospermum Ointment)

Main Herbs
    1000g sesame oil   25g lard
    380g flava wax   100g lithospermum
    100g *tang-kuei*

Effects
    Used for treating dryness of the skin, wrinkles, rhagades, ulceration and skin hyperplasia.

Uses
    Eczema, psoriasis, keratosis, athlete's foot, warts, corns, acne, frostbite, macules, prickly heat, body odor, baldness, external injuries, burns, hemorrhoids, rectal prolapse, and ulcerations.

Wei-cheng-fang
(Eucommia and Achyranthes Formula)

Main Herbs
    5.0g *tang-kuei*   3.0g achyranthes   4.0g rehmannia
    2.0g paeonia   2.0g astragalus   3.0g anemarrhena
    1.0g eucommia   3.0g atractylodes   1.0g phellodendron

Effects
    Good for treating the primary stage of weakness near the waist and in the feet when abdominal strength is normal.

Uses
    Weakness of the feet during convalescence, weak knees after childbirth, wasting of the spinal cord, inflammation of the spinal cord, paralysis of the legs due to beriberi, vertebral caries, and poliomyelitis.

Wei-feng-tang
(Atractylodes and Setaria Combination)

Main Herbs

3.0g tang-kuei   3.0g atractylodes
3.0g paeonia   4.0g hoelen
3.0g cnidium   2.0g cinnamon
3.0g ginseng   2.0g setaria (millet)

Effects

Used to treat chronic enteritis and persistent diarrhea in patients with a weak conformation.

Uses

Chronic enteritis, chronic proctitis, ulcerative colitis, proneness to rectal prolapse in the winter, tendency to hemorrhage in the winter, and chronic diarrhea.

Wei-ling-tang
(Magnolia and Hoelen Combination)

Main Herbs

2.5g atractylodes   2.5g white atractylodes
2.5g magnolia bark   2.5g hoelen
2.5g citrus   2.5g polyporus
1.5g jujube   2.5g alisma
1.5g ginger   2.0g cinnamon
1.0g licorice

Effects

Suitable for patients who often have water toxin or diarrhea on contraction of acute gastritis. Also for heat stroke with the accompanying symptoms of abdominal pain, abdominal distention, thirst, edema, and pain upon urination.

Uses

Acute gastritis, acute enteritis, colitis, acute nephritis, abdominal pain with diarrhea, edema, and neuralgia in the summer.

Wei-mai-i-chi-tang
(Schizandra and Ophiopogon Combination)

Main Herbs

4.0g astragalus	4.0g atractylodes	2.0g citrus
2.0g ginger	2.0g bupleurum	1.0g cimicifuga
4.0g ginseng	3.0g *tang-kuei*	2.0g schizandra
2.0g jujube	1.5g licorice	4.0g ophiopogon

Effects

Used for treating patients with a *Pu-chung-i-chi-tang* conformation accompanied by pulmonary tuberculosis and coughing.

Wen-ching-tang
(Tang-kuei and Evodia Combination)

Main Herbs

1.0g evodia	2.0g moutan
3.0g *tang-kuei*	1.0g ginger
2.0g cnidium	2.0g paeonia
2.0g ginseng	2.0g licorice
2.0g cinnamon	5.0g pinellia
2.0g gelatin	5.0g ophiopogon

Effects

Used for treating menstrual irregularity, uterine bleeding, annoying fever in the palms, dry lips and mouth, distention in the lower abdomen, cold waist, and abdominal pain.

Uses

Climacteric disorders, infertility, menstrual irregularity, uterine bleeding, leukorrhea, underdeveloped uterus, habitual abortion, neurotic symptoms, frostbite, eczema, and keratitis of the palms.

Wen-ching-yin
(Tang-kuei and Gardenia Combination)

Main Herbs

    4.0g *tang-kuei*   1.5g coptis
    4.0g rehmannia   3.0g scute
    3.0g paeonia   1.5g phellodendron
    3.0g cnidium   2.0g gardenia

Effects

Used for treating dark-brown, coarse skin; severe itching; ulcers of the mucous membrane; flushing up; nervous excitement; resistance in the abdomen; liver disorders; severe uterine bleeding; excessive menstrual bleeding; persistent abnormal leukorrhea; underweight due to internal bleeding; and a tendency to bleed.

Uses

Metrorrhagia, menorrhagia, abnormal leukorrhea, peptic and duodenal ulcers, hemorrhaging, itching, dermatitis, eczema, hives, psoriasis, neurotic symptoms and hypertension.

Wen-tan-tang
(Bamboo and Chih-shih Combination)

Main Herbs

    2.5g citrus   1.5g *chih-shih*   1.0g licorice
    6.0g hoelen   2.0g bamboo   1.0g coptis
    6.0g pinellia   3.0g ginger   3.0g zizyphus

Effects

Used for treating stomach diseases, gastroptosis, gastric atonia, and insomnia in patients having poor muscle tone and development.

Uses

Insomnia, terror, cardiac palpitations, melancholy, and gastrointestinal disorders.

Wu-chi-san
(Tang-kuei and Magnolia Formula)

Main Herbs

2.0g hoelen	1.2g angelica
2.0g white atractylodes	1.2g *chih-ko*
2.0g citrus	1.2g platycodon
2.0g pinellia	1.2g dried ginger
2.0g atractylodes	1.2g cinnamon
1.2g *tang-kuei*	1.2g *ma-huang*
1.2g paeonia	1.2g jujube
1.2g cnidium	1.2g licorice
1.2g magnolia	1.2g ginger

Effects

Used for treating stagnancies of *ch'i*, blood, sputum, cold, and food.

Uses

Acute and chronic gastroenteritis, gastric spasms, hernia, lower back pain, pain during menstruation, valvular diseases, neuralgia, rheumatism, beriberi, contusions, common colds in the elderly.

Wu-chu-yu-tang
(Evodia Combination)

Main Herbs

4.0g evodia	6.0g ginger
3.0g ginseng	3.0g jujube

Effects

Used for treating chills in the liver and stomach, vomiting, restlessness, headaches, subcardiac distention, cold hands and feet, and a submerged pulse.

Uses

Vomiting, eclampsia, acute vomiting and diarrhea, headaches, migraine, food poisoning, indigestion, prolapsed stomach, and beriberi.

Wu-ling-san
(Hoelen Five Herb Formula)

Main Herbs

4.5g polyporus   6.0g alisma
4.5g hoelen   3.0g cinnamon
4.5g atractylodes

Effects

Suitable for stagnant water in the stomach due to metabolic fluid disorders, thirst, vomiting, difficult urination, flushing up, palpitations, vertigo, anxiety, headaches, abdominal pain, diarrhea, edema, fever, and a floating and fast pulse.

Uses

Vomiting and diarrhea due to a common cold, acute gastroenteritis, gastrectasis, gastric atonia, gastroptosis, diabetes, seasickness, indigestion, toxemia during pregnancy, hypersalivation, nephritis, cardiac edema, hernia, uremia, migraines, recurrent headaches, trigeminal neuralgia, viral conjunctivitis, inflammation of the tear sac, night blindness, blisters, and chicken pox.

Wu-mei-wan
(Mume Formula)

Main Herbs

3.0g mume   3.0g ginseng
3.0g asarum   2.0g *tang-kuei*
3.0g aconite   2.0g zanthoxylum
3.0g cinnamon   5.0g ginger
3.0g phellodendron   7.0g coptis

Effects

Used for treating paroxysmal abdominal pain or anxiety due to pinworm infestation, cold hands and feet, vomiting, incessant diarrhea, and fever in the upper torso and chills in the lower torso.

Uses

Pinworms (ascariasis), gastritis, excessive stomach acid, gastric ulcer, intestinal colic, chronic diarrhea, psychoneurosis, insomnia, climacteric disorders.

Yen-nien-pan-hsia-tang
(Evodia and Pinellia Combination)

Main Herbs

5.0g pinellia	3.0g areca seed	1.0g evodia
3.0g platycodon	2.0g ginseng	3.0g peucedanum
2.0g ginger	3.0g tortoise shell	1.0g *chih-shih*

Effects

Used for treating chronic gastrointestinal disorders, pain in the chest, stiff shoulders, cold feet, prolapsed stomach, gastric distention, gastric ulcers, abdominal weakness, and lack of vigor.

Uses

Gastric ulcers, duodenal ulcers, chronic gastritis, intercostal neuralgia, stomach ailments, chronic pancreatitis, stiff shoulders, anxiety, chest pain, loss of appetite, abnormal appetite.

Yin-chen-hao-tang
(Capillaris Combination)

Main Herbs

4.0g capillaris	1.0g rhubarb
3.0g gardenia	

Effects

Used for treating jaundice, distention in the upper abdomen, discomfort in the chest cavity, nausea, thirst, difficult urination, constipation, and dark-colored urine.

Uses

Jaundice, acute hepatitis, nephritis, edema, beriberi, inflammation in the mouth, hives, itching, inflammation of the gums, pain in the eyes, and uterine bleeding other than menstrual bleeding.

Yin-chen-wu-ling-san
(Capillaris and Hoelen Formula)

Main Herbs
    6.0g capillaris   4.5g polyporus
    4.0g alisma   4.5g atractylodes
    4.5g hoelen   3.0g cinnamon

Effects
    Used to treat liver disturbances, jaundice, thirst, decreased urine, dark-colored urine, abdominal distention, excessive thirst, and fever.

Uses
    Jaundice, hepatitis, nephritis, renal cirrhosis, ascites.

Yueh-pi-chia-pan-hsia-tang
(Ma-huang, Gypsum, and Pinellia Combination)

Main Herbs
    6.0g *ma-huang*   3.0g jujube
    8.0g gypsum   2.0g licorice
    3.0g ginger   5.0g pinellia

Effects
    Used for treating stridor, cough, facial edema, excessive thirst, and a tendency toward decreased urine.

Uses
    Asthma, chronic bronchitis, pulmonary emphysema, pregnancy kidney, severe cough that causes facial edema, ocular swelling, extreme thirst, and decreased urine.

Yueh-pi-chia-chu-tang
(Atractylodes Combination)

Main Herbs

    6.0g *ma-huang*   2.0g licorice
    8.0g gypsum   4.0g atractylodes
    3.0g jujube   3.0g ginger

Effects

Used for treating edema, spontaneous perspiration, decreased urine due to the internal fluids overflowing to the surface (excessive sweating); skin and muscular problems; loss of the three humors, and weakness around the waist and in the feet.

Uses

Nephritis, dermatic nephritis, beriberi, arthritic rheumatism, hernia, skin eruptions, corneal opacity, eczema, fungal infections, polyps, athlete's foot, tired and aching feet, subcutaneous abscesses, and jaundice.

Yueh-pi-tang
(Ma-huang and Gypsum Combination)

Main Herbs

    6.0g *ma-huang*   2.0g licorice
    8.0g gypsum   3.0g ginger
    3.0g jujube

Effects

Used for treating the initial stage of dropsy in which there is a floating pulse, spontaneous perspiration, edema, anemophobia, asthmatic cough, decreased urine and excessive thirst.

Uses

Dropsy, primary nephritis, dermatic nephritis, arthritis of the legs, primary carbuncles, beriberi, and edema.

HERBS USED IN CHINESE MEDICINE

HERBS USED IN CHINESE MEDICINE

Names of Herbs

Herbs used in Chinese Medicine are essentially natural products, mostly derived from plants. In ancient times the name of the same herb differed from one medical school to another. A Chinese medical practitioner had to learn the various terms for the same herb. Some of the most important ones will be discussed in this section. (Note: the names used in Japan and China for the same herb also differ.)

Very often the name of an herb is prefixed with a character denoting the habitat, quality, or processing method of the herbs. Here is a list of the prefixes with their meanings.

Sheng (fresh). A fresh instead of dried herb.

Kan (dry). A dried instead of fresh herb.

Sheng kan (raw dried). The raw herb has been dried without further processing.

Shou (cooked). The herb has been processed by heating, cooking, or boiling.

Chih (processed). The herb has been processed by cutting, chopping, or heating.

Shan (mountain). The herb grows in a mountainous region,

the main habitat being Szechuan, China.
Chuan (abbreviation for Szechuan). Herb comes from Szechuan, China.
Shu (synonym of Szechuan). Same meaning as *Chuan*.
Tu (native). Native, local, or domestic product; generally denotes a local substitute.
Hu (Northwestern tribes of China). A product indigenous to the Northwest Region of China.
Ho (Japan). A Japanese substitute.
Chen (genuine). A Japanese product which is equal or similar to a Chinese drug.
Tang (China). An herb indigenous to China.
Ku tu (imported in ancient times). A superior quality product which was formerly imported.
Zou (flesh). The tender and fleshy part of a plant.
Shuang (frost). Burnt; white, frost-like ash.

Storage

Chinese herbals are readily subject to the growth of molds and insect infestation. Therefore, it is necessary to take preventative measures against these deleterious effects. In winter because the temperature and humidity are low, the danger of such attacks is greatly reduced. The moist air and higher temperatures of summer, however, create an environment in which molds and insects thrive. In recent years insecticides, fungicides, and air tight packaging in tins has eliminated much of the loss of herbals that used to occur. Carbon tetrachloride or trichloromethane are the most commonly used preservatives although carbon disulfide, which is highly flammable, is used occasionally.

Compounding

The herbs are first cut single handedly with a cutter into thin slices. Then they are shredded in a double handed cutter pan. The fine debris or chips are then removed and the chopped herb stored.

According to the requirements of the respective prescription, the herbs are processed by heating, cooking, washing with water, and removing the unwanted parts. Today drugstores provide compounded herbs which need no further processing.

Dispensing

If the regimen is to be one dose a day for ten days, each herb is weighed and divided into ten portions. One portion of each herb is combined with the others and packaged separately in ten bags. In the same manner if the regimen is three doses a day for ten days, the daily portions are equally divided into three parts and placed in thirty bags. Drugs such as aconite, gypsum, talc, mirabilitum, coix, and jade gelatin differ greatly in specific gravity and must be carefully weighed on a scale.

Decoction

The best decocting container is an earthenware pot; however an aluminum pot is also good. First the herbs are placed in the pot with twenty times their weight of water. Then they are cooked over a medium flame for about thirty minutes. Generally the water is then reduced by half. The dregs are removed then while the liquid is hot. A purgative preparation is cooked quickly while a tonic is cooked slowly. Herbs like aconite must be cooked for a long time in order to enable complete extraction of the effective ingredients.

Herb Properties

For centuries Chinese herbs have been classified as either chilly, hot, warm, cool, or bland. Generally these properties are considered when prescribing an herbal remedy, but the rules for use are very flexible.

General Notes

The following extensive charts list 451 herbs that are recommended in Chinese medical texts or used as folk remedies. They are arranged alphabetically according to their Chinese name. The first column names the herb. Immediately following the full name is the short form, the commonly used name. The second column gives botanical name, common name and sometimes a description of the herb and its habitat. In the third column the part of the plant that is used in the formulas is described. The fourth column tells how to select the correct herb and gives further information on the parts used. The fifth and sixth columns then give the herb's property, functions, and symptoms which indicate its use.

Chinese Name/ Common Name	Scientific Name/ Description	Part Used	Method of Selection and Processing	Property	Function/Symptoms
a-chiao 阿膠 (gelatin)	Gelatin produced from cooking the bones and skin of cattle		Depending on the methods of production and differences in raw materials, there are many different qualities. Gelatin produced in Shan Tung province, China, is the best. Commonly yellow gelatin (*huang-ming-chiao*) and jade gelatin (*yu-a-chiao*) are used.	bland	sedative, analgesic, hemostatic/pain, hemorrhage, dysuria, insomnia
a-hsien-yao 阿仙藥 (catechu)	*Acacia catechu* Willd./Leguminosae. A shrub indigenous to Malaysia.	leaves and young twigs	An extract containing some earth. Usually is formed into a rectangular mass.	mildly chilly	astringent, antipyretic, refrigerant/gastro-intestinal disturbance, hemorrhage, dysuria
a-pien 阿片 (opium)	*Papaver somniferum* L./ Papaveraceae; A perennial herb.	immature poppies		warm	analgesic, spasmolytic, sedative, sobering, antidiarrheal/diarrhea, abdominal pain, cough
a-wei 阿魏 (asafoetida)	*Ferula foetida* Reg./ Umbelliferae; A perennial herb indigenous to northern India and Iran.	resin exudated by the plant		bland	stomachic, intestinal corrective, carminative, anthelmintic/dyspepsia, abdominal pain, ascariasis

Chinese Name/ Common Name	Scientific Name/ Description	Part Used	Method of Selection and Processing	Property	Function/Symptoms
ai-yeh 艾葉 (artemisia)	Artemisia vulgaris L./ Compositae; common mugwort. A perennial wild herb found everywhere.	leaves that look silky and have small stems		warm	a warm astringent/ hemoptysis, hemorrhage, epistaxis, abdominal pain
an-hsi-hsiang 安息香 (benzoin)	Styrax benzoin/Styracaceae A tall plant indigenous to Sumatra and Thailand.	resin exudated from the trunk bark		bland	expectorant, preservative/ bronchitis, gastrointestinal disturbances
an-chien-tzu 菴蕳子 (keiskeana)	Artemisia keiskeana Miq./Compositae. A perennial wild herb found everywhere.	seeds		mildly chilly	tonic/impotence, menoxenia
cha-tai 鮓荅 (ma-pao) 馬寶 (horse bezoar)	Equus caballus L./Equidae	stones found in the intestines of a horse		chilly	spasmolytic, sedative, antidotal/infantile epilepsy, insomnia, hysteria
cha-yeh 茶葉 (tea)	Thea sinensis L./Theaceae; A commonly cultivated shrub.	leaves	This is green tea.	mildly chilly	diuretic, cardiotonic, anodyne, antidiarrheal/ fatigue, prostration, cardiac edema, neurosis
chai-hu 柴胡 (bupleurum)	Bupleurum falcatum L.; B chinence DC./Umbelliferae; sickle-leaved hare's ear. A	roots		mildly chilly	antipyretic/thoraco-costal distress, alternating chills and fever, and diseases of

Chinese Name/ Common Name	Scientific Name/ Description	Part Used	Method of Selection and Processing	Property	Function/Symptoms
	perennial herb that grows in the mountains.				the respiratory system
chan-su 蟾酥 (toad secrection)	*Bufo bufo gargarizans* Cantor/Bufonidae. An amphibious animal.	white secretion from the poisonous gland between the eyes	The commercial product is generally from China; often adulterated with flour.	warm	analgesic, cardiotonic, antitoxin/gastroenteritis, carcinoma
chan-tuei 蟬蛻 (cicada)	*Stenopsocus* sp./Psocidae *Cryptotympana atrata* Fabr./Cicadidae	skin that the cicada sheds after it comes out of the ground		chilly	febrifuge/common cold, headache, ocular diseases
chang-chu 蒼朮 (atractylodes)	*Atractylodes lancea* DC./ Compositae. A perennial wild herb found everywhere.	old roots of *chang-chu* or small-leafed *chang-chu* (*ku-li-chang-chu*)	Chinese *ku-li-chang-chu* is preferred. It has a mold-like white powder growing on the surface.	warm	warm diuretic, analgesic/ oliguria or frequency of urination due to renal insufficiency, generalized pain, intra-gastric water stagnancy, gastro-enteritis, edema
chang-nao 樟腦 (camphor)	*Cinnamomum camphora* Nees/Lauraceae; A tall plant cultivated in the warm southern lands.	after wooden cores are distilled with steam a solid substance,		hot	excitant, cardiotonic/acute cardiac failure

Herbs Used in Chinese Medicine

Chinese Name/ Common Name	Scientific Name/ Description	Part Used	Method of Selection and Processing	Property	Function/Symptoms
chang-shan 常山 (dichroa)	Dichroa febrifuga Lour./ Saxifragaceae; Szechuan varnish. A low plant indigenous to China.	roots; camphor, is obtained	In Japan this drug is replaced with tzu-yang-hua (Hydrangea macrophylla var. Otaka Makino).	chilly	febrifuge, emetic/seizures of malaria
che-chien-tsao 車前草 (plantago)	Plantago asiatica L./ Plantaginaceae; plantain. A perennial wild herb found everywhere.	whole herb		chilly	antiphlogistic, anticough, diuretic/ocular diseases, coughs
che-chien-tzu 車前子 (plantago seed)	Plantago asiatica L./ Plantaginaceae; plantain. A perennial wild herb found everywhere.	seeds		chilly	antiphlogistic, diuretic, antipyretic, tonic/ocular diseases
che-chung 䗪蟲 (eupolyphaga)	Eupolyphaga sinensis W./ Corydiidae. An insect.	whole body of the female insect		chilly	exsanguinative, emmenagogue/amenorrhea, abdominal pain, stale extravasated blood
che-ku-tsai 鷓鴣菜 (digenea)	Digenea simplex Agardh. /Rhodomelaceae. A sea weed found in the South Seas.	whole herb	Remove entrapped sand.	chilly	anthelmintic/ascariasis, pin worms, embryo toxin, abdominal pain, slobbering

Chinese Name/ Common Name	Scientific Name/ Description	Part Used	Method of Selection and Processing	Property	Function/Symptoms
chen-chu 眞珠 (pearl)	Pearls found in certain mussels, clams, and mollusks. Pteria martensii/Pteriidae; Cristaria plicata/Unionidae		Can be replaced by calcium carbonate.	chilly	antipyretic, sedative/ headache, insomnia (also used as an eye drop)
chen-hsiang 沈香 (aquilaria)	Aquilaria agallocha Roxb./Thymelaeaceae; gharuwood, lignum aloes, or "agar"	wood containing the plant resin	Use black-brown one that gives off a characteristic fragrance when burnt.	mildly warm	stomachic, analgesic, sedative/vomiting, abdominal pain
chen-sha 針砂 (iron powder)	Iron or steel filings.			bland	hemopoeitic, tonic, sedative/anemia, cardiac palpitations
cheng-liu 檉柳 (tamarisk)	Tamarix chinensis Lour. /Tamariacaceae; A delicate tall plant indigenous to China.	branches and leaves		bland	diaphoretic, diuretic, antidotal/measles, poxes, arthralgia, alcoholism
chi-kan 雞肝 (chicken liver)	Gallus domesticus Briss.; chicken.	liver		warm	nutrient tonic/ocular diseases
chi-li-tzu 蒺藜子 (tribulus)	Tribulus terrestris L. /Zygophyllaceae; calthrop. An annual wild herb found growing	fruit		warm	tonic/neurosis, ocular diseases

Chinese Name/ Common Name	Scientific Name/ Description	Part Used	Method of Selection and Processing	Property	Function/Symptoms
chi-lin-hsueh 騏驎血 (calamus gum)	Calamus draco Bl. / Palmae; dragon's blood. A vine indigenous to India and the tropical zone.	reddish resin exudated by the bark of the plant		bland	astringent, hemostatic, analgesic/hemorrhages, abdominal pain, cuts
chi-shih 芰實 (trapa)	Trapa natans L./Oenotheraceae; water chestnut. An annual herb growing in ponds.	fruit		cool	antiphlogistic, stomachic/ gastroenteritis, thirst, alcoholism
chi-tsao 蠐螬 (holotrichia)	The dried whole bodies of the larvae of scarab.			warm	exsanguinative/extravasated blood new or old
Chi-tzu-huang 雞子黃 (yolk)	The yolk of chicken eggs		Remove egg white.	bland	nutrient tonic/nutrition supplement
chiang-huang 薑黃 (turmeric)	Curcuma longa L./Zingiberacear; A perennial herb indigenous to China.	rhizomes		warm	aromatic, stomachic, hemostatic/jaundice, fever, gallbladder problems
chiang-huo 羌活 (chiang-huo)	Angelica sylvestris L./ Umbelliferae; angelica. Indigerous to Szechuan on the seashore.	roots		warm	diaphoretic, febrifuge, analgesic, spasmolytic/ common cold, edema,

Chinese Name/ Common Name	Scientific Name/ Description	Part Used	Method of Selection and Processing	Property	Function/Symptoms
	China. (See *tu-huo* 獨活 also.)				generalized pain
chiang-lang 蚚螂 (scarab beetle)	*Geotrupes laevistrialus* Motsch.	all		chilly	spasmolytic, antidotal/sores and swellings
chiang-tsan 殭蠶 (silk worm)	*Bombyx mori* L./Bombycidae.	dead larvae that have become white and stiff	Use bleached white and stiff larvae.	bland	sedative, lactogogue/ pediatric epilepsy or mania, infantile night crying
chiao-i 膠飴 (maltose)	Glutinous rice or ordinary rice which is cooked along with some malt and warm water to saccharize the rice. Resultant liquid is filtered and allowed to thicken by evaporation into a semi-solid mass.		Use the kind that is not adulterated with sugar—akaiame (red-syrup gel) or mizu ame (water-syrup gel). In preparing the decoction, first decoct all the herbs then dissolve the maltose gel in the decocted liquid.	warm	nutrient, lenitive, analgesic/ acute impetuous conditions, yin-weakness conditions
chieh-keng 桔梗 (platycodon)	*Platycodon grandiflorum* A, DC./Campanulaceae; A perennial wild herb found in mountainous areas.	roots	Prepared by drying the raw fresh roots called *sheng-kan* (生乾 raw dried). The solid and heavy ones are preferred.	mildly warm	expectorant, pus dispersant/ thick sputum, abscesses

Chinese Name/ Common Name	Scientific Name/ Description	Part Used	Method of Selection and Processing	Property	Function/Symptoms
chieh-ku-mu 接骨木 (sambucus)	Sambucus racemosa L./ Caprifoliaceae; red elderberry. A wild low plant found everywhere.	stems and leaves		bland	analgesic/aches and pains in the limbs and joints
chieh-tzu 芥子 (brassica)	Brassica juncea (L.) Coss.; Sinapis alba L./Cruciferae; white mustard. A biennial herb cultivated everywhere.	seeds		hot	acrid stomachic, anticough, expectorant, rubefacient/ chronic bronchitis
chien-hu 前胡 (peucedanum)	Peucedanum dercursivum Max./Umbelliferae. A perennial wild herb found everywhere.	roots		mildly chilly	antipyretic, anticough, expectorant/common cold, cough, headache
chien-niu-tzu 牽牛子 (pharbitis)	Ipomoea hederacea Jacq./ Convolvulaceae; morning glory. An annual herb cultivated everywhere.	seeds	Use variety with black seeds.	chilly	purgative, diuretic/anuria, edema, beriberi
chien-pai 鉛白 (ceruse)	Alkaline lead carbonate.		Use internally or externally.	chilly	anthelmintic/dermatosis
chien-shih 芡實 (euryale)	Euryale ferox Salisb./ Nymphaeaceae; foxnut. An annual aquatic plant	seeds		bland	nutrient, tonic, astringent, sedative/neuralgia, arthritis, impotence, diarrhea

Chinese Name/ Common Name	Scientific Name/ Description	Part Used	Method of Selection and Processing	Property	Function/Symptoms
chien-tan 鉛丹 (minium)	Red lead oxide. cultivated everywhere.		Use as a plaster.	chilly	preservative, pus dispersant
chien-tsao 茜草 (madder)	Rubia cordifolia L./ Rubiaceae; A perennial wild herb found everywhere.	roots		warm	hemostatic, emmenagogue, diuretic/amenorrhea, dysmenorrhea, hemorrhage
chih-hsiao-tou 赤小豆 (phaseolus)	Phaseolus calcaratus Roxb. /Leguminosae; mung bean. An annual herb cultivated everywhere.	seeds		bland	diuretic/edema, beriberi
chih-ko 枳殼 (chih-ko)	Citrus trifoliata L./Rutaceae; thorny lime bush. A delicate tall plant cultivated everywhere.	the pericarps of the immature fruit	May be used as a substitute of chih-shih.	mildly chilly	aromatic stomachic/thoracic distension, thoracic pain, cough, sputum
chih-mu 知母 (anemarrhena)	Anemarrhena asphodeloides Bunge./Liliaceae. A perennial herb cultivated everywhere; indigenous to China.	rhizomes	Chinese product.	chilly	cleansing and cooling, antipyretic, antithirst, diuretic, anticough/ extreme thirst

Herbs Used in Chinese Medicine

Chinese Name/ Common Name	Scientific Name/ Description	Part Used	Method of Selection and Processing	Property	Function/Symptoms
chih-shih 枳實 (chih-shih)	Same as chih-ko.	immature fruit	The small ones are broken up and dried. Those with a strong odor are preferred. The global shaped variety chu-yuan (Citrus medica L. var. sacrodactylis Swingle) has a milder odor.	chilly	Same as for chih-ko
chih-shih-chih 赤石脂 (kaolin)	The variety of kaolin that contains traces of iron oxides; the red bole (red variety of siliceous clay).			warm	astringent, hemostatic antidiarrheal/gastroenteritis, hemorrhage diarrhea
chin-chiu 秦艽 (chin-chiu)	Gentiana macrophylla Pall./Gentianaceae. A perennial herb indigenous to China.	roots		bland	febrifuge, diuretic, anodyne/ pulmonary tuberculosis, arthralgia, jaundice
chin-pi 秦皮 (fraxinus)	Fraxinus bungeana DC./ Oleaceae; shensi ash. A tall plant indigenous to China.	bark	Occasionally this drug is replaced by the bark of chin (Fraxinus pubinervus)	chilly	astringent, anti-diarrheal, stomachic/feverish diarrhea
chin-yin-hua 金銀花 (lonicera)	Lonicera japonica Thunb./ Caprifoliaceae; honey-suckle or woodbine. A perennial wild herb found everywhere.	flower bud	This drug is often substituted by jen-tung.	chilly	cleansing the blood, diuretic, antidotal/sores and swellings

Chinese Name/ Common Name	Scientific Name/ Description	Part Used	Method of Selection and Processing	Property	Function/Symptoms
ching-chieh 荊芥 (schizonepeta)	*Schizonepeta tenuifolia* Briq./Labiatae. An annual herb indigenous to China.	fruit spikes	Use those with less stems and leaves but with a strong odor.	warm	diaphoretic, febrifuge, antidotal/headache, vertigo, sores and swellings, dermatoses
ching-fen 輕粉 (calomel)	A steam-sublimed calomel (HgCl) in the form of a flaky powder.			chilly	diuretic, purgative, antisyphilitic/syphilis, scabies, dysuria, difficulty in defecation, oral treatment of dermatoses
ching-hao 青蒿 (ching-hao)	*Artemisia apiacea* Hce./ Compositae; southern wood. An annual wild herb found everywhere.	whole herb		chilly	antipyretic, anhidrotic/ debility, wasting fever, sores and swellings
ching-hsiang-tzu 青箱子 (celosia)	*Celosia argenta* L./ Amaranthaceae; cockscomb. An annual wild herb found everywhere.	seeds		mildly chilly	antipyretic, astringent, hemostatic, antidiarrheal/ hemorrhage of various conditions, liver and ocular diseases
ching-mu-hsiang 青木香 (birthwort)	*Aristolochia debilis* Sieb. et Zucc./Aristolochiaceae. A perennial wild creeping herb.	roots		chilly	astringent, analgesic/diarrhea, abdominal pain

Herbs Used in Chinese Medicine

Chinese Name/ Common Name	Scientific Name/ Description	Part Used	Method of Selection and Processing	Property	Function/Symptoms
ching-pi 青皮 (blue citrus peel)	*Citrus reticulata* Blanco./ Rutaceae; sweet peel tangerine. A shrub cultivated everywhere	the green pericarps of the fruit	Often the white inner layer is removed.	warm	aromatic stomachic, antiemetic, anticough, expectorant/gastroenteritis, emesis, bronchitis
ching-tai 青黛 (indigo)	*Polygonum tinctorium* Lour./Polygonaceae; indigo plant. An annual herb cultivated everywhere.	soak leaves in water and let ferment	Blue juice is yielded. A substance floats to the top of the liquid and forms into a cyanic powder.	chilly	antipyretic, antidotal/throat pain, stomatitis
chiu-lung-chung 九龍蟲 (exotic worm)	A kind of small oviparus insect living everywhere.	all	Usually the imago is swallowed live.		seminal tonic/impotence
chu 醋 (vinegar)	Rice vinegar containing about 4% acetic acid.		An extract for drugs.	warm	antiphlogistic, astringent
chu-chieh-jen-sheng 竹節人參 (chu-chieh ginseng)	*Panax repens* Maxim./ Araliaceae; ginseng. A wild perennial herb found in the mountains.	rhizomes	A substitute for *jen-sheng* (ginseng).	mildly chilly	stomachic, tonic, anticough, expectorant/degenerated metabolism due to deteriorated G.I.

Chinese Name/ Common Name	Scientific Name/ Description	Part Used	Method of Selection and Processing	Property	Function/Symptoms
chu-ju 竹茹 (bamboo)	Phyllostachys nigra Munro var. henonis Stapf ex Rendle/ Graminae; bamboo. Cultivated everywhere.	white flesh of bamboo	Take a fresh shoot with the green skin removed and scrape into thin strips.	mildly chilly	cleansing and cooling antifebrile, antithirst, anticough/feverish diseases
chu-hua 菊花 (chrysanthemum)	Chrysanthemum indicum L./Compositae; garden daisy. A wild perennial herb found everywhere.	yellow flowers	Use fragrant petals with the bracts removed as much as possible.	mildly chilly	cleansing and cooling, febrifuge, sedative/ headache, vertigo, ocular diseases
chu-li 竹瀝 (bamboo sap)	Brown colored liquid that comes out of a bamboo when placed above a fire.			very chilly	cleansing and cooling, antifebrile, anticough, cough supressant/feverish diseases
chu-ling 豬苓 (polyporus)	Grifola umbellata (Pers.) Pilat./Polyporaceae; Fungi; pig's dung. A fungus growing on the roots of trees.	fungus core		bland	diuretic, febrifuge, antithirst/dysuria, thirst, edema
chu-mai 瞿麥 (dianthus)	Dianthus superbus L./ Caryophyllaceae; pink. A perennial wild herb found everywhere.	seeds	Use those of disk shape which are heavy.	chilly	antiphlogistic, diuretic, promotes menstrual flow/ gonorrhea, edema

Chinese Name/ Common Name	Scientific Name/ Description	Part Used	Method of Selection and Processing	Property	Function/Symptoms
chu-pi 橘皮 (aurantium)	*Citrus nobilis* Lour./ Rutaceae; sweet peel tangerine. A tall plant cultivated everywhere.	yellow fruit peels	The fresh green peel called *ching-chu-pi*.	warm	aromatic stomachic, antiemetic, anticough, expectorant/vomiting, hiccups
chu-sha 朱砂 (cinnabar)	Red mercuric sulfide (HgS).		In ancient times native cinnabar was used. Often used as a coating material for pills.	mildly chilly	sedative, spasmolytic/ epilepsy
chu-shih 楮實 (broussonetia)	*Broussonetia papyrifera* Vent./Moraceae; paper mulberry. A tall plant cultivated everywhere.	fruit		chilly	diuretic, tonic/edema, impotence, strengthens the stomach
chu-tan 豬膽 (pig gall)	*Sus scrofa Domesticus*; the domestic pig.	gall bladder	Compress semi-dried variety (*chu-tan-chih*) until the bile juice exudes. Bear's gall is equally effective.	chilly	stomachic, intestinal corrective, analgesic, sedative, antispasm/ gastroenteritis, dyspepsia, abdominal ache, hepatitis
chu-yeh 竹葉 (bamboo leaves)	*Phyllostachys henonis* Mak./Gramineae. Cultivated everywhere.	leaves	All varieties of bamboo may be used. In China the leaves of Commelina communis L./Commelinaceae are used for this drug.	chilly	cleansing and cooling, antifebrile, antithirst, analgesic/feverish diseases

Natural Healing with Chinese Herbs

Chinese Name/ Common Name	Scientific Name/ Description	Part Used	Method of Selection and Processing	Property	Function/Symptoms
chuan-chiung 川芎 (cnidium)	*Cnidium officinale* Makino/ Umbelliferae. A perennial herb indigenous to China.	roots and stems		warm	a warm exsanguinative, hemopoeitic tonic, analgesic/anemia, chills, menoxenia, female disorders
chuan-ku 川骨 (nuphar)	*Nuphar japonicum* DC./ Nymphaeaceae; wild cardamon. A perennial water herb.	roots and stems			exsanguinative indicated in prepartum, postpartum, menoxenia, female disorders
chuan-shan-chia 穿山甲 (anteater scales)	*Manis pentadactyla* L./ Manidae. A mammal indigenous to Africa.	scales		mildly chilly	pus and toxin dispersant, emmenagogue/rheumatism
chueh-ming-tzu 决明子 (cassia seed)	*Cassia tora* L./ Leguminosae; foetid cassia. An annual herb cultivated everywhere	seeds		bland	antiphlogistic, laxative, diuretic/hepatic diseases, ocular diseases
chung-wei-tzu 茺蔚子 (leonurus fruit)	*Leonurus sibiricus* L./ Labiatae; Siberian mother wort or lion's tail. A biennial wild herb found everywhere.	fruit		mildly warm	diuretic/edema

Herbs Used in Chinese Medicine

Chinese Name/ Common Name	Scientific Name/ Description	Part Used	Method of Selection and Processing	Property	Function/Symptoms
chung-pai 葱白 (allium)	*Allium fistulosum* L./ Liliaceae; Chinese small onion. A perennial herb cultivated everywhere.	the white portion of the tubular leaves	Use it raw.	warm	diaphoretic, diuretic/common cold, edema
erh-chu 莪述 (zedoaria)	*Curcuma zedoaria* Rosc./ Zingiberaceae. A perennial herb indigenous to Eastern India; cultivated everywhere in the warm lands.	rhizomes soaked in hot water before use	Also called *hong-hua-shih-yu*.	warm	aromatic stomachic, stimulant, carminative/ dyspepsia, chest and abdominal pain
fan-hsing 番杏 (tetragonia)	*Tetragonia expansa* Murray/ Aizoaceae. A perennial wild herb found at the seashore.	all			stomachic/gastric cancer
fan-hung-hua 番紅花 (saffron)	*Crocus sativus* L./Iridaceae; saffron crocus. A perennial herb indigenous to Southern Europe and Asia Minor.	stigma		bland	sedative, cleansing the blood, emmenagogue/menoxenia, female diseases
fang-chi 防己 (stephania)	*Stephania tetrandra* S. Moore./Menispermaceae. A vine growing in the wilds everywhere.	rhizome or stem		very chilly	antiphlogistic, diuretic, analgesic/edema, neuralgia, arthritis, rheumatism
fang-feng 防風 (siler)	*Siler divaricatum* Benth et HK./Umbelliferae. A perennial herb indigenous	rhizomes	The Chinese product, *pi-fang-feng* is favored; *pin-fang-feng* may also be	chilly	diaphoretic, antipyretic, analgesic/common cold, headache, pain

Chinese Name/ Common Name	Scientific Name/ Description	Part Used	Method of Selection and Processing	Property	Function/Symptoms
fan-pi 反鼻 (viper)	Agkistrodon acutus Guenther. A snake indigenous to China.	all	used as a substitute.	warm	pus dispersant/carbuncles and swellings
fei-tzu 榧子 (torreya)	Torreya grandis Fort./ Taxaceae; kaya nut. A tall plant found in the wilds everywhere.	seeds	Japanese equivalent may also be used.	bland	anthelmintic/duodenal parasite
feng-hsien-tzu 鳳仙子 (garden balsam)	Impatiens balsamina L./ Balsaminaceae; touch-me-not or balsam. An annual herb cultivated everywhere.	seeds		warm	emmenagogue, antidotal/ amenorrhea, dysmenorrhea, carcinoma
feng-mi 蜂蜜 (mel)	Apis chinensis L./Apidae; bees.	honey		bland	nutrient, lenitive, flavoring, tonic/acute impetuous conditions, edema, and as a binder for the manufacture of pills.
fu-ling 茯苓 (hoelen)	Poria cocos (Schw.) Wolff/ Polyporaceae. A fungus growing on and covering the roots of wild pines.			bland	cardiotonic, diuretic, sedative/gastric water stagnancy, abnormal urination, cardiac palpitation, alternating muscular cramping, vertigo, thirst, cough, dyspnea

Herbs Used in Chinese Medicine

Chinese Name/ Common Name	Scientific Name/ Description	Part Used	Method of Selection and Processing	Property	Function/Symptoms
fu-pen-tzu 覆盆子 (rubus)	*Rubus coreanus* Miq./ Rosaceae; wild raspberry. A low plant cultivated everywhere.	fruit		warm	nutrient tonic, seminal tonic/impotence, spermatorrhea, polyuria
fu-ping 浮萍 (lemna)	*Lemna minor* L./Lemnaceae; duckweed. A perennial water weed floating on water everywhere.	all		chilly	diaphoretic, diuretic/edema, dysuria
fu-shih 浮石 (pumice)	Granite from a volcano composed almost entirely of vitreous substance.			bland	diuretic, anticough, anticoagulant/thirst, bronchitis, diabetes mellitus
fu-tzu 附子 (aconite)	*Aconitum carmichaeli* Debx./ Ranunculaceae; aconite. A perennial wild herb found everywhere. The chief root is called *wu-tou*, the autumn root or daughter root is called *fu-tzu*.	tuber	The roots are cut open longitudinally, soaked in saline water, then coated with lime and dried. It is called *pai-ho-fu-tzu*. The *fu-tzu* are wrapped in moist craft paper and heated in hot ashes or in a pressurized autoclave for 20 to 120 minutes and are called *pao-fu-tzu*. These two kinds of processed *fu-tzu* are	very hot	revives extremely degenerated metabolic function; diuretic, cardiotonic/limb arthralgia, heavy limbs, paralysis, chills

Chinese Name/ Common Name	Scientific Name/ Description	Part Used	Method of Selection and Processing	Property	Function/Symptoms
ha-ma 蝦蟆 (rana)	Rana temporaria chensinensis David.; frog.	all	commonly used because the processing reduces toxicity. Remove the intestine and roast the body.	cool	tonic, analgesic/pediatric Kan disease (tabes mesenteris
hai-chin-sha 海金沙 (lygodium)	Lygodium japonicum Sw./ Schizaeceae; climbing fern. A pteridophytic plant found everywhere.	spores on leaves	The reddish brown powder is preferred.	chilly	diuretic, analgesic/ urethral diseases
hai-ma 海馬 (hippocampus)	Hippocampus coronatus/ Syngnathidae; sea horse. A hard bone shell fish found everywhere.	all	The large variety is indigenous to China.	warm	tonic, aphrodisiac/geriatric individuals and postpartum women
hai-sung 海松 (hai-sung)	Pinus koraiensis S. et Z./ Pinaceae; Korean pine. A tall plant found everywhere.	seeds		warm	stomachic, diuretic, anticough/bronchitis
hai-tsao 海藻 (sargassum)	Sargassum siliquastrum Ag./ Sargassaceae; algae. A seaweed found everywhere			chilly	diuretic, alterative, anticough/dysuria, edema, asthma, cough
hai-tung-pi 海桐皮 (erythrina)	Erythrina indica Lam./ Leguminosae; Indian coral tree. A tall plant cultivated everywhere	bark of the tree	In Japan this drug is replaced by the bark of the Araiaceous tzu chiu, a wild tall plant cultivated	warm	astringent, analgesic/ gastroenteritis, dysentery or whitish diarrhea, knee and waist pain, sores and

Chinese Name/ Common Name	Scientific Name/ Description	Part Used	Method of Selection and Processing	Property	Function/Symptoms
han-shui-shih 寒水石 (calcite)	Native white marble.		everywhere. The whiter the better.	chilly	swellings febrifuge, diuretic/vexation, thirst, dysuria
hei-tou 黑豆 (glycine)	*Glycine soja* S. et Z./ Leguminosae; black soybean. An annual herb cultivated everywhere.	seeds		chilly	nutrient, tonic, diuretic, antidotal/poisoning from aconite
ho-shih 鶴虱 (carpesium fruit)	*Carpesium abrotanoides* L./Compositae; pig's head. A biennial herb found everywhere.	fruit		cool	anthelmintic/ascariasis, pin worms, tape worms
ho-shou-wu 何首烏 (ho-shou-wu)	*Polygonum multiflorum* Thunb./Polygonaceae. A wild perennial herb found everywhere.	root		warm	laxative, seminal tonic/ neurasthenia, adenoids
ho-tzu 訶子 (terminalia)	*Terminalia chebula* Retz./ Combretaceae; beleric myrobalans. A tall plant indigenous to Eastern India.	fruit		warm	astringent, sedative/ hemorrhage, cough, diarrhea, asthma

Chinese Name/ Common Name	Scientific Name/ Description	Part Used	Method of Selection and Processing	Property	Function/Symptoms
ho-yeh 荷葉 (lotus leaves)	*Nelumbo nucifera* Gaertn./ Nymphaeaceae; Indian lotus. A perennial water plant cultivated everywhere.	leaves		bland	astringent, hemostatic/ chronic diarrhea, melena
hou-pu 厚朴 (magnolia bark)	*Magnolia officinalis* Rehd. et Wils./Magnoliaceae. A tall plant indigenous to China.	bark of the branches and twigs		warm	astringent, stomachic, intestinal corrective/tension and distention of the chest or abdomen muscles, diarrhea, cough, vomiting
hsi-chiao 犀角 (rhinoceros)	*Rhinoceros unicornis* L./ Rhinocerotidae. The two-horned rhinoceros indigenous to Africa or India.	horn	Render into powder or chips. A species of unicorn rhinoceros indigenous to India named *wu hsi chiao* or *pen hsi* is the most expensive; often the horn of *shui hsi* is used in its place.	chilly	febrifuge, antidotal/measles, poxes
hsi-hsien 豨薟 (siegesbeckia)	*Siegesbeckia pubescens* Mak./ Compositae. A perennial wild herb found everywhere.	all		chilly	tonic, sedative, antidotal/ anemia, neuralgia, rheumatism paralysis, adynamia, hemiplegia
hsi-hsin 細辛 (asarum)	*Asarum sieboldi* Miq./ Aristolochiaceae. A perennial herb growing in the mountains.	root		warm	febrifuge, anticough, analgesic/cough, thoracic distention, thoracic ache

Chinese Name/ Common Name	Scientific Name/ Description	Part Used	Method of Selection and Processing	Property	Function/Symptoms
hsia-ku-tsao 夏枯草 (prunella)	*Prunella vulgaris* L./Labiatae; heal-all or carpenter weed. A perennial wild herb found everywhere.	flower spikes		chilly	antiphlogistic, diuretic/sores and swellings, scrofula, ocular diseases
hsiang-ju 香薷 (elsholtzia)	*Elsholtzia cristata* Willd./ Labiatae; lepechin. An annual wild herb found everywhere.	stem and leaves		mildly warm	antipyretic, diuretic/edema
hsiang-ho 蘘荷 (mioga)	*Zingiber mioga* Rosc./ Zingiberaceae; Japanese ginger. A perennial herb cultivated everywhere.	root		warm	antiphlogistic/cataract, eye injury
hsiang-shih 香豉 (soja)	This is also called insipid relish from fermented hispidia beans.		Often replaced by dried *na-tou*.	chilly	antiphlogistic, antipyretic, stomachic, digestant/thoracic vexation, melancholy
hsiang-fu-tzu 香附子 (cyperus)	*Cyperus rotundus* L./ Cyperaceae: nutgrass. A perennial wild herb found everywhere.	rhizomes		bland	aromatic stomachic, sedative, analgesic, exsanguinative/dyspepsia, diarrhea, abdominal pain, menoxenia, female diseases

Chinese Name/ Common Name	Scientific Name/ Description	Part Used	Method of Selection and Processing	Property	Function/Symptoms
hsiao-mai 小麥 (wheat)	Triticum vulgare Vill./ Gramineae; A cultivated biennial herb.	seeds	Most often the flour is used (wheat flour)	chilly	nutrient, antiphlogistic, paregoric, analgesic, antithirst/neurosis, spontaneous sweating, night sweats
hsiao-shih 硝石 (saltpeter)	Potassium Nitrate.			very chilly	antiphlogistic, diuretic
hsiao-tou-kou 小豆蔻 (elettaria)	Elettaria cardamomum Maton/Zingiberaceae; cardamon. A perennial herb indigenous to the Philippines.	fruit		warm	a fragrant stomachic, carminative/gastroenteritis, dyspepsia
hsieh 蠍 (scorpion)	Buthus martensi Karsch/ Buthidae.	all		bland	sedative/pediatric epilepsy, convulsive seizures
hsieh-pai 薤白 (bakeri)	Allium bakeri Regel/Liliaceae; garden shallot or baker's garlic. A perennial herb cultivated everywhere.	bulbs		warm	warm stomachic, intestinal corrective anticough, expectorant/ chronic gastritis, cardiac asthma, backache, thoracic pain
hsin-i (magnolia flower)	Magnolia liliflora Desr./ Magnoliaceae; magnolia. A tall plant cultivated	flower bud		warm	antipyretic, diaphoretic, analgesic/rhinitis, empyema, toothache, headache

Chinese Name/ Common Name	Scientific Name/ Description	Part Used	Method of Selection and Processing	Property	Function/Symptoms
	everywhere.				
hsing-jen 杏仁 (apricot seed)	*Prunus armeniaca* L./ Rosaceae; apricot. A perennial shrub cultivated everywhere.	kernel		warm	anticough, expectorant, diuretic/water toxin in chest, dyspnea, asthma, cough, thoracic distention, thoracic pain, edema
Hsiung-huang 雄黃 (realgar)	Native mineral disulphide of arsenic, As_2S_2.		The more transparent the better. Pulverized into a powder.	warm	antidotal, insecticidal/ dermatoses, noxious sores
hsiung-tan 熊膽 (bear gall)	*Ursus torquatus* Schinz./ Ursidae. Himalayan black bear.	dried content of gall bladder	Yellowish brown to dark yellowish brown, translucent or non-transparent solid masses. Many are counterfeit.	chilly	cholegogue, excitant, spasmolytic, analgesic/ emergent cases, acute disease, pediatric diseases
hsu-sui-tzu 續隨子 (lathyris)	*Euphorbia lathyris* L./ Euphorbiaceae; caperspurge, mole plant. A biennial herb cultivated everywhere.	seeds	poisonous	warm	diuretic, emmenagogue, purgative/edema, ascites, amenorrhea, poisoning
hsu-twan 續斷 (dipsacus)	*Dipsacus japonicus* Miq./ Dipsacaceae; teazel. A perennial wild herb found everywhere.	root		mildly warm	tonic, sedative, emmenagogue/ general pain

Chinese Name/ Common Name	Scientific Name/ Description	Part Used	Method of Selection and Processing	Property	Function/Symptoms
hsuan-fu-hua 旋覆花 (inula)	*Inula japonica* Thunb./Compositae; A perennial wild herb found everywhere.	flower	Those with the most petals.	warm	stomachic, antiemetic, analgesic, expectorant/ cough, eructation, abdominal pain
hsuan-sheng 玄參 (scrophularia)	*Scrophularia ningpoensis* Hemsley./Scrophulariaceae; figwort. A wild perennial herb found everywhere.	root		mildly chilly	antiphlogistic, antipyretic, sedative/venereal diseases, pharyngo-laryngeal ache
hsun-lu 薰陸 (mastic)	*Pistacea khinjuk* Stocks/ Anacardiaceae; Bombay mastic. A delicate tall plant indigenous to Eastern India.	resin exuded from the tree	Many similar articles are not the same.	warm	diuretic/edema used also as a fragrant fumigant
hu-chiao 胡椒 (pepper)	*Piper nigrum* L./Piperaceae; black pepper. A creeper indigenous to the philippines.	immature fruit		hot	aromatic and acrid stomachic, carminative/ anorexia, dyspepsia, abdominal pain
hu-huang-lien 胡黃蓮 (picrorrhiza)	*Picrorrhiza kurroa* Benth./ Scrophulariaceae. A perennial herb indigenous to China.	root	In Japan this drug is replaced by *tang yao* (swertia).	chilly	antiphlogistic, antipyretic, stomachic, intestinal corrective/hepatitis, ocular diseases, spontaneous sweating

Herbs Used in Chinese Medicine

Chinese Name/ Common Name	Scientific Name/ Description	Part Used	Method of Selection and Processing	Property	Function/Symptoms
hu-ku 虎骨 (tiger's shinbone)	*Felis tigris* L./Felidae; tiger.	tibia bones		warm	analgesic, spasmolytic/ pain in limbs, waist and back, convulsions, epilepsy
hu-lu-pa 胡蘆巴 (trigonella)	*Trigonella foenum-graecum* L./Leguminosae; fenugreek seed. An annual herb indigenous to China.	seeds		warm	nutrient, tonic, laxative/ gastroenteritis, abdominal distention, abdominal pain, nephritis
hu-ma 胡麻 (sesame)	*Sesamum indicum* L./Pedaliaceae; sesame. An annual herb cultivated everywhere.	seeds		bland	laxative, demulcent
hu-ma-yu 胡麻油 (sesame oil)	*Sesamum indicum* L./Pedaliaceae; sesame. An annual herb cultivated everywhere.	yellow oil	Seeds are heated and compressed.		raw material for plasters
hu-pi 槲皮 (quercus)	*Quercus dentata* Thunb./ Fagaceae; big leaf oak. In the wilds everywhere.	bark of the tree	Often used as a substitute for bark of the wild cherry.		astringent/skin diseases
hu-po 琥珀 (succinum)	Amber. Resin from Pinaceous plants indigenous to Africa and other regions; they become fossilized.			bland	astringent, diuretic, hemostatic, sedative/ hemorrhages from various conditions, urethritis,

Chinese Name/ Common Name	Scientific Name/ Description	Part Used	Method of Selection and Processing	Property	Function/Symptoms
hua-shih 滑石 (talc)	Argillaceous earth, the chief constituent of which is hydrous aluminum silicate.		Not the commonly used talc but the massive pieces of talc capable of being cut into ornamental figures. *Tang hua shih* imported from China is dirty and white and completely odorless.	chilly	cystitis, rheumatism, amenorrhea antiphlogistic, diuretic, antithirst/cystitis, urethral diseases
huai-chiao 槐角 (sophora fruit)	*Sophora japonica* L./Leguminosae; pagoda tree. A tall plant indigenous to China.	fruit		chilly	astringent, sedative hemostatic/hemorrhage of various conditions, hypertension, cerebral hemorrhage, metritis, hemorrhoids
huai-hua 槐花 (sophora flower)	*Sophora japonica* L./Leguminosae; pagoda tree. A tall plant indigenous to China.	flower buds		mildly chilly	astringent, hemostatic, analgesic/various kinds of hemorrhages, hypertension, cerebral hemorrhage, metritis, diarrhea
huang-chi 黃耆 (astragalus)	*Astragalus membranaceus* Bge./Leguminosae; yellow vetch. A perennial herb	root	Those with a soft texture and a slightly sweet taste (*mien huang chi*) are used.	mildly warm	antihidrotic, diuretic, tonic/water toxin on the body surface, weakness,

Herbs Used in Chinese Medicine

Chinese Name/ Common Name	Scientific Name/ Description	Part Used	Method of Selection and Processing	Property	Function/Symptoms
	indigenous to China.		(In Japan the so-called ho-huang-chi which is hard and bitter is a different herb.)		malnutrition, spontaneous sweating, night sweats, dysuria, dropsy
huang-chin 黃芩 (scute)	Scutellaria baicalensis Georgi/Labiatae; baical skullcap. A perennial herb indigenous to China.		Use the bright yellow, young roots. The old roots are yellowish green and look rigid.	chilly	antiphlogistic/congestive and phlogistic rigidity beneath the heart, thoracocostal distress, vexation in the heart, diarrhea
huang-ching 黃精 (sibiricum)	Polygonatum sibiricum Rehd./Liliaceae; deer bamboo. A perennial wild herb found everywhere.	rhizomes		bland	nutrient, tonic, febrifuge/ weakness after an illness
huang-chung 蝗蟲 (locusts)	Oxya velox Fab./Acridiae; locusts.	all	Often found clinging to rice.		spasmolytic, anticough/ bronchitis, asthma, whooping cough
huang-lien 黃連 (coptis)	Coptis teeta Wallich./Ranunculaceae; golden thread. A perennial herb cultivated or found in the mountain areas.	rhizomes		chilly	anti-inflammatory and bitter tasting stomachic/ congestion and inflammation with vexation and depression in the heart, dyspepsia, palpitation, mental distress, rigidity beneath the heart, vomiting, diarrhea,

Chinese Name/ Common Name	Scientific Name/ Description	Part Used	Method of Selection and Processing	Property	Function/Symptoms
huang-po 黃檗 (phellodendron)	*Phellodendron amurense* Rupr./Rutaceae; Amur cork tree. A wild tall plant found in the mountains.	bark with epidermis removed		chilly	antiphlogistic, stomachic, astringent/gastroenteritis, abdominal pain, jaundice, diarrhea.
huang-tu 黃土 (fu-lung-kan)	Burnt yellow earth found inside of ancient Chinese stoves. Today substitute coarse powder made from earthenware or pottery after the first coarse burn.		Used externally in powder form for contusions. Used as an eye wash when decocted in liquid.		abdominal pain
				mildly warm	warm antiemetic, astringent, hemostatic/ hemorrhage, hematemesis, epistaxis, morning sickness
hui-hsiang 茴香 (fennel)	*Foeniculum vulgare* Mill./ Umbelliferae; fennel. A perennial herb cultivated everywhere.	fruit	During the Edo era in Japan, this drug was called *ta-hui-hsiang*, while the name *hsiao-hui-hsiang* was ascribed to *shih-lo* (Umbelliferous *Peucedanum graveolens* Bth. Hk.).	warm	aromatic stomachic, expectorant/gastritis, stomachache, abdominal pain
hung-hua 紅花 (carthamus)	*Carthamus tinctorius* L./ Compositae; safflower. A biennial herb indigenous to India.	flower petals		warm	exsanguinative/female ailments, prepartum, postpartum illnesses abdominal pain, menoxenia

Herbs Used in Chinese Medicine

Chinese Name/ Common Name	Scientific Name/ Description	Part Used	Method of Selection and Processing	Property	Function/Symptoms
huo-hsiang 藿香 (agastache)	*Agastache rugosa* O. Kuntze; *Pogostemon cablin* (Blanco) Benth./Labiatae. A perennial wild herb found everywhere.	leaves		mildly warm	aromatic stomachic/ gastroenteritis, dyspepsia, vomiting, abdominal pain
i-chih 益智 (black cardamon)	*Amomum amarum* Lour./ Zingiberaceae; black or bitter cardamon. A perennial herb indigenous to China.	fruit		warm	aromatic bitter stomachic, intestinal corrective/gastroenteritis, dyspepsia, diarrhea
i-yi-jen 薏以仁 (coix)	*Coix lachryma-jobi* L./ Graminae; Job's tears. An annual herb cultivated everywhere.	seeds	When used with its hulls is called *chiu-mai* (dove's wheat), a folk medicine.	mildly chilly	nutrient, diuretic, analgesic, pus dispersant/dropsy, coarse skin, general pain, suppuration
i-mu-tsao 益母草 (leonurus)	*Leonurus sibiricus* L./ Labiatae; Siberian motherwort. A biennial wild herb found everywhere.	stem and leaves		mildly chilly	exsanguinative, tonic, emmenagogue, hemostatic/ menoxenia, female ailments
i-pao-tuo-la 伊保多螺 (ligustrum wax)	*Ligustrum obtusifolium* Sieb. et Zucc./Oleaceae; Waxtree. Found in the wilds.	wax secreted on the tree by male imagos of *Ericerus pela* Chavannes	Secreta are collected and melted to form a solid mass called ibota wax.		hemostatic, analgesic/ cuts (Also used as a lubricant for sliding doors)

Chinese Name/ Common Name	Scientific Name/ Description	Part Used	Method of Selection and Processing	Property	Function/Symptoms
i-tou-suo-sha 伊豆縮砂 (alpinia seed)	Alpinia japonica Miq./ Zingiberaceae; wild ginger. A perennial wild herb found in warm fields.	seeds			aromatic stomachic, a substitute of suo-sha
jen-sheng 人參 (ginseng)	Panax ginseng C.A. Meyer/ Araliaceae. A perennial herb indigenous to China and Korea and cultivated everywhere in Japan.	roots or rootlets	Small roots with a yellowish brown surface and longitudinal grooves are called chung-sheng. The thin roots called shu-sheng (whisker jen-sheng) are commonly used for the drug. Bulky white jen-sheng (Korean jen-sheng) after being steamed turns a yellowish red color and is called red jen-sheng. Sometimes Japanese jen-sheng is used as a substitute.	warm	stomachic, tonic, seminal tonic/degenerated metabolism due to weakened stomach and intestines, thoraco-costal distress and fullness, anorexia, lassitude, pain, diarrhea
jen-tung-teng 忍冬藤 (lonicera stem)	Lonicera japonica Thunb./ Caprifoliaceae; Japanese honeysuckle. A perennial wild herb found everywhere.	stem and leaves	This drug may be used in place of Lonicerae Flos.	chilly	cleanses the blood, diuretic, antidotal/arthritis, syphilis, pustulent diseases, sores and swellings
jou-tou-kou 肉豆蔻	Myristica fragrans Houtt. /Myristacaceae; nutmeg.	seeds		warm	aromatic stomachic, intestinal corrective/

Herbs Used in Chinese Medicine

Chinese Name/ Common Name	Scientific Name/ Description	Part Used	Method of Selection and Processing	Property	Function/Symptoms
(myristica)	A tall plant indigenous to the Philippines.				gastroenteritis (Also used as a food flavoring agent)
jou-tsung-jung 肉苁蓉 (cistanche)	Cistanche salsa (C.A. Mey.) G. Beck./Orobanchaceae; broomrape. A perennial herb indigenous to China.	all		mildly warm	tonic, aphrodisiac/impotence, spermatorrhea, chilly waist and feet
ju-hsiang 乳香 (mastic)	Boswellia carterii Birdw./ Burseraceae; Bombay mastic or terebinth tree. Indigenous to Africa.	resin exudated from the trunk of the tree		bland	analgesic, emmenagogue/ dropsical pains, abdominal pain (Also used as a deodorant)
jung-yen 戎鹽 (crystal salt)	Native salt; impure sodium chloride containing traces of ferric oxide which gives a reddish color or ferrous oxide which gives a blue color.		Use sodium chloride.	chilly	antiphlogistic, hemostatic/ toothache, hemorrhages from various conditions
kan-cha 甘茶 (Kan-cha)	Hydrangea thunberigii Sieb./Saxifragaceae; hydrangea. A low plant cultivated everywhere.	leaves		cool	a sweetening agent, a substitute for sugar
kan-chi 乾漆 (dried lacquar)	Rhus vernicifera DC./ Anacardiaceae. A tall varnish tree found	varnish exudated by tree		warm	exsanguinative, anthelmintic/ amenorrhea, ascariasis, chronic dermatoses

Chinese Name/ Common Name	Scientific Name/ Description	Part Used	Method of Selection and Processing	Property	Function/Symptoms
	everywhere.	and dried after long standing			
kan-chiang 乾薑 (dried ginger)	Zingiber officinale Rosc./Zingiberaceae. A perennial herb cultivated everywhere.	peeled rhizomes are soaked in lime juice and then dried	The so-called san-ho-kan-chiang or hei-chiang has been peeled and soaked in hot boiled water before drying.	hot	reviving metabolic functions/weakness confomation, water toxin that soars up, vomiting, cough, chills, vexation and irritation, chill and aches in chest and abdomen, low back pain
kan-sui 甘遂 (kan-sui)	Euphorbia sieboldiana Morr. et Dcne./Euphorbiaceae; Siebold's spurge. A perennial herb indigenous to China.	root		chilly	water dispersant, cathartic/difficulty in bowel movement and urination, edema, thoraco-abdominal pain
kan-sung 甘松 (spikenard)	Nardostachys chinensis Batal./Valerianaceae. A perennial herb indigenous to Himalayan mountains.	rhizomes		warm	aromatic stomachic, spasmolytic, analgesic/ headache, thoraco-abdominal pain
kan-tsao 甘草 (licorice)	Glycyrrhiza glabra L./ Leguminosae. A perennial herb indigenous	root	Those that are sweet with less bitterness, cylindrical in shape, and coarse and	bland	paregoric, anticough, expectorant, analgesic/ cramping, stomachache

Herbs Used in Chinese Medicine

Chinese Name/ Common Name	Scientific Name/ Description	Part Used	Method of Selection and Processing	Property	Function/Symptoms
	to China.		large in diameter are better. Generally backed.		arthralgia, pharyngeal pain, abdominal pain, diarrhea
kao-pen 藁本 (kao-pen)	*Ligusticum sinense* Oliv.; *Nothosmyrnium japonicum* Miq./Umbelliferae. A perennial wild herb found everywhere.	rhizomes		warm	spasmolytic, analgesic headace, abdominal pain
keng-mi 粳米 (oryza)	*Oryza sativa* L./Gramineae; rice. An annual herb cultivated everywhere.		Not polished.	cool	nutrient, tonic, lenitive, antithirst/thirst, vexation and irritation
ko-ken 葛根 (pueraria)	*Pueraria hirsuta* Schneid/ Leguminosae; ke hemp. A wild vine found everywhere.	root	Remove the outer skin and dice; now called *chiao-ko-ken*.	bland	diaphoretic, febrifuge, lenitive/feverish diseases, common cold, rigidity in the back and neck
kou-chi-tzu 枸杞子 (lycium fruit)	*Lycium chinense* Mill./ Solanaceae; Chinese wolfberry. A wild shrub found everywhere.	berry	May be used in the production of lycium wine.	bland	antiphlogistic, tonic, nutrient, seminal tonic, diuretic/ weakness, pulmonary diseases, diabetes mellitus
kou-chi-yeh 枸杞葉 (lycium leaves)	*Lycium chinense* Mill./ Solanaceae; Chinese wolfberry. A wild shrub found everywhere.	leaves	The cortices of the roots are called *ti-ku-pi*.	cool	cleansing and cooling, antipyretic, anticough, virilizing/vexatious fever, weakness fever

Chinese Name/ Common Name	Scientific Name/ Description	Part Used	Method of Selection and Processing	Property	Function/Symptoms
ku-ching-tsao 穀精草 (eriocaulon)	*Eriocaulon buergerianum* Koern./Eriocaulaceae; pipewort. An annual herb found near ponds.	all		mildly warm	antiphlogistic, cleansing and cooling/ocular diseases
ku-lien-pi 苦楝皮 (melia bark)	*Melia azedarach* L./Meliaceae; Persian lilac. A tall plant cultivated everywhere.	cortices of root and trunk		chilly	antipyretic, anthelmintic, ascariasis, pin worms, tape worms
ku-lien-tzu 苦楝子 (melia)	*Melia azedarach* L./Meliaceae; Persian lilac. A tall plant cultivated everywhere.	fruit		chilly	astringent, analgesic/ abdominal pain
ku-mu 苦木 (picrasma)	*Picrasma ailanthoides* Planchon/Simarubaceae. A tall wild plant found everywhere.	wood of the tree			a bitter stomachic/ gastroenteritis, dyspepsia
ku-sheng 苦參 (sophora)	*Sophora flavescens* Ait./ Leguminosae; sophora. A perennial wild herb found everywhere.	root		chilly	stomachic, diuretic; antipyretic, analgesic, insecticide/sores and swellings edema
kua-lou-ken 栝樓根 (trichosanthes root)	*Trichosanthes multiloba* Miq./Cucurbitaceae. A perennial wild herb found everywhere.	root	Pale and non-bitter roots are used.	mildly chilly	antipyretic, antithirst/ weakness conformation with thirst (Also used as a lactogogue)

Herbs Used in Chinese Medicine

Chinese Name/ Common Name	Scientific Name/ Description	Part Used	Method of Selection and Processing	Property	Function/Symptoms
kua-lou-shih 栝樓實 (trichosanthes seed)	*Trichosanthes multiloba* Miq./Cucurbitaceae. A perennial wild herb found everywhere.	seeds	Seeds that resemble persimmons. The kernels are called *kua-lu-jen*. Occasionally the seeds of *wang-kua* (*Kochia scoparia*) are substituted.	chilly	antiphlogistic, anticough, expectorant, analgesic/ cardiac, asthma, thoracic pain
kua-ti 瓜蒂 (melon pedicle)	*Cucumis melo* L./Cucurbitaceae; cataloup. A wild annual herb found everywhere.	peduncles of immature fruit	Use the very bitter ones. Burn and render into powder.	chilly	emetic indicated for toxin within chest
kuan-tung-hua 款冬花 (tussilago)	*Tussilago farfara* L./Compositae; coltsfoot. A perennial herb indigenous to China.	flower buds		warm	stomachic, anticough, expectorant/bronchitis
kuei-chih 桂枝 (cinnamon)	*Cinnamomum cassia* Bl./ Lauraceae; Chinese cinnamon. A tall plant indigenous to southern China, eastern India, and Indochina.	bark of twigs	Regardless of the thickness of the bark, select that with a strong pungent odor, a sweet but not harsh taste. Of the Japanese variety the cortices of the roots have a strong fragrance. Used in the preparation of the *tu su*.	very hot	diaphoretic, febrifuge, analgesic/headache, fever, flushing up, anemophobia, general aching

Chinese Name/ Common Name	Scientific Name/ Description	Part Used	Method of Selection and Processing	Property	Function/Symptoms
kuei-pan 龜板 (turtle shell)	*Chinemys reevesii* (Gary); *Clemmys japonica* Tem. et Sch.; terrapin.	plastron or back shell of the river terrapin		bland	hematonic strengthening agent, febrifuge/ pulmonary tuberculosis, debility before and after labor
kun-pu 昆布 (laminaria)	*Laminaria japonica* Aresch./Laminariaceae; sweet tangle.	all		chilly	diuretic, alterative, anticough/dysuria, edema, bronchitis
la-ku-shih 蝲蛄石 (shrimp stone)		spike-form stone of lime; each year two such are generated in the stomach of the shrimp			stomachic, antacid, diuretic/gastroenteritis
lai-fu-tzu 萊菔子 (raphanus)	*Raphanus sativus* L./ Cruciferae; radish. A biennial herb cultivated everywhere.	seeds		bland	stomachic, expectorant/ gastritis, bronchitis
lan-shih 藍實 (indigo fruit)	*Polygonum tinctorium* Lour./Polygonaceae; indigo plant. An annual	fruit		chilly	febrifuge, antidotal/ feverish diseases

Chinese Name/ Common Name	Scientific Name/ Description	Part Used	Method of Selection and Processing	Property	Function/Symptoms
lan-tsao 蘭草 (thoroughwort)	*Eupatorium chinense* L./ Compositae; Chinese thoroughwort. A perennial wild herb. herb cultivated everywhere.	all		bland	diaphoretic, febrifuge, diuretic/feverish diseases, menoxenia, jaundice, rheumatism
lang-tang 莨菪 (hyoscyamus)	*Hyoscyamus niger* L./ Solanaceae; henbane. A perennial herb indigenous to China.	rhizomes		warm	analgesic, spasmolytic, sedative/abdominal pain, neuralgia, whooping cough, asthma, hyperhidrosis, tenesmus; externally for hemorrhoids
lei-wan 雷丸 (omphalia)	*Omphalia lapidescens* Schroet./ Polyporaceae. Fungi; thunder pills. A fungus growing on the roots of bamboo.			chilly	anthelmintic/tape worms
li-ching 瀝青 (asphalt)	Native asphalt.				preservative, a material for plasters.
li-ken-pi 李根皮 (communis)	*Prunus communis* Huds./ Rosaceae; plum. A tall plant cultivated everywhere.	cortices of roots		chilly	antiphlogistic, sedative/ neurosis

Chinese Name/ Common Name	Scientific Name/ Description	Part Used	Method of Selection and Processing	Property	Function/Symptoms
li-lu 藜蘆 (veratrum)	*Veratrum nigrum* L./Liliaceae; black veratrum. Perennial wild herb found everywhere.	root and rhizomes	In Europe white veratrum is used, in the U.S. green veratrum. Both varieties are extremely poisonous.	chilly	rendering emesis, antidotal, hypotensive, sedative/hypertension
liang-chiang 良薑 (galanga)	*Alpinia officinarum* Hance./Zingiberaceae; lesser galangal. A perennial herb indigenous to China.	rhizomes		hot	aromatic stomachic, analgesic/gastritis, dyspepsia, gastralgia, abdominal pain
liao-shih 蓼實 (hydropiper)	*Polygonum hydropiper* L./Polygonaceae; smartweed or water pepper. An annual herb found in the wilds everywhere.	fruit		warm	antiphlogistic, diuretic/ocular diseases
lien-chiao 連翹 (forsythia)	*Forsythia suspensa* Vahl./Oleaceae; forsythia. A low plant indigenous to China.	fruit		mildly chilly	antiphlogistic, diuretic, pus dispersant/sores and swellings, scrofulosis
lien-chien-tsao 連錢草 (glechoma)	*Glechoma hederacea* L./Labiatae; ground ivy or field balm. A perennial wild herb found everywhere.	all			febrifuge, tonic/children's tabes mesenteris

Herbs Used in Chinese Medicine

Chinese Name/ Common Name	Scientific Name/ Description	Part Used	Method of Selection and Processing	Property	Function/Symptoms
lien-jou 蓮肉 (lotus seed)	*Nelumbo nucifera* Gaertn./ Nymphaeaceae; Indian lotus. A perennial herb cultivated everywhere.	seeds	Remove the black outer skin.	bland	nutrient tonic, seminal tonic/ gastroenteritis, impotence, neurasthenia
ling-yang-chiao 羚羊角 (antelope horn)	*Saiga tatarica* L./Bovidae; A mammal indigenous to the North of China and Mongolia.	horn	In Japan this drug is replaced by *tan lu* (blanket deer) horns.	chilly	febrifuge, antidotal, analgesic/feverish diseases
liu-chi-nu-tsao 劉寄奴草 (anomala)	*Artemisia anomala* S. Moore; *Solidago virga-aurea* L./ Compositae; goldenrod. A perennial wild herb found everywhere.	all		warm	exsanguinative, analgesic, hemostatic, rendering menstrual flow, prepartum and postpartum/hemorrhage from all conditions, headache
liu-huang 硫黃 (sulfur)	Native sulfur. Often the sublimed sulfur is used.			warm	laxative/used externally in dermatosis
lou-lu 漏蘆 (rhaponticum)	*Rhaponticum uniflorum* DC.; *Echinops dahuricus* Fisch. /Compositae; globe thistle.	root		chilly	pus dispersant, hemostatic/ hemorrhage of all kinds, sores and swellings, hemorrhoids
lu-chiao 鹿角 (deer horn)	*Cervus sika* Tmm.; sika deer. A mammal living everywhere.	horn	Horns are made into powder and burnt black; called *lu-chiao-shuan*.	warm	tonic, dispelling pus/sores and swellings

691

Chinese Name/ Common Name	Scientific Name/ Description	Part Used	Method of Selection and Processing	Property	Function/Symptoms
lu-fan 綠礬 (melanterite)	Alum of ferrous sulfate.			chilly	astringent, hematonic/ anemia, yellow emaciation
lu-feng-fang 露蜂房 (wasps nest)	Hornets' and wasps' nests exposed to wind and dew.			bland	spasmolytic, antidotal, emmenagogue/ pediatric terrors and convulsion
lu-huei 蘆薈 (aloe)	*Aloe vulgaris* Lam./Liliaceae. A perennial herb indigenous to Africa.	juice contained in leaves	Dried to solid extract form.	chilly	antiphlogistic, diuretic, antidotal/thirst, jaundice, rheumatism, liver ailments
lu-jung 鹿茸 (young deer horn)	*Cervus sika* Tmm.; *C. nippon* Temminck/Cervidae; sika deer.	newly grown young horns covered with velvety hair	Cut into thin slices.	warm	tonic, aphrodisiac/ neurasthenia, impotence, spermatorrhea, night sweats
lu-kan-shih 爐甘石 (zinc-bloom)	A mixture of impure zinc carbonate and zinc oxide, or the zinc bloom.		May be replaced with a mixture of zinc oxide and 1% of ferric sulfate.	warm	antiphlogistic, astringent, preservative/ external uses and as an eye drop
lu-ken 蘆根 (phragmites)	*Phragmites communis* (L.) Trin./Gramineae; common reed. A perennial wild herb	rhizomes	Rhizomes are used raw.	chilly	antiphlogistic, diuretic, antidotal/ feverish diseases with

Herbs Used in Chinese Medicine

Chinese Name/ Common Name	Scientific Name/ Description	Part Used	Method of Selection and Processing	Property	Function/Symptoms
	found everywhere.				thirst, jaundice, arthritis, liver ailments
luan-fa-shuang 亂髮霜 (human hair)	Loose strands of human hair collected from combs or brushes.		Burn black.	mildly warm	diuretic, hemostatic/ hematuria
lung-ku 龍骨 (dragon bone)	Fossilized bones of ancient mammoths.			bland	astringent, sedative/ palpitation at the navel, hysteria and terror, vexation and irritation, spermatorrhea, insomnia
lung-nao 龍腦 (borneol)	*Dryobalanops aromatica* Gaertn./Dipterocarpaceae; A tall plant indigenous to Borneo and the Philippines.	exudated solid substance from trunk	Often *pien-nao* is subjected to chemical purification.	mildly chilly	antiphlogistic, anodyn/cardiac palpitation
lung-tan 龍膽 (gentiana)	*Gentiana scabra* Bge./ Gentianaceae; gentian. A perennial herb indigenous to China.	root		very chilly	febrifuge, bitter stomachic, diuretic/ dyspepsia, gastritis, jaundice
lung-yen-jou 龍眼肉 (longan)	*Nephelium longana* Lamb./ Sapindaceae. A tall plant indigenous to China.	pseudocarp (mesocarp) of fruit with the		warm	nutrient tonic/ neurasthenia, insomnia

Chinese Name/ Common Name	Scientific Name/ Description	Part Used	Method of Selection and Processing	Property	Function/Symptoms
ma-chien-tzu 馬錢子 (nux vomica)	*Strychnos nux-vomica* L./ Loganiaceae. A tall plant indigenous to India and the Philippines.	epicarp (shell) and kernels removed seeds		chilly	bitter stomachic, tonic/chronic gastro-intestinal disturbances
ma-huang 麻黃 (ma-huang)	*Ephedra sinica* Stapf/ Ephedraceae; ephedra. A low wild plant indigenous to Mongolia, China.	stem above ground	Remove roots which are anhidrotic. Nodes are numerous and hence not easy to eliminate.	warm	diaphoretic, febrifuge, anticough, water dispersant/dyspnea due to disturbance in the skin's excretion function, cough, asthma, anhidrosis
ma-ming-tuei 馬明退 (silkworm molt)	*Bombyx mori* L.	molts of silkworms		bland	hemostatic/gastric and uterine hemorrhage
ma-tou-ling 馬兜鈴 (aristolochia)	*Aristolochia debilis* S. et Z./ Aristolochiaceae. A perennial wild creeper found everywhere.	fruit		chilly	febrifuge, anticough, expectorant, antidotal/bronchitis, asthma

Herbs Used in Chinese Medicine

Chinese Name/ Common Name	Scientific Name/ Description	Part Used	Method of Selection and Processing	Property	Function/Symptoms
ma-tzu-jen 麻子仁 (linum)	*Cannabis sativa* L./Moraceae; hemp. An annual herb cultivated everywhere.	fruit	Remove hulls before use.	bland	demulcent, diuretic, anticough, analgesic/constipation
mai-men-tung 麥冬門 (ophiopogon)	*Ophiopogon spicata* Ker.-Gawl./Liliaceae; black leek. A perennial herb cultivated everywhere.	swollen tubers (or tubers) from thin roots of small-leafed species *Ophiopogon japonica*		mildly chilly	antiphlogistic, febrifuge, nutrient, tonic, anticough, expectorant, antithirst/cough pharyngitis or laryngitis, pulmonary tuberculosis
mai-ya 麥芽 (malt)	*Hordeum vulgare* L./Gramineae; barley. An annual herb cultivated everywhere.	sprouts of seeds		warm	stomachic, nutrient, tonic, digestion
man-ching-tzu 蔓荊子 (vitex)	*Vitex trifolia* L. var. *ovata* Mak./Verbenaceae. A wild low plant found everywhere.	fruit		mildly chilly	sedative, antiphlogistic, analgesic/ear ache, headache, eye ache, neuralgia, convulsive pains
man-tuo-luo-hua 曼陀羅花 (datura)	*Datura alba* Nees.; *D. metel* L./Solanaceae. An annual herb found in the wild everywhere.	flower		warm	anesthetic, analgesic, spasmolytic, anticough/ bronchitis, asthma

Chinese Name/ Common Name	Scientific Name/ Description	Part Used	Method of Selection and Processing	Property	Function/Symptoms
mang-hsiao 芒硝 (mirabilitum)	Side product of table salt, crude magnesium sulfate.		In the past regarded as sodium sulfate but it has been re-identified as magnesium sulfate.	very chilly	cathartic, diuretic/ distention in chest and abdomen, constipation, extravasation, jaundice
mao-ken 茅根 (imperata)	Imperata cylindrica (L.) Beauv. var. major (Nees) Hubb./Gramineae; floss grass. A perennial wild herb found everywhere.	rhizomes		chilly	antiphlogistic, diuretic, cleansing the blood/gonorrhea, nephroses, metritis
meng-chung 虻蟲 (tabanus) (gadfly)	Tabanus bivittatus Matsumura/ Tabanidae; bi-wing insect family.	entire body of females		mildly chilly	exsanguinative/stale extravasation, dysmenorrhea, distention in lower abdomen
mi-la 蜜蠟 (yellow wax)	Apis chinensis L./Apidae; honey bee.	yellowish wax from bee's nests	If the wax has been subject to sunlight bleaching, it is called sun-bleached beeswax.	mildly warm	used as an ointment
mi-tuo-seng 密陀僧 (litharge)	Lead monoxide.			bland	astringent, hemostatic/ raw material for the manufacture of plaster
mien-ma 綿馬 (aspidium)	Aspidium falcatum Sw./ Polypodiaceae; wood fern.	root	The Chinese name is kuan-chung.	chilly	astringent, hemostatic, anthelmintic/hemorrhage

Herbs Used in Chinese Medicine

Chinese Name/ Common Name	Scientific Name/ Description	Part Used	Method of Selection and Processing	Property	Function/Symptoms
	A perennial wild herb found everywhere.				from various conditions, tape worms
mo-yao 沒藥 (myrrh)	Commiphora myrrha Engl. Burseraceae. A shrub found along the banks of the Red Sea.	resin from the bark		bland	stomachic, analgesic/ sores and swellings, also used as an astringent when applied externally to the lips
mu-chin-hua 木槿花 (hibiscus flower)	Hibiscus syriacus L./ Malvaceae; shrubby althaea. A low plant cultivated everywhere.	white flowers		cool	demulcent, astringent, hemostatic/diarrhea, melena
mu-hsiang 木香 (saussurea)	Saussurea lappa Clarke/ Compositae. A perennial wild herb indigenous to India.	root		warm	stomachic, intestinal corrective/gastroenteritis, vomiting, diarrhea, abdominal pain
mu-kua 木瓜 (chaenomeles)	Chaenomeles lagenaria Koidz./ Rosaceae; Chinese quince. A low plant cultivated everywhere.	fruit		warm	diuretic, intestinal corrective, analgesic/ beriberi, rheumatism
mu-la 木蠟 (white wax)	Rhus succedanea L./ Anacardiaceae; Hungarian fustic. A tall tree found everywhere.	white wax, a solid fatty resin compressed	Although called a wax, it is a fat.		base of an ointment

Chinese Name/ Common Name	Scientific Name/ Description	Part Used	Method of Selection and Processing	Property	Function/Symptoms
mu-li 牡蠣 (oyster shell)	Ostrea talienwhanensis Crosse/Ostreidae; a shelled mollusk.	from pericarpium of fruit and bleached by sunlight shell	Grind into a coarse powder.	mildly chilly	sedative, astringent, antacid, antithirst/ thoracic and abdominal palpitation, hysteria, vexation, irritation, spermatorrhea
mu-tan-pi 牡丹皮 (moutan)	Paeonia moutan Sims/ Ranunculaceae; tree peony. A shrub cultivated everywhere.	cortices of roots	Remove wooden core.	mildly chilly	exsanguinative, analgesic, sedative/headache, abdominal ache, menoxenia, appendicitis, female ailments
mu-pieh-tzu 木鱉子 (momordica)	Momordica cochinchinensis Spr./Cucurbitaceae; wild cucumber. A perennial creeper indigenous to China.	seeds		warm	antiphlogistic, antidotal/sores and swellings
mu-tien-liao 木天蓼 (actinidia)	Actinidia Polygama Miq./ Actinidiaceae. A perennial herb found everywhere.	galls formed at center of		warm	tonic, cardiotonic, diuretic, analgesic/ colic, low back pain

Chinese Name/ Common Name	Scientific Name/ Description	Part Used	Method of Selection and Processing	Property	Function/Symptoms
mu-tsei 木賊 (equisetum)	*Equisetum hiemale* L./ Equisetaceae. A wild perennial herb found everywhere.	flower by fly during summer all		warm	astringent, hemostatic, diuretic/hemorrhage, edema
mu-tung 木通 (akebia)	*Akebia quinata* Decne./ Lardizabalaceae. A wild vine found everywhere.	stem		mildly chilly	antiphlogistic, diuretic/nephritis, edema
nan-tien-chu 南天燭 (nandina)	*Nandina domestica* Thunb./ Berberidaceae. A shrub cultivated everywhere.	fruit	White variety is preferred but sometimes substituted with *chih-nan-tien*, red variety bleached with sulfate.		anticough/asthma, whooping cough
niu-pang-tzu 牛蒡子 (arctium)	*Arctium lappa* L./Compositae; Great Burdock. A cultivated biennial herb.	seeds		chilly	antipyretic, antidotal, diuretic/ edema, sores, and swellings
niu-hsi 牛膝 (achyranthes)	*Achyranthes bidentata* Blume/Amaranthaceae. A perennial herb found everywhere.	root		bland	diuretic, tonic/ menoxenia

Chinese Name/ Common Name	Scientific Name/ Description	Part Used	Method of Selection and Processing	Property	Function/Symptoms
niu-huang 牛黃 (bos) (cow bezoar)	Cow bezoar, a coagulated mass formed as a result of some illness in the gall bladder of cows, goats or antelopes.		A global shaped, brittle soft mass that stains the nails a yellow color when it is touched.	cool	antipyretic, sedative, spasmolytic, antidotal, cardiotonic/ pediatric epilepsy
niu-pi-hsiao 牛皮消 (caudatum)	Cynanchum caudatum Maxim./Asclepiadaceae. A perennial wild herb found everywhere.	root			diuretic/edema
niu-pien-tsao 牛扁草 (geranium)	Geranium wilfordii Maxim. /Geraniaceae; geranium. A wild perennial herb found everywhere.	stem and leaves	Those with profuse leaves.	bland	abdominal pain, diarrhea
niu-tan 牛膽 (cow gall)	Cow's gall bladder.			very chilly	stomachic, peptic, intestinal corrective, purgative/gastro- enteritis, dyspepsia, chronic constipation, jaundice, sores and abscesses
nu-chen 女貞 (ligustrum)	Ligustrum lucidum Ait./ Oleaceae; white wax tree. A low plant growing everywhere in the wild.	fruit		bland	antipyretic, tonic/ pulmonary tuberculosis edema

Herbs Used in Chinese Medicine

Chinese Name/ Common Name	Scientific Name/ Description	Part Used	Method of Selection and Processing	Property	Function/Symptoms
pa-chi 菝葜 (pa-chi)	Smilax china L./Liliaceae; Chinese sarsaprilla. A perennial wild herb found everywhere.	rhizomes		bland	antipyretic, tonic/ pulmonary tuberculosis, edema
pa-chi-tien 巴戟天 (morinda)	Morinda officinalis How./ Rubiaceae. A vine plant indigenous to China.	root		mildly warm	tonic, seminal tonic/ impotence, premature ejaculation, disturbances in genitalia, menoxenia
pa-chiao 芭蕉 (musa)	Musa sapientum L./Musaceae; banana or plantain. A perennial herb cultivated everywhere.	root, stem, and leaves		chilly	diuretic/edema, beriberi
pa-mu-man 八目鰻 (lamprey)	Entosphenus japonicus Martens. A sea fish living in cold water.			chilly	diuretic, nutrient, tonic, seminal tonic/ edema, impotence
pa-tou 巴豆 (croton)	Croton tiglium L./Euphorbiaceae. A low plant of the tropical zone.	seeds	Remove the seed coat.	hot	purgative, emetic/ distention in chest and abdomen, constipation, abdominal pain
pai-chang 白菖 (calamus)	Acorus calamus L./Araceae; sweet flag or calamus. A cultivated perennial herb found everywhere.	rhizomes	Chang-pu used in Chinese medicine is generally shih-chang-pu.		aromatic stomachic, analgesic/gastroenteritis

Chinese Name/ Common Name	Scientific Name/ Description	Part Used	Method of Selection and Processing	Property	Function/Symptoms
pai-chi 白芨 (bletilla)	Bletilla hyacinthina R. Br.; B.striata/Orchidaceae. A perennial herb cultivated everywhere.	root		mildly chilly	a glutinous hemostatic, hematemesis/hemoptysis gastric ulcer
pai-chiang 敗醬 (thlaspi)	Thlaspi arvense L./Cruciferae; Patrinia scabiosaefolia Link./Valerianaceae. A perennial wild herb found everywhere.	root	Sometimes this drug is substituted with chi-tsao (Valeriana officinale L.).	chilly	antiphlogistic, anti-coagulant, diuretic, pus dispersant, exsanguinative/gastro-enteritis, carbuncular swellings
pai-chih 白芷 (angelica)	Angelica anomala Lall./ Umbelliferae; angelica. A perennial wild or cultivated herb.	root		warm	sedative, analgesic/ headache, vertigo, neuralgia
pai-chiu 白酒 (wine)	Ordinary wine sold in the market.	rhizomes of young herb	Any variety.	hot	tonic, excitant
pai-chu 白朮 (white atractylodes)	Atractylodes ovata Thunb./ Compositae. A wild or cultivated herb found everywhere.			warm	a warm diuretic
pai-chu-chai 白屈菜	Chelidonium majus L. var. asiaticum Ohwl./Papawild	leaves	Poisonous leaves.		analgesic/gastric cancer

Herbs Used in Chinese Medicine

Chinese Name/ Common Name	Scientific Name/ Description	Part Used	Method of Selection and Processing	Property	Function/Symptoms
pai-fan 白礬 (alum) (celandine)	A perennial wild herb found everywhere. Naturally occurring potash alum or potassium sulfate.			chilly	astringent, hemostatic, preservative
pai-fen 白粉 (pai-fen)	Oryza sativa L./Gramineae; rice.	pulverized starch of rice			paregoric, nutrient
pai-fu-tzu 白附子 (korean aconite)	Aconitum coreanum (Leveil.) Leveil/Ranunculaceae. A perennial herb indigenous to China.	tuber	Sometimes white lead is used instead.	very warm	analgesic, spasmolytic, expectorant/neuralgia, rheumatism, headache, facial nerve paralysis
pai-ho 百合 (lily)	Lilium brownii Spae./ Liliaceae. A perennial wild herb found everywhere.	bulb		bland	nutrient, tonic, anticough expectorant/bronchitis, pulmonary tuberculosis, neurasthenia
pai-hsien 白蘚 (fraxinella)	Dictamnus albus L./Rutaceae. A perennial herb cultivated everywhere.	cortices of roots		chilly	alterative/sores and swellings, scabies, jaundice
pai-kuo 白果 (ginkgo)	Ginkgo biloba L./Ginkgoaceae; maiden hair tree. A tall tree cultivated everywhere.	seeds		bland	diuretic, anticough, expectorant/asthma, bronchitis

703

Chinese Name/ Common Name	Scientific Name/ Description	Part Used	Method of Selection and Processing	Property	Function/Symptoms
pai-pien-tou 白扁豆 (dolichos)	*Dolichos lablab* L./ Leguminosae; hyacinth bean. A wild annual herb found everywhere.	seeds		mildly warm	stomachic, intestinal corrective, antidotal/ gastroenteritis, diarrhea, stomachache
pai-pu 百部 (stemona)	*Stemona tuberosa* Lour./ Stemonaceae. A perennial herb indigenous to China.	tuber		mildly chilly	insecticidde/scabies, lice, mosquitos, flies
pai-shih-chih 白石脂 (white kaolin)	One kind of kaolin, i.e. aluminum silicate hydrous.			warm	astringent, hemostatic, antidiarrheal/acute gastroenteritis, chronic diarrhea
pai-tan 白檀 (santalum)	*Santalum album* L./Santalaceae; sandal wood. A tall plant indigenous to India.	core of the wood		warm	diuretic, bactericidal/ gonorrhea
pai-tao-hua 白桃花 (persica flower)	*Prunus persica* S. et Z. var. *vulgaris* Maxim./ Rosaceae; peach. A tall plant cultivated everywhere.	white blossoms	Use fresh ones.	bland	diuretic, purgative/ difficulty in bowel movement and urination, edema
pai-ting-hsiang 白丁香 (sparrow faeces)	*Passer rutilans* Brisson/ Ploceidae; a tree sparrow.	male sparrow's feces			diuretic/ocular diseases

Herbs Used in Chinese Medicine

Chinese Name/ Common Name	Scientific Name/ Description	Part Used	Method of Selection and Processing	Property	Function/Symptoms
pai-tou-kou 白豆蔻 (cluster)	*Amomum cardamomum* L./ Zingiberaceae; Siam cardamon. A perennial herb indigenous to the Philippines.	fruit		hot	aromatic stomachic, carminative/gastro-enteritis, dyspepsia
pai-tou-weng 白頭翁 (anemone)	*Anemone cernua* Th./Ranunculaceae; pulsatilla. A perennial wild herb found everywhere.	root		chilly	antiphlogistic, astringent, hemostatic/feverish diarrhea, tenesmus
pai-wei 白薇 (pai-wei)	*Cynanchum atratum* Bge./ Asclepiadaceae. A perennial wild herb found everywhere.	root		chilly	antipyretic, diuretic, tonic/malaria, edema, pulmonary tuberculosis, dysuria
pai-yu 白魚 (lepisma)	*Lepisma saccharina* L; silver fish or fish mot'..	all	May be replaced with a carp.		diuretic indicated for edema, jaundice; a lactogogue
pan-hsia 半夏 (pinellia)	*Pinellia tuberifera* Ten./ Araceae. A perennial wild herb found everywhere.	bulb		warm	antiemetic, antiretching, sedative, expectorant/intragastric stagnant water that adversely flushes up causing nausea and vomiting, cough, vertigo, cardiac

Natural Healing with Chinese Herbs

Chinese Name/ Common Name	Scientific Name/ Description	Part Used	Method of Selection and Processing	Property	Function/Symptoms
斑蝥 pan-wu (cantharides)	*Mylabris sidae* Fab./Meloidae. A winged insect abundant everywhere.	all		chilly	palpitation, pharyngeal and laryngeal pain stimulative diuretic/ rubefacient, or a blistering agent; used in promoting the growth of hair
萆薢 pei-chieh (tokoro)	*Dioscorea tokoro* Mak./ Dioscoreaceae; fish poison yam. A perennial herb found everywhere in the wild.	rhizomes		bland	diuretic, antidotal/ sores and swellings
貝母 pei-mu (fritillaria)	*Fritillaria roylei* Hook./ Liliaceae; fritillary. A perennial herb indigenous to China but cultivated everywhere.	bulb	Szechuan species are smaller in size; the Pekinese species are larger.	mildly chilly	anticough, expectorant, pus dispersant/carbuncles, swellings (also used as a lactogogue)
硼砂 peng-sha (borax)	This is the native sodium biborate.			cool	preservative/ external use
蓖麻 pi-ma (ricinus)	*Ricinus communis* L./ Euphorbiaceae; castor oil plant. A low plant	seeds	Poisonous.	bland	used externally for abscesses; oil compressed from seeds

Herbs Used in Chinese Medicine

Chinese Name/ Common Name	Scientific Name/ Description	Part Used	Method of Selection and Processing	Property	Function/Symptoms
	or annual herb indigenous to tropical regions.				as laxative
pi-pa-yeh 枇杷葉 (eriobotrya)	*Eriobotrya japonica* Lindl./Rosaceae; loquat. A tall plant cultivated everywhere.	leaves			cleansing and cooling, stomachic, antiemetic, anticough, dissolving summer hotness/bronchitis
pi-po 蓽茇 (piper)	*Piper longum* L./Piperaceae; long pepper. A perennial herb found everywhere.	fruit		hot	aromatic stomachic, analgesic/gastralgia, abdominal pain, toothache
pieh-chia 鱉甲 (tortoise shell)	*Amyda sinensis* Weigmann.; *Trionyx tuberculatus* Cantor; fresh water turtle.	lower shell	The *tai-mao* that is used in tools is another species *Eretmochelys squamosa* Girard.	bland	antipyretic, antidotal, tonic/pulmonary tuberculosis
pien-hsu 萹蓄 (polygonum)	*Polygonum aviculare* L./ Polygonaceae; knot or gooseweed. An annual wild herb found everywhere.	stem and leaves		bland	antiphlogistic, diuretic, antidiarrheal. anthelmintic/gastroenteritis, diarrhea, ascariasis

Chinese Name/ Common Name	Scientific Name/ Description	Part Used	Method of Selection and Processing	Property	Function/Symptoms
pin-fang-feng (glehnia)	*Glehnia littoralis* Fr. Schmidt/Umbelliferae; an Umbelliferous perennial herb found at the seashore.	root	Can be used in place of *Siler divaricatum* Bth. et Hk. in the prescription *Tu-su-san*.	mildly chilly	diaphoretic, febrifuge, analgesic
pin-lang 檳榔 (areca seed)	*Areca catechu* L./Palmae; areca nut or betel palm. A tall plant indigenous to the tropical zone.	seeds		warm	stomachic, astringent, anthelmintic, intestinal corrective/beriberi, tape worms
po-ho 薄荷 (mentha)	*Mentha arvensis* L./Labiatae; field mint. A perennial herb cultivated everywhere.	leaves		cool	cleansing and cooling, diaphoretic, febrifuge, stomachic/gastroenteritis, common cold
po-tzu-jen 柏子仁 (biota)	*Thuja orientalis* L./ Cupressaceae; arbor vitae. A low plant cultivated everywhere.	kernel of fruit		bland	nutrient, tonic/ impotence
pu-huang 蒲黃 (bulrush)	*Typha latifolia* L./ Typhaceae; cattail. A perennial wild herb found everywhere.	pollen		bland	astringent, diuretic, hemostatic/hematemesis, melena, hemoptysis, hematuria, metrorrhagia, hemorrhoidal bleeding
pu-ku-chih 補骨脂 (psoralea)	*Psoralea corylifolia* L./ Leguminosae; scurfy pea. An annual indigenous	seeds		very warm	tonic, seminal tonic/ feebleness, impotence, menoxenia, bed wetting

Herbs Used in Chinese Medicine

Chinese Name/ Common Name	Scientific Name/ Description	Part Used	Method of Selection and Processing	Property	Function/Symptoms
pu-kung-ying 蒲公英 (dandelion)	Taraxacum officinale Web./Compositae. A perennial herb found in the wilds everywhere to China.	all		chilly	antiphlogistic, bitter stomachic, alterative, emmenagogue/gastritis, dyspepsia, sores and swellings
san-ling 三稜 (scirpus)	Scirpus maritimus L./ Cyperaceae; bulrush. A perennial wild herb found everywhere.	tuber		bland	exsanguinative, analgesic, lactogogue/ amenorrhea, menoxenia, postpartal abdominal pain, metropathy
sang-chi-sheng 桑寄生 (loranthus)	Loranthus yadoriki S. et Z., L. parasiticus (L.) Merr./ Loranthaceae; mulberry epiphyte. Found growing on tall plants.	twigs and leaves	The epiphytes found on Morus alba L. (mulberry) are preferred. In Japan the mulberry plant is a shrub and low so the epiphytes on other plants such as juniper and peach trees are used.	bland	tonic, antidotal, anodyne, emmenagogue/ neuralgia, rheumatism, arteriosclerosis, hypertension, sores and swellings, prepartum and postpartum
sang-pai-pi 桑白皮 (morus)	Morus alba L./Moraceae; mulberry. A tall plant cultivated everywhere.	cortices of roots	Remove the reddish epidermal skin. Sometimes replaced by bark of tzu (Catalpa kaempferi L.).	chilly	antiphlogistic, diuretic, febrifuge, anticough/ bronchitis, cough, stridor

Chinese Name/ Common Name	Scientific Name/ Description	Part Used	Method of Selection and Processing	Property	Function/Symptoms
sha-sheng 沙參 (adenophora)	Adenophora tetraphylla (Thunb.) Fisch./ Campanulaceae; blue bell. A perennial wild herb found everywhere.	root		mildly chilly	anticough, expectorant/ bronchitis
sha-tang 砂糖 (brown sugar)	Saccharum officinarum L./Gramineae; sugar cane. A perennial herb cultivated in warm regions. Another source for this drug is the sweet carrot cultivated in cold regions.	stem	Sugar compressed from these plants is used.	chilly	nutrient, diuretic, sweetening agent/thirst, cough with sputum
shan-cha-hua 山茶花 (camellia)	Camellia japonica L./ Theaceae; camelia or tea oil tree. A tall plant in the wilds.	flower	Shan-cha oil is the fatty oil squeezed from seeds, used as an ointment.	chilly	astringent, hemostatic/ bleeding from various conditions
shan-cha-tzu 山楂子 (crataegus)	Crataegus pinnatifida Bge. var. major N.E. Br./Rosaceae. Indigenous to China.	fruit		mildly warm	stomachic, digestant, intestinal corrective/ anorexia, abdominal pain, diarrhea
shan-chiao 山椒 (zanthoxylum)	Zanthoxylum piperitum D.C./Rutaceae; Japanese pepper.	pericarpia of immature fruit	Cultivated variety has no thorns on branches and fruit is large and even in size; contains very few	hot	a warm stomachic, intestinal corrective, diuretic, carminative, anthelmintic/chronic

Chinese Name/ Common Name	Scientific Name/ Description	Part Used	Method of Selection and Processing	Property	Function/Symptoms
			seeds and has a very pleasant flavor; hence it is highly prized. The seeds are called *chiao mu*.		gastroenteritis, gastric laxation, gastroptosis, gastric atonia, ascariasis
shan-chih-tzu 山梔子 (gardenia)	*Gardenia jasminoides* L./ Rubiaceae; Cape jasmine. A shrub found in the wilds everywhere.	fruit		chilly	antiphlogistic, antipyretic, diuretic, hemostatic/congestion, epistaxis, hematemesis, jaundice
shan-chu-yu 山茱萸 (cornus)	*Cornus officinalis* S. et Z./Cornaceae; dogwood. A tall plant indigenous to China.	fruit	Take out seeds and retain the tender fleshy part of the fruit, which tastes sour and acrid.	mildly warm	an astringent tonic/ impotence, spermatorrhea, frequency of urination
shan-pien-tou 山扁豆 (mimosoides)	*Cassia mimosoides* L./ Leguminosae. An annual wild herb found everywhere.	stem, fruit, and leaves			stomachic, diuretic/ gastroenteritis, edema, nephrosis
shan-tou-ken 山豆根 (subprostrata)	*Sophora subprostrata* Chun et T. Chen./Leguminosae; *Menispermum dauricum* DC./ Menispermaceae; pigeon pea. A low plant	roots which taste very bitter		chilly	anti-inflammatory, antipyretic, antidotal/ throat pain, toxic swellings, sores and ulcers, abdominal pain,

Chinese Name/ Common Name	Scientific Name/ Description	Part Used	Method of Selection and Processing	Property	Function/Symptoms
shan-tzu-ku 山慈姑 (pleione)	*Pleione sp.*/Orchidaceae; *Tulipa edulis* Bak./Liliaceae; edible tulip. A perennial found in the wilds everywhere. native to China.	bulb		bland	diarrhea, carcinoma nutrient, tonic, cardiotonic, antidotal/ cardiac diseases
shan-yao 山藥 (dioscorea)	*Dioscorea batatas* Decne./ Dioscoreaceae; Chinese yam. A perennial wild herb found everywhere.	root		bland	nutrient, tonic, anti-thirst, anti-diarrhea/enteritis, bed wetting, night sweats, spermatorrhea
shang-lu 商陸 (phytolacca)	*Phytolacca esculenta* Van Hout./Phytolaccaceae; poke root. A perennial wild herb found everywhere.	root		chilly	diuretic, water dispersant/nephritis, edema
shao-yao 芍藥 (paeonia or peony)	*Paeonia albiflora* Pall./ Ranunculaceae; Chinese peony. A perennial herb cultivated everywhere.	root	Use as much as posible of the root with cortices attached.	mildly chilly	astringent, paregoric, spasmolytic, analgesic/ abdominal distention, abdominal ache, limb spasms, diarrhea
she-chuang-tzu 蛇床子 (selinum)	*Selinum japonicum* Miq./ Umbelliferae. An annual herb indigenous to China.	fruit	In Japan the fruit of *chueh-i* (*Torilis japonica*) is substituted. The hook hair on the fruit is removed.	warm	antiphlogistic, astringent, aphrodisiac/impotence, strong vaginal itching

Chinese Name/ Common Name	Scientific Name/ Description	Part Used	Method of Selection and Processing	Property	Function/Symptoms
she-hsiang 麝香 (musk)	*Moschus moschiferus* Linn./ Cervidae. Musk deer indigenous to China and found in the mountains.	musk contained in a sack located between the navel and testicles	The musk appears dark brown and has an ammonia-like odor.	warm	excitant, cardiac tonic, spasmolytic/ acute diseases
shen-chu 神麯 (shen-chu)	This spirit leaven is produced from flour, red mung beans, apricot, the juices of *Artemisia apiacea* (southern wood), *Xanthium strumarium* (cocklebur or clotbur), *Polygonum hydropiper* (smart weed or water pepper) which are blended and fermented until a yellowish white mold grows.		Often the Chinese product, rectangular cubes of 3–4cm in length, is used. Sometimes wine leaven is used as a substitute.	warm	stomachic, digestant/ gastroenteritis
sheng-chiang 生薑 (ginger)	*Zingiber officinale* Rosc./Zingiberaceae. A perennial herb cultivated everywhere.	rhizomes	Formerly *sheng-chiang* was raw, fresh, old ginger. In view of difficulty in storage, skin of old ginger was peeled and it was coated with lime	warm	stomachic, antiemetic/regurgitation of water toxin causing vomiting, cough, hiccup, nausea, eructation. This drug is referred to

Herbs Used in Chinese Medicine

Chinese Name/ Common Name	Scientific Name/ Description	Part Used	Method of Selection and Processing	Property	Function/Symptoms
			juice for preservation. This drug is now replaced by *kan-sheng-chiang* (dry, raw ginger) called *kan-chiang*. When *kan-chiang* is used dosage is one-third that of *sheng-chiang*. Fresh raw ginger acquires a strong smell and taste; its medicinal effect is different from that of *kan-sheng-chiang*. *Sheng-chiang-chih* (*sheng-chiang* juice) is obtained from compressing raw old ginger.		as the "sacred drug for vomiting." It also acts as a flavoring agent to modify tastes and odors of other herbs so as to increase the appetite and make them more acceptable to the stomach.
sheng-ma 升麻 (cimicifuga)	*Cimicifuga foetida* L./ Ranunculaceae. A wild perennial herb found everywhere.	rhizomes	Black, hard and light tubers with a bitter taste are preferred. The reddish brown type is *chih-sheng-ma*, another species.	mildly chilly	antipyretic, antidotal, analgesic/generalized fever, anhidrosis, headache, pharyngeal or laryngeal ache, measles, sores and swellings

Herbs Used in Chinese Medicine

Chinese Name/ Common Name	Scientific Name/ Description	Part Used	Method of Selection and Processing	Property	Function/Symptoms
sheng-sheng-ju 生生乳 (sheng-sheng-ju)	A sublimate of mercurials or mercuric chloride. It is poisonous.				syphilis
shih-chang-pu 石菖蒲 (acorus)	*Acorus gramineus* Soland./ Araceae. A perennial herb found everywhere.	rhizomes		warm	aromatic, stomachic, diuretic, analgesic/ gastroenteritis, abdominal pain
shih-chueh-ming 石決明 (haliotis)	*Haliotis gigantea* Chem./ Haliotidae; a shellfish whose name is more commonly rendered as *pao-yu*.		Render into coarse powder.	bland	antipyretic, diuretic, sedative/ocular diseases, pulmonary tuberculosis
shih-chun-tzu 使君子 (quisqualis)	*Quisqualis indica* L./ Combretaceae; Rangoon creeper. Indigenous to India.	fruit		warm	anthelmintic/ ascariasis
shih-hu 石斛 (dendrobium)	*Dendrobium nobile* Lindl./ Orchidaceae. A wild perennial herb found everywhere.	all		chilly	antipyretic, analgesic, tonic/thirst, impotence, arthralgia
shih-kao 石膏 (gypsum)	Native soft gypsum or calcium sulfate dihydrate, $CaSO_4 \cdot 2H_2O$, which is		Pulverize into a coarse powder.	very chilly	cooling, antipyretic, antithirst, sedative/ generalized fever

Chinese Name/ Common Name	Scientific Name/ Description	Part Used	Method of Selection and Processing	Property	Function/Symptoms
	a crude gypsum and will lose one and a half molecules of water upon heating at 100-120° and become the so-called burnt gypsum.				with a white fur on the tongue, dry mouth and tongue, great thirst
shih-liu-pi 石榴皮 (punica)	Punica granatum L./Punicaceae; pomegranate. A tall plant cultivated everywhere.	bark and root cortices	Root cortices are better.	warm	anthelmintic/tapeworms, ascariasis
shih-luo 蒔蘿 (graveolens)	Peucedanum graveolens Bth. et Hk./Umbelliferae; dill. A perennial herb cultivated everywhere.	fruit		bland	stomachic, carminative, expectorant/gastroenteritis
shih-nan 石南 (photinia)	Photinia serrulata Lindl./Rosaceae; Rhododendron Metternichi S. et Z./Ericaceae. A shrub indigenous to China.	leaves		bland	diuretic, antipyretic, analgesic/generalized aches, adynamia, impotence, menoxenia
shih-ping-yu 矢柄魚 (pipe fish)	This fish is found in warm seas. It is identified as Fistularia serrata Bleek				tonic/carcinomous swellings—to be taken orally
shih-suan 石蒜 (lycoris)	Lycoris radiata Herb./Amaryllidaceae.	bulb	Poisonous.	warm	expectorant/cough, carcinoma,

Chinese Name/ Common Name	Scientific Name/ Description	Part Used	Method of Selection and Processing	Property	Function/Symptoms
	A perennial herb found everywhere.				carbuncles
shih-ti 柿蒂 (kaki)	Diospyros kaki L. f./ Ebenaceae; persimmon or date fig. A tall plant cultivated everywhere.	calyces of the fruit		warm	hiccups
shih-wei 石葦 (pyrrosia)	Pyrrosia lingua (Thunb.) Far./Polypodiaceae. A wild perennial herb found everywhere.	leaves		mildly chilly	diuretic, hemostatic/ cystitis, urethritis, gonorrhea
shih-yao 十藥 (houttuynia)	Houttuynia cordata Th./ Saururaceae.	part found above ground in flowering season		mildly chilly	antiphlogistic, diuretic, antidotal/ fetal toxicosis, sores and swellings
shu-chi 蜀漆 (dichroa)	Dichroa febrifuga Lour./ Saxifragaceae; Szechuan varnish. A low plant indigenous to China.	stem and leaves	In Japan this drug is replaced by tzu-yang-hua (Hydrangea macrophylla var. otaksa Makino).	bland	febrifuge, emetic/ malarial seizures
shu-fu 鼠婦 (wood louse)	Oniscus ascellus Millepeda; a tiny insect of the Crustacea.	all			diuretic, exsanguinative/ dysuria, edema

Chinese Name/ Common Name	Scientific Name/ Description	Part Used	Method of Selection and Processing	Property	Function/Symptoms
shu-li-tzu 鼠李子 (rhamnus)	Rhamnus dahuricus Pall./ Rhamnaceae; Japanese buckthorn, rat plum. A shrub found everywhere in the wild.	fruit			laxative
shui-chih 水蛭 (leech)	Hirudo nipponica Whitman/ Hirudinidae; a leech found in pools or rivers	all	The whole body is dried by placing it in burnt ashes.	bland	exsanguinative, dissolving blood clots, anticoagulant/stale extravasated blood, dysmenorrhea, and uterine myoma
shui-yang 水楊 (salix)	Salix purpurea L. var. serica Wimm./Salicaceae; purple willow. A low wild plant growing everywhere.	bark	The branches and leaves are boiled and used for a bath.	bland	antipyretic, astringent/sores and swellings
su 酥 (milk scum)	Scum formed on milk that has been heat-evaporated and then cooled in a shallow container.				nutrient, digestant/ thirst
su-ho-hsiang 蘇合香 (styrax)	Liquidambar orientalis Mill./Hamamelidaceae; rose mallows. A tall plant indigenous to	resinous juice from the bark		warm	expectorant, excitant, anthelmintic, preservative/cough, asthma, ascariasis,

Herbs Used in Chinese Medicine

Chinese Name/ Common Name	Scientific Name/ Description	Part Used	Method of Selection and Processing	Property	Function/Symptoms
	Asia Minor.				externally for scabies
su-mu 蘇木 (sappan wood)	*Caesalpinia sappan* L./ Leguminosae. A tall plant indigenous to India, Malaysia, and tropical areas.			bland	astringent, hemostatic/ hemorrhage
su-tieh 蘇鐵 (phoenix)	*Phoenix dactylifera* L./ Palmae; date palm. A low plant cultivated everywhere.	fruit		warm	astringent, antitussive, expectorant/cough
suan-tsao-jen 酸棗仁 (zizyphus)	*Zizyphus sativa* var. *spinosa* (Bge.) Schneid./ Rhamnaceae; wild jujube. A low plant indigenous to China.	seeds		bland	astringent neurotonic, sedative/neurotic insomnia, somnolence
sun-tai-lang-chung 孫大郎蟲 (hermes)	*Hermes grandis*; an insect.	larvae			tonic, spasmolytic
sung-chih 松脂 (pinus resin)	*Pinus* species of the Pinaceae. A tall plant found everywhere.	Resin from the trunk of tree is distilled	Native resin always contains some water. Often the imported resins are used.	warm	antiphlogistic The unguent character of this drug makes it suitable for use as

719

Chinese Name/ Common Name	Scientific Name/ Description	Part Used	Method of Selection and Processing	Property	Function/Symptoms
		to drive off the turpentine; remainder is used for drug			the base of ointment. It is indicated for carbuncles and furuncles.
sung-luo 松蘿 (usnea)	*Usnea longissima* Ach./ Usneaceae; pine lichen. A filiform lichen growing as an epiphyte on the bark of tall trees.	all		bland	diuretic, anticough, expectorant/bronchitis
suo-sha 縮砂 (cardamon)	*Amomum xanthioides* Wall./ Zingiberaceae; bastard cardamon. A perennial herb indigenous to Eastern India.	fruit	Remove skin of the seeds. This drug can also be substituted with *i-tou-suo-sha*.	warm	aromatic stomachic/ anorexia, eructation, vomiting, abdominal pain, diarrhea
ta-chi 大薊 (cirsium)	*Cirsium japonicum* DC./ Compositae; tiger thistle. A perennial wild herb found everywhere.			cool	astringent, hemostatic, diuretic/bleeding from various causes, sores or abscesses
ta-chi 大戟 (euphorbia)	*Euphorbia pekinensis* Rupr./Euphorbiaceae; Peking spurge. A	root		chilly	cathartic, diuretic/ thoracic pain, edema, dysuria

Herbs Used in Chinese Medicine

Chinese Name/ Common Name	Scientific Name/ Description	Part Used	Method of Selection and Processing	Property	Function/Symptoms
	perennial herb indigenous to China.				
ta-feng-tzu 大風子 (hydnocarpus)	Hydnocarpus anthelmintica Pierre/Flacourtiaceae; Chinese chaulmoogra. A tall plant found in the tropical areas of Asia.	seeds	Often the seed oil is used.	hot	leprosy
ta-fu-pi 大腹皮 (areca)	Areca catechu L./Palmae. A tall plant indigenous to the Philippines.	pericarpia of fruit		mildly warm	stomachic, intestinal corrective, diuretic/ ascites
ta-huang 大黃 (rhubarb)	Rheum officinale Baill./ Polygonaceae. A perennial herb indigenous to China.	root and stem	Tong-ta-huang, which is light in weight with a dark brown surface and yellowish brown interior of sponge-like holes, is often used. Chin-weng-ta-huang, of excellent quality, is not often used in Japan. The other variety, called ho-ta-huang, is not a true Rheum.	chilly	antiphlogistic, stomachic, exsanguinative, diuretic, purgative, cathartic/bound toxins, thoracic and abdominal distention, abdominal pain, constipation, dysuria, jaundice, extravasation, swollen abscesses

Chinese Name/ Common Name	Scientific Name/ Description	Part Used	Method of Selection and Processing	Property	Function/Symptoms
ta-huei-hsiang 大茴香 (illicium)	*Illicium verum* Hook. F./ Magnoliaceae; star or Chinese anise. A tall plant indigenous to the Philippines.	fruit	*Illicium religiosum* S. et Z. (bastard or Japanese anise) is a tall magnoliaceaous plant whose fruit is poisonous and cannot be used in place of this drug.	warm	aromatic stomachic, expectorant, exsanguinative, lactogogue/gastroenteritis, abdominal pain
ta-kan 獺肝 (otter liver)	*Lutra lutra* L./Mustelidae; fresh water otter.	liver		warm	nutrient, tonic, hemopoeitic/pulmonary tuberculosis, cough, night blindness
ta-suan 大蒜 (garlic)	*Allium sativum* L. forma *pekinense* Mak./Liliaceae. A perennial herb indigenous to China.	bulb		warm	stomachic, intestinal corrective, excitant, strengthening agent, seminal tonic, antidotal/gastroenteritis, dysentery, arteriosclerosis, diseases of old age
ta-tsao 大棗 (jujube)	*Zizyphus vulgaris* Lam./ Rhamnaceae; jujube. A tall plant cultivated everywhere.	fruit	Fruit full of flesh with small kernels is the best. Chinese variety is preferred.	warm	paregoric, tonic, diuretic, analgesic/ muscular cramping and dragging pains, hypersensitivity, cough,

Chinese Name/ Common Name	Scientific Name/ Description	Part Used	Method of Selection and Processing	Property	Function/Symptoms
tai-che-shih 代赭石 (hematite)	Red hematite Fe_2O_3 contaminated with some soil.			chilly	vexation, irritation, convulsive pain, abdominal pain
tan-fan 膽礬 (bluestone)	Copper sulfate; blue vitriol.		Use kind with blue crystals.	chilly	hemopoeitic, astringent, hemostatic/hemorrhage, eructation, vomiting
					astringent, emetic/ rendition of emesis in poisoning; (also used as a caustic agent)
tan-sheng 丹參 (salvia root)	Salvia multiorrhiza Bge./ Labiatae. A wild perennial herb found everywhere.	root		mildly chilly	exsanguinative, tonic, sedative/ menoxenia, metrorrhagia, abdominal pain, arthralgia
tang-kuei 當歸 (tang-kuei)	Angelica sinensis (Oliv.) Diels /Umbelliferae. A perennial herb found everywhere.	root	Big and tender roots with strong fragrance.	warm	exsanguinative, sedative, tonic/ anemia, abdominal pain, overall chills, pain, dysmenorrhea

Chinese Name/ Common Name	Scientific Name/ Description	Part Used	Method of Selection and Processing	Property	Function/Symptoms
tang-yao 當藥 (swertia)	*Swertia japonica* Makino/ Gentianaceae. A biennial wild herb found everywhere.	whole herb harvested during flowering season	Use those with strong bitter taste.		bitter stomachic, intestinal corrective/ gastroenteritis, abdominal pain
tao-jen 桃仁 (persica)	*Prunus persica* S. et Z. var. *vulgaris* Maxim/ Rosaceae; peach. A tall plant cultivated everywhere.	seed kernels	Use fat ones. Recently the apex and skin of the kernels from China have not been removed.	bland	antiphlogistic, exsanguinative/fullness in the lower abdomen, menoxenia, appendicitis
teng-hsin-tsao 燈心草 (juncus)	*Juncus effusus* L./Juncaceae; common rush. A perennial wild or cultivated herb found everywhere.	all		chilly	diuretic/dysuria, nephritis
ti-fu-tzu 地膚子 (kochia)	*Kochia scoparia* (L.) Schrad./ Chenopodiaceae; pigweed or goosefoot. A wild annual herb found everywhere.	fruit		chilly	antiphlogistic, diuretic, astringent/ gonorrhea, edema
ti-huang 地黃 (rehmannia)	*Rehmannia glutinosa* (Gaertner.) Lib./ Scrophulariaceae. A perennial herb cultivated everywhere but indigenous	root	Raw fresh ones are called *sheng-ti-huang* (raw rehmannia); dry ones, *kan-ti-huang* (dry rehmannia); and	chilly	hemopoeitic tonic, antipyretic, hemo- static/anemia, feebleness

Herbs Used in Chinese Medicine

Chinese Name/ Common Name	Scientific Name/ Description	Part Used	Method of Selection and Processing	Property	Function/Symptoms
	to China		the steam dried ones *sho-ti-huang* (cured rehmannia). Usually dry rehmannia is used.		
ti-ku-pi 地骨皮 (lycium bark)	*Lycium chinense* Mill./ Solanaceae; Chinese wolfberry. A wild shrub found everywhere.	cortices of roots	Use with the leaves.	chilly	cleansing and cooling, antipyretic, tonic, anticough/vexatious fever
ti-lung 地龍 (earthworm)	*Pheretima asiatica*; *Lumbricus terrestris* L./ Lumbricidae; an insect.	all	Use those retaining some earth within the stomach after being dried.	chilly	antifebrile/common cold
ti-yu 地榆 (sang'isorba)	*Sanguisorba officinalis* L./Rosaceae; burnet. A perennial wild herb found everywhere.	root		mildly chilly	astringent, hemo-static/hemoptysis, hematemesis, melena, dysentery
tiao-teng-kou 釣藤鈎 (gambir)	*Uncaria rhynchophylla* (Miq.) Jacks./Rubiaceae.		Mostly imported from China.	mildly chilly	sedative, analgesic/ headache, dizziness, infantile night crying
tien-hsiung 天雄	*Aconitum hemsleyanum* Pritz./Ranunculaceae;	tuber	Long single root of Aconitum fischeri,	very hot	revives extremely de-generated metabolic

Chinese Name/ Common Name	Scientific Name/ Description	Part Used	Method of Selection and Processing	Property	Function/Symptoms
(tien-hsiung)	aconite. A wild perennial herb found everywhere.		i.e. the autumn roots that do not bear daughter roots.		function, diuretic, cardiotonic/limb arthralgia, heavy limbs, paralysis, chills
tien-ling-kai 天靈蓋 (human skull)	A human skull.				indicated in pulmonary tuberculosis
tien-ma 天麻 (gastrodia)	Gastrodia elata Bl./ Orchidaceae. A rare, wild perennial herb.	rhizomes	In the market this herb is often adulterated with dried potato.	bland	spasmolytic, analgesic/ headache, vertigo, aching in arms and legs, pediatric epilepsy and spasms
tien-men-tung 天門冬 (asparagus)	Asparagus lucidus Lindl./ Liliaceae. A wild perennial herb found everywhere.	root		very chilly	antipyretic, tonic, anticough, diuretic, antithirst/gout, edema
tien-ming-ching 天名精 (carpesium)	Carpesium abrotanoides L./Compositae; pig's head. A wild biennial herb found everywhere.	stem and leaves			hemostatic/extravasated blood, melena, hematuria
tien-nan-hsing 天南星	Arisaema thunbergii Bl./Araceae; jack-in-the-	rhizomes		warm	spasmolytic, sedative, expectorant/infantile

Chinese Name/ Common Name	Scientific Name/ Description	Part Used	Method of Selection and Processing	Property	Function/Symptoms
(arisaema)	pulpit. A wild perennial herb found everywhere.				spasms
ting-li 葶藶 (lepidium)	*Lepidium apetalum* Willd; *Draba nemorosa* L./Cruciferae. An annual or biennial herb indigenous to China.	seeds		very chilly	laxative, diuretic, cough suppressant, expectorant/fullness in chest and abdomen, cough, asthma, edema
ting-hsiang 丁香 (clove)	*Eugenia caryophyllata* Thunb. /Myrtaceae; clove. Indigenous to the Philippines.	flower buds	Fat buds with a strong fragrance.	warm	aromatic stomachic, strengthening agent, carminative/gastroenteritis, abdominal pain
tsan-sha 蠶砂 (silkworm excreta)	*Bombyx mori* L./Bombycidae; larvae of the silkworm.	excreta of the larvae		warm	sedative, analgesic/ headache, rheumatism, metrorrhagia
tsang-erh 蒼耳 (xanthium)	*Xanthium strumarium* L./ Compositae; cocklebur or clotbur. A perennial wild herb found everywhere.			warm	diaphoretic, febrifuge, diuretic, analgesic/ headache, neuralgia, edema, arthralgia
tsao-chia 皂莢 (gleditsia)	*Gleditsia sinensis* Lam./Leguminosae: soap	fruit	The Chinese variety *chu-ta-tsao-chia* is	warm	stimulant, expectorant/ cough with sputum

Chinese Name/Common Name	Scientific Name/Description	Part Used	Method of Selection and Processing	Property	Function/Symptoms
	bean tree. A tall plant found everywhere.		preferred.		
tsao-chiao-chih 皂角刺 (gleditsia spine)	Gleditsia sinensis Lam./Leguminosae; soap bean tree. A tall plant found everywhere.	thorns on plant	Due to similarity in pronunciation of this drug to that of tsao-chiao-tzu, this drug is commonly called tsao-chiao-li for discrimination.	warm	stimulant, expectorant/used in place of tsao-chia owing to its mild action
tsao-chiao-tzu 皂角子 (gleditsia seed)	Gleditsia sinensis Lam./Leguminosae; soap bean tree. A tall plant found everywhere.	seeds		warm	expectorant/also used in place of tsao-chia owing to its mild action
tsao-kuo 草果 (tsao-kuo)	Amomum tsao-ko Crevost et Lemaire./Zingiberaceae; Chinese cardamon. A perennial herb indigenous to the Philippines.	fruit		warm	aromatic stomachic, digestant/gastro-enteritis, malaria
tsao-tou-kou 草豆蔻 (tsao-tou-kou)	Alpinia katsumadai Hay./Zingiberaceae; wild cardamon. A perennial herb indigenous to the Philippines.	fruit		warm	aromatic stomachic, digestant, carminative/gastroenteritis

Chinese Name/ Common Name	Scientific Name/ Description	Part Used	Method of Selection and Processing	Property	Function/Symptoms
tse-chi 澤漆 (helioscopia)	*Euphorbia helioscopia* L./Euphorbiaceae; wart weed. A perennial wild herb found everywhere.	rhizomes		chilly	febrifuge, diuretic/ malaria, edema
tse-hsieh 澤瀉 (alisma)	*Alisma platago-aquatica* L./ Alismataceae; water plantain. A perennial herb found in ponds.	tuber	Chinese product with a global shape is preferred.	chilly	diuretic, antithirst, analgesic/dysuria, vertigo, thirst
tse-lan 澤蘭 (tse-lan)	*Eupatorium japonicum* Thunb. /Compositae; Chinese thorough wort. A perennial wild herb found everywhere.	all		mildly warm	diuretic, exsanguinative/ amenorrhea, edema, sores and swellings
tse-po-yeh 側柏葉 (biota leaves)	*Thuja orientalis* L./Pinaceae; arbor vitae. A low plant cultivated everywhere.	leaves		chilly	stomachic, astringent, hemostatic/hemoptysis, hematemesis, epistaxis, cerebral hemorrhage, hematuria, metrorrhagia
tsin-hsieh 津蟹 (eriocheir)	*Eriocheir japonicus* de Haan/Decapoda	whole body is burnt black for medicinal use; called *tsin-hsieh-shuan*	This drug is often replaced with *yen-shu-shuan* (burnt black of Mogera wogura).	chilly	pus dispersant, tonic/sores and swellings

Chinese Name/ Common Name	Scientific Name/ Description	Part Used	Method of Selection and Processing	Property	Function/Symptoms
tsung-ken 棕根 (aralia)	*Aralia canescens* S. et Z./Araliaceae; angelica tree or prickly elder. A low plant found in the wild everywhere.	cortices of roots.			stomachic, diuretic, analgesic/edema, diabetes mellitus, gatric ulcer
tsung-lu 棕櫚 (trachycarpus)	*Trachycarpus fortunei* H. Wendl./Palmae; hemp or windmill palm. A tall plant cultivated everywhere.	leaves		bland	astringent, hemostatic/hematemesis, epistaxis, uterine bleeding, gastric or intestinal bleeding
tu-chung 杜仲 (eucommia)	*Eucommia ulmoides* Oliv./ Eucommiaceae; hardy rubber tree. A tall plant indigenous to China.	bark	Use those yielding white lustrous threads like silk worm threads between the fractured surfaces when the bark is broken.	warm	sedative, analgesic, tonic/neuralgia, generalized aching
tu-fu-ling 土茯苓 (smilax)	*Smilax glabra* Roxb./ Liliaceae; China root. A low plant indigenous to China.	tuber	Chinese kind has bland tender texture.	bland	as a diuretic with anticoagulant property, antidotal/syphilis, scrofulosis, sores and abscesses
tu-heng 杜衡 (blumei)	*Asarum blumei* Duch./ Aristolochiaceae. A Perennial wild herb found	root		warm	antipyretic, anticough, analgesic

Chinese Name/ Common Name	Scientific Name/ Description	Part Used	Method of Selection and Processing	Property	Function/Symptoms
tu-huo 獨活 (tu-huo)	Angelica laxiflora Diels/ Umbelliferae. A perennial wild herb found everywhere.	root		warm	diaphoretic, febrifuge, analgesic, spasmolytic/ common cold, generalized pain, edema
tu-kua-ken 土瓜根 (cucumeroides)	Trichosanthes cucumeroides (Ser.) Maxim./Cucurbitaceae. Found in the wilds everywhere.	root	Use bitter ones.	chilly	exsanguinative, diuretic, pus dispersant/ menoxenia, cough, hematemesis
tu-kua-shih 土瓜實 (cucumeroides seed)	Trichosanthes cucumeroids (Ser.) Maxim./Cucurbitaceae. Found in the wilds everywhere.	seeds	Seeds resembling a cockroach's head.	chilly	antiphlogistic, antipyretic, expectorant, analgesic
tu-mu-hsiang 土木香 (elecampane)	Inula helinium L./Compositae. A perennial herb cultivated everywhere.	root		warm	stomachic, diuretic, diaphoretic/gastro-enteritis, bronchitis
tu-szu-tzu 菟絲子 (cuscuta)	Cuscuta japonica Chois./ Convolvulaceae; dodder. A wild annual herb found everywhere.	seeds		bland	nutrient tonic, aphrodisiac/ impotence
tu-tung-tsao 土通草 (galeola)	Galeola septentrionalis/ Orchidaceae. A perennial cultivated herb.	fruit		bland	diuretic, seminal tonic/edema, gonorrhea

Chinese Name/ Common Name	Scientific Name/ Description	Part Used	Method of Selection and Processing	Property	Function/Symptoms
tun-chih 豚脂 (lard)	Sus scrofa domesticus; the domestic pig.	pig fat			ointment base
tung-kua-tzu 冬瓜子 (benincasa)	Benincasa cerifera Savi./ Cucurbitaceae; white gourd or gourd melon. A perennial herb cultivated everywhere.	seeds		mildly chilly	antiphlogistic, diuretic, laxative, pus dispersant/ carbuncular swellings
tung-kuei-tzu 冬葵子 (abutilon)	Abutilon avicennae Gaertn.; Malva verticillata L./ Malvaceae; Chinese mallow. A perennial herb cultivated everywhere.	seeds		chilly	demulcent, diuretic/dysuria
tung-pien 童便 (boys' urine)	Human urine from healthy boys under age twelve.			chilly	tonic, hemostatic/ hemoptysis, chronic respiratory diseases, debility after an illness
tzu-ho-che 紫河車 (placenta)	Human placenta obtained after delivery.			warm	tonic, aphrodisiac, organ therapeutic, lactogogue/neurasthenia, impotence, pulmonary tuberculosis, progressive weak pains

Herbs Used in Chinese Medicin

Chinese Name/ Common Name	Scientific Name/ Description	Part Used	Method of Selection and Processing	Property	Function/Symptoms
tzu-hua-ti-ting 紫花地丁 (viola)	*Viola patrinii* DC./Violaceae. A perennial wild herb found everywhere.	all		chilly	antiphlogistic, antidotal/ sores and swellings, suppurative diseases
tzu-ken 紫根 (lithospermum)	*Lithospermum officinale* L. var. *erythrorizon* Clarke./Boraginaceae; groomwell. A perennial wild herb found everywhere.	root	Used as an ingredient of the external ointment, *tzu-yun-kao*.	chilly	febrifuge, antidotal, diuretic/sores and swellings
tzu-kuang 紫礦 (shellac)	*Laccifer lacca* Kerr./ Lacciferidae; female insects. A parasite found in aggregation on the branches and twigs of various kinds of trees. They excrete a reddish resin-like substance.		Pigment separated from this substance can be used as an industrial dye.		cleansing the blood/a substitute for *mo-yao* (*Commiphora myrrha myrrha* Engl./ Burseraceae).
tzu-pai-pi 梓白皮 (catalpa bark)	*Catalpa bungei* C.A. Mey./Bignoniaceae. A tall plant indigenous to China.	bark of tree	In Japan they replace this herb with the bark of *Morus alba* L., mulberry.	chilly	febrifuge, diuretic, anthelmintic/ocular diseases, pin worms, ascariasis
tzu-pai-yeh 梓白葉 (catalpa leaves)		leaves			stomachic, astringent, antidotal/gastric ulcer, sores and swellings

Chinese Name/ Common Name	Scientific Name/ Description	Part Used	Method of Selection and Processing	Property	Function/Symptoms
tzu-shih-ying 紫石英 (fluorite)	Amethyst.		In China called *ying shih*, "irridescent stone" which is calcium fluoride.	warm	antiphlogistic, diuretic/impotence
tzu-su-tzu 紫蘇子 (perilla fruit)	*Perilla frutescens* (L.) Britt. /Labiatae. An annual herb cultivated everywhere.	fruit		warm	antipyretic, antitussive, stomachic/cough
tzu-su-yeh 紫蘇葉 (perilla)	*Perilla frutescens* (L.) Britt./ Labiatae. An annual herb cultivated everywhere.	leaves	Violet on both sides of the leaves. Use fresh ones.	warm	diaphoretic, febrifuge, anticough, diuretic/ common cold, neurosis, asthma, cough
tzu-tan 紫檀 (pterocarpus)	*Pterocarpus santalinus* Rolfe/ Leguminosae; red sanders wood. A tall plant indigenous to India.	core of the wood		bland	stomachic, hemostatic/ gastroenteritis, various sores
tzu-wei 紫葳 (campsis)	*Campsis grandiflora* (Thunb.) K. Schum./Bignoniaceae. A vine found everywhere.	flower		chilly	febrifuge, emmenagogue, diuretic/dysmenorrhea, diuretic/dysmenorrhea, abdominal pain
tzu-wan 紫菀 (aster)	*Aster tataricus* L. f./Compositae; purple aster. A perennial herb cultivated everywhere.	root	Use those of purplish black color that are tender. The Japanese variety is stiff.	warm	cough suppressant, expectorant, sedative/ chronic bronchitis, pulmonary tuberculosis

Chinese Name/Common Name	Scientific Name/Description	Part Used	Method of Selection and Processing	Property	Function/Symptoms
tzu-yang-hua 紫陽花 (hydrangea)	*Hydrangea macrophylla* var. *otaksa* Makino/ Saxifragaceae. A low plant cultivated everywhere.	leaves	In Japan this drug is substituted with *chang-shan* (*Orixa japonica* Th., Szechuan varnish).	chilly	febrifuge, emetic/malarial seizures
wang-chiang-nan 望江南 (coffee senna)	*Cassia occidentalis* L./ Leguminosae. An annual herb found everywhere.	seeds			stomachic, intestinal corrective/diarrhea, abdominal pain
wang-pu-liu-hsing 王不留行 (vaccaria)	*Saponaria vaccaria* L./ Caryophyllaceae; cow herb. An annual or biennial herb cultivated everywhere.	seeds		bland	exsanguinative, sedative, diuretic/menoxenia, sores and swellings (also effective as a lactogogue)
wei-ching 葦莖 (phragmites stem)	*Phragmites communis* (L.) Trin/Gramineae; common reed. A perennial wild herb found everywhere.	young stem at roots	Rhizomes are named *lu-ken*.	chilly	antiphlogistic, diuretic, antidotal/thirst, jaundice, arthritis, hepatic diseases
wei-jui 萎蕤 (polygonatum)	*Polygonatum officinale* All./Liliaceae; Solomon's seal. A perennial wild herb found everywhere	rhizomes		bland	nutrient tonic/impotence, diabetes mellitus

Chinese Name/ Common Name	Scientific Name/ Description	Part Used	Method of Selection and Processing	Property	Function/Symptoms
wei-ling-hsien 威靈仙 (clematis)	*Clematis chinensis* Retz./ Ranunculaceae; Chinese clematis. A perennial wild herb found everywhere.	root		warm	diuretic, analgesic, emmenagogue/headache, neuralgia, rheumatism, arthralgia, gout
wei-mao 衛矛 (thimble tree)	*Euonymus alatus* (Thunb.) Regel./Celastraceae. A wild low plant found everywhere.	leaves and twigs		chilly	exsanguinative/ menoxenia, prepartum– postpartum ailments, amenorrhea
wen-ke 文蛤 (meretrix)	*Meretrix meretrix* L./Veneridae.	shell		chilly	antipyretic, diuretic, antithirst/ dysuria
wen-na-chi 膃肭臍 (callorhinus)	*Callorhinus ursinus* L./ Otarridae; beaver or fur seal. Found in northern seas.	dried follicles or penis with testicles and umbilicus		hot	nutrient tonic, seminal tonic/impotence and weakness in the male, pulmonary diseases
wu-chia-pi 五加皮 (acanthopanax)	*Acanthopanax spinosum* Miq./Aralicaceae. A wild low plant found everywhere.	bark		warm	analgesic, tonic/ muscular and bone aches, abdominal pain, impotence
wu-chiu 烏桕 (sapium)	*Sapium sebiferum* Roxb./ Euphorbiaceae; tallow tree. A tall plant cultivated	leaves and cortices of roots		cool	febrifuge, diuretic, laxative/sores and swellings

Chinese Name/ Common Name	Scientific Name/ Description	Part Used	Method of Selection and Processing	Property	Function/Symptoms
	everywhere, indigenous to China.				
wu-chu-yu 吳茱萸 (evodia)	*Evodia rutaecarpa* (Juss.) Bth./Rutaceae. A shrub cultivated everywhere, indigenous to China.	fruit	Use those harvested more than one year ago, free from stench. Small fruit with pungent odor preferred.	very hot	stomachic, diuretic, analgesic/headache, vomiting, thoracic distention and chest pain
wu-i 蕪荑 (ulmus)	*Ulmus macrocarpa* Hce./Ulmaceae; stinking elm. A low plant indigenous to China.	seeds		bland	anthelmintic/pin worms, tape worms, ascariasis, hemorrhoids
wu-mei 烏梅 (mume)	*Prunus mume* S. et Z./Rosaceae; dark plum. A tall plant cultivated everywhere.	smoke black unripe fruit	Black ones with a strong, sour taste.	warm	cleansing and cooling, antipyretic, anthelmintic/gastroenteritis, diarrhea, abdominal pain, ascariasis
wu-pei-tzu 五倍子 (nutgalls)	*Rhus javanica* L./Anacardiaceae; nut-gall tree. A tall plant found in the wilds everywhere.	galls are produced on leaves or leaf stalks by an insect, probably the aphid		bland	astringent, hemostatic/bleeding from various causes, diarrhea

Chinese Name/ Common Name	Scientific Name/ Description	Part Used	Method of Selection and Processing	Property	Function/Symptoms
wu-tou 烏頭 (wu-tou)	Same as fu-tzu.				
wu-tse-ku 烏賊骨 (cuttlebone)	Sepia esculenta Hoyle./ Sepiidae	back bone of cuttle fish		mildly warm	astringent, antacid, hemostatic/gastritis, gastric ulcer, gastric hyperacidity, melena, leukorrhea
wu-wei-tzu 五味子 (schizandra)	Schizandra chinensis Baill./Magnoliaceae. A wild vine plant.	fruit		warm	astringent, anticough, expectorant/cough, thirst
wu-yao 烏藥 (lindera)	Lindera strychnifolia F. Vill./Lauraceae. A low plant indigenous to China.	root		warm	aromatic, stomachic, analgesic, intestinal corrective/headache, abdominal pain, diarrhea
yai-chiao 崖椒 (yai-chiao)	Zanthoxylum schinifolium S. et Z./Rutaceae. A wild shrub found everywhere.	leaves			antiphlogistic/ external wounds (applied in powder form)
yang-mei-pi 楊梅皮 (myrica)	Myrica rubra S. et Z./ Myricaceae; box myrtle. A tall plant cultivated everywhere.	bark of tree		warm	astringent, hemostatic/ diarrhea, contusion

Herbs Used in Chinese Medicine

Chinese Name/ Common Name	Scientific Name/ Description	Part Used	Method of Selection and Processing	Property	Function/Symptoms
yang-ti 羊蹄 (rumex)	*Rumex crispus* L./Polygonaceae; yellow dock. A perennial wild herb found everywhere.	root		chilly	insecticide/scabies, alopecia, dermatoses; used externally
yeh-kan 射干 (belamcanda)	*Belamcanda chinensis* (L.) DC./Iridaceae; blackberry lily. A perennial wild herb found everywhere.	rhizomes		chilly	antiphlogistic, anticough, expectorant/bronchitis, pulmonary emphysema, sore throat
yen-ming-pi 延命皮 (sapindus)	*Sapindus mukorossi* Gaertner/Sapindaceae; bodhi seeds. A tall wild plant found everywhere.	fleshy part of fruit	A detergent.		antiseptic
yen-ming-tsao 延命草 (isodon)	*Isodon japonicus*/Labiatae. A perennial wild herb found everywhere.	leaves			bitter stomachic/ gastroenteritis
yen-hu-suo 延胡索 (corydalis)	*Corydalis bulbosa* DC./ Papaveraceae. A perennial herb indigenous to China.	tuber		warm	analgesic, emmenagogue/ headache, abdominal pain, menorrhagia
yen-shu-shuang 鼹鼠霜 (talpa)	*Talpa longirostris* M. Edw.; mole.	whole animal burnt black	May be used in place of *tsin-hsieh-shuan* (the burnt black of *Eriocheir japonicus*		tonic, excitant, pus dispelling agent/ carcinomas

Chinese Name/ Common Name	Scientific Name/ Description	Part Used	Method of Selection and Processing	Property	Function/Symptoms
yen-tsao 煙草 (tabacco)	*Nicotiana tabacum* L./ Solanaceae. A perennial herb indigenous to South America and cultivated everywhere.	leaves	de Haan.) in the formula *po-chou-san*.	hot	insecticidal/externally used in dermatosis
yin-chen 茵陳 (capillaris)	*Artemisia capillaris* Thunb./Compositae; evergreen artemisia. A perennial wild herb found everywhere.	spikes of fruit or young stalks and leaves (*mien-yin-chen*)	Usually the fruit spikes are used. In China the downy mass (*mien-yin-chen*) is used.	mildly chilly	antiphlogistic, antipyretic, diuretic, capable of promoting bile excretion (as a cholegogue)/the sacred herb for jaundice
yin-yang-huo 淫羊藿 (epimedium)	*Epimedium macranthum* Morr. et Dcne./Berberidaceae. A perennial wild herb found everywhere.	leaves		warm	tonic, aphrodisiac/ impotence
yin-yu 茵芋 (skinmia)	*Skimmia japonica* Thunb./ Rutaceae. A shrub found in the wilds everywhere.	stem and leaves		mildly warm	analgesic/rheumatism, arthralgia, paralysis
ying-pi 櫻皮	*Prunus pseudocerasus*	bark of	Often replaced by		anticough, astringent/

Herbs Used in Chinese Medicine

Chinese Name/ Common Name	Scientific Name/ Description	Part Used	Method of Selection and Processing	Property	Function/Symptoms
(cherry bark)	Lindl./Rosaceae; cherry. A tall plant cultivated everywhere.	tree	the bark of *pu-su*, *Quercus*, oak.		sores and swellings
ying-shih 營實 (ying-shih)	*Rosa multiflora* Miq./ Rosaceae; rambling rose. A low plant found everywhere in the wild.	fruit		warm	purgative, diuretic/ constipation, edema, sores and swellings
ying-su-ke 罌粟殼 (papaver)	*Papaver somniferum* L./ Papaveraceae; opium poppy. A biennial herb.	hulls of poppies after the opium content is removed	Now treated as a narcotic; sale is prohibited.	mildly chilly	anticough, analgesic, antidiarrheal/ abdominal pain
yu-chiao 魚膠 (isinglass)	Sturgeon fish found in the Mediterranian Sea.	swimming bladder	Processed by dissolving in water to form a glue. Such fish glue is called Isinglass.	saline, bland	used as the coating material for adhesive plasters
yu-chin 鬱金 (curcuma)	*Curcuma aromatica* Salisb./ Zingiberaceae; tumeric. A perennial herb indigenous to China.	rhizomes		chilly	stomachic, intestinal corrective, hemostatic, analgesic/gastro- enteritis, abdominal pain, emmenagogue, jaundice, hepatitis

Chinese Name/ Common Name	Scientific Name/ Description	Part Used	Method of Selection and Processing	Property	Function/Symptoms
yu-li-jen 郁李仁 (prunus)	*Prunus japonica* Thunb./ Rosaceae. A shrub cultivated everywhere.	kernel of the seed		bland	laxative, diuretic/ edema, dysuria
yu-pai-pi 榆白皮 (elm bark)	*Ulmus campestris* L./ Ulmaceae; English elm. A tall plant cultivated everywhere.	cortices of roots		bland	mucilage, paregoric, diuretic, purgative/ dysuria, prepartum and postpartum ailments
yu-yu-liang 禹餘糧 (limonite)	Solid mass of brown hematite.			bland	astringent, hemostatic, antidiarrheal/ hemorrhage, diarrhea
yuan-chih 遠志 (polygala)	*Polygala tenuifolia* Willd./Polygalaceae; Japanese senega. A perennial herb indigenous to China.	root		warm	tonic, sedative, expectorant/bronchitis, palpitation
yuan-hua 芫花 (genkwa)	*Daphne genkwa* S. et Z./ Thymelaeaceae; fish poison. A shrub indigenous to China.	flower		warm	antidiarrheal, water dispersant, diuretic/ cardiac asthma, cough, edema
yueh-chu 越橘 (vaccinium)	*Vaccinium vitis-idaea* L./ Ericaceae. A low plant found in the wilds everywhere.	leaves			preservative, astringent/urethritis, cystitis

HERB INDEX

A

abutilon 732
acanthopanax 736
achyranthes 699
aconite 669
acorus 715
actinidia 698
adenophora 710
agastache 681
akebia 699
alisma 729
allium 667
aloe 692
alpinia seed 682
alum 703
anemarrhena 660
anemone 705
angelica 702
anomala 691
anteater scales 666
antelope horn 691

apricot seed 675
aquilaria 656
aralia 730
arctium 699
areca 721
areca seed 708
arisaema 727
aristolochia 694
artemisia 653
asafoetida 652
asarum 672
asparagus 726
asphalt 689
aspidium 696
aster 734
astragalus 678
atractylodes 654
aurantium 665

B

bakeri 674

bamboo 664
bamboo leaves 665
bamboo sap 664
bear gall 675
belamcanda 739
benincasa 732
benzoin 653
biota 708
biota leaves 729
birthwort 662
black cardamon 681
bletilla 702
blue citrus peel 663
bluestone 723
blumei 730
borax 706
borneol 693
bos 700
boy's urine 732
brassica 659
broussonetia 665
brown sugar 710
bulrush 708
bupleurum 653

C

calamus 701
calamus gum 657
calcite 671
callorhinus 736
calomel 662
camellia 710
camphor 654
campsis 734
cantharides 706
capillaris 740
cardamon 720
carpesium 726
carpesium fruit 671

carthamus 680
cassia seed 666
catalpa bark 733
catalpa leaves 733
catechu 652
caudatum 700
celandine 703
celosia 662
ceruse 659
chaenomeles 697
cherry bark 741
chiang-huo 657
chicken liver 656
chin-chiu 661
chih-ko 660
chih-shih 661
ching-hao 662
chrysanthemum 664
chu-chieh ginseng 663
cicada 654
cimicifuga 714
cinnabar 665
cinnamon 687
cirsium 720
cistanche 683
clematis 736
clove 727
cluster 705
cnidium 666
coffee senna 735
coix 681
communis 689
coptis 679
cornus 711
corydalis 739
cow bezoar 700
cow gall 700
crataegus 710
croton 701
crystal salt 683

cucumeroides 731
cucumeroides seed 731
curcuma 741
cuscuta 731
cuttlebone 738
cyperus 673

D

dandelion 709
datura 695
deer horn 691
dendrobium 715
dianthus 664
dichroa 655, 717
digenea 655
dioscorea 712
dipsacus 675
dolichos 704
dragon bone 693
dried ginger 684
dried lacquar 683

E

earthworm 725
elecampane 731
elettaria 674
elm bark 742
elsholtzia 673
epimedium 740
equisetum 699
eriobotrya 707
eriocaulon 686
eriocheir 729
erythrina 670
eucommia 730
erphorbia 720
eupolyphaga 655
euryale 659
evodia 737

exotic worm 663

F

fennel 680
fluorite 734
forsythia 690
fraxinella 703
fraxinus 661
fritillaria 706
fu-lung-kan 680

G

galanga 690
galeola 731
gambir 725
garden balsam 668
gastrodia 726
gardenia 711
garlic 722
gelatin 652
genkwa 742
gentiana 693
geranium 700
ginger 713
ginkgo 703
ginseng 682
glechoma 690
gleditsia 727
gleditsia seed 728
gleditsia spine 728
glehnia 708
glycine 671
graveolens 716
gypsum 175

H

hai-sung 670
haliotis 715

helioscopia 729
hematite 723
hermes 719
hibiscus flower 697
hippocampus 670
ho-sou-wu 671
hoelen 668
holotrichia 657
horse bezoar 653
houttuynia 717
human hair 693
human skull 726
hydnocarpus 721
hydrangea 735
hydropiper 690
hyoscyamus 689

I

illicium 722
imperata 696
indigo 663
indigo fruit 688
inula 676
iron powder 656
isinglass 741
isodon 739

J

jujube 722
juncus 724

K

kaki 717
kan-cha 683
kan-sui 684
kaolin 661
kao-pen 685
keiskeana 653
kochia 724

korean aconite 703

L

laminaria 688
lamprey 701
lard 732
lathyris 675
leech 717
lemna 669
leonurus 681
leonurus fruit 666
lepidium 727
lepisma 705
licorice 684
ligustrum 700
ligustrum wax 681
lily 703
limonite 742
linum 695
lindera 738
litharge 696
lithospermum 733
locusts 679
longan 693
lonicera 661
lonicera stem 682
loranthus 709
lotus leaves 672
lotus seed 691
lycium bark 725
lycium fruit 685
lycium leaves 685
lycoris 716
lygodium 670

M

madder 660
magnolia bark 672

magnolia flower 674
ma-huang 694
malt 695
maltose 658
mastic 676, 683
mel 668
melanterite 692
melia 686
melia bark 686
melon pedicle 687
mentha 708
meretrix 736
milk scum 718
mimosoides 711
minium 660
mioga 673
mirabilitum 696
momordica 698
morinda 701
morus 709
moutan 698
mume 737
musa 701
musk 713
myrica 738
myristica 683
myrrh 697

N

nandina 699
nuphar 666
nutgalls 737
nux vomica 694

O

omphalia 689
ophiopogon 695
opium 652

oryza 685
otter liver 722
oyster shell 698

P

pa-chi 701
paeonia (peony) 712
pai-fen 703
pai-wei 705
papaver 741
pearl 656
pepper 676
perilla 734
perilla fruit 734
persica 724
persica flower 704
peucedanum 659
pharbitis 659
phaseolus 660
phellodendron 680
phoenix 719
photinia 716
phragmites 692
phragmites stem 735
phytolacca 712
picrasma 686
picrorrhiza 676
pig gall 665
pinellia 705
pinus resin 719
pipe fish 716
piper 707
placenta 732
plantago 655
plantago seed 655
platycodon 658
pleione 712
polygala 742
polygonatum 735

polygonum 707
polyporus 664
prunella 673
prunus 742
psoralea 708
pterocarpus 734
pueraria 685
pumice 669
punica 716
pyrrosia 717

Q

quercus 677
quisqualis 715

R

rana 670
raphanus 688
realgar 675
rehmannia 724
rhamnus 717
rhaponticum 691
rhinoceros 672
rhubarb 721
ricinus 706
rubus 669
rumex 739

S

saffron 667
salix 718
saltpeter 674
salvia root 723
sambucus 659
sanguisorba 725
santalum 704

sapindus 739
sapium 736
sappan wood 719
sargassum 670
saussurea 697
scarab bettle 658
schizandra 738
schizonepeta 662
scirpus 709
scorpion 674
scrophularia 676
scute 679
selinum 712
sesame 677
sesame oil 677
shellac 733
shen-chu 713
sheng-sheng-ju 715
shrimp stone 688
sibiricum 679
siegesbeckia 672
siler 667
silkworm 658
silkworm excreta 727
silkworm molt 694
skimmia 740
smilax 730
soja 673
sophora 686
sophora flower 678
sophora fruit 678
sparrow faeces 704
spikenard 684
stemona 704
stephania 667
styrax 718
subprostrata 711
succinum 677
sulfur 691
swertia 724

T

tabacco 740
tabanus 696
talc 678
talpa 739
tamarisk 656
tang-kuei 723
tea 653
terminalia 671
tetragonia 667
thimble tree 736
thlaspi 702
thoroughwort 689
tien-hsiung 726
tiger's shinbone 677
toad secretion 654
tokoro 706
torreya 668
tortoise shell 707
trachycarpus 730
trapa 657
tribulus 656
trichosanthes root 686
trichosanthes seed 687
trigonella 677
tsao-kuo 728
tsao-tou-kou 728
tse-lan 729
tu-huo 731
turmeric 657
turtle shell 688
tussilago 687

U

ulmus 737
usnea 720

V

vaccaria 735
vaccinium 742
veratrum 690
vinegar 663
viper 668
viola 733
vitex 695

W

wasps' nest 692
wheat 674
white atractylodes 7
white kaolin 704
white wax 697
wine 702
wood louse 717
wu-tou 738

X

xanthium 727

Y

yai-chiao 738
yellow wax 696
ying-shih 741
yolk 657
young deer horn 692

Z

zanthoxylum 710
zedoaria 667
zinc-bloom 692
zizyphus 719

GLOSSARY OF CHINESE MEDICAL TERMINOLOGY

A

Absolute yin disease
chueh yin ping 厥陰病
Shang han lun: "Chueh means cold limbs caused by the separation of yin and yang. The elevation of yang ch'i and the sinking of yin ch'i lengthens the distance between them, resulting in cold limbs. Absolute yin disease has the symptoms of upper fever and lower chills, a feeling of aching and burning in the chest, and vomiting after intake of food. If purgatives are misused, prolonged diarrhea will occur.

Abundance
tun fu 敦阜
Obesity.

Accumulation
chi chu 積聚
Abdominal neoplasm.

Acupuncture point; locus
ching hsueh 經穴

Any of the points in the human body where acupuncture can be applied.

Acute lower abdominal pain
hsiao fu chi chieh 小腹急結
The symptom of abdominal blood stagnation; the abdominal conformation of *Tao-ho-cheng-chi-tang* (Persica and Rhubarb Combination).

Adverse cough
ke ni shang chi 咳逆上氣
Asthmatic cough.

Adverse menses
ni ching 逆經
Vicarious menstruation, that is, bleeding from the mouth and nose at the time of the menstrual cycle.

Affected disease
so sheng ping 所生病
An illness which originates in the organs and affects the meridian belonging to the organ.

Agitated heart
hsin chung 心悰
Trembling with fear; trepidation.

Air (*chi*) agent
chi chi 氣劑
An agent used for the treatment of *chi* diseases (diseases caused by air stagnation) or air flushing-up after illness; it has the effect of calming the disturbance. Gonson Goto said: "All diseases are caused by the stagnation of *chi* in the body."

Air (*chi*) haste
chi chi 氣急
Rapid respiration.

Air (chi) share swelling
chi fen chung 氣分腫
Swelling due to poor air circulation in the body.

Air (*chi*) weakness
chi hsu 氣虛
Lack of vitality; physical weakness. A conformation of *Szu-chun-tzu-tang* (Major Four Herb Combination) or *pu-chung-i-chi-tang* (Ginseng and Astragalus Combination).

Altering fever
pien cheng 變蒸
A non-periodical fever or fever of children when wisdom teeth are coming in.

Alternate chilling and fever
wang lai han je 往來寒熱
Alternating onset of severe chills and fever; as the severe chills stop, the fever rises, and vice versa. It often occurs in lesser yang disease. *Chai-hu-chi* (Bupleurum-containing Formula) is prescribed as treatment.

Alternate conformation
pien cheng 變證
A diagnosis secondary to *cheng cheng* (exact conformation). Changing symptoms of the disease cause a shift from *cheng cheng* to *pien cheng*.

Alternating chills and fevers
nueh 瘧
Malaria or malaria-like diseases.

Ancestral muscle
tzung chin 宗筋
Muscle inside the penis. The penis.

Ancient prescriptions
ku fang 古方
Medical prescriptions from *Shang han lun* and *Chin kuei yao lueh*. These texts include all treatments recommended before the Tang dynasty.

Anemophobia
eh feng 惡風
Fear of cold arising from the external air or a blowing wind. Anemophobia is a symptom of greater yang disease. *Shang han lun*: "In greater yang disease, the duration of perspiration due to fever, anemophobia, and slow pulse is termed *chung feng*." Under the condition of severe chills and anemophobia, purgatives are prohibited from being administered, so it is essential for physicians to question the patient about these points.

Anesthetic boiling soup
ma fei san 麻沸散
A Chinese anesthetic: *Ma-fei-san* (Datura and Angelica Formula).

Annoyance and palpitation
fan chi 煩悸
Heart palpitation with chest distress.

Annoyance and restlessness
fan tsao 煩躁
Two conditions of distress. *Shang han lun*: "Patients with a feeling of vexation but without restlessness are curable; those with restlessness but no vexation will die."

Anuria
lung pi 癃閉
Anuresis or dysuria with distention in the lower abdomen.

Anxiousness under the heart
hsin hsia chi 心下急
A feeling of an impetuous mild pain, distention, and discomfort under the heart.

Appointed middle
wei chung 委中
Acupuncture point in the direct center of the popliteal fossa; it belongs to the greater yang bladder meridian of the feet.

Appointed middle toxin
wei chung tu 委中毒
Pain or tumor at the popliteal fossa due to fever condition in the liver and gall bladder which originated in the urinary bladder.

Ascariasis coldness
yu chueh 蚘厥
Cold limbs caused by a roundworm infection.

Attacked viscera
chung tsang 中臟
A type of apoplexy characterized by sudden loss of consciousness.

B

Back disease
fa pei 發背
Furunculosis on the back.

Bed fatigue
ju lao 蓐勞
Puerperal tuberculosis.

Bed fever
ju je 蓐熱
Puerperal fever.

Bedroom fatigue
fang lao 房勞
Fatigue caused by excessive sexual activities.

Behind schedule
chien chi 愆期
Irregular menses.

Big head plague
ta tou wen 大頭瘟
Also called the "big head wind" because it is caused by evil wind; characterized by flushing and/or painful swelling of the eyes, face, and head (hence the name), deafness, and tonic spasm of the jaw muscles. When the condition becomes serious, loss of consciousness occurs.

Bird's eyes
chueh mu 雀目
Night blindness.

Black eyeball
wu ching 烏睛
The irises.

Blockage of urine
pi lung 閉癃
A disease name. *Pi* means obstruction of urine and *lung* is a urinary stuttering condition that occurs more than ten times each day.

Blood abnormality
hsieh pi 血癖
Blood stagnation.

Blood block
hsieh chia 血瘕
Stagnant blood in the lower abdomen which forms an impalpable hematoma causing acute pain of no definite location.

Blood compartment
hsieh shih 血室
1. Area of blood storage.
2. Uterus.

Blood conformation
hsieh cheng 血證
The presence of blood stagnation.

Blood course
hsieh chih tao 血之道
A neurotic disorder occurring in women after menopause.

Blood drip
hsieh lin 血淋
Painful hematuria (bloody urination).

Blood-dripping pain
hsieh li tung 血瀝痛
Low back pain due to difficult menstruation.

Blood fever
hsieh je 血熱
A feverish symptom, especially observed in women after labor, which causes an unwillingness to place hands and feet under the bedding.

Blood paralysis
hsieh pi 血痺
Numbness and insensitivity to pain caused by poor blood circulation.

Blood poison
hsieh ku 血蠱
1. Enlarged abdomen due to mixture of blood and chi.
2. Myometrium myoma.

Blood weakness
hsieh hsu 血虛
Anemia; a deficiency in the amount of red blood cells in the blood.

Bloody feces
hsia hsieh 下血
Intestinal hemorrhage; enterorrhagia.

Blossom tumor
fan hua chuang 飜花瘡
Severe malignant tumor that is exacerbating.

Body fever
shen je 身熱
Generalized fever resembling tidal fever but without perspiration and not occurring at regular intervals; symptom of lesser yang or sunlight yang disease.

Bone choke
ku keng 骨哽
Choking from a piece of fish bone lodged in the throat.

Bone steam fever
ku cheng je 骨蒸熱
Fever of tuberculosis; an exhausting fever.

Bone trough
ku tsao 骨槽
Alveolus socket of a tooth.

Bone trough wind
ku tsao feng 骨槽風
Inflammation of the lower jawbone.

Bow drawn in the reverse direction
chiao kung fan chang 角弓反張
This describes the individual with a stiff neck bent in the shape of a drawn bow as is often seen in tetanus.

Breast's center
shan chung 膻中
An acupuncture point on the conception vessel; it is even with the fourth intercostal space and midway between the nipples.

Breast rock
ju yen 乳岩
Breast cancer.

Breast wind
ju feng 乳風
Swelling disease of the breast.

Bulging flesh clinging to the eyeball
nu jou pan ching 胬肉攀睛
Wing-shaped swollen tissue around the eyes; pterygium.

Burning swelling
hsin chung 焮腫
Swelling induced by inflammation.

Burning fever
hsin je 焮熱
Inflammation.

C

Cancrum oris
tsou ma kan 走馬疳
Oral ulcerations; oral cancer.

Capped dizziness
mao hsuan 冒眩
Sensation of dizziness with a feeling that the head is covered.

Catching cold
chung han 中寒
1. Catching a common cold.
2. Chill in the middle *chiao* due to lack of yang.

Catching evil
chung eh 中惡
Disease caused by "evil air."

Catching wetness
chung shih 中濕
Diseases caused by humidity.

Catching wind
chung feng 中風
In *Chin kuei yao lueh* means hemiplegia caused by cerebral hemorrhage and cerebromalacia. In *Shang han lun* means fever induced by influenza.

Ceased drink
ting yin 停飲
The stagnation of water in the stomach.

Change clothes
keng i 更衣
To discharge feces.

Chest paralysis
hsiung pi 胸痺
Chest discomfort and achiness; appears in cardiac and thoracic diseases as well as in stomach diseases.

Chi 氣
An invisible and rheological entity in Chinese medicine. It plays a very important role and has the abstract meaning of vitality and energy. In Chinese medical terminology the word "air" is frequently used, such as in air flushing-up, air dispersion, air stagnation, and air diseases.

Chi drip
chi lin 氣淋
Frequent urination due to neurosis.

Chi weakness
chi hsu 氣虛
Lack of vitality; physical weakness. A conformation of *Szu-chun-tzu-tang* (Major Four Herb Combination) or *Pu-chung-i-chi-tang* (Ginseng and Astragalus Combination).

Child pillow disease
erh chen ping 兒枕病
Labor (childbirth) pain and afterpain.

Chill drink
han yin 寒飲
Water disease; water toxin.

Chilling hernia
han shan 寒疝
Abdominal pain induced by the intake of cold foods; chills.

Chilling purgatives
han hsia chih chi 寒下之劑
Purgatives are divided into two types: chilling and warming. Chilling purgatives are prescriptions to which are added such chilling agents as rhubarb *(ta-huang)*, mirabilitum *(mang-hsiao)*, and similar drugs. Warm purgatives are

prescriptions to which are added chilling agents such as rhubarb (*ta-huang*) and warming agents such as asarum (*hsi-hsin*). aconite (*fu-tzu*), and cinnamon (*Kuei-chih*).

Chillphobia
eh han 惡寒

Fear of cold and feeling cold even under heavy bedding. Occurs with greater yang and lesser yin diseases. *Shang han lun*: "Diseases accompanied by fever and severe chills originate in yang; diseases with severe chills but no fever originate in yin."

Chills
han 寒

A slow metabolism and chill conformation. Indicated by cold limbs; a submerged, slow, and weak pulse; clear urine; and pallor. Chills and fever may occur simultaneously in a complicated manner, as when there is surface fever with inside chills or upper-half body fever with lower-half body chills. The many variations of the symptoms make it difficult to diagnose a chills and fever conformation. In the Chinese classics, *Han* also means "evil chills" and "outside chills" as in "*shang han*" (injured by evil chills).

Chills and fever
han je 寒熱

There are several interpretations for *han* and *je*. *Han* can be interpreted as slow metabolism, chills, water, evil, and severe chills. *Je* stands for fast metabolism, fire, on an increase in body temperature.

Chronic drink
pi yin 癖飲

Same as *liu yin*-retaining drink. Water toxin disease in the broad sense and stagnant water in the stomach in the narrow sense.

Chronic swellings
ku chia 痼瘕

Abdominal mass, myoma, malignant tumor.

Clear-off feces
ching pien 清便

Fecal excreta.

Clear-off grain
ching ku 清穀

Watery diarrhea of undigested food.

Clear-off pus and blood
ching nung hsieh 清膿血

Bloody feces.

Closed-mouth diarrhea
chin kou li 噤口痢

Diarrhea with anorexia.

Cold medicine
leng yao 冷藥

Antiphlogistics and analgesics: coptis (*huang-lien*), rhubarb (*ta-huang*), gardenia (*chih-tzu*), and scute of skullcap (*huang-chin*).

Collapsing leak
peng lou 崩漏

Massive uterine hemorrhage.

Combined formula
ho fang 合方

A formula made up two or more other formulas. Before use, a careful quantitative adjustment of each ingredient is made. When one herb is prescribed in two or more formulas, the greater amount is used in the combination.

Complex formula
fu fang 複方

A formula consisting of many herbs.

Conception vessel
jen mo 任脈

The main vessel in the body; originates at the pubic area and extends in a line to the umbilicus, sternum, throat, and lips. There are twenty-three acupuncture points along the path of this vessel.

Conflict between wind and moisture
feng shih hsiang po 風濕相搏
A complication of water toxin and the wind of the outside evils. Wind and moisture in conflict may cause disease.

Conformation
cheng 證
Cheng has two different meanings: syndrome (set of symptoms) or a treatment. In modern diagnosis, the categorization of a disease is based on its nature and causative factors. But in Chinese medicine, disease is also segregated by treatment. If, for example, it has been proven that a disease can be partially or totally cured with *Ko-ken-tang* (Pueraria Combination) then the disease is said to be the conformation of *Ko-ken-tang* (Pueraria Combination). Therefore, patients suffering from the same disease may have a different conformation due to different physiques; conversely, patients with different diseases but like conformations may take the same formula.

Congealed blood
pei hsieh 怀血
Stagnant blood.

Congested chest conformation
chieh hsiung cheng 結胸證
Swelling, a feeling of hardness, and aching under the heart.

Congested kernel
chieh ho 結核
Swollen lymph glands.

Congested toxin
chieh tu 結毒
Secondary and tertiary syphilis.

Convenient mind
pien hsin 便心
Continuous urge to move the bowels.

Convulsion and relaxation
chi tsung 瘈瘲
Clonic muscle spasms.

Convulsive disease
ching ping 痙病
Tetanus and similar diseases with mild and severe muscle spasms.

Cramps in the lower abdomen
hsiao fu chu chi 小腹拘急
Tension and twitching of the abdominal muscles; belongs to the abdominal conformation of *Pa-wei-wan* (Rehmannia Eight Formula).

Crane's knee wind
ho hsi feng 鶴膝風
Tuberculous arthritis and related diseases.

D

Decadent sound
cheng sheng 鄭聲
Soft-voiced, repetitious statements of the very ill.

Deeper the fever is, the colder the limbs become.
je sheng chueh sheng 熱深厥深
A warm febrile disease with persistent high fever, limbs that become suddenly cold, and loss of consciousness. The deeper the "warm evil" attacks, the colder the limbs get.

Depressing covering
yu mao 鬱冒
Impaired consciousness.

Devil's attack
kuei chi 鬼擊
Unconsciousness caused by "evil air."

Devil's back
kuei pei 鬼背
Hunchback.

Devil's infusion
kuei chu 鬼疰
Infectious diseases which pass from one family member to another.

Diaphoretics
fa piao chi 發表劑
Formulas that produce perspiration to eliminate "body surface disease": *Kuei-chih-tang* (Cinnamon Combination), *Ma-huang-tang* (Ma-huang Combination), and *Ko-ken-tang* (Pueraria Combination).

Diaphragm choke
ke yeh 膈噎
Hiccups.

Difficulty in fecal excretion
ta pien nan 大便難
Constipation.

Digesting agent
hsiao tao chi 消導劑
Medication to assist food remaining in the digestive tract to pass into the excretory system.

Digesting grain
hsiao ku 消穀
Strong digestive action that increases the frequency of hunger pangs.

Digesting thirst
hsiao ke 消渴
Excessive water drinking due to severe thirst, but without increased urination.

Directing
tao yin 導引
Treatment by self-massage.

Discharged poison
pien tu 便毒
Inguinal bubo; inguinal lymphogranulomatosis.

Dispensary prescriptions
chu fang 局方
Short name for *Ho chi chu fang* (Experimental Prescriptions of Physicians) compiled by Chen En-fang in the Sung dynasty.

Distant blood
yuan hsieh 遠血
Bleeding distant to the anus after the fecal excretion; enterorrhagia.

Distention of the lower abdomen
hsiao fu chung pi 小腹腫痞
Swelling of the lower abdomen with resistance when pressure is applied. The abdominal conformation of *Ta-huang-mu-tan-pi-tang* (Rhubarb and Moutan Combination).

Distention swelling
cheng chang 膪脹
Distention of the upper abdomen.

Distressed chest
hsiung hsieh ku man 胸脇苦滿
A distressed feeling from the upper chest to the lower part of the ribs. The patient has a distended feeling with resistance and pain when pressed. *Chai-hu-chi* (Bupleurum-containing Formula) is used.

Dragging pain
cheh tung 掣痛
Pain induced by spasm.

Drink
yin 飲
Same as (*tan*) sputum; water diseases.

Drink patient
yin chia 飲家
Patients with chronic water diseases.

Drink propensity
yin pi 飲癖
Chronic stagnant water diseases.

Dry beriberi
kan chiao chi 乾脚氣
Beriberi without edema.

Dry blood
kan hsieh 乾血
Dry blood clot.

Dry fever
tsao je 燥熱
Fever without a decrease in urination.

Dry stool
tsao shih 燥屎
Dry and hard stools.

Dry vomiting
kan ou 乾嘔
Retching without vomitus.

Duck's fluidity
ya tang 鴨溏
Soft, fluid feces.

E

Eggplant
chieh tzu 茄子
Prolapse of the uterus.

Epidemic eye
i yen 疫眼
Epidemic conjunctivitis.

Epilepsy
chien 癇
Convulsions that occur at regular intervals.

Erosion
kan 疳
Cancrum oris, venereal ulcer, or a type of infantile disease caused by digestive trouble and malnutrition, nervous system instability, or tuberculosis.

Exhausting malaria
tan nueh 癉瘧
A type of malaria caused by "thriving fever"; characterized by periodicity, high fever, vexation, labored breathing, chest distress, thirst, and frequent nausea.

Exsanguinatives
chu yu hsieh chi 驅瘀血劑
Formulas used to remove stagnant blood in the body, such as *Tao-ho-cheng-chi-tang* (Persica and Rhubarb Combination), *Ta-huang-mu-tan-pi-tang* (Rhubarb and Moutan Combination), *Kuei-chih-fu-ling-wan* (Cinnamon and Hoelen Formula), and *Ti-tang-tang* (Rhubarb and Leech Formula).

Externally infected
wai kan 外感
Diseases caused by the outside evils, such as colds, intestinal fever, and influenza.

F

Faint
chueh 厥
1. Sudden unconsciousness due to various causes.
2. Cold extremities.
3. Adverse ascension of *chi*, usually from the abdomen upward to the heart and ribs, caused by chill toxin in most cases.

Faint adverseness
chueh ni 厥逆
Shang han lun: "Lesser yin disease displays the symptoms of diarrhea of undigested food particles, inside cold with outside fever, cold limbs, and a feeble pulse. *Szu-ni-tang* (Aconite and G.L. Combination) is the major formula."

Fatigue relapse
lao fu 勞復
Disease which recurs due to overwork after recovery.

Fear of fever
eh je 惡熱
The fever of sunlight yang disease not accompanied by either severe chills or anemophobia. The patient has an intolerable feeling of warmth accompanied by general malaise.

Fetal hindrance
pao tsu 胞阻
Frequent aching in the abdomen and vaginal bleeding after conception.

Fetus leakage
tai lou 胎漏
Bloody vaginal discharge without abdominal pain during pregnancy.

Fetus poison
tai tu 胎毒
Eczema on the face and head of an infant; it is caused by toxin carried over from the parents. Rhubarb (*ta-huang*) and cnidium (*chuan-chiung*) are taken orally.

Fever
fa je 發熱
Fever in *Shang han lun* refers to the fever on the body "surface." A fever accompanied by severe chills and anemophobia; it is the fever of greater yang disease.

Fever faint
je chueh 熱厥
Thriving fever accompanied by cold limbs.

Fever flush
huo ni 火逆
An adverse alteration of disease as a consequence of erroneous treatment by the fire method: burning needle, fumigation, fomentation, moxibustion, ... etc.

Feverish diarrhea
je li 熱痢
Diarrhea with a burning sensation at the anus.

Feverish painful feeling in the heart
hsin chung teng je 心中疼熱
A sensation of severe distress in the chest accompanied by pain and fever.

Fever with diarrhea
hsieh je li 瀉熱痢
Diarrhea accompanied by "fever on the surface." It is a conformation of *Kuei-chih-jen-sheng-tang* (Cinnamon and Ginseng Combination).

"Fifth watch" diarrhea
wu ching hsieh 五更瀉
Diarrhea which occurs in the early morning between four and six.

Five elements
wu hsing 五行
Wood, fire, earth, metal, and water.

Flesh climax
jou chi 肉極
1. Protuberance of a part of flesh.
2. Polypus.
3. Pterygium.

Fluidity
tang 溏
Fluid feces.

Flushing up
shang chung 上衝
A sensation of congestion in the abdomen and chest as if air is pushing up. *Shang han lun*: "*Kuei-chih-tang* (Cinnamon Combination) is administered to patients suffering from flushing up after greater yang disease. Those without air congestion should not

be treated with *Kuei-chih-tang* (Cinnamon Combination)."

Food relapse
shih fu 食復
The relapse of an illness due to a lack of proper diet therapy during the convalescent period.

Food toxicosis
shih tu 食毒
Toxicity in the intestine due to intake of unwholesome foods.

Forceful fire
wu huo 武火
Strong fire; heat; high fever.

Four adversities
szu ni 四逆
Chilling of the limbs.

Four diagnoses
szu chen 四診
The Chinese physician makes a diagnosis using four general methods: observing, listening and smelling, questioning, and touching. Observing: visible manifestations - the physical appearance including the color of the face and skin, and the condition of the nails, eyes, and tongue. Listening and smelling: body sounds, breathing, coughing, body odor, mouth odor, and odor of excretions. Questioning: patients feelings and subjective symptoms. Touching: palpation of the patient's body such as the pulses, the abdomen, and the back.

Fox bewildering disease
hu huo ping 狐惑病
A mental illness. *Chin kuei yao lueh:* "Fox bewildering disease has symptoms similar to those of typhus, such as drowsiness, restlessness of the eyes, uneasiness, disgust at the smell of food, and complexion color change to red, black, or white. *Kan-tsao-hsieh-hsin-tang* (Pinellia and Licorice Combination) is the major formula for the treatment."

Fragile time
tsui shih 脺時
One full day; same as "one round time."

Fright
hsin chieh 心怯
Panic, fear, or nervousness.

Frost
shuang 霜
Medications that are burned into ashes for application.

G

Gathering emptiness
tso kung 撮空
The strange behavior of mentally ill patients who engage in purposeless activities such as gathering nonexistent objects.

Goosefoot wind
er chang feng 鵞掌風
Cornification on the palm.

Goose wind
er yen feng 鵞雁風
Sudamina; vesicular cutaneous eruption.

Grain duct
ku tao 穀道
Rectum and anus.

Grain-like sores
ku tsui chuang 穀嘴瘡
Pimples and acne.

Greater yang disease
tai yang ping 太陽病
Shang han lun: "Greater yang disease has as its main symptoms floating pulse, headache, stiff neck, and severe chills." In the process of contracting

a febrile disease, the patient suffers first from greater yang disease, the first stage of all febrile diseases. Muscle relaxants, such as *Kuei-chih-tang* (Cinnamon Combination), and diaphoretics such as *Ma-huang-tang* (Ma-huang Combination) and *Ko-ken-tang* (Pueraria Combination) are often administered.

Greater yang meridian
tai yang ching 太陽經
Greater yang bladder meridian of the feet.

Greater yin disease
tai yin ping 太陰病
Shang han lun: "The main symptoms of greater yin disease are distended abdomen, vomiting, loss of appetite, diarrhea, and occasional stomachache. If purgatives are prescribed, hardness under the chest will occur and diarrhea will become more serious." The abdominal distention of greater yin disease belongs to the "weak" type, as distinguished from the "strong" abdominal distention of sunlight yang disease. If these special symptoms are not evident, the diagnosis of abdomen conformation and pulse feeling need to be done.

Greater yin meridian
tai yin ching 太陰經
Greater yin lung meridian of the hands.

Greasy wind
yu feng 油風
Alopecia areata: loss of hair in circumscribed patches with little or no inflammation.

Green blindness
lu mang 綠盲
Glaucoma.

Guest conformation
ke cheng 客證
In contrast to the major conformation, the guest conformation indicates the minor symptoms not always present in a disease. It may appear and disappear from time to time and is not specifically responsible for the disease determination.

Guest obstinacy
ke wu 客忤
Unconsciousness due to extreme fear of unusual or unknown things.

Guiding medicine to the meridian
yin ching pao shih 引經報使
To direct the medication to the specific reactive site on one of the twelve meridians existing in the human body.

Gum-boils
ya kan 牙疳
Gingival ulcer or abscess; stomatitis; cancrum oris. Gangrenous stomatitis may be induced when the gum abscess worsens.

H

Half-out, half-in conformation
pan wai pan li 半外半裏
The middle conformation of lesser yang disease with symptoms of a bitter taste in the mouth, thirst, dizziness, tinnitus, cough, chest fullness, and chest ache.

Harmful swelling
ku chang 蠱脹
Same as tympany in the intestines (*ku-chang*).

Head covering
tou mao 頭冒
A heavy head.

Head necrosis
nao chu 腦疽
Brain tumor.

Head wind
tou feng 頭風
Habitual headaches.

Heartache
hsin tung 心痛
Chest ache.

Heart annoyance
hsin fan 心煩
Vexation and discomfort in the heart.

Heart chi disease
hsin chi ping 心氣病
Neurosis.

Heart wind
hsin feng 心風
Neurosis, neurasthenia.

Heavenly acts
tien hsing 天行
Epidemic diseases and pestilence. Diseases such as leprosy, cholera, plague, and smallpox were thought to be a punishment sent by heaven.

Heavenly snake poison
tien she tu 天蛇毒
Swelling disease of the fingers; felon.

Heavenly water
tien kuei 天葵
Menses.

Hernia
shan 疝
Abdominal pain, colic.

Hernia fullness
shan chi 疝氣
The protrusion of part of the intestine through the abdominal muscles. *Chu ping yuan hou lun* (On Symptoms and Causes of Diseases): "*Shan* means pain, especially lower abdominal pain."

Hidden air
fu chi 伏氣
A pathogen hidden inside the body which eventually causes illness.

Hidden menses
an ching 暗經
Amenorrhea.

Hidden water
fu yin 伏飲
Water toxin that is not apparent.

Hollow pulse
ming men 命門
Acupuncture point below the spinous process of the second lumbar vertebra.

Hope gateway
chi men 期門
Acupuncture point on absolute yin liver meridian of the feet. Located in the sixth intercostal space, two ribs below the nipple. In the *Shang han lun*, it is described as the site of fever intrusion into the "blood compartment." When this happens, *Hsiao-chai-hu-tang* (Minor Bupleurum Combination) should be prescribed, and acupuncture on point *chi men* performed.

Hot medicine
je yao 熱藥
Herbs that stimulate metabolism such as aconite.

Hotness
je 熱
Fever, hot feeling, and inflammation.

I

Immortal labor
shen hsien lao 神仙勞
Loss of appetite that occurs in nervous diseases.

Impaired cold intoxication
shang leng tu 傷冷毒
Rheumatism and related diseases.

Imperial fire
chun huc 君火
The functions of the heart on which all physiological activities are based.

Imperial, ministerial, assistant, and servant herbs
chun chen tso shih 君臣佐使
The principle of formulation and administration of herbal drugs: Imperial herbs (superior herb drugs) are the major herbs for a disease; ministerial herbs (general herb drugs) are the herbs used to assist the imperial herbs; assistant herbs (inferior herb drugs) are the herbs for supplementary functions; servant herbs are the herbs for functional catalysis.

Incomplete delivery
pan chan 半產
Miscarriage.

Incomplete pan
chien p'en 欠盆
Middle of the superior border of the clavicle, in a direct line up from nipple.

Individual joint disease
li chieh feng 歷節風
Polyarthritis.

Inhalation
chu pi 搐鼻
Insufflation of an herb medication ground into a powder.

Insensible paralysis
wan pi 瘖痺
Insensibility; loss of feeling.

Inside abdominal contraction
fu li chu chi 腹裏拘急
A nervous condition; excessive intestinal contractions or paralytic ileus.

Inside chills
li han 裏寒
Internal chills accompanied by diarrhea, stomachache, water flushing-up or diluted saliva in the mouth, cold limbs, and submerged-slow pulse. Tonics such as *Jen-sheng-tang* (Ginseng and Ginger Combination) are recommended.

Inside conformation
li cheng 裏證
Internal symptoms of stomachache and constipation or diarrhea; treated with *Pai-hu-tang* (Gypsum Combination), *Cheng-chi-tang* (Rhubarb-containing formulas) and similar formulas. An inside chills conformation should be treated with *Szu-ni-tang* (Aconite and G.L. Combination), *Jen-sheng-tang* (Ginseng and Ginger Combination), *Cheng-wu-tang* (Vitality Combination), and similar formulas.

Inside fever
li je 裏熱
Internal fever.

Inside strong
li shih 裏實
A strong and elastic abdomen, a strong pulse, and a tendency toward constipation. Sunlight yang disease is of the inside strong conformation.

Inside weak
li hsu 裏虛
Weak abdomen with a lack of elasticity; or a stiff abdomen without resistance, plus a weak pulse. Greater yin disease belongs to the inside weak conformation.

Internal injury
nei shang 內傷
In contrast to diseases resulting from external causes, internal injury is caused by physical exhaustion and negligence of good health measures. It is sometimes difficult to distinguish internal

injury from diseases due to external causes because they are so interrelated.

Intestinal carbuncle
chang yung 腸癰
Appendicitis.

Intestinal dirt
chang kou 腸垢
Feces containing mucus.

Intestinal wash
chang pi 腸澼
Enteritis.

Intestinal wind
chang feng 腸風
Intestinal hemorrhage.

Inward attack
nei kung 內攻
An assault on the internal viscera by external toxins (possibly due to accumulated toxins) causing a disease or disorder.

Ironing
yun 熨
Fomentation, a poultice.

K

Kidney accumulation
shen chi 腎積
Same as "*pen tun*" (running pig), *Chin kuei yao lueh*: "*Pen tun* has the symptoms of air flushing-up, chest and abdominal ache, and alternate chills and fever; it should be treated mainly with *Pen-tun-tang* (Pueraria and Ginger Combination)."

Kidney locus
shen yu 腎俞
Acupuncture point on greater yang bladder meridian of the feet.

Kidney meridian
shen ching 腎經
The lesser yin kidney meridian of the feet.

Kidney water
shen shui 腎水
Semen, the origin of vitality.

L

Leaking-off
lou hsia 漏下
Metrorrhagia.

Leaning breathing
i hsi 倚息
Difficult breathing; gasping.

Lesser yang disease
shao yang ping 少陽病
Shang han lun: "Lesser yang disease exhibits the symptoms of a bitter taste in mouth, thirst, and dizziness." Detection of these symptoms depend on questioning, since they are subjective symptoms. In addition to symptoms mentioned above, chest pain, fretfulness, cough, palpitations, gasping respirations, nausea, vomiting, and loss of appetite are also present. The symptoms of a distressed chest and swelling under the heart can be felt by palpating the abdomen. *Chai-hu-chi* (Bupleurum-containing Formulas), *Chih-tzu-chi* (Gardenia-containing Formulas), and *Hsieh-hsin-tang* (Pinellia-containing Combination) are frequently prescribed.

Lesser yin disease
shao yin ping 少陰病
Shang han lun: "Lesser yin disease has as its main symptoms a weak and small pulse and drowsiness." Weakness causes the patient to desire rest. In addition to the above symptoms, generalized aches, headache, severe chills, and cold feet will be present if the patient is of the "surface chill" type.

A stomachache, anxiety, diarrhea, constipation, urinary incontinence, and clear urine will appear if the patient is of the "inside chill" type. *Ma-huang-fu-tzu-kan-tsao-tang* (*Ma-huang*, Aconite, and Licorice Combination) is prescribed for the "surface chill" type patient tending towards the strong conformation, and *Ma-huang-hsi-hsin-fu-tzu-tang* (*Ma-huang*, Aconite, and Asarum Combination) is prescribed for the patient with a tendency towards the weak conformation. For the "inside chill" type of strong conformation, *Ta-huang-fu-tzu-tang* (Rhubarb and Aconite Combination) is prescribed, and for those of weak conformation, *Szu-ni-tang* (Aconite and G.L. Combination) is prescribed.

Liver conformation
kan cheng 肝證
Epilepsy, neurosis, or psychosis.

Liver depression
kan yu 肝鬱
Neurosis, mental depression.

Liver epilepsy and muscle spasm
kan chi chin luan 肝癇筋攣
Epilepsy with muscle convulsion.

Liver-faint headache
kan chueh tou tung 肝厥頭痛
Headache caused by an abnormality in the liver.

Liver meridian
kan ching 肝經
One of the fourteen meridians in the human body: the absolute-yin meridian of the feet.

Liver spots
kan pan 肝斑
Liver spots (chloasma hepaticum).

Liver vessel
kan yu 肝俞
Acupuncture point of the greater yang bladder meridian of the feet.

Liver weakness
kan hsu 肝虛
Symptoms caused by weakness of the liver meridian. *Su wen:* "Liver weakness affects the eyesight and hearing and makes the patient susceptible to attacks of panic."

Look talk
chan yu 譫語
Delirium.

Longitudinal and latitudinal meridians
ching lo 經絡
Vessels for the passage of *ch'i* within the human body: the greater yin lung meridian of the hands, sunlight yang stomach meridian of the feet, greater yin spleen meridian of the feet, lesser yin heart meridian of the hands, greater yang small intestine meridian of the hands, greater yang bladder meridian of the feet, lesser yin kidney meridian of the feet, absolute yin pericardium meridian of the hands, lesser yang triple warmer meridian of the hands, lesser yang gall meridian of the feet, absolute yin liver meridian of the feet. Those meridians that travel in the longitudinal direction are called *ching*, while those that crisscross and intersect the longitudinal meridians are called *lo* or latitudinal meridians.

Losing excrement
i sou 遺溲
Incontinence of urine and feces.

Losing feces
i shih 遺屎
Fecal incontinence.

Losing health
shih jung 失榮
Malignant tumor, cancer, and related conditions.

Losing semen
shih ching 失經
Spermatorrhea.

Losing sweat
to han 脫汗
Emission of sweat just before dying.

Loss of yang
to yang 脫陽
Collapse.

Lost blood
wang hsieh 亡血
Anemia caused by bleeding due to various causes.

Lost yang
wang yang 亡陽
A lack of vitality.

Lower abdomen
hsiao fu 小腹
Hypogastrium.

Lower heaviness
hsia chung 下重
Diarrhea with cramping.

Lower stomach
hsia kuan 下脘
An acupuncture point on the conception vessel; located on the lower part of stomach, 2 *tsun* (1 *tsun* is about an inch) above the umbilicus.

Lower *yuan*
hsia yuan 下元
Same as lower *chiao* (the lower gastrointestinal tract).

Lung atrophy
fei wei 肺痿
The distinction between lung atrophy and lung carbuncle was made in the *Chin kuei yao lueh*. The former is "weak" and the latter is the "strong" lung disease.

M

Major conformation
chu cheng 主證
Major symptoms as opposed to minor symptoms. Distinguishing between the major conformations of diseases is important in determining which prescription will be used. For example, swelling and a sensation of hardness beneath the heart is the major conformation for *Pan-hsia-hsieh-hsin-tang* (Pinellia Combination), while vomiting with diarrhea is the minor conformation. Therefore, if only vomiting and diarrhea occur (without the major conformation of swelling and hardness beneath the heart), it is not the conformation of *Pan-hsia-hsieh-hsin-tang*.

Malaria
mu nueh 母瘧
Malaria with high fever.

Malaria origin
nueh mu 瘧母
Swelling of the spleen due to chronic malaria.

Mastication
fu chu 咬咀
The ancient practice of chewing an herb to reduce it to small pieces.

Membrane field
mu yuan 募原
Mu is the diaphragm, *yuan* is the area between the heart and diaphragm.

Menstrual water
ching shui 經水
Menstruation.

Mercury agent
kung chi 汞劑
Mercury preparation.

Middle of ruler
chih chung 尺中
Inner stomach.

Middle warmer
chung chiao 中焦
1. The stomach.
2. The epigastrium.

Middle stomach
chung kuan 中脘
Acupuncture point on the conception vessel, 4 *tsun* above the umbilicus.

Mild fever
wei je 微熱
In *Shang han lun*, weak mild fever means "hidden fever" or "inside fever." Modern diagnosis considers a body temperature around 37.2°C (99°F) to be a mild fever.

Ministerial fire
hsiang huo 相火
Often mentioned as a relative entity to imperial fire with respect to the coordination of the two "fires", one to warm the viscera and the other to promote vitality.

Miscellaneous diseases
tsa ping 雜病
Diseases other than chilling and feverish diseases recorded in *Shang han lun*; they are discussed in *Chin kuei yao lueh*.

Moisture of rule
chih tse 尺澤
An acupuncture point at the elbow crease on the lateral border of the tendon of the biceps brachii muscle.

Mole cricket boils
lou ku chieh 螻蛄癤
A furuncular skin infection affecting children, usually on the head; impetigo.

Monthly pain
yueh hsin tung 月信痛
Painful menstruation.

Mouth and eyes obliquity
kou yen k'uai hsieh 口眼喎斜
Facial neuroparalysis.

Moving air
tung chi 動氣
Palpitation.

Moving air or *chi* between the kidneys
shen chien tung chi 腎間動氣
Air that originates in the kidney and moves around the umbilicus; it can be felt by touching the abdomen.

Moving disease
shih tung ping 是動病
Diseases occurring at the meridian which itself is the primary source of the disease.

Muscle texture
tsou li 腠理
Skin and mucous membrane including any membrane of internal organs.

N

Nasal deep
pi yuan 鼻淵
Pararhinitis.

Natural micturition
tzu li 自利
Normal excretion of urine; free micturition.

Neck scrofula
ma tao hsia ying 馬刀俠瘻
A reddish swelling on the neck.

Nine cavities
chiu chiao 九竅
The nine openings in the human body: the ears, eyes, nostrils, mouth, anus, and urethra. *Ling shu:* "There are nine regions on earth and nine cavities in the human body."

No damage to purpose
yu ku wu sun 有故無損
This describes a treatment that is not suggested under normal circumstances, but can be used when necessary without causing harmful effects. For example, purgatives are not routinely prescribed for the condition of severe vomiting, but they can be administered safely when it is essential to the treatment.

Nose fan
pi shan 鼻扇
Difficult breathing; respiration with movement of the alanasi.

Numbness of the lower abdomen
hsiao fu pu jen 小腹不仁
Hyposensitivity of numbness of the lower abdomen; an abdominal conformation of the *Pa-wei-wan* (Rehmannia Eight Formula). It is likely that adynamia of the lower abdomen will occur at the same time.

Numbness of the mouth
kou pu jen 口不仁
No sense of taste in the mouth. *Shang han lun:* "It is a combination of three yang symptoms: distention of the stomach and heaviness of the body, difficulty in turning, and no sense of taste. This should be treated mainly with *Pai-hu-tang* (Gypsum Combination)."

Numbness of throat
hou pi 喉痺
Acute tonsillitis or diphtheria.

Nourishment
jung 榮
1. Nutrients taken, digested, and incorporated into the blood.
2. Blood vessels.

Nourishment and nursing
tiao li 調理
Nourishment and nursing carried out in period of convalescence during which drugs necessary for health care are sometimes administered.

Nourishment and protection
jung wei 榮衛
Physical nutrition; protection against "evils." *Jung* circulates within the blood vessels and *wei* outside the vessels. The former is equivalent to the blood stream and the latter to lymph and body fluids.

O

Obstructive chronicity
cheng ku 癥痼
Mass in the abdomen.

Obstructive disease
cheng ping 癥病
Same as *"cheng chieh"* (obstructive knot); bowel obstruction.

Obstructive knot
cheng chieh 癥結
Obstruction of the bowels with distention and hardness of the abdomen.

Obstructive swelling
cheng chia 癥瘕
Same as *cheng ku*-chronic obstruction; benign tumor. *Cheng* denotes a neoplasm or mass that is fixed in position and grows at definite times while *chia* is a movable tumor that does not occur

at definite times.

Offspring organ
tzu tsang 子臟
The uterus.

Old grain
su ku 宿穀
Undigested food particles in the stomach.

One round time
chou shih 周時
One full day.

Osteonecrosis
fu ku chu 附骨疽
Necrosis of the bones.

Overflowing drink
i yin 溢飲
A kind of edema.

Overnight drunkenness
su tsui 宿醉
Drunkenness of two days' duration. Hangover.

P

Palpation of pulses
mo chen 脈診
The important pulses are briefly described as follows:
1. Floating pulse: The fingers experience a floating sensation while palpating lightly. It appears when the patient is suffering from an evil febrile disease. If he has a floating-strong pulse with fever and severe chills, he is of the surface strong conformation. If he has a floating-weak pulse, he is of the surface weak conformation.
2. Submerged pulse: Appears to be deeply submerged and only reveals itself when pressure is firmly applied to the artery. This means that the illness is situated very deep in the body. If the patient has a submerged-strong pulse, he is of the inside strong conformation. If he has a submerged-weak pulse, he is of the inside weak conformation.
3. Slow pulse: Appears with chilling disease. A slow and strong pulse goes with a sputum disease; a slow pulse with aching signifies a condition of chilling ache; a slow-weak pulse belongs to the weak chilling conformation.
4. Fast pulse: A pulse of high frequency which often occurs with febrile diseases. A fast and strong pulse belongs to the strong fever conformation, while a fast and feeble pulse is of the weak fever conformation.
5. Empty pulse: The weak and feeble pulse of a patient who has lost his vigor. It belongs to the weak conformation.
6. Full pulse: A strong pulse, the sign of vitality and health.
7. Tight pulse: Similar to the "chordal pulse", it is a sign of competition between the normal and evil. Those with severe pain in the body may have a floating, tight pulse. Those with chest and abdominal pain will have a submerged tight pulse. Tight pulse also appears with water intoxication, chilling, and feverish diseases.
8. Chordal pulse: The pulse is like the taut string of a drawn bow; it often appears with water intoxication diseases. Those with fever and a tense-large-chordal pulse are of the weak conformation. A chordal-small pulse indicates a muscle spasm.
9. Large pulse: The range is wide and large. The presence of a large pulse indicates an increase in both normal and evil *chi*.
10. Lively pulse: A lively pulse in one who is seriously ill is a good prognosis; on the other hand, the prognosis is poor if the pulse is not lively, even though no serious symptoms of illness are apparent.

Palpitation
chi 悸
Cardiac palpitation.

Pattern prescriptions
tao chi 套劑
Frequently used prescriptions.

Paralysis
pi 痹
A temporary condition in which pain, numbness, or loss of voluntary motion occur. *Pi* in *Su wen* (Familiar Conversations) refers to a disease combining the three elements of "wind", chill, and wet.

Paralytic numbness
hsien pi 痃癖
Stiffness and pain in the shoulders and back; also, muscle spasm in the abdomen.

Paralytic weakness
wei jo 痿弱
Permanent loss of sensation and voluntary motion in the entire body.

Partial dryness
pien ku 偏枯
Unilateral paralysis, hemiplegia.

Pen stone
pi ching 筆磬
Calcification of the joints.

Pestilence
wen 瘟
General term for acute infectious diseases.

Petal-like gums
chih yin chieh pan 齒齦結瓣
Gingival inflammation resembling a red petal and accompanied by bleeding, aching ulceration, and fetid breath.

Pigeon tail
chiu wei 鳩尾
The region at the substernum; an acupuncture point on the conception vessel.

Pimples
ke ta 疙瘩
A general term for warts, pustules, and macules.

Plum kernel air
mei ho chi 梅核氣
The feeling of having a round object in the throat; often observed in patients with neurotic disorders.

Posterity school
hou shih pai 後世派
A school of Chinese medicine established by Dosan Manase in the middle of the Tokugawa era in Japan. It followed the theories of yin and yang and the Five Elements Arrangement and primarily used prescriptions developed after the Sung dynasty.

Pregnancy cough
tzu sou 子嗽
"Maternal cough"; persistent cough during pregnancy resulting in fretfulness and untimely contractions.

Pregnancy swelling
tzu chung 子腫
Edema during pregnancy.

Prolonged aphonia
chiu yin 久瘖
Losing one's voice gradually and intermittently. The condition is aggravated by using the voice.

Prolonged chills
chiu han 久寒
Water toxin caused by prolonged chilling.

Protection
wei 衛
Body defenses (against "evils").

Pseudo-fever
chia je 假熱
Not a true fever; the sensation of feverishness without a rise in body temperature; referred to in the phrase "real chilling and pseudo-fever."

Pulse feeling area
tsun kou 寸口
The broad definition of *"tsun kou"* is the site of the radial arteries on the wrists, the same site modern Western medicine uses for pulse taking; the narrow definition, the pulse area by the middle, and ring fingers of the wrist. The index finger rests on *tsun kou*, the middle finger on *kuan shang*, and the ring finger on *chih chung*.

Puncture the vessels
tzu lo 刺絡
To cause discharge of blood by puncturing the acupuncture point with a needle.

Purgatives
hsieh chi 瀉劑
An attacking agent; agents that evacuate the bowels.

Purulence leaking
nung lou 膿漏
Paranasal sinusitis.

Push and grasp
tuei na 推拿
A method used in bone-setting; also a type of massage.

Q

Quiet placenta
hsi pao 息胞
Retained placenta.

R

Reddish tumor
ying liu 癭瘤
A reddish tumor occurring on the neck and shoulders.

Red moving wind
chih yu feng 赤油風
Erysipelas.

Regurgitation of stomach
wei fan 胃反
Persistent emesis; gastrectasis; or narrow pylorus.

Remorse and anger from the heart
hsin chung ao nao 心中懊惱
Distressed feeling inside the heart accompanied by anxiety.

Remove stomach
chu chung 除中
Chung, the "stomach evil air," increases intensely before death; it removes "stomach air" and induces the need for food in the stomach which is attempting to save itself. This may be an explanation for the increase in appetite felt before death.

Retaining drink
liu yin 留飲
The general term for water toxin diseases; specifically refers to stagnant water in the stomach.

Resting diarrhea
hsiu hsi li 休息痢
Chronic paroxysmal diarrhea.

Return of yang
hwei yang 回陽
Recovery of vitality.

Reverse joint pulse
fan kuan mo 反關脈
Abnormal location of arterial pulsa-

tion, on the back of the hand rather than on the wrist.

Rich pregnancy
sheng tai 盛胎
The continuation of menses during pregnancy.

Ribbon-like excretion
tai hsia 帶下
Leukorrhea.

Rock symptom
yen cheng 岩證
Cancer.

Rotten eyelid wind
lan hsien feng 爛弦風
Belpharitis marginalis.

Rough skin
pi fu chia tso 皮膚甲錯
Rough skin caused by blood stagnation and malnutrition.

Running pig
pen tun 奔豚
Air flushing up from the lower abdomen. It appears in neurotic disorders, particularly hysteria.

Running pig symptoms
pen tun cheng 奔豚症
Heart palpitation, hysteria, air flushing up from the lower abdomen to the heart, and difficulty in breathing.

Running sore
lou chuang 漏瘡
A fistula.

Rush gasping
chuan chi 喘氣
Difficult breathing, dyspnea.

S

School of ancient prescriptions
ku fang pai 古方派
A school of Chinese medicine in the seventeenth century which proposed that the methods described in the *Shang han lun* and *Chin kuei yao lueh* be used instead of the Five Elements Arrangement as the standard for disease diagnosis.

Self sweating, spontaneous sweating
tzu han 自汗
Sweating that is not induced by a disphoretic.

Severe chills; chillphobia
eh han 惡寒
Fear of cold and feeling cold even under heavy bedding. Occurs with greater yang and lesser yin diseases. *Shang han lun:* "Diseases accompanied by fever and severe chills originate in yang; diseases with severe chills but no fever originate in yin."

Severe leaky orbit
ta tzu lou 大眥漏
Inflammation of the tear sac.

Severe orbital inflammation
ta tzu chih yen 大眥赤眼
Keratitis.

Severe wind air
li feng chi 厲風氣
Edema of the feet.

Sheng--a unit of volume measurement 升
One *sheng* in *Shang han lun* is equal to approximately 1 *ho* and 1 *shao* strong. One *ho* is equal to 1/10 of the present unit of 1 *sheng* (31.6 cubic inches).

Shoulder breath
chien hsi 肩息
To gasp with the shoulders shrugged.

Shuddering sweat
chan han 戰汗
Sweating accompanied by trembling; cold sweat.

Sickening heart
eh hsin 噁心
Nausea.

Sick eyes
kan yen 疳眼
Acute eye disorder in which there is dryness of the cornea and white spots caused by sensitivity to tuberculosis.

Side conformation
chien cheng 兼證
Same as guest (minor) conformation.

Sighing air
ai chi 噯氣
Belching; eructation.

Single formula
tan fang 單方
A prescription containing only one herb.

Six meridians
liu ching 六經
The six channels of *chi* in the human body: greater yang, sunlight yang, lesser yang, greater yin, absolute yin, and lesser yin.

Skin nuts
jou shang su chi 肉上粟起
Goose flesh.

Skin water
pi shui 皮水
Edema.

Slip-out of uterus
yin ting hsia to 陰挺下脫
Prolapse of the uterus.

Slow wind
huan feng 緩風
Beriberi.

Smelling method
hsiu fa 齅法
Same as *hsun fa*, smoking method. Treatment by inhalation or fumigation with burning herbs.

Smoking method
hsun fa 薰法
Treatment in which the smoke of a heated medication is inhaled or used as a fumigant. For example, the fumes from burning *shui-yin-chi* (mercury-containing formulas) can be used to treat syphilis, and those of realgar (*hsiung-huang*) to treat oxyuriasis (pinworm disease).

Soaking agent
pao chi 泡劑
A method of preparation of herbs; maceration; percolation.

Sore patients
chuang chia 瘡家
Those with chronic swelling and external injuries.

Sore tuberculosis
chuang lao 瘡癆
Osteoarthritic tuberculosis.

Soup burn
tang fa 湯發
Burned by hot water; scalded.

Spleen ache
pi teng 脾疼
Stomachache.

Spleen disease
pi tan 脾癉
A persistent desire to eat or suck on sweets.

Spoiled blood
pei hsieh 怀血
Stagnant blood.

Spontaneous sweating, self sweating
tzu han 自汗
Sweating that is not induced by a diaphoretic.

Sputum
tan 痰
Water diseases; congestion.

Sputum drink
tan yin 痰飲
A general term for "water diseases" caused by the water changes in the body or stagnant water in the stomach.

Sputum kernel
tan ho 痰核
Swollen lymphglands.

Stagnancy under the heart
hsin hsia pi 心下痞
A feeling of stagnancy under the heart; the area is soft and painless when pressed.

Stagnancy and hardness under the heart
hsin hsia pi pien (ying) 心下痞鞕
A feeling of both stagnancy and hardness in the epigastic area; both a subjective and an objective symptom.

Stagnant blood
yu hsieh 瘀血
Symptoms of dryness in the mouth and a desire to rinse the mouth with water without swallowing. Patients have a sensation of fullness in the abdomen that can not be detected by abdominal palpation. Other symptoms are general or local fever accompanied by anxiety, purple spots (petechiae) on the skin and mucous membrane, greenish blood vessels, rough skin, dark purple tongue-edge, pale lips, black stools, and a submerged-harsh pulse, submerged-knotted pulse, submerged-harsh-feeble pulse, or large-slow pulse. Lower abdominal resistance with pain is the main abdominal symptom shown in palpation.

Stagnant cheeks
chih i 滯頤
Erosion at the corners of the mouth and the chin due to continuous drooling.

Stagnant water
chih yin 支飲
Excess fluid in the cardiac area, lungs, or stomach. Diseases caused by stagnant water under the heart, such as valvular diseases, nephritis, and pulmonary edema. *Chin kuei yao lueh*: "Stagnant water is an illness accompanied by a cough, dyspnea, restlessness, and edema." *Mu-fang-chi-tang* (Stephania and Ginseng Combination) is usually prescribed.

Startling wind
ching feng 驚風
Infantile convulsion due to cerebral meningitis, polio, high fever, or similar diseases.

Steel needle eyes
tou chen yen 偷針眼
Hordeolum; stye.

Stomach *chi*
wei chi 胃氣
Digestive functions; vitality.

Stomach family
wei chia 胃家
A term referring to the gastrointestinal system.

Stomach grumbling
fu chung lei ming 腹中雷鳴
Borborygmus; a symptom appearing

in the conformations of *Pan-hsia-hsieh-hsin-tang* (Pinellia Combination), *Kan-tsao-hsieh-hsin-tang* (Pinellia and Licorice Combination), and *Sheng-chiang-hsieh-hsin-tang* (Pinellia and Ginger Combination).

Stomach retardation
na tai 納呆
Retardation of the stomach function: indigestion and lack of appetite.

Sticky sputum
chiao tan 膠痰
Thick saliva.

Stone drip
shih lin 石淋
Vesicle calculus.

Stored drink
hsu yin 蓄飲
Water stagnation in the stomach.

Stored fever
hsu je 蓄熱
Same as stagnant fever, *yu je*.

Straw bed
tsao ju 草蓐
The period of confinement in childbirth; puerperium.

Striking agents
kung chi chi 攻擊劑
Purgatives, emetics, and diaphoretics.

Strong adverse flushing-up
ta ni shang chi 大逆上氣
Severe accumulation and ascension of air in the body; feeling of congestion.

Strong diarrhea
shih li 實痢
Diarrhea of the strong conformation. *Ta-chai-hu-tang* (Major Bupleurum Combination) and *Ta-cheng-chi-tang* (Major Rhubarb Combination) are suitable for its treatment.

Strong fever
shih je 實熱
Same as strong fire (*shih huo*).

Strong fever
chuang je 壯熱
High fever; high body temperature.

Strong fire
shih huo 實火
The inflammation, congestion, and fever in a strong conformation. Gypsum (*shih-kao*), rhubarb (*ta-huang*), and coptis (*huang-lien*) are used for treatment.

Strong menses
chi ching 激經
Also called "rich pregnancy"; refers to the continuation of menses from the beginning of pregnancy until the fetus is near term. The phenomenon is not harmful to either the mother or the fetus.

Strong wind
ta feng 大風
Leprosy.

Sudden blindness
pao mang 暴盲
Bleeding at the optic fundus.

Sudden disorder with cramps
huo luan chuan chin 霍亂轉筋
Excessive fluid loss due to severe vomiting and diarrhea which causes a spasm of the gastrocnemius muscle.

Sudden faintness
pao chueh 暴厥
An ancient term, this refers to the sudden faintness caused by sharp flushing-up of air in the body and a rapid pulse.

Sudden loss
pao to 暴脫
Apoplexy; the sudden and excessive

loss of sweat, blood, or semen; acute diarrhea, etc. Results in a great loss of vitality and separation of yin and yang.

Sudden restraint
chu chi 拘急
A muscular spasm.

Summer-directed disease
chu hsia ping 注夏病
Symptoms that are associated with the summer season, such as fatigue and lack of appetite.

Summer faint
shu chueh 暑厥
A disease due to heat stroke in the summer; symptoms of sudden fainting, cold limbs, dirty complexion, dry teeth, and obstructed urine and feces.

Sun dawn
yang tan 陽旦
Another name for cinnamon (*kuei-chih*).

Sunlight yang disease
yang ming ping 陽明病
Shang han lun: "Sunlight yang disease shows the symptom of a strong, full stomach." Fullness or distention of the stomach can be felt by palpating the abdomen. The patient has a tendency toward constipation.

Sunlight yang stomach meridian
yang ming wei ching 陽明胃經
A meridian of the feet.

Surface conformation
piao cheng 表證
Denotes the symptoms appearing on the surface of the body, such as chill-phobia, anemophobia, fever, headache, generalized aching, a floating pulse, ... etc.
Apparent greater yang disease conformations such as severe chills, evil wind, fever, headache, generalized achiness, and floating pulse. If also accompanied by spontaneous sweating and a floating weak pulse, it is the surface weak conformation and *Kuei-chih-tang* (Cinnamon Combination) should be used. When sweating does not occur but there is a floating tight pulse, it is the surface strong conformation and *Ma-huang-tang* (*Ma-huang* Combination) should be used.

Surface and inside
piao li 表裏
Surface: the surface of the body. Inside: the internal organs.

Suspending ache
hsuan tung 懸痛
Cramps.

Suspending drink
hsuan yin 懸飲
A type of "sputum drink" (*tan yin*).

Swelling of blood
Hsieh fen chung 血分腫
Edema caused by the suppression of menses.

Swollen cheek
cha sai 痄腮
Parotitis.

Syphilis poison
yang mei chuang tu 楊梅瘡毒
Syphilis lesions on the skin, bone, and other areas of the body (secondary stage).

Systematic gateway
chang men 章門
Acupuncture point of absolute yin liver meridian on the feet.

T

Take a break
chiang hsi 將息
To take proper care of oneself during the recovery stage of an illness in order to make a good recovery.

Tartar's smell
hu chou 狐臭
Armpit odor.

Tension below the umbilicus
chi hsia chu chi 臍下拘急
An abdominal conformation of *Pa-wei-wan* (Rehmannia Eight Formula) in which there is tension between the abdominal muscle and the umbilicus.

Terminate sweat
chueh han 絕汗
Same as "*to han*" (losing sweat).

Thick medicine
hou yao 厚藥
Medicine with a strong odor and taste.

Thin medicine
po yao 薄藥
Herbs with mild odor and taste.

Three yang and three yin
san yang san yin 三陽三陰
Six stages of disease – the greater, lesser, and sunlight yang; greater, lesser, and absolute yin.

Thunderhead wind
lei tou feng 雷頭風
Glaucoma.

Tidal fever
chao je 潮熱
Sunlight yang disease fever which rises and falls like the tide with perspiration of the whole body but no severe chills.

Tight pulse
chin mo 緊脈
Rapid pulse.

Time air
shih chi 時氣
Diseases related to seasonal weather changes.

Time plague
shih i 時疫
Epidemic febrile diseases.

Time toxin
shih tu 時毒
Epidemic diseases.

Toad epidemic
hsia ma wen 蝦蟆瘟
Parotitis, erysipelas, and diphtheria.

To cause a disturbance (internally)
ming hsuan 瞑眩
Any reaction due to detoxification by medication; an indication that recovery is imminent.

Tongue lameness
she chien 舌蹇
Difficulty in moving the tongue which results in speaking disability.

Tonic agents
pu chi 補劑
Medicines used to enhance physical strength rather than purge the disease.

Traveling ache
tsou tung 走痛
Aching that moves from one part of the body to another.

Triple stomach
san kuan 三脘
1. The upper abdomen (epigastrium), middle abdomen, and lower abdomen.
2. (a) the diaphragm, (b) the heart, and (c) the umbilicus.

Triple warmer
san chiao 三焦
Upper *chiao*, the portion of the body from the diaphragm up to the head. Middle chiao, the epigastrium. Lower chiao, the portion from the umbilicus down to the feet.

True chilling and pseudo-fever
chen han chia je 眞寒假熱
Not actually a febrile disease. If patient's pseudo-fever is mistaken for true fever and treated with cooling agents, the patient's condition will grow worse. *Szu-ni-tang* (Aconite and G.L. Combination) is used to warm the chill, after which the pseudo-fever will recede. Clear urine and a late, weak pulse accompany the symptoms of "real chilling and pseudo-fever."

True heartache
chen hsin tung 眞心痛
Angina pectoris.

Turbid drink
cho yin 濁飲
Water toxin; stagnant water in the stomach.

Turbid drink adversity
cho yin shang ni 濁飲上逆
Headache, dizziness, and vomiting cause by stagnant water toxin in the stomach.

Turning yellow
fa huang 發黃
Jaundice.

Tympany (within the) intestines
ku chang 鼓腸
Distended abdomen due to flatus in the intestine with, or without, water stagnation in the abdomen.

Twitching ureter
chuan pao 轉胞
Suppression of urine; *Pa-wei-wan* (Rehmannia Eight Formula) is the treatment.

U

Underworld spring
chung chuan 重泉
Underground; hades.

Uneasy feeling in the heart
hsin chung tan tan 心中憺憺
"*Tan*" means emptiness and vibration. Refers to intense heart palpitations and a feeling of emptiness.

Upper stomach
shang kuan 上脘
An acupuncture point on the conception vessel located on the upper part of the stomach 5 *tsun* (1 *tsun* is about 1 inch) above the umbilicus.

Upper warmer
shang chiao 上焦
The portion of the body above the diaphragm.

Unstable mind
cheng chung 怔忡
A condition resembling neurosis with symptoms of heart palpitation, nervousness, and a feeling of tightness in the chest.

Ureteral tangle
pao hsi liao li 胞系了戾
Convolution of the ureter caused by forced retention of urine; results in anuria or dysuria.

V

Vanish sore
chi chuang 漆瘡
A skin condition induced by contact with varnish.

Verruca
hou tzu 猴子
A kind of excrescence; a wart.

Vexation and fever of the five viscera
wu hsin fan je 五心煩熱
Oppressive fever of the entire body.

Visceral irritation
tsang tsao 臟躁
A type of nervous condition (occurring mainly in women) in which the primary symptoms are depression, delusions, mania, and hypersensitivity or hyposensitivity. When the episode begins, the patient feels irritable, depressed, and restless. This is followed by sighing, sadness, crying, and sometimes even muscle spasms. However, the complexion is not pale and consciousness not impaired.

Viscera toxin
tsang tu 臟毒
Malignant tumor in the rectum; rectal cancer.

Vomiting infant
tu erh 吐兒
Regurgitation of milk in infants.

Vomiting red
tu hung 吐紅
Vomiting blood; hemoptysis.

W

Wai Tai 外台
One of three ministries in ancient China; the censor's ministries.

Wandering yellow
tsou huang 走黃
A migratory toxin which penetrates the heart via the blood vessels and causes heart distress, vomiting, alternate chills and fever, and unconsciousness.

Warm and chill
shang han 傷寒
Diseases induced by external causes; febrile diseases. A narrow meaning is malignant diseases.

Warm disease
wen i 瘟疫
A febrile disease resembling typhoid fever.

Warm medicine
wen yao 溫藥
Chinese medicines are divided into five categories—warm, chill, hot, cool or cold, and even. Warm medicine has a warming effect. Cinnamon (*kuei-chih*), ginger (*sheng-chiang*), dry ginger (*kan-chiang*), zanthoxylum (*shu-chiao*), asarum (*shi-hsin*), *tang-kuei*, and cnidium (*chuan-chiung*) are warm medicines.

Warm tonics
wen pu 溫補
Warm medicines are for yin conformation diseases; tonics are for weak conformation diseases. If the disease belongs to both the yin and weak conformations, then a warm tonic is administered, such as *Jen-sheng-tang* (Ginseng and Ginger Combination), *Fu-tzu-li-chung-tang* (Aconite, Ginseng, and Ginger Combination), *Szu-ni-tang* (Aconite and G.L. Combination), and *Chen-wu-tang* (Vitality Combination).

Washed bag
pi nang 澼囊
Stagnant water stomach diseases such as gastroptosis, stomach atony, and gastrectasis.

Water
shui 水
Loss of taste, phlegm, drinking, and sputum diseases. According to Chinese medical theories, phlegm means water,

not merely expectoration. Ancient people said: "To deal with strong diseases, one should begin by treating phlegm."

Water adversity
shui ni 水逆

Severe thirst with a strong desire to drink. However, vomiting occurs as the result of drinking water, so the patient remains thirsty and has dysuria. Vomiting can be stopped by taking *Wu-ling-san* (Hoelen Five Herb Formula).

Water disease
shui yin 水飲
1. Sputum disease.
2. Gastric stagnant water.

Water toxin
shui tu 水毒
Edema.

Weak and strong
hsu shih 虛實

In general, weak denotes a condition of weak resistance and strong denotes a strong resistance. However, those considered weak or strong in normal health may not be diagnosed as such when they are ill. For example, those normally thought to be of the weak conformation may surprisingly change to a strong conformation when they are sick, or vise versa. In addition, there are surface-weak and inside-strong or upper-half weak and lower-half strong conformations. The determination of weak or strong is the basis of disease diagnosis in Chinese medicine, and it requires at least a year's experience to make the correct judgment since there are various stages and phases in weak or strong conformation concepts. The weak and strong states are represented by the following conformations in sequence from weak to strong. *Kuei-chih-tang* (Cinnamon Combination), *Kuei-chih-erh-ma-huang-i-tang* (Cinnamon Two and *Ma-huang* One Combination), *Kuei-chih-ma-huang-ke-pan-tang* (Cinnamon and *Ma-huang* Combination), *Ko-ken-tang* (Pueraria Combination), and *Ma-huang-tang* (*Ma-huang* Combination) are formulas of surface conformation. *Hsiao-ching-lung-tang* (Minor Blue Dragon Combination) is the prescription for "surface evil" and inside chill conformation. *Ta-ching-lung-tang* (Major Blue Dragon Combination) is of the "surface evil" and inside fever conformation. *Chai-hu-chiang-kuei-tang* (Bupleurum, Cinnamon, and Ginger Combination), *Chai-hu-kuei-chih-tang* (Bupleurum and Cinnamon Combination), *Hsiao-chai-hu-tang* (Minor Bupleurum Combination), *Szu-ni-san* (Bupleurum and Chih-shih Formula), *Chai-hu-chia-lung-ku-mu-li-tang* (Bupleurum and Dragon-Bone Combination), and *Ta-chai-hu-tang* (Major Bupleurum Combination) are formulas of half-out half-in evil conformation. *Tiao-wei-cheng-chi-tang* (Rhubarb and Mirabilitum Combination), *Hsiao-cheng-chi-tang* (Minor Rhubarb Combination), and *Ta-cheng-chi-tang* (Major Rhubarb Combination) are formulas of inside strong conformation. Therefore, to make the disease diagnosis simply by judging the differences between weak and strong is not enough; the concepts of surface and inside, upper and lower, etc., are also important. A detailed study of this subject can be found in *Shang han lun* (Treatise of Febrile Diseases).

Weak annoyance
hsu fan 虛煩

Weak vitality with discomfort and a dragging ache in chest.

Weak bladder *chi*
pao chi pu ku 脬氣不固

A weak bladder resulting in urinary incontinence and enuresis.

Weak diarrhea
hsu li 虛痢
Diarrhea of the weak conformation belonging to *Chen-wu-tang* (Vitality Combination).

Weakening hernia
tuei shan 癩疝
Inguinal hernia; scrotal hernia.

Weak fever
hsu je 虛熱
Same as weak fire (*hsu huo*).

Weak fire
hsu huo 虛火
Fever, inflammation, and blood congestion caused by fatigue and trauma. Tonics such as ginseng (*jen-sheng*), astragalus (*huang-chi*), and hoelen (*fu-ling*) are remedies.

Weak inside movement
hsu li chih tung 虛裏之動
The heartbeat at the *hsu li* point (equivalent to the location of the heart apex).

Weak spleen and stomach
pi wei hsu jo 脾胃虛弱
Poor digestion. The "spleen" in Chinese medicine refers to the co-digestive organs, not just the spleen itself; it can be deemed to be equivalent to the pancreas.

Wearing eyes
tai yen 戴眼
A condition characterized by up-turned and motionless eyes; a cerebro-neurotic symptom appearing in the severe stage of a disease.

Wearing yang
tai yang 戴陽
Cold feet and a red face; this symptom appears in weak-yang-flushing-up or tuberculosis.

Weary wet
lao shih 勞濕
Chronic wet toxin disease resulting in physical weakness.

Wetness
shih 濕
Wet air and water toxin (water diseases); syphilis; certain skin diseases.

Wet fever
shih je 濕熱
Fever with decrease of urination; the same as "stagnant fever."

Wet patient
shih chia 濕家
Chin kuei yao lueh: "Patients with long-term wet disease have a general body aching, fever, and smoky yellowish skin."

Wet toxin
shih tu 濕毒
Syphilis.

White drink
pai yin 白飲
Thick rice soup.

White excess
pai yin 白淫
1. Leukorrhea containing white or grayish semi-solid material.
2. Spermatorrhea.

White fertility
pai wo 白沃
Leukorrhea.

White tiger wind
pai hu feng 白虎風
Swollen and painful joints; polyarthritis.

White turbidity
pai cho 白濁
White and turbid urine with proteinuria such as occurs in gonorrhea.

Wild duck's fluidity
wu tang 鶩溏
Same as *ya tang* (duck's fluidity); soft or fluid feces.

Will compartment
chih shih 志室
Acupuncture point of the greater yang bladder meridian of the feet.

Wind disease
feng wen 風溫
A kind of acute febrile disease induced by the "spring wind evil."

Wind eyes
feng yen 風眼
Purulent conjunctivitis.

Wind moisture
feng shih 風濕
Wind means "outside evils"; moisture means "water toxins"; wind moisture is a disease caused by the combination of these two factors. Its symptoms resemble rheumatism.

Wind water
feng shui 風水
Edema of a surface conformation.

Withered wax
ku la 枯臘
Underweight with dry, rough skin due to malnutrition.

Worm accumulation
chung chi 蟲積
Chronic ascariasis.

Y

Yellow obese disease
huang pang ping 黃胖病
Heart palpitation and wheezing due to anemia; also intestinal parasites.

Yellow sweat disease
huang han 黃汗
Symptoms of yellow sweat, fever, and edema.

Yang conformation
yang cheng 陽證
An active, sporadic, febrile condition accompanied by rapid metabolism. It manifests the symptoms of facial redness, mouth dryness, discolored urine, and a massive-large or rapid-slippery pulse.

Yin conformation
yin cheng 陰證
Quiescent, sinking, chilling types of disease in which metabolism is retarded. The patient has light colored urine, cold limbs, a submerged-slow-small pulse, pallor, and low vitality. Formulas containing dry ginger (*kan-chiang*) and aconite (*fu-tzu*) are used.

Yin thrives and dispels yang
yin sheng ke yang 陰盛格陽
Occurs when yang *chi* has been eliminated by excessive yin chills within the body causing the symptoms of "real chill inside and pseudo-fever outside."

Yin weakened fire moving
yin hsu huo tung 陰虛火動
Water belongs to yin and is governed by the kidneys. Fire belongs to yang and is governed by the heart. Water and fire are mutually destructive to each other. Therefore, if one engages in excessive sexual activity, the water of the kidneys will decrease and the fire of the heart will increase and result in umbilical palpitation. *Ti-huang-chi* (Rehmannia-containing formulas) and *Tzu-yin-chiang-huo-tang* (Phellodendron Combination) are the common prescriptions.

Yin weakness
yin hsu 陰虛
Impotence.

Yin yang 陰陽
The meaning of yin and yang is complicated and varies with time and place. The confusion concerning yin and yang becomes a great obstacle in the study of Chinese medicine. A comprehensive medical classification of yin yang is shown below:

Yin	Yang
The organs	The body surface
Ventral side	Dorsal side
The five viscera (heart, lungs, liver, kidneys, and spleen). Of these five viscera, the heart and lungs belong more to yang and the kidneys more to yin.	The six "bowels" (gall bladder, stomach, large intestine, small intestine, three warmers, and bladder).
	Upper half of the body
Lower half of the body	*Chi*
	Mental matters
	Fire
Blood	Fever
Physical matters	Sporadic diseases
	Floating pulse
	Fast pulse
	Rapid metabolism

One point of clarification that needs to be made is that there is no pure yin or pure yang because they are interrelated and intermixed. So, although yang represents the male element and yin represents the female element, there is female (hormone) in the male body and male (hormone) in the female body. Therefore, the determination of yin or yang is based mainly on how many of the natural characteristics of one or the other predominate. The ancient Chinese theory about yin yang is described in the *Annals of Lu Pu-Wei*: "The union of yin and yang creates life; lack of coordination between yin and yang leads to illness; and the separation of yin and yang results in death." The philosophical view of the world in the *I Ching* (The Classic of Changes) was based on yin yang, and Chinese medical theories were based on the *I Ching*. In addition to yin yang, however, the concept of weak and strong is also very important to disease diagnosis. However, because of the proliferation of schools of Chinese medicine, every explanation of weak and strong conformation differs from one another.

Yin yang yi 陰陽易
1. Sickness in healthy people after having sexual intercourse with a person who has just recovered from illness. (Sickness belongs to yin; health belongs to yang.)
2. Sexual intercourse, (the female and male exchange yin and yang; the female represents the source of yin, and male the source of yang).

GLOSSARY OF CHINESE HERBAL FORMULAS

Ah-chiao-fu-tzu-tang 阿膠附子湯
(Gelatin and Aconite Combination)

gelatin	5.0	licorice	2.5	aconite	0.5-1

Chai-hu-chih-chieh-tang 柴胡枳桔湯
(Bupleurum, *Chih-shih,* and Platycodon Combination)

bupleurum	5.0	pinellia	5.0	ginger	3.0
Scute	3.0	trichosanthes seed	3.0	platycodon	3.0
licorice	1.0	*chih-shih*	1.5		

Chai-hu-chiung-kuei-tang 柴胡芎歸湯
(Bupleurum, Cnidium, and *Tang-kuei* Combination)

tang-kuei	4.0	saussurea	3.0	paeonia	4.0
cardamon	3.0	cnidium	4.0	gentiana	1.0
bupleurum	4.0	*chih-ko*	1.0	cyperus	3.0
licorice	1.0	citrus	3.0	ginger	1.0

Chai-hu-chu-pan-hsia-chia-kua-lu-tang 柴胡去半夏加瓜呂湯
(Bupleurum and Trichosanthes Root Combination)

bupleurum	6.0	trichosanthes root	5.0	ginseng	3.0
scute	3.0	licorice	3.0	jujube	3.0
ginger	3.0				

Chai-hu-hou-pu-tang 柴胡厚朴湯
(Bupleurum and Magnolia Combination)

bupleurum	5.0	hoelen	5.0	magnolia bark	3.0
citrus	3.0	areca seed	3.0	perilla	1.5

Chai-hu-pieh-chia-tang 柴胡鱉甲湯
(Bupleurum and Tortoise Shell Combination)

bupleurum	5.0	atractylodes	4.0	paeonia	3.0
areca seed	3.0	tortoise shell	2.0	chih-shih	2.0
licorice	1.5				

Chai-hu-shu-kan-san 柴胡疏肝散
(Bupleurum and Gardenia Formula)

bupleurum	4.0	paeonia	4.0	chih-shih	3.0
licorice	2.0	cyperus	3.0	cnidium	3.0
blue citrus peel	2.0	gardenia	3.0	ginger	1.0

Chai-hu-shu-kan-tang 柴胡疏肝湯
(Bupleurum and Cyperus Combination)

bupleurum	4.0	paeonia	4.0	chih-shih	3.0
licorice	2.0	cyperus	3.0	cnidium	3.0
blue citrus peel	2.0				

Chai-keng-pan-hsia-tang 柴梗半夏湯
(Bupleurum, Platycodon, and Pinellia Combination)

bupleurum	4.0	jujube	2.5	pinellia	4.0
ginger	2.5	platycodon	2.0	chih-shih	1.5
apricot seed	2.0	blue citrus peel	1.5	trichosanthes seed	2.0
licorice	1.0	scute	2.5		

Chang-pin-tang 常檳湯
(Dichroa and Areca Seed Combination)

| dichroa | 12.0 | areca seed | 6.0 | licorice | 3.0 |

Chang-shan-tang 常山湯
(Dichroa Combination)

| dichroa | 3.0 | anemarrhena | 3.0 | areca seed | 3.0 |

Put above herbs into 200 ml. of water. Decoct it until the content remains 100 ml. Then put it outdoor in the evening in order to get the dew. Take of potion in next morning.

Chang-yung-tang 腸癰湯
(Coix and Persica Combination)

| coix | 9.0 | benincasa | 6.0 | persica | 5.0 |
| moutan | 4.0 | | | | |

Che-ku-tsai-tang 鷓鴣菜湯
(Digenea and Rhubarb Combination)

| digenea | 3.0 | rhubarb | 1.5 | licorice | 1.5 |

Same as *San-wei-che-ku-tsai-tang* (Digenea and Rhubarb Combination).

Chen-hsiang-chiang-chi-tang 沈香降氣湯
(Aquilaria and Cyperus Combination)

| aquilaria | 2.0 | cardamon | 3.0 | cyperus | 5.0 |
| licorice | 1.5 | | | | |

Chen-jen-yang-tsang-tang 眞人養臟湯
(Paeonia and Papaver Combination)

paeonia	4.0	tang-kuei	2.0	ginseng	2.0
atractylodes	2.0	myristica	2.0	licorice	1.0
cinnamon	1.0	saussurea	4.0	terminalia	4.0
papaver	8.0				

Chen-sha-tang 鍼砂湯
(Iron Powder Combination)

oyster shell	4.0	atractylodes	4.0	hoelen	6.0
cinnamon	4.0	ginseng	2.0	iron powder	1.5
licorice	1.5				

Chen-wu-tang-ho-sheng-mo-san 眞武湯合生脈散
(Vitality Combination with Ginseng, Schizandra, and Ophiopogon Combination)

This is a combination of *Chen-wu-tang* (Vitality Combination) with 8.0 g of ophiopogon, 2.0 g of schizandra, and 3.0 g of ginseng.

Cheng-hsin-tang 正心湯
(Antelope Horn and Zizyphus Combination)

tang-kuei	4.0	hoelen	4.0	rehmannia	4.0
antelope horn	3.0	zizyphus	3.0	ginseng	2.0
platycodon	2.0	licorice	1.0		

Cheng-yen-i-fang 蒸眼一方
(Alum and Licorice Formula)

alum	2.0	licorice	2.0	coptis	2.0
phellodendron	2.0	carthamus	2.0		

Put the above herbs into 300 ml of water. Boil it until the content remains 200 ml. Use it to wash eyes frequently.

Chi-fei-wan 起廢丸
(Lacca and Persica Formula)

lacca	1.0	persica	1.0	rhubarb	2.0

Po-chou-san (Eriocheir and Viper Formula) 1.0

Chi-hsien-san 七賢散
(Hoelen and Rehmannia Formula)

hoelen	6	rehmannia	5	dioscorea	3
moutan	3	cornus	2	ginseng	2
astragalus	2				

Chi-kan-wan 鷄肝丸
(Chicken Liver Formula)

To dry and grind a chicken liver into powder. Then put it with dioscorea into pill. Take 3 pills for each time, and three times a day.

Chi-ming-san-chia-fu-ling 鶏鳴散加茯苓
(Areca Seed and Chaenomeles Formula with Hoelen)

areca seed	4.0	chaenomeles	3.0	ginger	3.0
aurantium	2.5	platycodon	2.5	perilla leaves	1.0
evodia	1.0	hoelen	6.0		

Chi-wei-che-ku-tsai-tang 七味鷓鴣菜湯
(Cinnamon and Digenea Combination)

coptis	1.5	rhubarb	1.5	licorice	1.5
ginger	1.5	cinnamon	4	pinellia	6
digenea	3				

Chi-wei-ching-pi-tang 七味清脾湯
(Pinellia and Mume Combination)

magnolia	3	blue citrus peel	3	pinellia	5
galanga	1	mume	2.5	tsao-ko	2.5
licorice	2	jujube	2	ginger	2

Chi-wei-pai-chu-san 七味白朮散
(Ginseng, Pueraria, and Atractylodes Formula)

hoelen	3	ginseng	3	pueraria	3
atractylodes	3	licorice	1.5	agastache	1.5
saussurea	1.5	chih-ko	1	schizandra	1
bupleurum	3				

Chia-chien-hsiao-chai-hu-tang 加減小柴胡湯
(Minor Bupleurum Combination Modified)

bupleurum	2.0	scute	2.0	gardenia	2.0
kaki	2.0	cardamon	2.0	pinellia	2.0
citrus	2.0	agastache	2.5	fennel	1.0
saussurea	1.0	aquilaria	1.0	licorice	1.0
mume	2.5	ginger	2.5		

Chia-chien-hsieh-pai-san 加減瀉白散
(Morus and Lycium Formula Modified)

morus	3.0	lycium bark	1.0	anemarrhena	1.0
citrus	1.0	platycodon	1.0	blue citrus peel	2.0
asarum	2.0	scute	2.0	licorice	2.0

Chia-chien-liang-ke-san 加減涼膈散
(Forsythia and Paeonia Formula)

forsythia	3.0	scute	3.0	gardenia	3.0
platycodon	3.0	coptis	1.0	mentha	1.0
tang-kuei	3.5	paeonia	3.5	rehmannia	3.5
chih-shih	1.0	licorice	1.0		

Chia-tzu-tang 甲字湯
(Ginger, Cinnamon, and Hoelen Combination)

cinnamon	4.0	hoelen	4.0	moutan	4.0
persica	4.0	paeonia	4.0	licorice	1.5
ginger	3.0				

Chia-wei-cheng-chi-tang 加味承氣湯
(Rhubarb and Mirabilitum Combination)

rhubarb	3.0	mirabilitum	5.0	*chih-shih*	3.0
magnolia bark	3.0	*tang-kuei*	3.0	carthamus	2.0
licorice	2.0				

Chia-wei-chieh-tu-tang 加味解毒湯
(Coptis and Talc Combination)

coptis	2.0	scute	2.0	phellodendron	2.0
gardenia	2.0	bupleurum	2.0	capillaris	2.0
gentiana	2.0	akebia	2.0	talc	3.0
cimicifuga	1.5	licorice	1.5	juncus	1.5
rhubarb	1.5				

Chia-wei-hsi-chiao-ti-huang-tang 加味犀角地黃湯
(Rhinoceros and Rehmannia Combination Modified)

rhinoceros	3.0	rehmannia	4.0	paeonia	4.0
moutan	3.0	*tang-kuei*	3.0	coptis	2.0
scute	2.0				

Chia-wei-hsiao-hsien-hsiung-tang 加味小陷胸湯
(Pinellia and Trichosanthes Combination)

pinellia	6.0	trichosanthes seed	3.0	*chih-shih*	2.0
gardenia	2.0	coptis	1.5		

Chia-wei-szu-wu-tang 加味四物湯（回春）
(Platycodon and *Tang-kuei* Four Combination)

tang-keui	2.0	phellodendron	2.0	anemarrhena	2.0
cnidium	2.0	trichosanthes root	2.0	platycodon	4.0
licorice	4.0	rehmannia	3.0	paeonia	3.0

Chia-wei-wen-tan-tang 加味温胆湯
(Bamboo and Citrus Combination Modified)

pinellia	6.0	hoelen	6.0	ginger	3.0
citrus	2.5	bamboo	2.0	*chih-shih*	1.5
licorice	1.0	zizyphus	2.0-5.0	coptis	1.5

Chiang-fan-wan 絳礬丸
(Melanterite and Citrus Formula)

melanterite	10.0	magnolia bark	5.0	citrus	5.0
scirpus	5.0	zedoaria	5.0	coptis	5.0
sophora	5.0	licorice	2.0	cyperus	1.5

Grind above herbs into powder. Make them to pills with vinegar. Take 1 pill each time and two or three times a day.

Chiang-huo-yu-feng-tang 羌活愈風湯
(Ginger and *Chianghuo* Combination)

atractylodes	2.0	cnidium	1.2	chrysanthemum	1.2
eucommia	1.2	gypsurm	2.0	asarum	1.2
mentha	1.2	*chin-chiu*	1.2	rehmannia	2.0
astragalus	1.2	lycium fruit	1.2	scute	1.2
chianghuo	1.2	*chih-ko*	1.2	bupleurum	1.2
paeonia	1.2	siler	1.2	ginseng	1.2
anemarrhena	1.2	licorice	1.2	*tang-kuei*	1.2
ma-huang	1.2	lycium bark	1.2	cinnamon	1.2
vitex	1.2	angelica	1.2	*tuhuo*	1.2
ginger	3.0				

Chiang-shen-tang 強神湯
(Carthamus and Silkworm Combination)

carthamus	1.5	silkworm	3.0	trachycarpus	2.0
licorice	1.0				

Chia-wei-hsiao-ke-tang 加味消渴湯
(Atractylodes and Licorice Combination)

hoelen	3.0	white atractylodes	3.0	alisma	3.0
rehmannia	3.0	paeonia	3.0	atractylodes	3.0
citrus	3.0	licorice	0.5		

Chia-wei-liang-ke-san 加味涼膈散
(Forsythia and Gypsum Formula)

scute	3.0	platycodon	3.0	gypsum	10.0
mentha	2.0	forsythia	3.0	gardenia	3.0
rhubarb	1.0	licorice	1.0		

Chia-wei-ning-hsien-tang 加味寧癇湯
(Aquilaria and Hoelen Combination)

aquilaria	2.0	cardamon	2.0	evodia	2.0
cyperus	3.0	aurantium	3.0	licorice	1.5
coptis	1.0	hoelen	4.0		

Chia-wei-pa-mo-san 加味八脈散
(Hoelen, Polyporus, and Alisma Formula)

polyporus	3.0	alisma	3.0	hoelen	3.0
akebia	3.0	rehmannia	3.0	apricot seed	3.0
kao-pen	2.0	gardenia	2.0	anemarrhena	2.0
phellodendron	2.0				

Chia-wei-ping-wei-san 加味平胃散
(Magnolia and Ginger Formula Modified)

atractylodes	4.0	magnolia bark	3.0	citrus	3.0
jujube	2.0	licorice	1.0	ginger	1.0
malt	2.0	shen-chu	2.0		

Chia-wei-szu-wu-tang 加味四物湯（正傳）
(Paeonia and *Tang-kuei* Four Combination)

tang-kuei	3.0	cnidium	3.0	paeonia	3.0
rehmannia	3.0	atractylodes	3.0	ophiopogon	5.0
ginseng	2.0	achyranthes	2.0	phellodendron	1.5
schizonepeta	1.5	coptis	1.5	anemarrhena	1.5
eucommia	1.5				

Chiao-mei-hsieh-hsin-tang 椒梅瀉心湯
(Pinellia, Mume, and Zanthoxylum Combination)

Pan-hsia-hsieh-hsin-tang (Pinellia Combination) with 2.0 grams each of mume and zanthoxylum.

Chiao-mei-tang 椒 梅 湯
(Mume and Zanthoxylum Combination)

mume	2.0	zanthoxylum	2.0	areca seed	2.0
chih-shih	2.0	saussurea	2.0	cardamon	2.0
cyperus	2.0	cinnamon	2.0	melia	2.0
magnolia bark	2.0	licorice	2.0	ginger	2.0

Chieh-hsien-yu-yao-fang 疥癬浴藥方
(Paeonia and Lonicera Formula)

rhubarb	38	smilax	19.0	*tang-kuei*	38
cinnamon	15.0	*tuhuo*	19	lonicera	90.0
bupleurum	19	atractylodes	19	perilla	57.0
magnolia bark	19	paeonia	150.0		

Chieh-keng-chieh-tu-tang 桔梗解毒湯
(Platycodon and Smilax Combination)

smilax	3.0	platycodon	3.0	cnidium	3.0
paeonia	3.0	rhubarb	1.0	astragalus	2.0
licorice	1.5				

Chieh-keng-tang (for lung gangrene) 桔 梗 湯
(Platycodon Combination)

platycodon	3.0	rehmannia	4.0	*tang-kuei*	4.0
saussurea	1.0	licorice	2.0	thlaspi	2.0
morus	2.0	coix	8.0		

Chieh-lao-san 解 勞 散
(Tortoise Shell, Bupleurum, and *Chih-shih* Formula)

Szu-ni-san (Bupleurum and *Chih-shih* Formula) with 3.0 g each of tortoise shell and hoelen, and 2.0 g each of jujube and ginger.

Chien-chin-chi-ming-san 千金雞鳴散
(*Tang-kuei*, Persica, and Rhubarb Formula)

tang-kuei	5.0	persica	5.0	rhubarb	2.0

Chien-chin-kua-lu-tang (Kua-lu-tang) 千金瓜呂湯（與瓜呂湯同）
(Trichosanthes Seed Combination)

| Trichosanthes seed | 2 | pinellia | 6 | bakeri | 4 |
| chih-shih | 2 | ginger | 2 | | |

Chien-chin-pan-hsia-tang 千金半夏湯
(Pinellia, Ginger, and Evodia Combination)

| pinellia | 5.0 | ginger | 3.0 | aconite | 0.6 |
| evodia | 2.0 | | | | |

Chih-chuan-i-fang 治喘一方
(Hoelen, Magnolia, and Apricot Formula)

| hoelen | 6.0 | magnolia bark | 3.0 | cinnamon | 3.0 |
| apricot seed | 4.0 | perilla fruit | 2.0 | licorice | 2.0 |

Chih-hsiao-erh-ai-chih-ni-fang 治小兒愛吃泥方
(Gypsum, Citrus, and Quisqualis Formula)

scute	2.0	citrus	2.0	atractylodes	2.0
hoelen	2.0	quisqualis	2.0	licorice	2.0
picrorrhia	1.0	gypsum	5.0		

Chih-hsiao-tou-tang 赤小豆湯（東洋）
(Phaseolus and Phytolacca Combination)

phaseolus	6.0	phytolacca	4.0	*ma-huang*	4.0
cinnamon	4.0	forsythia	4.0	viper	1.5
rhubarb	1.5	ginger	3.0		

Chih-hsiao-tou-tang 赤小豆湯（濟生）
(Phaseolus and Alisma Combination)

phaseolus	4.0	*tang-kuei*	4.0	phytolacca	4.0
alisma	2.0	forsythia	2.0	paeonia	2.0
stephania	2.0	polyporus	2.0	helioscopia	2.0
morus	1.5				

Chih-lei-pu-kan-tang 止淚補肝湯
(Equisetum and Tribulus Combination)

| *tang-kuei* | 3.0 | paeonia | 3.0 | cnidium | 3.0 |

rehmannia	3.0	equisetum	2.0	tribulus	2.0
prunella	2.0				

Chih-mu-fu-ling-tang 知母茯苓湯
(Anemarrhena and Hoelen Combination)

bupleurum	3.0	gelatin	2.0	anemarrhena	2.0
atractylodes	2.0	hoelen	2.0	ginseng	2.0
schizandra	2.0	platycodon	2.0	scute	2.0
pinellia	2.0	cnidium	1.0	mentha	1.0
tussilago	1.0	ophiopogon	1.0	ginger	1.0

Chih-pang-wan 治胖丸
(Atractylodes and Citrus Formula)

atractylodes	3.0	magnolia bark	3.0	citrus	3.0
licorice	2.0	melanterite	1.0	jujube	1.0

Chih-shih-chih-tzu-shih-tang 枳實梔子豉湯
(*Chih-shih*, Gardenia, and Soja Combination)

chih-shih	2.0	gardenia	2.0	soja	2.0

Chih-ta-pu-i-fang 治打撲一方
(Cinnamon and Nuphar Formula)

nuphar	3.0	quercus	3.0	cnidium	3.0
cinnamon	3.0	rhubarb	1.0	clove	1.0
licorice	1.5				

Chih-tzu-hou-pu-tang 梔子厚朴湯
(Gardenia and Magnolia Combination)

gardenia	3.0	magnolia bark	4.0	*chih-shih*	2.0

Chih-tzu-kan-chiang-tang 梔子乾薑湯
(Gardenia and Ginger Combination)

gardenia	2.0	ginger	2.0

Chih-tzu-kan-lien-tang 梔子甘連湯
(Gardenia, Licorice, and Coptis Combination)

gardenia	3.0	licorice	4.0	coptis	1.0

Chin-chiu-chiang-huo-tang 秦艽羌活湯
(*Chin-chiu* and *Chiang-huo* Combination)

chiang-huo	5.0	chin-chiu	3.0	astragalus	3.0
siler	2.0	cimicifuga	1.5	licorice	1.5
ma-huang	1.5	bupleurum	1.5	hao-pen	0.5
asarum	0.5	carthamus	0.5		

Chin-chiu-fang-feng-tang 秦艽防風湯
(*Chin-chiu* and Siler Combination)

chin-chiu	2.0	alisma	2.0	citrus	2.0
bupleurum	2.0	siler	2.0	tang-kuei	3.0
atractylodes	3.0	licorice	1.0	phellodendron	1.0
cimicifuga	1.0	rhubarb	1.0	persica	3.0
carthamus	1.0				

Chin-suo-shih 金鎖匙
(Borax and Realgar Formula)

saltpeter	1.5	borax	5.0	borneol	1.0
indigo	1.0	silk worm	1.0	cinnabar	1.0
realgar	3.0	phellodendron	3.0		

Ching-chi-an-huei-tang 清肌安蚘湯
(Bupleurum and Digenea Combination)

This is a combination of *Hsiao-chai-hu-tang* (Minor Bupleurum Combination) without jujube, then add 3.0 grams each of digenea and ophiopogon into it.

Ching-chieh-lien-chiao-tang 荊芥連翹湯 (一貫堂)
(Schizonepeta and Forsythia Combination)

tang-kuei	1.5	paeonia	1.5	cnidium	1.5
rehmannia	1.5	coptis	1.5	scute	1.5
phellodendron	1.5	gardenia	1.5	forsythia	1.5
siler	1.5	mentha	1.5	schizonepeta	1.5
licorice	1.5	chih-ko	1.5	bupleurum	2.0
angelica	2.0	platycodon	2.0		

Ching-chung-an-huei-tang 清中安蛔湯
(Coptis and Mume Combination)

coptis	2.0	phellodendron	2.0	*chih-shih*	2.0
mume	3.0	zanthoxylum	2.0		

Ching-fei-tang (for hemorrhoid bleeding) 清肺湯
(Rehmannia and Sanguisorba Combination)

rehmannia	3.0	*tang-kuei*	3.0	sanguisorba	2.0
cnidium	2.0	scute	2.0	gardenia	2.0
phellodendron	2.0	paeonia	1.5	coptis	1.5
biota leaves	1.5	sophora flower	1.5	gelatin	1.5

Ching-je-chieh-yu-tang 清熱解鬱湯
(Cyperus and Ginger Combination)

gardenia	3.0	atractylodes	3.0	cnidium	2.0
cyperus	2.0	citrus	2.0	coptis	1.0
licorice	1.0	*chih-ko*	1.0	dried ginger	0.5
ginger	0.5				

Ching-liang-yin 清涼飲
(Gardenia and Mentha Combination)

gardenia	2.5	*chih-ko*	2.5	forsythia	2.5
siler	2.5	scute	2.0	*tang-kuei*	2.0
ginger	2.0	platycodon	2.0	coptis	1.0
licorice	1.0	mentha	1.0		

Ching-shang-yin 清上飲
(Bupleurum and Gardenia Combination)

bupleurum	3.0	pinellia	3.0	scute	2.0
paeonia	2.0	gardenia	2.0	curcuma	2.0
blue citrus peel	2.0	rhubarb	2.0	mirabilitum	2.0
magnolia bark	1.5	*chih-shih*	1.5	ginger	1.5
coptis	1.0	licorice	1.0		

Ching-shih-tang 清濕湯
(*Tuhuo* and Stephania Combination)

tuhuo	2.0	siler	3.0	alisma	3.0
stephania	3.0	paeonia	3.0	scute	3.0
coix	9.0	phellodendron	1.5	licorice	1.5

Ching-wei-hsieh-huo-tang 清胃瀉火湯
(Scute and Mentha Combination)

forsythia	2.0	platycodon	2.0	scute	2.0
gardenia	2.0	rehmannia	2.0	pueraria	2.0
coptis	1.0	scrophularia	1.0	cimicifuga	1.0
mentha	1.0	licorice	1.0		

Chiu-ni-tang 救逆湯
(Cinnamon, Dichroa, Oyster Shell, and Dragon-bone Combination)

Same as *Kuei-chih-chu-shao-yao-chia-shu-chi-lung-ku-mu-li-tang* (Cinnamon, Dichroa, Oyster Shell, and Dragon-bone Combination).

Chiu-wei-ching-pi-tang 九味清脾湯
(Hoelen and Citrus Combination)

blue citrus peel	2.0	magnolia bark	2.0	bupleurum	3.0
scute	3.0	pinellia	3.0	atractylodes	3.0
hoelen	4.0	licorice	1.0	jujube	1.5
ginger	1.5	*tsao-ko*	1.5		

Chiu-wei-pan-hsia-tang 九味半夏湯
(Pinellia, Aurantium, and Polyporus Combination)

pinellia	3	aurantium	3	licorice	3
bupleurum	3	polyporus	3	ginger	2
cimicifuga	2	alisma	4	hoelen	4

Chiung-huang-san 芎黃散
(Cnidium and Rhubarb Formula)

rhubarb	1.0	cnidium	2.0

Chiung-kuei-tang 芎歸湯
(Cnidium and *Tang-kuei* Combination)

cnidium	4.5	*tang-kuei*	6.0

Chu-feng-chieh-tu-san 驅風解毒散
(Siler and Forsythia Formula)

siler	3.0	arctium	3.0	schizonepeta	1.5
chiang-huo	1.5	licorice	1.5	forsythia	5.0
platycodon	3.0	gypsum	5.0		

Chu-feng-chu-tung-tang 驅風觸痛湯
(Ophiopogon and Asarum Combination)

ophiopogon	5.0	scute	4.0	chiang-huo	3.0
tu-huo	3.0	siler	3.0	atractylodes	3.0
tang-kuei	3.0	cnidium	3.0	angelica	3.0
vitex	2.0	hao-pen	1.5	asarum	1.0
licorice	1.0				

Chu-feng-pai-tu-san 祛風敗毒散
(*Chih-shih* and *Tu-huo* Formula)

chih-shih	2.0	paeonia	2.0	peucedanum	2.0
bupleurum	2.0	schizonepeta	2.0	mentha	2.0
arctium	2.0	atractylodes	2.0	tu-huo	2.5
silkworm	2.5	forsythia	2.5	cnidium	2.5
chiang-huo	2.5	cicada	1.0	licorice	1.0

Chu-lan-shui 除爛燧
(*Tang-kuei*, Coptis, and Schizonepeta Combination)

tang-kuei	5.0	schizonepeta	1.0	phellodendron	1.5
coptis	1.2	mentha	0.4	carthamus	0.6
chrysanthemum	0.6	alum	0.2		

Chu-ling-tang-ho-szu-wu-tang 猪苓湯合四物湯

This is a combination of *Chu-ling-tang* (Polyporus Combination) with *Szu-wu-tang* (*Tang-kuei* Four Combination).

Chu-pi-pan-hsia-tang 橘皮半夏湯
(Aurantium and Pinellia Combination)

aurantium	3.0	bupleurum	3.0	apricot seed	3.0
platycodon	3.0	cyperus	3.0	pinellia	4.0
hoelen	4.0	morus	1.5	perilla	1.5
dried ginger	0.5				

Chu-pi-ta-huang-pu-hsiao-tang 橘皮大黃朴硝湯
(Aurantium, Rhubarb, and Mirabilitum Combination)

aurantium	2.0	rhubarb	2.0	mirabilitum	3.0

Chu-pi-ta-wan
(Gypsum and Bamboo Formula)   竹皮大丸

bamboo	3.0	gypsum	10.0	cinnamon	4.0
licorice	3.0	*pai-wei*	3.0	jujube	5.0

Chu-pi-tang
(Aurantium Combination)   橘皮湯

aurantium	3.0	ginger	6.0

Chu-shih-pu-chi-tang
(Bupleurum, Citrus, and Anemarrhena Combination)   除濕補氣湯

citrus	3.0	bupleurum	3.0	anemarrhena	3.0
astragalus	1.5	phellodendron	1.5	atractylodes	5.0
tang-kuei	5.0	schizandra	1.0	licorice	1.0
hao-pen	2.0	cimicifuga	2.0		

Chu-yang-ho-hsueh-tang
(*Tang-kuei*, Siler, and Astragalus Combination)   助陽和血湯

astragalus	3.0	*tang-kuei*	3.0	siler	3.0
bupleurum	3.0	licorice	2.0	angelica	1.0
vitex	1.0	cimicifuga	1.0		

Chuan-li-chung-tang
(Cinnamon and Cardamon Combination)   喘理中湯

perilla fruit	3.0	cardamon	3.0	magnolia bark	3.0
cinnamon	3.0	aquilaria	1.5	saussurea	1.5
aurantium	1.5	licorice	1.5	ginger	1.5

Chang-yuan-tang
(Ginseng and Psoralea Combination)   壯原湯

ginseng	4.0	aconite	0.5-1	atractylodes	4.0
ginger	2.0	hoelen	4.0	cardamon	2.0
psoralea	3.0	citrus	2.0	cinnamon	3.0

Chui-feng-wan
(*Ho-shou-wu* and Schizonepeta Formula)   追風丸

ho-shou-wu	4.0	schizonepeta	4.0	sophora	4.0
atractylodes	4.0	gleditsia	4.0		

Chung-cheng-tang　　　　　　　　　　　　　　中正湯
(Pinellia and Agastache Combination)

pinellia	5.0	atractylodes	4.0	agastache	3.0
aurantium	3.0	dried ginger	3.0	magnolia bark	3.0
rhubarb	3.0	coptis	2.0	saussurea	1.0
licorice	1.0				

Chung-huang-kao　　　　　　　　　　　　　　中黃膏
(Phellodendron and Curcuma Ointment)

sesame oil　100 ml　　flava wax　　　380　curcuma　　　40
phellodendron　20

Erh-hsien-tang　　　　　　　　　　　　　　二仙湯
(Paeonia and Scute Combination)

Scute　　　　3.0　　　　　　Paeonia　　　　3.0

Fa-sheng-san　　　　　　　　　　　　　　髮生散
(Adiantum and Viper Formula)

adiantum　　4.0　viper　　　1.0　bat　　　　1.0

　　Make above herbs into frost. Add sesame oil into it and stir up to a muddy form. Spred it over the infection part.

Fan-pi-chiao-kan-tan　　　　　　　　　　　　反鼻交感丹料
(Hoelen and Viper Formula)

| hoelen | 5.0 | cyperus | 3.0 | viper | 2.0 |
| ginger | 1.5 | | | | |

Fei-kan-fang　　　　　　　　　　　　　　肺疳方
(Akebia and Pinellia Formula)

akebia	3.0	areca seed	3.0	stephania	3.0
polyporus	3.0	alisma	3.0	pinellia	5.0
platycodon	2.0	saussurea	1.0	clove	1.0

Feng-yin-tang　　　　　　　　　　　　　　風引湯
(Rhubarb and Dragon-Bone Combination)

| rhubarb | 1.2 | ginger | 1.2 | dragon bone | 1.2 |
| cinnamon | 0.9 | licorice | 0.6 | oyster shell | 0.6 |

calcite	1.8	kaolin	1.8	white kaolin	1.8
fluorite	1.8	gypsum	1.8	talc	1.8

Fei-yung-tang 肺癰湯
(Platycodon and Scute Combination)

platycodon	3.0	scute	3.0	apricot seed	4.0
fritillaria	4.0	trichosanthes root	2.0	brassica	2.0
licorice	2.0				

Fu-ling-pu-hsin-tang 茯苓補心湯
(Hoelen Heart Tonic Combination)

tang-kuei	1.5	cnidium	1.5	paeonia	1.5
rehmannia	1.5	*chih-shih*	1.5	pinellia	1.5
hoelen	1.5	platycodon	1.5	perilla leaves	1.5
bupleurum	2.0	citrus	2.0	pueraria	2.0
ginseng	2.0	saussurea	1.0	licorice	1.0
ginger	1.0				

Fu-ling-yin-ho-pan-hsia-hou-pu-tang 茯苓飲合半夏厚朴湯

This is a combination of *Fu-ling-yin* (Hoelen Combination) with *Pan-hsia-hou-pu-tang* (Pinellia and Magnolia Combination).

Fu-pi-sheng-mo-san-chia-pai-chi 扶脾生脈散加白及
(Ginseng and Bletilla Formula)

ginseng	2.0	aster	2.0	atractylodes	2.0
schizandra	1.5	licorice	1.5	*tang-kuei*	4.0
bletilla	4.0	ophiopogon	6.0	paeonia	3.0

Ho-kou-san 和口散
(Bulrush and Cinnabar Formula)

bulrush	2.0	cinnabar	5.0

Ho-li-leh-wan 訶梨勒丸
(Terminalia Formula)

terminalia	3.0	citrus	3.0	magnolia bark	3.0

Grind above herbs into powder and make it with mel to pill. Take 3 pills each time.

Hou-pu-ma-huang-tang 厚朴麻黃湯
(Magnolia and *Ma-huang* Combination)

magnolia bark	4.0	schizandra	3.0	*ma-huang*	3.0
gypsum	10.0	apricot seed	4.0	pinellia	4.0
ginger	1.5	asarum	1.5	wheat	10.0

Hou-shih-hei-san 侯氏黑散
(Chrysanthemum and Siler Formula)

chrysanthemum	12.0	alum	0.9	siler	3.0
atractylodes	3.0	*tang-kuei*	0.9	asarum	0.9
ginger	0.9	hoelen	0.9	cnidium	0.9
oyster shell	0.9	cinnamon	0.9	ginseng	0.9
platycodon	2.4				

Hsi-kan-ming-mu-san 洗肝明目散
(Nandina and Gardenia Formula)

nandina	1.5	forsythia	1.0	gypsum	1.0
equisetum	1.5	*tang-kuei*	1.0	bupleurum	1.0
hoelen	1.0	cnidium	1.0	rhubarb	0.5
scute	1.0	gardenia	1.0	licorice	0.5
coptis	1.0	platycodon	1.0		

Hsi-kan-ming-mu-tang 洗肝明目湯
(Gardenia and Vitex Combination)

tang-kuei	1.5	forsythia	1.5	*chiang-huo*	1.0
cnidium	1.5	siler	1.5	vitex	1.0
paeonia	1.5	cassia seed	1.5	chrysanthemum	1.0
rehmannia	1.5	coptis	1.0	platycodon	1.0
scute	1.5	schizonepeta	1.0	tribulus	1.0
gardenia	1.5	mentha	1.0	licorice	1.0
gypsum	3.0				

Hsia-ku-tsao-tang 夏枯草湯
(Prunella Combination)

prunella	5.0	licorice	1.5

Hsia-pin-tang 夏檳湯
(Pinellia and Areca Combination)

pinellia	2.0	atractylodes	2.0	areca seed	1.2
citrus	1.2	chaenomeles	1.2		

Hsiang-chiung-tang 香芎湯
(Cyperus and Cnidium Combination)

gypsum	12.0	cinnamon	4.5	licorice	2.0
mentha	1.0	cyperus	5.0	cnidium	5.0

Hsiang-pu-tang 香朴湯
(Saussurea and Magnolia Combination)

magnolia bark	5.0	saussurea	1.0	aconite	0.5-1

Hsiang-sha-ping-wei-san 香砂平胃散
(Cyperus, Cardamon, and Atractylodes Formula)

atractylodes	4.0	magnolia bark	3.0	citrus	3.0
ginger	2.0	jujube	2.0	licorice	1.0
cyperus	4.0	agastache	1.0	cardamon	1.5

Hsiao-chai-hu-chia-chieh-keng-shih-kao-tang 小柴胡湯加桔梗、石膏
(Bupleurum, Platycodon, and Gypsum Combination)

bupleurum	7	pinellia	5	ginger	4
scute	3	jujube	3	ginseng	3
licorice	2	platycodon	3	gypsum	10

Hsiao-pai-chung-yin 小百中飲
(Ginseng and Smilax Combination)

smilax	1.5	ginseng	0.5	tang-kuei	0.5
cnidium	0.5	hoelen	0.5	coptis	0.5
achyranthes	0.3	licorice	0.3		

Hsiao-pin-pen-tun-tang 小品奔豚湯
(Licorice and Pueraria Combination)

baked licorice	3.0	cummunis	5.0	pueraria	5.0
scute	2.5	cinnamon	2.5	trichosanthes seed	2.5
ginseng	2.5	cnidium	2.5		

Hsiao-shih-ta-yuan 滑石大圓
(Saltpeter and Rhubarb Formula)

saltpeter	6.0	rhubarb	8.0	ginseng	2.0
licorice	2.0	*tang-kuei*	1.0		

Hsiao-tu-wan 滑毒丸
(Saltpeter and Forsythia Formula)

saltpeter	3.0	forsythia	3.0	akebia	3.0
scute	3.0	dianthus	3.0	rhubarb	1.0
licorice	1.0	cicada	1.0		

Hsieh-hsin-tao-chih-san 瀉心導赤散
(Ophiopogon and Hoelen Formula)

gardenia	2.0	scute	2.0	ophiopogon	4.0
coptis	1.5	anemarrhena	3.0	talc	3.0
ginseng	3.0	rhinoceros	3.0	hoelen	3.0
rehmannia	3.0	licorice	2.0		

Hsieh-pi-tang 瀉脾湯
(Hoelen and Pinellia Combination)

hoelen	5.0	pinellia	5.0	magnolia bark	2.5
cinnamon	3.0	ginger	3.0	ginseng	3.0
scute	3.0	licorice	2.0		

Hsieh-tao-jen-ta-huang-tang 謝導人大黃湯
(Paeonia and Rhubarb Combination)

rhubarb	1.5	licorice	1.5	asarum	1.5
scute	5.0	paeonia	4.0		

Hsieh-wei-tang 瀉胃湯
(Rhubarb and Pueraria Combination)

rhubarb	1.0	pueraria	6.0	*chih-shih*	2.0
platycodon	3.0	peucedanum	3.0	apricot seed	3.0
ginger	4.0				

Hsien-feng-kao 先鋒膏
(Resin and Flava Wax Ointment)

resin	200	flava wax	160	sesame oil	600 ml
spikemoss	30				

Hsien-hsiung-tang 陷胸湯
(Rhubarb and Trichosanthes Combination)

rhubarb	1.0	coptis	2.0	licorice	1.0
trichosanthes seed	3.0				

Hsin-i-ching-fei-tang 辛夷清肺湯
(Magnolia Flower and Gypsum Combination)

magnolia flower	2.0	anemarrhena	3.0	lily	3.0
scute	3.0	gardenia	3.0	ophiopogon	5.0
gypsum	5.0	cimicifuga	1.0	eriobotrya	2.0

Hsing-ho-shao-yao-san 行和芍藥散
(Paeonia, Tang-kuei, and Coptis Formula)

paeonia	6.0	tang-kuei	3.0	coptis	3.0
rhubarb	1.0	areca seed	1.0	saussurea	1.0
cinnamon	1.0	licorice	1.0	scute	3.0

Hsing-shih-pu-chi-yang-hsieh-tang 行濕補氣養血湯
(Ginseng and Lygodium Combination)

ginseng	2.5	atractylodes	2.5	hoelen	2.5
tang-kuei	2.0	paeonia	2.0	cinidium	2.0
akebia	1.5	magnolia bark	1.5	citrus	1.5
raphanus	1.5	lygodium	1.5	saussurea	1.0
licorice	1.0	areca	1.0	perilla	1.0

Hu-po-san 琥珀散
(Succinum and Lygodium Formula)

succinum	2.0	lygodium	2.0	talc	3.0

Grind above herbs into powder and mix. Each time take 2.0 grams and three times daily.

Hua-shih-yang-pi-tang 化食養脾湯
(Cardamon and Six Major Herb Combination)

ginseng	4.0	atractylodes	4.0	hoelen	4.0
pinellia	4.0	licorice	1.0	citrus	2.0
ginger	2.0	jujube	2.0	cardamon	1.5
shen-chu	2.0	malt	2.0	crataegus	2.0

Hua-tu-wan 化毒丸
(Mastic and Realgar Formula)

mastic	10	calomel	1.0	rhubarb	3.0
realgar	3.0	hair ash	3.0		

Huan-hsien-tang 緩痃湯
(Bupleurum, Scute, and Licorice Combination)

bupleurum	6.0	cinnamon	3.0	trichosanthes seed	3.0
scute	3.0	oyster shell	3.0	tortoise shell	3.0
paeonia	3.0	ginger	2.0	licorice	2.0

Huang-chieh-san 黃解散
(Coptis and Scute Formula)

coptis	3.0	scute	2.0	phellodendron	2.0
gardenia	1.0				

Grind above herbs into powder. Take 1.0 gram for each time. Three times a day.

Huang-chieh-wan 黃解丸
(Scute and Coptis Formula)

Make *Huang-lien-chieh-tu-tang* (Scute and Coptis Combination) into pill.

Huang-chin-chia-pan-hsia-sheng-chiang-tang 黃芩加半夏生薑湯
(Scute, Pinellia, and Ginger Combination)

Huang-chin-tang (Scute and Licorice Combination) with pinellia 5.0, ginger 3.0.

Huang-chi-tang 黃耆湯
(Astragalus and Ginger Combination)

astragalus	1.0	ginseng	1.5	rana	1.5
quisqualis	1.5	tortoise shell	2.0	citrus	2.0
cnidium	2.0	paeonia	2.0	ginger	2.0
bupleurum	2.5	*tang-kuei*	3.0	rehmannia	3.0
hoelen	3.0	pinellia	3.0		

Huang-lien-chu-pi-tang 黃連橘皮湯
(Coptis and Aurantium Combination)

coptis	1.5	aurantium	3.0	apricot seed	3.0
ma-huang	3.0	pueraria	5.0	*chih-shih*	2.0
magnolia bark	3.0	licorice	1.0		

Huang-lien-hsiao-tu-yin 黃連消毒飲
(Coptis and Stephania Combination)

coptis	1.5	*chianghuo*	1.5	scute	1.5
phellodendron	1.5	*hao-pen*	1.5	stephania	1.5
platycodon	1.5	*tang-kuei*	1.5	rehmannia	1.5
anemarrhena	1.5	*tu-huo*	1.5	siler	1.5
astragalus	1.5	forsythia	1.5	ginseng	1.0
licorice	1.0	citrus	1.0	sappan wood	1.0
alisma	1.0				

Hui-shou-san 回首散
(Lindera and Chaenomeles Formula)

lindera	2.5	citrus	2.5	silk worm	2.5
ginger	2.5	*ma-huang*	2.5	cnidium	2.5
platycodon	2.5	*chih-ko*	2.0	angelica	1.5
licorice	1.5	chaenomeles	3.0		

Huo-hsieh-san-yu-tang 活血散瘀湯
(Cnidium and Persica Combination)

cnidium	2.5	*tang-kuei*	2.5	paeonia	2.5
sappan wood	2.5	moutan	2.5	*chih-ko*	2.5
benincasa	2.5	persica	2.5	areca seed	2.5
rhubarb	2.5				

I-chi-yang-jung-tang 益氣養榮湯
(Ginseng, *Tang-kuei,* and Cyperus Combination)

astragalus	2.0	atractylodes	2.0	hoelen	2.0
ginseng	2.0	*tang-kuei*	2.0	cnidium	2.0
paeonia	2.0	rehmannia	2.0	citrus	2.0
fritillaria	2.0	cyperus	2.0	bupleurum	1.5
platycodon	1.0	licorice	1.0		

I-kan-fu-pi-san 抑肝扶脾散
(Bupleurum and Atractylodes Formula)

ginseng	2.0	atractylodes	2.0	hoelen	2.0
gentiana	1.0	brassica	2.0	crataegus	2.0
citrus	2.0	blue citrus peel	2.0	*shen-chu*	2.0
picrorrhiza	1.0	coptis	1.0	bupleurum	1.0
licorice	1.0				

I-yi-jen-san 薏苡仁散
(Coix Formula)

benincasa	6.0	moutan	4.0	persica	4.0
coix	8.0	paeonia	3.0		

Jen-sheng-hu-tao-tang 人參胡桃湯
(Ginseng and Walnut Combination)

ginseng	3.0	walnut	3.0

Jen-sheng-san (Sheng-hui-jen-sheng-san) 人參散（聖惠人參散同）
(Ginseng and Ophiopogon Formula)

ophiopogon	6.0	bupleurum	3.0	hoelen	3.0
paeonia	2.0	oyster shell	2.0	astragalus	2.0
ginseng	2.0	tortoise shell	2.0	licorice	1.5

Jen-sheng-shun-chi-san 人參順氣散
(Ginseng, Cnidium, and Platycodon Formula)

ginseng	2.0	cnidium	2.0	platycodon	2.0
atractylodes	2.0	angelica	2.0	citrus	2.0
chih-shih	2.0	*ma-huang*	2.0	lindera	2.0
silkworm	2.0	licorice	2.0		

Jen-sheng-yin-tzu 人參飲子
(Ginseng and Bamboo Leaves Combination)

bupleurum	7.0	scute	3.0	pinellia	5.0
ginseng	3.0	jujube	3.0	licorice	2.0
ginger	4.0	ophiopogon	5.0	bamboo leaves	3.0

Kan-chiang-fu-tzu-tang 乾薑附子湯
(Ginger and Aconite Combination)

ginger 1.0 aconite 0.5-1.0

Put these two herbs into 250 ml. of water. Boil it until the content remains 100 ml. and take of potion.

Kan-chiang-huang-chin-huang-lien-tang 乾薑黃芩黃連湯
(Ginger, Scute, and Coptis Combination)

ginger	3.0	coptis	3.0	scute	3.0
ginseng	3.0				

Kan-lien-chih-tzu-tang 甘連梔子湯
(Licorice, Coptis, and Gardenia Combination)

licorice 4.0 coptis 2.0 gardenia 2.0

Kan-tsao-ma-huang-tang 甘草麻黃湯
(Licorice and *Ma-huang* Combination)

licorice 1.0 *ma-huang* 3.0

Ku-sheng-tang 苦參湯
(Sophora Combination)

sophora 6.0

Kua-lu-chu-mai-wan 瓜呂瞿麥丸
(Trichosanthes and Dianthus Formula)

trichosanthes root	2.0	hoelen	3.0	dioscorea	3.0
aconite	0.5-1.0	dianthus	1.0		

Kua-lu-hsieh-pai-pai-chu-tang 瓜呂薤白白酒湯
(Trichosanthes, Bakeri, and Vinegar Combination)

  trichosanthes seed 2.0 bakeri 6.0 vinegar 400 ml. (Decoct trichosanthes seed 2.0 grams, and bakeri 6 grams with 400 ml. of vinegar until 150 ml remains. t.i.d.)

Kua-lu-hsieh-pai-pan-hsia-tang 瓜呂薤白半夏湯
(Pinellia, Bakeri, and Trichosanthes Combination)

| trichosanthes seed | 3.0 | bakeri | 4.5 | pinellia | 6.0 |

Decoct Trichosanthes seed 3.0 grams, bakeri 4.5 grams, Pinellia 6.0 grams with 40 ml. of vinegar, and 400 ml. H_2O until 200 ml. t.i.d.

Kua-lu-kuei-chih-tang 瓜呂桂枝湯
(Trichosanthes and Cinnamon Combination)

| cinnamon | 4.0 | paeonia | 4.0 | jujube | 4.0 |
| ginger | 4.0 | licorice | 2.0 | trichosanthes root | 3.0 |

Kua-lu-mu-li-san 瓜呂牡蠣散
(Trichosanthes and Oyster Shell Formula)

trichosanthes root   oyster shell

Kua-lu-tang 瓜 呂 湯
(Trichosanthes Combination)

| trichosanthes seed | 3.0 | pinellia | 6.0 | bakeri | 4.0 |
| chih-shih | 2.0 | ginger | 2.0 | | |

Kua-tzu-jen-tang 瓜子仁湯
(Benincasa Combination)

| coix | 9.0 | persica | 6.0 | moutan | 4.0 |
| benincasa | 3.0 | | | | |

Kuei-chi-chien-chung-tang 歸耆建中湯
(Tang-kuei, Astragalus, and Paeonia Combination)

Tang-kuei-chien-chung-tang (Tang-kuei, Cinnamon, and Paeonia Combination) with astragalus 2.0.

Kuei-chiang-tsao-tsao-huang-hsin-fu-tang 桂薑棗草黃辛附湯
(Cinnamon and Six Herb Combination)

| cinnamon | 3.0 | ginger | 3.0 | jujube | 3.0 |

| licorice | 2.0 | *ma-huang* | 2.0 | asarum | 2.0 |
| aconite | 0.5-1.0 | | | | |

Kuei-chih-chia-ling-chu-fu-ching-chieh-tang 桂枝加苓朮附荊芥湯
(Cinnamon, Aconite, and Schizonepeta Combination)

This is a combination of *Kuei-chih-chia-ling-chu-fu-tang* (Cinnamon and Aconite Combination) with 2.0 grams of schizonepeta.

Kuei-chih-chia-ling-chu-tang 桂枝加苓朮湯
(Cinnamon, Heoeln, and Atractylodes Combination)

cinnamon	4.0	ginger	3.0	jujube	3.0
paeonia	3.0	licorice	1.5	hoelen	5.0
atractylodes	5.0				

Kuei-chih-chia-shao-yao-sheng-chiang-jen-sheng-tang 桂枝加芍藥生薑人參湯
(Cinnamon and P. G. G. Combination)

This is a combination of *Kuei-chih-tang* (Cinnamon Combination) with 1.5 g each of paeonia and ginger, and 4.5 g of ginseng.

Kuei-chih-chu-shao-yao-tang 桂枝去芍藥湯
(Cinnamon minus Paeonia Combination)

This is a combination of *Kuei-chih-tang* (Cinnamon Combination) without paeonia.

Kuei-chih-fu-ling-tang 桂枝茯苓湯
(Cinnamon and Hoelen Combination)

| cinnamon | 4.0 | hoelen | 4.0 | moutan | 4.0 |
| persica | 4.0 | paeonia | 4.0 | | |

Kuei-chih-erh-ma-huang-i-tang 桂枝二麻黃一湯
(*Ma-huang* and Double Cinnamon Combination)

cinnamon	4.5	paeonia	3.0	ginger	3.0
jujube	3.0	*ma-huang*	1.5	apricot seed	1.5
licorice	2.5				

Kuei-chih-erh-yueh-pei-i-tang 桂枝二越婢一湯
(Cinnamon, *Ma-huang,* and Gypsum Combination)

cinnamon	2.5	paeonia	2.5	licorice	2.5
ma-huang	2.5	ginger	3.5	jujube	3.0
gypsum	3.0				

Kuei-chih-kan-tsao-lung-ku-mu-li-tang 桂枝甘草龍骨牡蠣湯
(Cinnamon, Licorice, Dragon Bone, and Oyster Shell Combination)

cinnamon	4.0	licorice	2.0	dragon-bone	2.0
oyster shell	2.0				

Kuei-chih-kan-tsao-tang 桂枝甘草湯
(Cinnamon and Licorice Combination)

cinnamon 4.0 licorice 2.0

Kuei-chih-tao-jen-tang 桂枝桃仁湯
(Cinnamon, Persica, and Rehmannia Combination)

This is a combination of *Kuei-chih-tang* (Cinnamon Combination) with 5.0 grams of persica and 4.0 grams of rehmannia.

Kuei-pan-tang 龜板湯
(Turtle Shell Combination)

turtle shell	4.0	paeonia	4.0	cnidium	4.0
tang-kuei	5.0	rehmannia	5.0	haliotis	4.0

Kuei-tzu-fu-ling-san 葵子茯苓散
(Abutilon and Hoelen Formula)

abutilon 8.0 hoelen 1.5

Grind above herbs into powder. Take 2.0 grams for each time.

Kun-tan-wan 滾痰丸
(Rhubarb and Aquilaria Formula)

rhubarb	8.0	chlorite	1.0	aquilaria	0.5
scute	8.0				

Li-hsiao-san
(Asarum and Cimicifuga Formula)　　　　　立效散

asarum	2.0	cimicifuga	2.0	siler	2.0
licorice	1.5	gentiana	1.0		

Li-tse-tung-chi-tang
(Angelica and Siler Combination)　　　　　麗澤通氣湯

chiang-huo	3.0	tu-huo	3.0	siler	3.0
pueraria	3.0	atractylodes	3.0	allium	3.0
cimicifuga	1.0	ma-huang	1.0	zanthoxylum	1.0
licorice	1.0	angelica	4.0	ginger	1.0
jujube	1.0	astragalus	4.0		

Lien-chiao-tang (for sudamina)
(Forsythia and Akebia Combination)　　　　連翹湯

platycodon	2.0	licorice	1.0	carthamus	1.0
forsythia	3.0	akebia	3.0		

Lien-chiao-tang (for ophthalmology)
(Forsythia and Scute Combination)　　　　連翹湯

forsythia	3.0	scute	3.0	ma-huang	3.0
cnidium	3.0	licorice	2.0	rhubarb	2.0
chih-shih	2.0				

Lien-chiao-tang (for erysipelas)
(Forsythia and Cimicifuga Combination)　　連翹湯

forsythia	1.5	scute	1.5	ma-huang	1.5
cimicifuga	1.5	cnidium	1.5	licorice	1.5
rhubarb	2.0	chih-shih	2.0		

Lien-li-tang
(Ginseng, Ginger, and Coptis Combination)　　連理湯

　　This is a combination of *Li-chung-tang* (Ginseng and Ginger Combination) with coptis 1.5 and hoelen 3.0.

Ling-yang-chiao-san
(Antelope Horn Formula)　　　　　羚羊角散

antelope horn	3.0	scute	3.0	cimicifuga	3.0

| licorice | 3.0 | plantago | 3.0 | gardenia | 2.0 |
| gentiana | 2.0 | cassia seed | 5.0 | | |

Ling-yang-chiao-tang 羚羊角湯
(Antelope Horn Combination)

tang-kuei	3.0	gambir	3.0	cnidium	3.0
hoelen	4.0	atractylodes	4.0	bupleurum	2.0
antelope horn	2.0	licorice	1.5		

Liu-shen-wan 六神丸
(Bear Gall and Pearl Formula)

toad secretion	5.0	musk	25.0	bos	13.0
bear gall	17.0	pearl	17.0	cinnabar	12.0
borneol	3.0				

Liu-tu-chien 六度煎
(Paeonia and Tiger's Shinebone Formula)

| paeonia | 4.0 | tang-kuei | 4.0 | astragalus | 2.0 |
| limonite | 4.0 | aconite | 0.3 | tiger's shinebone | 3.0 |

Liu-wei-hai-jen-tang 六味海人湯
(Digenea Six Combination)

| digenea | 5.0 | quisqualis | 3.0 | cinnamon | 3.0 |
| areca seed | 3.0 | melia bark | 3.0 | rhubarb | 2.0 |

Liu-wu-fu-tzu-tang 六物附子湯
(Aconite Six Combination)

| aconite | 0.5-1.0 | licorice | 1.0 | cinnamon | 3.0 |
| stephania | 3.0 | atractylodes | 5.0 | hoelen | 5.0 |

Liu-wu-pai-tu-tang 六物敗毒湯
(Lonicera and Coix Combination)

| limonite | 4.0 | lonicera | 5.0 | cnidium | 3.0 |
| chaenomeles | 3.0 | coix | 5.0 | rhubarb | 1.0 |

Lu-fan-wan
(Melanterite Formula) 綠礬丸

atractylodes	8.0	shen-chu	8.0	citrus	8.0
magnolia bark	8.0	jujube	8.0	licorice	5.0
melanterite	4.0				

Luan-fa-shuang
(Human Hair Formula) 亂髮霜

Burned the human hair. And take 1.0 gm each time. Three times a day.

Lung-ku-tang
(Dragon Bone Combination) 龍骨湯

dragon bone	3.0	hoelen	4.0	cinnamon	3.0
polygala	3.0	ophiopogon	3.0	oyster shell	3.0
licorice	1.5	ginger	1.0		

Lung-liu-wan
(Dragon Bone and Sulfur Formula) 龍硫丸

dragon bone	2.0	sulfur	3.0

Ma-huang-tso-cning-tang
(*Ma-huang* and *Chianghuo* Combination) 麻黃左經湯

chianghuo	3.0	siler	3.0	ma-huang	3.0
cinnamon	3.0	atractylodes	3.0	hoelen	3.0
asarum	2.0	stephania	5.0	ginger	1.5
licorice	1.5				

Ma-ming-tang
(Silkworm Molt Combination) 馬明湯

silkworm molt	1.0	carthamus	1.0	licorice	1.0
gypsum	5.0	curcuma	4.0	rhubarb	0.5

Man-chien-tang
(Aconite and Oyster Shell Combination) 曼倩湯

This is a combination of *Szu-ni-tang* (Aconite and G. L. Combination) with 2.0 grams of evodia and 4.0 grams of oyster shell.

Man-ching-tzu-san 蔓荊子散
(Vitex Formula)

vitex	1.5	paeonia	3.0	bupleurum	3.0
ophiopogon	3.0	hoelen	3.0	rehmannia	3.0
akebia	1.0	morus	1.0	chrysanthemum	1.0
cimicifuga	1.0	jujube	1.0	ginger	1.0
licorice	1.0				

Miao-kung-san 妙功散
(Astragalus and Hoelen Formula)

astragalus	4.0	dioscorea	4.0	polygala	4.0
ginseng	2.0	platycodon	2.0	licorice	2.0
cinnabar	0.3	musk	0.1	saussurea	2.5
hoelen	8.0				

Miao-kung-shih-i-wan 妙功十一丸
(Clove and Aquilaria Formula)

clove	saussurea	aquilaria
mastic	musk	scirpus
zedoria	pharbitis	coptis
omphalia	carpesium	picrorrhiza
scute	rhubarb	blue citrus peel
realgar	licorice	bear gall
phaseolus	calomel	croton

Ming-lang-yin 明朗飲
(Hoelen, Licorice, and Plantago Combination)

hoelen	6.0	cinnamon	4.0	atractylodes	3.0
licorice	2.0	plantago	3.0	asarum	1.5
coptis	1.5				

Ming-yen-i-fang 明眼一方
(Siler and Plantago Formula)

siler	3.0	chrysanthemum	1.5	plantago	3.0
talc	3.0	platycodon	3.0		

Mu-hsiang-tiao-chi-yin 木香調氣飲
(Saussurea and Cardamon Combination)

saussurea	1.0	santalum	1.0	cluster	1.0
clove	1.0	cardamon	1.5	agastache	1.5
licorice	1.5	ginger	3.0	salt	2.0

Mu-li-san 牡蠣散
(Oyster Shell Formula)

oyster shell	4.0	ma-huang	4.0	astragalus	4.0
wheat	8.0				

Mu-li-tang 牡蠣湯
(Oyster Shell Combination)

oyster shell	4.0	ma-huang	4.0	licorice	2.0
dichroa	3.0				

Mu-li-tse-hsieh-san 牡蠣澤瀉散
(Oyster Shell and Alisma Formula)

oyster shell	alisma	trichosanthes root
dichroa	lepidium	phytolacca
sargassum	equal potion	

Mu-tan-pi-san 牡丹皮散
(Moutan Formula)

ginseng	2.0	persica	2.0	saussurea	1.0
moutan	2.0	angelica	2.0	cinnamon	1.0
paeonia	2.0	tang-kuei	2.0	coix	5.0
hoelen	2.0	cnidium	2.0	astragalus	2.0
licorice	1.0				

Nei-shu-huang-lien-tang 內疏黃連湯
(Coptis and Saussurea Combination)

saussurea	1.0	coptis	1.0	gardenia	1.0
mentha	1.0	licorice	1.0	rhubarb	1.0
tang-kuei	4.0	forsythia	4.0	paeonia	3.0
scute	3.0	areca seed	3.0	platycodon	3.0

Nei-tuo-san 內托散
(Astragalus and Platycodon Formula)

ginseng	2.5	astragulus	2.0	cnidium	1.0
siler	1.0	platycodon	1.0	magnolia bark	2.0
cinnamon	2.0	*tang-kuei*	3.0	angelica	1.0
licorice	1.0				

Niang-ju-wan 釀乳丸
(Silkworm and Glutinous Rice Formula)

Put silk-worm and glutinous rice into pill, 9 pills are a daily dosage and three times a day.

Niu-hsi-san 牛膝散
(Achyranthes Formula)

achyranthes	3.0	cinnamon	3.0	paeonia	3.0
persica	3.0	*tang-kuei*	3.0	moutan	3.0
corydalis	3.0	saussurea	1.0		

Niu-pang-tzu-tang 牛蒡子湯
(Arctium Combination)

bupleurum	5.0	blue citrus peel	2.5	citrus	2.5
gardenia	2.5	scute	2.5	trichosanthes root	2.5
forsythia	2.0	arctium	2.0	lonicera	2.0
gleditsia	1.0	benincasa	4.0	licorice	1.5

Pa-wei-hsiao-yao-san 八味逍遙散
(*Tang-kuei,* Paeonia, and Bupleurum Formula)

tang-kuei	3.0	paeonia	3.0	bupleurum	3.0
atractylodes	3.0	hoelen	3.0	licorice	1.5
ginger	1.0	mentha	1.0		

Pa-wei-shan-chi-fang 八味疝氣方
(Cinnamon and Akebia Formula)

cinnamon	3.0	corydalis	3.0	akebia	3.0
lindera	3.0	moutan	3.0	pharbitis	3.0
persica	6.0	rhubarb	1.0		

Pa-wei-shun-chi-san 八味順氣散
(Atractylodes and Lindera Formula)

atractylodes	3.0	hoelen	3.0	blue citrus peel	3.0
angelica	3.0	citrus	3.0	lindera	3.0
ginseng	3.0	licorice	1.0		

Pa-wei-ti-huang-tang 八味地黃湯
(Rehmannia Eight Combination)

rehmannia	5.0	dioscorea	3.0	cornus	3.0
alisma	3.0	hoelen	3.0	moutan	3.0
cinnamon	1.0	aconite	1.0		

Pai-ho-ku-chin-tang 百合固金湯
(Lily Combination)

lily	4.0	*tang-kuei*	4.0	rehmannia	4.0
paeonia	3.0	fritillaria	3.0	scrophularia	3.0
platycodon	2.0	licorice	1.5	ophiopogon	6.0

Pai-tou-weng-chia-kan-tsao-ah-chiao-tang 白頭翁加甘草阿膠湯
(Anemone, Licorice, and Gelatin Combination)

anemone	2.0	licorice	2.0	gelatin	2.0
coptis	3.0	phellodendron	3.0	fraxinus	3.0

Pai-yun-kao 白雲膏
(White Wax and Calomel Ointment)

sesame oil	100 ml	white wax	380	ceruse	300
coconu oil	7.5	camphor	7.5	calomel	7.5

Pan-hsia-san-liao 半夏散料
(Pinellia Formula)

pinellia	3.0	cinnamon	3.0	licorice	3.0

Pan-hsia-ti-yu-tang 半夏地楡湯
(Pinellia and Sanguisorba Combination)

pinellia	5.0	sanguisorba	3.0

Pei-chi-tan 備急丹
(Rhubarb, Ginger, and Croton Formula)

Put equal portion of rhubarb, ginger and croton with mel into pills. Take 0.5 gram for each time.

Pei-mu-tang 貝母湯
(Fritillaria Combination)

schizandra	2.5	fritillaria	2.0	ginger	1.0
morus	2.5	cinnamon	2.0	saussurea	1.0
aurantium	2.5	apricot seed	2.0	scute	2.5
bupleurum	7.0	dried ginger	2.0	licorice	1.0

Pen-tun-tang 奔豚湯
(Pueraria and Ginger Combination)

pueraria	5.0	communis	5.0	ginger	4.0
pinellia	4.0	licorice	2.0	cnidium	2.0
tang-kuei	2.0	scute	2.0	paeonia	2.0

Pieh-chia-chien-wan 鱉甲煎丸
(Tortoise Shell Formula)

tortoise shell	12.0	rhubarb	3.0	paeonia	5.0
magnolia bark	3.0	cinnamon	3.0	pyrrosia	3.0
belamcanda	3.0	gelatin	3.0	eupolyphaga	5.0
scute	3.0	bupleurum	6.0	dianthus	2.0
wood louse	3.0	scarab-lang	6.0	persica	2.0
ginger	3.0	moutan	5.0	lepidium	1.0
pinellia	1.0	ginseng	1.0	mirabilitum	12.0
wasp's nest	4.0	campsis	3.0		

Ping-kan-liu-chi-yin 平肝流氣飲
(Pinellia and Coptis Combination)

tang-kuei	3.0	pinellia	3.0	hoelen	3.0
citrus	3.0	gardenia	2.0	cyperus	2.0
paeonia	2.0	cnidium	2.0	bupleurum	2.0
magnolia bark	2.0	coptis	1.0	blue citrus peel	1.0
evodia	1.0	licorice	1.0	ginger	1.0

Po-kuan-tang 破棺湯
(Persica and Apricot Seed Combination)

| persica | 3.0 | apricot seed | 3.0 | morus | 3.0 |

Po-ti-kao 破敵膏

This is a combination of *Ching-she-kao* with *Tso-tu-hao* (Asphalt Ointment).

Po-yeh-tang 柏葉湯
(Biota Leaves Combination)

| biota leaves | 1.0 | ginger | 1.0 | artemisia | 1.0 |

Pu-chung-chih-shih-tang 補中治濕湯
(Ginseng and Akebia Combination)

ginseng	3.0	atractylodes	3.0	hoelen	3.0
aurantium	3.0	ophiopogon	3.0	tang-kuei	3.0
akebia	3.0	scute	3.0	magnolia bark	3.0
cimicifuga	1.0				

Pu-fei-tang 補肺湯
(Jujube and Ophiopogon Combination)

ophiopogon	4.0	schizandra	3.0	cinnamon	3.0
jujube	3.0	oryza	3.0	morus	3.0
tussilago	2.0	ginger	2.0		

Pu-kan-san 補肝散
(Gypsum and Gastrodia Formula)

tang-kuei	1.5	cnidium	1.5	white atractylodes	5
atractylodes	1.5	lycium fruit	1.5	buddleia	1.5
chianghuo	1.5	gastrodia	1.5	bupleurum	1.5
hao-pen	1.5	forsythia	1.5	asarum	1.5
platycodon	1.5	siler	1.5	gypsum	2.0
mentha	1.0	equisetum	1.0	schizonepeta	1.0
licorice	1.0	gardenia	1.0	angelica	1.0

Pu-yang-huan-wu-tang 補陽還五湯
(Astragalus and Paeonia Combination)

| astragalus | 5.0 | tang-kuei | 3.0 | paeonia | 3.0 |

cnidium   2.0 persica   2.0 carthamus 2.0
earthworm   2.0

San-huang-chih-mu-tang 三黃知母湯
(Rhubarb, Scute, Coptis, and Anemarrhena Combination)
rhubarb   1.0 scute   1.0 coptis   1.0
anemarrhena 3.0 gypsum   1.0 licorice   1.5

San-huang-wan 三黃丸
(Rhubarb, Scute, and Coptis Formula)
rhubarb   scute   coptis
             in equal portions

San-pin-i-tiao-chiang 三品一條鎗
(Alum and Arsenic Formula)
alum   3   arsenic   1.5 realgar   0.3
mastic 0.2

San-sheng-wan 三聖丸
(Limonite Three Formula)
serpent's bezoar 3.0 limonite 3.0 iron powder 5.0

San-sheng-yin 三生飲
(Aconite and Arisaema Combination)
arisaema   6.0 wu-tou   0.5-1 aconite   0.5-1
saussurea   2.0 ginger   2.0

San-wei-che-ku-tsai-tang 三味鷓鴣菜湯
(Digenea and Rhubarb Combination)
digenea   3.0 rhubarb 1.5 licorice   1.5

Shan-hsiung-tang 芅凶湯
(Digenea and Bulrush Combination)
digenea   5.0 rhubarb 1.5 bulrush   1.5
melica bark 1.5

Shao-yao-szu-wu-chieh-tu-tang   芍藥四物解毒湯
(Paeonia Four Combination)

paeonia	2.0	scute	2.0	cimicifuga	2.0
pueraria	2.0				

She-chuang-tzu-tang   蛇床子湯
(Selinum Combination)

selinum	10.0	tang-kuei	10.0	clematis	10.0
sophora	10.0				

Put above herbs into 1000 ml. of water. Boil it until the content remains 700 ml. Use it wash the infected part.

Shen-hsiao-tang   神效湯
(*Tang-kuei* and Saussurea Combination)

atractylodes	2.0	cyperus	2.0	tang-kuei	2.0
saussurea	2.0	fennel	2.0	corydalis	2.0
black cardamon	2.0	lindera	2.0	gardenia	2.0
cardamon	2.0	juncus	2.0	licorice	2.0
ginger	1.0	evodia	1.0		

Shen-kung-nei-tuo-san   神功內托散
(*Tang-kuei*, Atractylodes, and Jujube Formula)

tang-kuei	3.0	hoelen	3.0	atractylodes	3.0
astragalus	2.0	ginseng	2.0	paeonia	2.0
cnidium	2.0	citrus	2.0	saussurea	1.0
licorice	1.0	anteater scales	1.0	ginger	1.0
jujube	1.0	aconite	0.5-1.0		

Shen-tan-tang   腎疸湯
(Hoelen and *Hao-pen* Combination)

chianghuo	2.0	siler	2.0	hao-pen	2.0
tu-huo	2.0	pueraria	2.0	bupleurum	2.0
alisma	2.0	ginseng	2.0	polyporus	2.0
shen-chu	2.0	atractylodes	2.0	white atractylodes	2.0
hoelen	3.0	phellodendron	1.5	licorice	1.0
cimicifuga	1.0				

Shen-ying-yang-shen-tan 神應養神丹
(*Tang-kuei* and Gastrodia Formula)

tang-kuei	3.0	cnidium	3.0	paeonia	3.0
gastrodia	3.0	*chiang-huo*	3.0	rehmannia	3.0
chaenomeles	3.0	cuscuta	3.0		

Shen-shui-kao 神水膏
(Mercury and Lard Ointment)

mercury	10.0	lard	100.0

Sheng-chin-tang 生津湯
(Ophiopogon and Rehmannia Combination)

ophiopogon	3.0	anemarrhena	3.0	astragalus	3.0
ginseng	3.0	oyster shell	3.0	trichosanthes root	3.0
licorice	1.5	coptis	1.0	rehmannia	4.0

Sheng-lien-tang 參連湯
(*Chu-chieh* Ginseng and Coptis Combination)

chu-chieh ginseng	5.0	coptis	3.0

Sheng-shih-yin 勝勢飲
(Cyperus and Hoelen Combination)

cyperus	4.0	*tang-kuei*	3.0	cnidium	2.5
hoelen	2.5	atractylodes	2.5	cinnamon	2.5
adenophora	2.5	akebia	2.0	clove	2.0
licorice	1.0				

Sheng-yang-san-huo-tang 升陽散火湯
(Bupleurum and Ginseng Combination)

ginseng	3.0	*tang-kuei*	3.0	paeonia	3.0
scute	4.0	bupleurum	4.0	ophiopogon	4.0
atractylodes	3.0	citrus	3.0	hoelen	3.0
licorice	1.5	ginger	1.5		

Shih-liu-ken-tang 石榴根湯
(Punica Combination)

punica	40	melia bark	3.0	areca seed	6.0

Sou-feng-chieh-tu-tang 搜風解毒湯
(Stephania and Smilax Combination)

stephania	3.0	smilax	3.0	lonicera	3.0
akebia	3.0	coix	3.0	chaenomeles	3.0
gleditsia seed	2.0	fraxinella	2.0		

Shou-lei-yin 收淚飲
(Schizonepeta and Scute Combination)

schizonepeta	3.0	siler	3.0	*tuhuo*	3.0
coptis	3.0	scute	3.0	gardenia	3.0
cnidium	3.0	equisetum	3.0	chrysanthemum	3.0
mentha	3.0	prunella	3.0	rehmannia	3.0

Szu-ling-tang 四苓湯
(Hoelen and Polyporus Combination)

alisma	4.0	hoelen	4.0	atractylodes	4.0
polyporus	4.0				

Szu-shun-ching-liang-yin 四順清涼飲
(Siler and Gardenia Combination)

forsythia	4.0	paeonia	3.0	siler	3.0
chianghuo	2.0	*tang-kuei*	5.0	gardenia	2.0
licorice	1.5	rhubarb	1.5		

Szu-shun-tang 四順湯
(Fritillaria and Aster Combination)

fritillaria	3.0	platycodon	3.0	aster	3.0
licorice	2.0				

Szu-wu-i-huang-tang 四物一黃湯
(Tang-kuei and Bulrush Combination)

tang-kuei	3.0	paeonia	3.0	cnidium	3.0
rehmannia	3.0	bulrush	5.0		

Szu-wu-tang-chiao-chi-chai-chien 四物湯脚氣加減
(*Tang-kuei* Four Combination Modified)

tang-kuei	3.0	cnidium	3.0	paeonia	3.0
rehmannia	3.0	chaenomeles	3.0	atractylodes	3.0
coix	6.0				

Ta-hsu-ming-tang 大續命湯（續命湯）
(*Ma-huang* and Ginseng Combination)

ma-huang	3.0	cinnamon	3.0	ginseng	3.0
tang-kuei	3.0	cnidium	3.0	dried ginger	2.0
licorice	2.0	apricot seed	4.0	gypsum	6.0

Ta-huang-hsiao-shih-tang 大黃消石湯
(Rhubarb and Saltpeter Combination)

rhubarb	4	phellodendron	4	saltpeter	4
gardenia	2				

Ta-kan-wan 大甘丸
(Rhubarb and Licorice Formula)

rhubarb	10	licorice	5.0

Ta-pai-chung-yin 大百中飲
(Achyranthes and Smilax Combination)

smilax	3.0	achyranthes	3.0	aquilaria	2.0
cnidium	3.0	licorice	1.5	coptis	1.5
areca seed	3.0	ginseng	2.0	rhubarb	2.0
cinnamon	3.0	scute	3.0	eucommia	2.0

Ta-pan-hsia-tang 大半夏湯
(Pinellia, Ginseng, and Mel Combination)

pinellia	7.0	ginseng	3.0	mel	20.0

Ta-san-chi-wu-san 大三七五散
(Hoelen and Cornus Formula)

cornus	2.0	ginger	2.0	hoelen	6.0
asarum	1.5	siler	4.0	aconite	0.5-1

Tang-chih-chung-i-fang 唐痔中一方
(Areca Seed and Ginger Formula)

areca seed	4.0	ginger	3.0	aurantium	3.0
chaenomeles	3.0	evodia	2.0	perilla leaves	2.0

Tang-kuei-hsu-san 當歸鬚散
(Tang-kuei and Lindera Formula)

tang-kuei	5.0	paeonia	4.0	lindera	4.0
cyperus	4.0	persica	2.5	sappan wood	2.5
carthamus	2.5	licorice	2.5	cinnamon	2.5

Tang-kuei-lien-chiao-tang 當歸連翹湯
(Tang-kuei and Forsythia Combination)

tang-kuei	1.5	forsythia	1.5	siler	1.5
scute	1.5	schizonepeta	1.5	angelica	1.5
paeonia	1.5	rehmannia	1.5	gardenia	1.5
atractylodes	1.5	ginseng	1.5	gelatin	1.5
sanguisorba	1.5	mume	1.0	licorice	1.0
jujube	1.0				

Tang-kuei-liu-huang-tang 當歸六黃湯
(Tang-kuei and Six Yellow Combination)

tang-kuei	3.0	dried rehmannia	3.0	cured rehmannia	3.0
phellodendron	3.0	scute	3.0	coptis	3.0
astragalus	3.0				

Tang-kuei-pai-chu-tang 當歸白朮湯
(Tang-kuei and Atractylodes Combination)

atractylodes	4.0	hoelen	4.0	tang-kuei	4.0
apricot seed	4.0	pinellia	4.0	polyporus	2.5
capillaris	1.5	chih-shih	1.5	peucedanum	3.0
licorice	1.0				

Tang-kuei-pei-mu-ku-sheng-wan-liao 當歸貝母苦參丸料
(Tang-kuei, Fritillaria, and Sophora Formula)

tang-kuei	3.0	fritillaria	3.0	sophora	3.0

Tang-kuei-san-liao 當歸散料
(Tang-kuei Formula)

tang-kuei	3.0	paeonia	3.0	cnidium	3.0
scute	3.0	atractylodes	1.5		

Tang-kuei-tang 當 歸 湯
(Tang-kuei Combination)

tang-kuei	5.0	pinellia	5.0	paeonia	3.0
magnolia bark	3.0	cinnamon	3.0	ginseng	3.0
ginger	1.5	astragalus	1.5	zanthoxylum	1.5
licorice	1.0				

Tang-kuei-yang-hsieh-tang 當歸養血湯
(Tang-kuei, Paeonia, and Rehmannia Combination)

paeonia	3.0	cured rehmannia	3.0	hoelen	3.0
tang-keui	3.0	fritillaria	1.5	trichosanthes	1.5
chih-shih	1.5	magnolia bark	1.5	cyperus	1.5
cnidium	1.5	perilla fruit	1.5	aquilaria	1.0
coptis	1.0				

Tao-chih-tung-ching-tang 導滯通經湯
(Atractylodes and Alisma Combination)

saussurea	1.0	atractylodes	5.0	alisma	5.0
morus	1.5	citrus	3.0	hoelen	6.0

Tao-jen-tang 桃 仁 湯
(Persica Combination)

persica	5.0	talc	5.0	moutan	3.0
tang-kuei	3.0	paeonia	3.0	gelatin	3.0

Ti-kang-san 提 肛 散
(Tang-kuei and Kaolin Formula)

cnidium	3.0	tang-kuei	3.0	atractylodes	3.0
ginseng	3.0	astragalus	3.0	citrus	3.0
licorice	3.0	cimicifuga	1.5	bupleurum	1.5
scute	1.5	coptis	0.7	angelica	0.7
kaolin	0.7				

Tiao-jung-tang 調 榮 湯
(Ginseng, Tang-kuei, and Rehmannia Combination)

ginseng	1.5	tang-kuei	5.0	rehmannia	5.0
cnidium	3.0	paeonia	3.0	caudatum	3.0
nuphar	3.0	atractylodes	3.0	hoelen	1.0
licorice	1.0				

Tien-hsiung-san 天雄散
(Aconite and Dragon Bone Formula)

| aconite | 0.5-1 | atractylodes | 8.0 | cinnamon | 6.0 |
| dragon bone | 3.0 | | | | |

Ting-chi-yin 定悸飲
(Hoelen and Evodia Combination)

hoelen	6.0	cinnamon	3.0	atractylodes	3.0
oyster shell	3.0	licorice	1.5	evodia	1.5
communis	2.0				

Ting-fu-li-chung-tang 丁附理中湯
(Clove and Aconite Combination)

| ginseng | 3.0 | licorice | 3.0 | atractylodes | 3.0 |
| ginger | 3.0 | clove | 1.0 | aconite | 0.5-1.0 |

Tsao-chia-wan 皂莢丸
(Gleditsia Formula)

Bake and grind gleditsia into powder then put it with mel and decoct with jujube. Take 2.0 grams for each time and three times a day.

Tsuei-ju-fang 催乳方
(Wasp's Nest and Rehmannia Formula)

Burn the equal portion of wasp's nest and rehmannia. Make it into pill as large as firmiana seed. Take 50 pills each time.

Tso-tu-kao 左突膏
(Asphalt Ointment)

| asphalt | 800 | flava wax | 220 | lard | 58 |
| sesame oil | 1000 | | | | |

Tu-hsien-san 禿癬散
(Sulfur and Rhubarb Formula)

| realgar | 0.6 | sulfur | 1.2 | bluestone | 0.3 |
| rhubarb | 0.9 | | | | |

Tu-huo-ko-ken-tang 獨活葛根湯
(*Tu-huo* and Pueraria Combination)

pueraria	5.0	rehmannia	4.0	cinnamon	3.0
paeonia	3.0	*ma-huang*	2.0	*tu-huo*	2.0
jujube	1.0	licorice	1.0	dried ginger	1.0

Tu-huo-tang 獨活湯
(*Tu-huo* Combination)

tu-huo	2.0	*chiang-huo*	2.0	siler	2.0
cinnamon	2.0	rhubarb	2.0	alisma	2.0
tang-kuei	3.0	persica	3.0	forsythia	3.0
stephania	5.0	phellodendron	5.0	licorice	1.5

Tu-sheng-tang 獨參湯
(Ginseng Combination)

ginseng 8.0

Tuan-li-tang 斷痢湯
(Pinellia and Jujube Combination)

pinellia	4.0	ginger	2.0	ginseng	2.0
coptis	2.0	aconite	0.5	jujube	3.0
hoelen	3.0	licorice	1.5		

Tung-hsien-wan 通仙丸
(Fogopyrum and Rhubarb Formula)

Put equal portion of fogopyrum and rhubarb into pill. Take 3 pills for each time.

Tzu-hsieh-jun-chang-tang 滋血潤腸湯
(*Tang-kuei*, Rehmannia, and Persica Combination)

tang-kuei	4.0	rehmannia	4.0	persica	4.0
paeonia	3.0	*chih-shih*	2.0	bakeri	2.0
rhubarb	1.5	carthamus	1.0		

Tzu-yin-chih-pao-tang 滋陰至寶湯
(*Tang-kuei* and Lycium Combination)

tang-kuei	3.0	paeonia	3.0	atractylodes	3.0
hoelen	3.0	citrus	3.0	bupleurum	3.0

anemarrhena	3.0	cyperus	3.0	lycium bark	3.0
ophiopogon	3.0	fritillaria	2.0	mentha	1.0
licorice	1.0				

Wei-ching-tang 葦莖湯
(Phragmites Stem Combination)

| phragmites stem | 3.0 | coix | 10.0 | persica | 4.0 |
| benincasa | 7.0 | | | | |

Wu-hu-tang 五虎湯
(Gypsum and Apricot Seed Combination)

| ma-huang | 4.0 | apricot seed | 4.0 | licorice | 2.0 |
| gypsum | 10.0 | morus | 3.0 | | |

Wu-ling-tang 五苓湯
(Hoelen Five Herb Combination)

| alisma | 6.0 | polyporus | 4.5 | atractylodes | 4.5 |
| hoelen | 4.5 | cinnamon | 2.5 | | |

Wu-ling-tung-chi-san 烏苓通氣散
(Lindera and Hoelen Formula)

lindera	2.0	tang-kuei	2.0	paeonia	2.0
cyperus	2.0	crataegus	2.0	citrus	2.0
ginger	2.0	hoelen	1.0	atractylodes	1.0
areca seed	1.0	corydalis	1.0	alisma	1.0
saussurea	0.5	licorice	0.5		

Wu-shen-tang 巫神湯
(Hoelen and Saussurea Combination)

hoelen	6.0	atractylodes	3.0	polyporus	3.0
alisma	3.0	cinnamon	3.0	coptis	2.0
ginger	1.0	saussurea	1.0		

Wu-tou-chih-shih-wan 烏頭赤石丸
(*Wu-tou* and Kaolin Formula)

| zanthoxylum | 2.0 | kaolin | 2.0 | wu-tou | 1.0 |
| aconite | 1.0 | ginger | 1.0 | | |

Grind above herbs into powder and make it with mel to pill. Take 0.5 gram for each time and three times daily.

Wu-tou-tang 烏頭湯
(*Wu-tou* Combination)

Ma-huang	3.0	paeonia	3.0	astragalus	3.0
licorice	3.0	*wu-tou*	0.5-1	mel	20

Wu-wu-chieh-tu-tang 五物解毒湯
(Cnidium and Lonicera Combination)

cnidium	5.0	lonicera	2.0	rhubarb	1.0
schizonepeta	1.5	houttuynia	2.0		

Yang-fei-tang 養肺湯
(Fritillaria and Hoelen Combination)

bupleurum	3.0	fritillaria	3.0	hoelen	4.0
apricot seed	4.0	gelatin	2.0	platycodon	2.0
morus	2.0	ginseng	2.0	*chih-shih*	1.5
schizandra	1.5	licorice	1.5		

Yang-hsieh-an-shen-tang 養血安神湯
(*Tang-kuei*, Rehmannia, and Hoelen Combination)

tang-kuei	3.0	rehmannia	3.5	cnidium	3.0
paeonia	3.0	coptis	1.5	biota	1.5
citrus	2.5	hoelen	3.5	atractylodes	3.5
zizyphus	3.5	licorice	1.5		

Yang-hsieh-tang 養血湯
(*Tang-kuei*, Rehmannia, and *Chin-chiu* Combination)

tang-kuei	4.0	rehmannia	4.0	*chin-chiu*	4.0
eucommia	4.0	cinnamon	4.0	limonite	4.0
cnidium	2.0	licorice	1.0		

Yang-po-san 楊柏散
(Myrica and Phellodendron Formula)

myrica	2.0	phellodendron	2.0	zanthoxylum	1.0

Grind above three herbs into powder and mix up. Then put it with vinegar into muddy form. Spread it over infected part. If patient is uncomfortable for vinegar, add wheat powder and spread it with water.

Yen-ling-tang 延齡湯
(Saussurea and Mastic Formula)

cinnamon	30	cardamon	30	clove	30
cinnabar	30	piper	3	santalum	3
saussurea	14	platycodon	14	mastic	14
terminalia	14	licorice	18	musk	6
borneol	5	aquilaria	30		

Yeh-kan-ma-huang-tang 射干麻黃湯
(Belamcanda and *Ma-huang* Combination)

belamcanda	2.5	ma-huang	3.0	ginger	3.0
schizandra	3.0	asarum	2.0	aster	2.0
tussilago	2.0	jujube	2.0	pinellia	4.0

Yin-chen-san 茵陳散
(Capillaris and Talc Formula)

capillaris	2.0	alisma	3.0	chih-shih	2.0
atractylodes	3.0	gardenia	2.0	hoelen	5.0
magnolia bark	2.0	coptis	1.5	polyporus	
talc	2.0	juncus	1.5		3.0

Yin-chen-szu-ni-tang 茵陳四逆湯
(Capillaris and Aconite Combination)

capillaris	2.0	licorice	3.0	ginger	2.0
aconite	0.5				

Yin-ching-tang 茵荊湯
(Capillaris and Schizonepeta Combination)

capillaris	2.0	schizonepeta	2.0	bulrush	2.0
iron powder	2.0	atractylodes	3.0	polyporus	3.0
alisma	3.0	hoelen	5.0		

Ying-chung-san 應鐘散
(Cnidium and Rhubarb Formula)

Same as *Chiung-huang-san* (Cnidium and Rhubarb Formula)

Yu-tse-san 羽澤散
(Alum and Apricot Seed Formula)

Alum	2.0	Apricot seed	2.0	Licorice	2.0
clove	1.0	borneol	1.0		

FORMULA INDEX
ENGLISH TO CHINESE

A

Abutilon and Hoelen Formula   *813*
(Kuei-tzu-fu-ling-san)   葵子茯苓散

Achyranthes and Smilax Combination   *827*
(Ta-pai-chung-yin)   大百中飲

Achyranthes Formula   *819*
(Niu-hsi-san)   牛膝散

Aconite and Arisaema Combination   *823*
(San-sheng-yin)   三生飲

Aconite and Dragon Bone Formula   *830*
(Tien-hsiung-san)   天雄散

Aconite and G. L. Combination   *625*
(Szu-ni-tang)   四逆湯

Formula Index

Aconite and Oryza Combination   571
(Fu-tzu-keng-mi-tang)   附子粳米湯

Aconite and Oyster Shell Combination   816
(Man-chien-tang)   曼倩湯

Aconite Combination   571
(Fu-tzu-tang)   附子湯

Aconite Six Combination   815
(Liu-wu-fu-tzu-tang)   六物附子湯

Adiantum and Viper Formula   801
(Fa-sheng-san)   髮生散

Agastache Formula   582
(Huo-hsiang-cheng-chi-san)   藿香正氣散

Akebia and Pinellia Formula   801
(Fei-kan-fang)   肺疳方

Alisma, Hoelen, and Ginger Combination   570
(Fu-ling-tse-hsieh-tang)   茯苓澤瀉湯

Alum and Apricot Seed Formula   834
(Yu-tse-san)   羽澤散

Alum and Arsenic Formula   823
(San-pin-i-tiao-chiang)   三品一條槍

Alum and Licorice Formula   788
(Cheng-yen-i-fang)   蒸眼一方

Anemarrhena and Hoelen Combination   795
(Chih-mu-fu-ling-tang)   知母茯苓湯

Anemone, Licorice, and Gelatin Combination   820
(Pai-tou-weng-chia-kan-tsao-ah-chiao-tang)   白頭翁加甘草阿膠湯

836

Formula Index

Angelica and Siler Combination 814
(Li-tse-tung-chi-tang) 麗澤通氣湯

Antelope Horn and Zizyphus Combination 788
(Cheng-hsin-tang) 正心湯

Antelope Horn Combination 815
(Ling-yang-chiao-tang) 羚羊角湯

Antelope Horn Formula 814
(Ling-yang-chiao-san) 羚羊角散

Aquilaria and Cyperus Combination 787
(Chen-hsiang-chiang-chi-tang) 沈香降氣湯

Aquilaria and Hoelen Combination 791
(Chia-wei-ning-hsien-tang) 加味寧瘤湯

Arctium Combination 819
(Niu-pang-tzu-tang) 牛蒡子湯

Areca and Evodia Combination 614
(Pien-chih-hsin-chi-yin) 變製心氣飲

Areca Seed and Chaenomeles Formula with Hoelen 789
(Chi-ming-san-chia-fu-ling) 雞鳴散加茯苓

Areca Seed and Ginger Formula 827
(Tang-chih-chung-i-fang) 唐痔中一方

Areca Seed Nine Combination
(Chiu-wei-ping-lang-tang) 九味檳榔湯

Asarum and Cimicifuga Formula 814
(Li-hsiao-san) 立效散

Asphalt Ointment 830
(Tso-tu-kao) 左突膏

Formula Index

Astragalus and Ginger Combination   807
(Huang-chi-tang)   黃耆湯

Astragalus and Hoelen Formula   817
(Miao-kung-san)   妙功散

Astragalus and Paeonia Combination   822
(Pu-yang-huan-wu-tang)   補陽還五湯

Astragalus and Platycodon Formula   558
(Chien-chin-nei-tuo-san)   千金內托散

Astragalus and Platycodon Formula   819
(Nei-tuo-san)   內托散

Astragalus and Tortoise Shell Combination   579
(Huang-chi-pieh-chia-tang)   黃耆鱉甲湯

Astragalus Combination   578
(Huang-chi-chien-chung-tang)   黃耆建中湯

Atractylodes and Alisma Combination   829
(Tao-chih-tung-ching-tang)   導滯通經湯

Atractylodes and Citrus Formula   795
(Chih-pan-wan)   治胖丸

Atractylodes and Hoelen Combination   601
(Ling-kuei-chu-kan-tang)   苓桂朮甘湯

Atractylodes and Licorice Combination   791
(Chia-wei-hsiao-ke-tang)   加味消渴湯

Atractylodes and Lindera Formula   820
(Pa-wei-shun-chi-san)   八味順氣散

Atractylodes and Setaria Combination   639
(Wei-feng-tang)   胃風湯

Formula Index

Atractylodes Combination   646
(Yueh-pi-chia-chu-tang)   越婢加朮湯

Aurantium and Pinellia Combination   799
(Chu-pi-pan-hsia-tang)   橘皮半夏湯

Aurantium Combination   800
(Chu-pi-tang)   橘皮湯

Aurantium, Rhubarb, and Mirabilitum Combination   799
(Chu-pi-ta-huang-pu-hsiao-tang)   橘皮大黃朴硝湯

B

Baked Licorice Combination   559
(Chih-kan-tsao-tang)   炙甘草湯

Bamboo and Chih-shih Combination   641
(Wen-tan-tang)   溫膽湯（千金方）

Bamboo and Citrus Combination Modified   792
(Chia-wei-wen-tan-tang)   加味溫膽湯

Bamboo Leaves and Gypsum Combination   567
(Chu-yeh-shih-kao-tang)   竹葉石膏湯

Bear Gall and Pearl Formula   815
(Liu-shen-wan)   六神丸

Belamcanda and Ma-huang Combination   834
(Yeh-kan-ma-huang-tang)   射干麻黃湯

Benincasa Combination   811
(Kua-tzu-jen-tang)   瓜子仁湯

Biota Leaves Combination   822
(Po-yeh-tang)   柏葉湯

Borax and Realgar Formula   796
(Chin-suo-shih)   金鎖匙

Formula Index

Bulrush and Cinnabar Formula   802
(Ho-kou-san)   和口散

Bupleurum and Atractylodes Formula   809
(I-kan-fu-pi-san)   抑肝扶脾散

Bupleurum and Chih-shih Formula   624
(Szu-ni-san)   四逆散

Bupleurum and Cinnamon Combination   554
(Chai-hu-kuei-chih-tang)   柴胡桂枝湯

Bupleurum and Cyperus Combination   786
(Chai-hu-shu-kan-tang)   柴胡疏肝湯

Bupleurum and Digenea Combination   796
(Ching-chi-an-huei-tang)   清肌安蛔湯

Bupleurum and Dragon Bone Combination   552
(Chai-hu-chia-lung-ku-mu-li-tang)   柴胡加龍骨牡蠣湯

Bupleurum and Gardenia Combination   797
(Ching-shang-yin)   清上飲

Bupleurum and Gardenia Formula   786
(Chai-hu-shu-kan-san)   柴胡疏肝散

Bupleurum and Ginseng Combination   825
(Sheng-yang-san-huo-tang)   升陽散火湯

Bupleurum and Paeonia Formula   557
(Chia-wei-hsiao-yao-san)   加味逍遙散

Bupleurum and Pinellia Combination   635
(Tsing-fu-tang)   淨腑湯

Bupleurum and Pueraria Combination   555
(Chai-ko-chieh-chi-tang)   柴葛解肌湯

Bupleurum and Rehmannia Combination　　553
(Chai-hu-ching-kan-tang)　　柴胡清肝湯

Bupleurum and Schizonepeta Combination　　621
(Shih-wei-pai-tu-tang)　　十味敗毒湯

Bupleurum and Tortoise Shell Combination　　786
(Chai-hu-pieh-chia-tang)　　柴胡鼈甲湯

Bupleurum and Trichosanthes Root Combination　　786
(Chai-hu-chu-pan-hsia-chia-kua-lu-tang)　　柴胡去半夏加瓜呂湯

Bupleurum, Chih-shih, and Platycodon Combination　　785
(Chai-hu-chih-chieh-tang)　　柴胡枳桔湯

Bupleurum, Cinnamon, and Ginger Combination　　554
(Chai-hu-kuei-chih-kan-chiang-tang)　　柴胡桂枝乾薑湯

Bupleurum, Citrus, and Anemarrhena Combination　　800
(Chu-shih-pu-chi-tang)　　除濕補氣湯

Bupleurum, Cnidium, and Tang-kuei Combination　　785
(Chai-hu-chiung-kuei-tang)　　柴胡芎歸湯

Bupleurum Formula　　583
(I-kan-san)　　抑肝散

Bupleurum, Paeonia, and Six Major Herb Combination　　555
(Chai-shao-liu-chun-tzu-tang)　　柴芍六君子湯

Bupleurum, Pinellia, and Citrus Formula　　583
(I-kan-san-chia-chen-pi-pan-hsia)　　抑肝散加陳皮半夏

Bupleurum, Platycodon, and Gypsum Combination　　804
(Hsiao-chai-hu-chia-chieh-keng-shih-kao-tang)
　　小柴胡加桔梗、石膏湯

Bupleurum, Platycodon, and Pinellia Combination　　786
(Chai-keng-pan-hsia-tang)　　柴梗半夏湯

Bupleurum, Scute, and Licorice Combination   807
(Huan-hsien-tang)   緩痃湯

C

Capillaris and Aconite Combination   834
(Yin-chen-szu-ni-tang)   茵陳四逆湯

Capillaris and Hoelen Formula   645
(Yin-chen-wu-ling-san)   茵陳五苓散

Capillaris and Schizonepeta Combination   834
(Yin-ching-tang)   茵荊湯

Capillaris and Talc Formula   834
(Yin-chen-san)   茵陳散

Capillaris Combination   644
(Yin-chen-hao-tang)   茵陳蒿湯

Cardamon and Fennel Formula   551
(An-chung-san)   安中散

Cardamon and Shen-chu Combination   576
(Hsiao-kan-yin)   消疳飲

Carthamus and Silkworm Combination   792
(Chiang-shen-tang)   強神湯

Cardamon and Six Major Herb Combination   806
(Hua-shih-yang-pi-tang)   化食養脾湯

Chicken Liver Formula
(Chi-kan-wan)   雞肝丸

Chih-shih and Tu-huo Formula   799
(Chu-feng-pai-tu-san)   祛風敗毒散

Formula Index

Chih-shih, Gardenia, and Soja Combination   795
(Chih-shih-chih-tzu-shih-tang)   枳實梔子豉湯

Chin-chiu and Chiang-huo Combination   796
(Chin-chiu-chiang-huo-tang)   秦艽羌活湯

Chin-chiu and Siler Combination   796
(Chin-chiu-fang-feng-tang)   秦艽防風湯

Chin-chiu and Tortoise Shell Combination   562
(Chin-chiu-pieh-chia-tang)   秦艽鱉甲湯

Chrysanthemum and Siler Formula   803
(Hou-shih-hei-san)   侯氏黑散

Chu-chieh Ginseng and Coptis Combination   825
(Sheng-lien-tang)   參連湯

Cimicifuga Combination   584
(I-tzu-tang)   乙字湯

Cinnamon, Aconite, and Schizonepeta Combination   812
(Kuei-chih-chia-ling-chu-fu-ching-chieh-tang)   桂枝加苓朮附荊芥湯

Cinnamon and Aconite Combination   591
(Kuei-chih-chia-fu-tzu-tang)   桂枝加附子湯

Cinnamon and Akebia Formula   819
(Pa-wei-shan-chi-fang)   八味疝氣方

Cinnamon and Astragalus Combination   592
(Kuei-chih-chia-huang-chi-tang)   桂枝加黃耆湯

Cinnamon and Atractylodes Combination   593
(Kuei-chih-chia-ling-chu-fu-tang)   桂枝加苓朮附湯

Cinnamon and Cardamon Combination   800
(Chuan-li-chung-tang)   喘理中湯

Formula Index

Cinnamon and Digenea Combination   789
(Chi-wei-che-ku-tsai-tang)
七味鷓鴣菜湯

Cinnamon and Dragon Bone Combination   593
(Kuei-chih-chia-lung-ku-mu-li-tang)
桂枝加龍骨牡蠣湯

Cinnamon and Ginseng Combination   596
(Kuei-chih-jen-sheng-tang)
桂枝人參湯

Cinnamon and Hoelen Formula   596
(Kuei-chih-fu-ling-wan)
桂枝茯苓丸

Cinnamon and Licorice Combination   813
(Kuei-chih-kan-tsao-tang)
桂枝甘草湯

Cinnamon and Nuphar Formula
(Chih-ta-pu-i-fang)
治打撲一方

Cinnamon and Pueraria Combination   592
(Kuei-chih-chia-ko-ken-tang)
桂枝加葛根湯

Cinnamon and Six Herbs Combination   811
(Kuei-chiang-tsao-tsao-huang-hsin-fu-tang)
桂薑棗草黃辛附湯

Cinnamon Combination   597
(Kuei-chih-tang)
桂枝湯

Cinnamon, Dichroa, Oyster Shell, and Dragon Bone Combination
    595, 798
(Kuei-chih-chu-shao-yao-chia-shu-chi-lung-ku-mu-li-chiu-ni-tang)
桂枝去芍藥加蜀漆龍骨牡蠣救逆湯
(Chiu-ni-tang)
救逆湯

Cinnamon, Hoelen, and Atractylodes Combination   812
(Kuei-chih-chia-ling-chu-tang)
桂枝加苓朮湯

Cinnamon, Licorice, Dragon Bone, and Oyster Shell Combination 813
(Kuei-chih-kan-tsao-lung-ku-mu-li-tang) 桂枝甘草龍骨牡蠣湯

Cinnamon and Paeonia Combination 594
(Kuei-chih-chia-shao-yao-tang) 桂枝加芍藥湯

Cinnamon and P.G.G. Combination 812
(Kuei-chih-chia-shao-yao-sheng-chiang-jen-sheng-tang)
桂枝加芍藥生薑人參湯

Cinnamon, Ma-huang, Aconite, and Asarum Combination 595
(Kuei-chih-chu-shao-yao-chia-ma-huang-fu-tzu-hsi-hsin-tang)
桂枝去芍藥加麻黃附子細辛湯

Cinnamon, Ma-huang, and Gypsum Combination 813
(Kuei-chih-erh-yueh-pei-i-tang) 桂枝二越婢一湯

Cinnamon minus Paeonia Combination 812
(Kuei-chih-chu-shao-yao-tang) 桂枝去芍藥湯

Cinnamon, Paeonia, and Rhubarb Combination 594
(Kuei-chih-chia-shao-yao-ta-huang-tang) 桂枝加芍藥大黃湯

Cinnamon, Persica, and Rehmannia Combination 813
(Kuei-chih-tao-jen-tang) 桂枝桃仁湯

Citrus and Pinellia Combination 551
(Erh-chen-tang) 二陳湯

Clematis and Stephania Combination 622
(Shu-ching-huo-hsieh-tang) 疏經活血湯

Clove and Aconite Combination 830
(Ting-fu-li-chung-tang) 丁附理中湯

Clove and Aquilaria Formula 817
(Miao-kung-shih-i-wan) 妙功十一丸

Formula Index

Cnidium and Lonicera Combination 833
(Wu-wu-chieh-tu-tang) 五物解毒湯

Cnidium and Moutan Combination 564
(Ching-je-pu-hsieh-tang) 清熱補血湯

Cnidium and Persica Combination 808
(Huo-hsieh-san-yu-tang) 活血散瘀湯

Cnidium and Rhubarb Formula 798
(Chiung-huang-san) 芎黃散

Cnidium and Rhubarb Formula 834
(Ying-chung-san) 應鐘散

Cnidium and Tang-kuei Combination 798
(Chiung-kuei-tang) 芎歸湯

Coix, Aconite, and Thlaspi Combination 584
(I-yi-fu-tzu-pai-chiang-tang) 薏苡附子敗醬湯

Coptis and Aurantium Combination 808
(Huang-lien-chu-pi-tang) 黃連橘皮湯

Coptis and Gelatin Combination 580
(Huang-lien-ah-chiao-tang) 黃連阿膠湯

Coptis and Mume Combination 796
(Ching-chung-an-huei-tang) 清中安蛔湯

Coix and Persica Combination 787
(Chang-yung-tang) 腸癰湯

Coptis and Saussurea Combination 818
(Nei-shu-huang-lien-tang) 內疏黃連湯

Coptis and Scute Combination 581
(Huang-lien-chieh-tu-tang) 黃連解毒湯

846

Formula Index

Coptis and Scute Formula   807
(Huang-chieh-san)   黃解散

Coptis and Stephania Combination   808
(Huang-lien-hsiao-tu-yin)   黃連消毒飲

Coptis and Talc Combination   790
(Chia-wei-chieh-tu-tang)   加味解毒湯

Coptis and Rhubarb Combination   617
(San-huang-hsieh-hsin-tang)   三黃瀉心湯

Coptis Combination   581
(Huang-lien-tang)   黃連湯

Coix Combination   585
(I-yi-jen-tang)   薏苡仁湯

Coix Formula   809
(I-yi-jen-san)   薏苡仁散

Croton and Apricot Seed Combination   635
(Tsou-ma-tang)   走馬湯

Croton and Hematite Formula   637
(Tzu-yuan)   紫 圓

Cyperus and Cardamon Combination   572
(Hsiang-sha-liu-chun-tzu-tang)   香砂六君子湯

Cyperus and Cnidium Combination   804
(Hsiang-chiung-tang)   香芎湯

Cyperus and Ginger Combination   797
(Ching-je-chieh-yu-tang)   清熱解鬱湯

Cyperus and Hoelen Combination   825
(Sheng-shih-yin)   勝勢飲

Formula Index

Cyperus and Perilla Formula   572
(Hsiang-su-san)
香蘇散

Cyperus, Cardamon, and Atractylodes Formula   804
(Hsiang-sha-ping-wei-san)
香砂平胃散

D

Dichroa and Areca Seed Combination   787
(Chang-pin-tang)
常檳湯

Dichroa Combination   787
(Chang-shan-tang)
常山湯

Digenea and Bulrush Combination   823
(Shan-hsiung-tang)
苂凶湯

Digenea and Rhubarb Combination   787
(Che-ku-tsai-tang)
鷓鴣菜湯

Digenea and Rhubarb Combination   823
(San-wei-che-ku-tsai-tang)
三味鷓鴣菜湯

Digenea Six Combination   815
(Liu-wei-hai-jen-tang)
六味海人湯

Dragon Bone and Sulfur Formula   816
(Lung-liu-wan)
龍硫丸

Dragon Bone Combination   816
(Lung-ku-tang)
龍骨湯

E

Equisetum and Tribulus Combination   794
(Chih-lei-pu-kan-tang)
止淚補肝湯

Eucommia and Achyranthes Formula   638
(Wei-cheng-fang)
痿證方

Evodia and Pinellia Combination   644
(Yen-nien-pan-hsia-tang)   延年半夏湯

Evodia Combination   642
(Wu-chu-yu-tang)   吳茱萸湯

F

Fogopyrum and Rhubarb Formula   831
(Tung-hsien-wan)   通仙丸

Forsythia and Akebia Combination   814
(Lien-chiao-tang) (for sudamina)   連翹湯

Forsythia and Cimicifuga Combination   814
(Lien-chiao-tang) (for erysipelas)   連翹湯

Forsythia and Gypsum Formula   791
(Chia-wei-liang-ke-san)   加味涼膈散

Forsythia and Lonicera Formula   560
(Chih-tou-chuang-i-fang)   治頭瘡一方

Forsythia and Paeonia Formula   790
(Chia-chien-liang-ke-san)   加減涼膈散

Forsythia and Scute Combination   814
(Lien-chiao-tang) (for ophthalmology)   連翹湯

Four Major Herb Combination   623
(Szu-chun-tzu-tang)   四君子湯

Fritillaria and Aster Combination   826
(Szu-shun-tang)   四順湯

Fritillaria and Hoelen Combination   833
(Yang-fei-tang)   養肺湯

Fritillaria Combination   821
(Pei-mu-tang)   貝母湯

Fu-lung-kan Combination　　*582*
(Huang-tu-tang)　　黃土湯

G

Galanga and Chih-shih Combination　　*598*
(Liang-chih-tang)　　良枳湯

Gambir Formula　　*590*
(Kou-teng-san), (Tiao-teng-san)　　鈎藤散，釣藤散

Gardenia and Ginger Combination　　*795*
(Chih-tzu-kan-chiang-tang)　　梔子乾薑湯

Gardenia and Magnolia Combination　　*795*
(Chih-tzu-hou-pu-tang)　　梔子厚朴湯

Gardenia and Mentha Combination　　*797*
(Ching-liang-yin)　　清涼飲

Gardenia and Soja Combination　　*561*
(Chih-tzu-shih-tang)　　梔子豉湯

Gardenia and Vitex Combination　　*803*
(Hsi-kan-ming-mu-tang)　　洗肝明目湯

Gardenia, Ginger, and Soja Combination　　*561*
(Chih-tzu-sheng-chiang-shih-tang)　　梔子生薑豉湯

Gardenia, Licorice, and Coptis Combination　　*795*
(Chih-tzu-kan-lien-tang)　　梔子甘連湯

Gardenia, Licorice, and Soja Combination　　*560*
(Chih-tzu-kan-tsao-shih-tang)　　梔子甘草豉湯

Gelatin and Aconite Combination　　*785*
(Ah-chiao-fu-tzu-tang)　　阿膠附子湯

Gentiana Combination　　*603*
(Lung-tan-hsieh-kan-tang)　　龍膽瀉肝湯

Ginger and Aconite Combination   810
(Kan-chiang-fu-tzu-tang)   乾薑附子湯

Ginger and Chianghuo Combination   729
(Chiang-huo-yu-feng-tang)   羌活愈風湯

Ginger and Hoelen Combination   599
(Ling-chiang-chu-kan-tang)   苓薑朮甘湯

Ginger, Cinnamon, and Hoelen Combination   790
(Chia-tzu-tang)   甲字湯

Ginger, Scute, and Coptis Combination   810
(Kan-chiang-huang-chin-huang-lien-tang)   乾薑黃芩黃連湯

Ginseng and Akebia Combination   822
(Pu-chung-chih-shih-tang)   補中治濕湯

Ginseng and Astragalus Combination   616
(Pu-chung-i-chi-tang)   補中益氣湯

Ginseng and Atractylodes Formula   620
(Sheng-ling-pai-chu-san)   參苓白朮散

Ginseng and Bamboo Leaves Combination   809
(Jen-sheng-yin-tzu)   人參飲子

Ginseng and Bletilla Formula   802
(Fu-pi-sheng-mo-san-chia-pai-chi)   扶脾生脈散加白及

Ginseng and Ginger Combination   585
(Jen-sheng-tang)   人參湯

Ginseng and Gypsum Combination   610
(Pai-hu-chia-jen-sheng-tang)   白虎加人參湯

Ginseng and Longan Combination   597
(Kuei-pi-tang)   歸脾湯

Formula Index

Ginseng and Lygodium Combination   806
(Hsing-shih-pu-chi-yang-hsieh-tang)   行濕補氣養血湯

Ginseng and Ophiopogon Formula   809
(Jen-sheng-san) (Sheng-hui-jen-sheng-san) 人聖散（聖惠人聖散同）

Ginseng and Psoralea Combination   800
(Chang-yuan-tang)   壯原湯

Ginseng and Smilax Combination   804
(Hsiao-pai-chung-yin)   小百中飲

Ginseng and Tang-kuei Ten Combination   620
(Shih-chuan-ta-pu-tang)   十全大補湯

Ginseng and Walnut Combination   809
(Jen-sheng-hu-tao-tang)   人參胡桃湯

Ginseng, Cnidium, and Platycodon Formula   809
(Jen-sheng-shun-chi-san)   人參順氣散

Ginseng Combination   831
(Tu-sheng-tang)   獨參湯

Ginseng, Ginger, and Coptis Combination   814
(Lien-li-tang)   連理湯

Ginseng, Pueraria, and Atractylodes formula   789
(Chi-wei-pai-chu-san)   七味白朮散

Ginseng, Tang-kuei, and Cyperus Combination   808
(I-chi-yang-jung-tang)   益氣養榮湯

Ginseng, Tang-kuei, and Rehmannia Combination   829
(Tiao-jung-tang)   調榮湯

G. L. and Aconite Combination with Ginseng   624
(Szu-ni-chia-jen-sheng-tang)   四逆加人參湯

Gleditsia Combination　　634
(Tuo-li-hsiao-tu-yin)　　　　　　　　　　　托裏消毒飲

Gleditsia Formula　　830
(Tsao-chia-wan)　　　　　　　　　　　　　皂莢丸

Gypsum and Apricot Seed Combination　　832
(Wu-hu-tang)　　　　　　　　　　　　　　五虎湯

Gypsum and Bamboo Formula　　800
(Chu-pi-ta-wan)　　　　　　　　　　　　　竹皮大丸

Gypsum and Cinnamon Combination　　611
(Pai-hu-chia-kuei-chih-tang)　　　　　　　　白虎加桂枝湯

Gypsum and Gastrodia Formula　　822
(Pu-kan-san)　　　　　　　　　　　　　　補肝散

Gypsum, Citrus, and Quisqualis Formula　　794
(Chih-hsiao-erh-ai-chih-ni-fang)　　　　　　治小兒愛吃泥方

Gypsum Combination　　611
(Pai-hu-tang)　　　　　　　　　　　　　　白虎湯

H

Hoelen and Alisma Combination　　568
(Fen-hsiao-tang)　　　　　　　　　　　　分消湯

Hoelen and Citrus Combination　　798
(Chiu-wei-ching-pi-tang)　　　　　　　　　九味清脾湯

Hoelen and Cornus Formula　　827
(Ta-san-chi-wu-san)　　　　　　　　　　　大三七五散

Hoelen and Evodia Combination　　830
(Ting-chi-yin)　　　　　　　　　　　　　　定悸飲

Hoelen and Hao-pen Combination　　824
(Shen-tan-tang)　　　　　　　　　　　　　腎疸湯

Formula Index

Hoelen and Pinellia Combination   805
(Hsieh-pi-tang)   瀉脾湯

Hoelen and Polyporus Combination   826
(Szu-ling-tang)   四苓湯

Hoelen and Rehmannia Formula   788
(Chi-hsien-san)   七賢散

Hoelen and Saussurea Combination   832
(Wu-shen-tang)   巫神湯

Hoelen and Schizandra Combination   600
(Ling-kan-chiang-wei-hsin-hsia-jen-tang)   苓甘薑味辛夏仁湯

Hoelen and Viper Formula   801
(Fan-pi-chiao-kan-tan)   反鼻交感丹料

Hoelen Combination   570
(Fu-ling-yin)   茯苓飲

Hoelen Combination with Pinellia and Magnolia Combination   802
(Fu-ling-yin-ho-pan-hsia-hou-pu-tang)   茯苓飲合半夏厚朴湯

Hoelen Five Herb Combination   832
(Wu-ling-tang)   五苓湯

Hoelen Five Herb Formula   643
(Wu-ling-san)   五苓散

Hoelen, G.L. and Aconite Combination   569
(Fu-ling-szu-ni-tang)   茯苓四逆湯

Hoelen Heart Tonic Combination   802
(Fu-ling-pu-hsin-tang)   茯苓補心湯

Hoelen, Licorice, and Jujube Combination   601
(Ling-kuei-kan-tsao-tang)   苓桂甘棗湯

Hoelen, Licorice, and Plantago Combination   *817*
(Ming-lang-yin)   明朗飲

Hoelen, Licorice, and Schizandra Combination   *602*
(Ling-kuei-wei-kan-tang)   苓桂味甘湯

Hoelen, Magnolia, and Apricot Formula   *794*
(Chih-chuan-i-fang)   治喘一方

Hoelen, Polyporus, and Alisma Formula   *791*
(Chia-wei-pa-mo-san)   加味八脈散

Hoelen, Schizandra, and Rhubarb Combination   *600*
(Ling-kan-chiang-wei-hsin-hsia-jen-huang-tang)   苓甘薑味半夏仁黃湯

Ho-shou-wu and Schizonepeta Formula   *800*
(Chui-feng-wan)   追風丸

Human Hair Formula   *816*
(Luan-fa-shuang)   亂髮霜

I

Inula and Hematite Combination   *578*
(Hsuan-fu-hua-tai-che-shih-tang)   旋覆花代赭石湯

Iron Powder Combination   *787*
(Chen-sha-tang)   鍼砂湯

J

Jujube and Ophiopogon Combination   *822*
(Pu-fei-tang)   補肺湯

K

Kaolin Combination   *559*
(Chih-shih-chih-tang)   赤石脂湯

L

Lacca and Persica Formula   788
(Chi-fei-wan)   起廢丸

Licorice, Aconite, and Ginger Pulse Combination   636
(Tung-mo-szu-ni-tang)   通脈四逆湯

Licorice and Aconite Combination   587
(Kan-tsao-fu-tzu-tang)   甘草附子湯

Licorice and Ginger Combination   588
(Kan-tsao-kan-chiang-tang)   甘草乾薑湯

Licorice and Jujube Combination   586
(Kan-mai-ta-tsao-tang)   甘麥大棗湯

Licorice and Ma-huang Combination   810
(Kan-tsao-ma-huang-tang)   甘草麻黃湯

Licorice and Pinellia Combination   587
(Kan-tsao-hsieh-hsin-tang)   甘草瀉心湯

Licorice and Pueraria Combination   804
(Hsiao-pin-pen-tun-tang)   小品奔豚湯

Licorice Combination   588
(Kan-tsao-tang)   甘草湯

Licorice, Coptis, and Gardenia Combination   810
(Kan-lien-chih-tzu-tang)   甘連梔子湯

Lily Combination   820
(Pai-ho-ku-chin-tang)   百合固金湯

Limonite Three Formula   823
(San-sheng-wan)   三聖丸

Lindera and Chaenomeles Formula   808
(Hui-shou-san)   回首散

856

Lindera and Hoelen Formula   832
(Wu-ling-tung-chi-san)   烏苓通氣散

Linum and Apricot Seed Formula   606
(Ma-tzu-jen-wan)   麻子仁丸

Linum and Rhubarb Combination   586
(Jun-chang-tang)   潤腸湯

Lithospermum and Oyster Shell Combination   636
(Tzu-ken-mu-li-tang)   紫根牡蠣湯

Lithospermum Ointment   638
(Tzu-yun-kao)   紫雲膏

Lonicera and Coix Combination   815
(Liu-wu-pai-tu-tang)   六物敗毒湯

Lotus and Citrus Combination   556
(Chi-pi-tang)   啓脾湯

Lotus Seed Combination   563
(Ching-hsin-lien-tzu-yin)   清心蓮子飲

M

Magnolia and Alisma Combination   615
(Pu-chi-chien-chung-tang)   補氣健中湯

Magnolia and Bupleurum Combination   786
(Chai-hu-hou-pu-tang)   柴胡厚朴湯

Magnolia and Ginger Formula   615
(Ping-wei-san)   平胃散

Magnolia and Ginger Formula Modified   791
(Chia-wei-ping-wei-san)   加味平胃散

Magnolia and Hoelen Combination   639
(Wei-ling-tang)   胃苓湯

Formula Index

Magnolia and Ma-huang Combination　803
(Hou-pu-ma-huang-tang)　　　　　　　　　厚朴麻黃湯

Ma-huang, Aconite, and Asarum Combination　605
(Ma-huang-hsi-hsin-fu-tzu-tang)　　　　　麻黃細辛附子湯

Ma-huang and Apricot Seed Combination　604
(Ma-hsing-kan-shih-tang)　　　　　　　　麻杏甘石湯

Ma-huang and Atractylodes Combination　604
(Ma-huang-chia-chu-tang)　　　　　　　　麻黃加朮湯

Ma-huang and Chianghuo Combination　816
(Ma-huang-tso-ching-tang)　　　　　　　麻黃左經湯

Ma-huang and Coix Combination　603
(Ma-hsing-i-kan-tang)　　　　　　　　　麻杏薏甘湯

Ma-huang and Double Cinnamon Combination　812
(Kuei-chih-erh-ma-huang-i-tang)　　　　桂枝二麻黃一湯

Ma-huang and Ginseng Combination　577, 827
(Hsu-ming-tang)　　　　　　　　　　　　續命湯
(Ta-hsu-ming-tang)　　　　　　　　　　大續命湯

Ma-huang and Gypsum Combination　646
(Yueh-pi-tang)　　　　　　　　　　　　越婢湯

Ma-huang and Magnolia Combination　619
(Shen-mi-tang)　　　　　　　　　　　　神秘湯

Ma-huang Combination　605
(Ma-huang-tang)　　　　　　　　　　　麻黃湯

Ma-huang, Gypsum, and Pinellia Combination　645
(Yueh-pi-chia-pan-hsia-tang)　　　　　越婢加半夏湯

Major Blue Dragon Combination　627
(Ta-ching-lung-tang)　　　　　　　　　大青龍湯

858

Major Rhubarb Combination   626
(Ta-cheng-chi-tang)   大承氣湯

Major Siler Combination   627
(Ta-fang-feng-tang)   大防風湯

Major Zanthoxylum Combination   626
(Ta-chien-chung-tang)   大建中湯

Mastic and Realgar Formula   807
(Hua-tu-wan)   化毒丸

Melanterite and Citrus Formula   792
(Chiang-fan-wan)   絳礬丸

Melanterite Formula   816
(lu-fan-wan)   綠礬丸

Mercury and Lard Ointment   825
(Shen-shui-kao)   神水膏

Minor Blue Dragon Combination   574
(Hsiao-ching-lung-tang)   小青龍湯

Minor Blue Dragon Combination incorporating Gypsum   574
(Hsiao-ching-lung-chia-shih-kao-tang)   小青龍加石膏湯

Minor Bupleurum Combination   573
(Hsiao-chai-hu-tang)   小柴胡湯

Minor Bupleurum Combination Modified   789
(Chia-chien-hsiao-chai-hu-tang)   加減小柴胡湯

Minor Cinnamon and Paeonia Combination   574
(Hsiao-chien-chung-tang)   小建中湯

Minor Pinellia and Hoelen Combination   577
(Hsiao-pan-hsia-chia-fu-ling-tang)   小半夏加茯苓湯

859

Formula Index

Minor Rhubarb Combination   573
(Hsiao-cheng-chi-tang)   小承氣湯

Minor Trichosanthes Combination   575
(Hsiao-hsien-hsiung-tang)   小陷胸湯

Morus and Lycium Formula Modified   789
(Chia-chien-hsieh-pai-san)   加減瀉白散

Moutan and Persica Combination   632
(Teng-lung-tang)   騰龍湯

Moutan Formula   818
(Mu-tan-pi-san)   牡丹皮散

Mume and Zanthoxylum Combination   793
(Chiao-mei-tang)   椒梅湯

Mume Formula   643
(Wu-mei-wan)   烏梅丸

Myrica and Phellodendron Formula   833
(Yang-po-san)   楊柏散

N

Nandina and Gardenia Formula   803
(Hsi-kan-ming-mu-san)   洗肝明目散

O

Ophiopogon and Asarum Combination   799
(Chu-feng-chu-tung-tang)   驅風觸痛湯

Ophiopogon and Hoelen Formula   805
(Hsieh-hsin-tao-chih-san)   瀉心導赤散

Ophiopogon and Rehmannia Combination   825
(Sheng-chin-tang)   生津湯

Ophiopogon and Trichosanthes Combination   606
(Mai-men-tung-yin-tzu)   麥門冬飲子

Ophiopogon Combination   606
(Mai-men-tung-tang)   麥門冬湯

Oyster Shell and Alisma Formula   818
(Mu-li-tse-hsieh-san)   牡蠣澤瀉散

Oyster Shell Combination   818
(Mu-li-tang)   牡蠣湯

Oyster Shell Formula   818
(Mu-li-san)   牡蠣散

P

Paeonia and Licorice Combination   618
(Shao-yao-kan-tsao-tang)   芍藥甘草湯

Paeonia and Lonicera Formula   793
(Chieh-hsien-yu-yao-fang)   疥癬浴藥方

Paeonia and Papaver Combination   787
(Chen-jen-yang-tsang-tang)   眞人養臟湯

Paeonia and Rhubarb Combination   805
(Hsieh-tao-jen-ta-huang-tang)   謝導人大黃湯

Paeonia and Scute Combination   801
(Erh-hsien-tang)   二仙湯

Paeonia and Tang-kuei Four Combination   791
(Chia-wei-szu-wu-tang)   加味四物湯（正傳）

Paeonia and Tiger's Shinebone Formula   815
(Liu-tu-chien)   六度煎

Paeonia Four Combination   824
(Shao-yao-szu-wu-chieh-tu-tang)   芍藥四物解毒湯

Formula Index

Paeonia, Licorice, and Aconite Combination 618
(Shao-yao-kan-tsao-fu-tzu-tang) 芍藥甘草附子湯

Paeonia, Tang-kuei, and Coptis Formula 806
(Hsing-ho-shao-yao-san) 行和芍藥散

Persica and Morus Combination 822
(Po-kuan-tang) 破棺湯

Persica and Rhubarb Combination 631
(Tao-ho-cheng-chi-tang) 桃核承氣湯

Persica Combination 829
(Tao-jen-tang) 桃仁湯

Perilla Fruit Combination 622
(Su-tzu-chiang-chi-tang) 蘇子降氣湯

Phaseolus and Alisma Combination 794
(Chih-hsiao-tou-tang) 赤小豆湯（濟生）

Phaseolus and Phytolacca Combination 794
(Chih-hsiao-tou-tang) 赤小豆湯（東洋）

Phellodendron and Curcuma Ointment 801
(Chung-huang-kao) 中黃膏

Phellodendron Combination 637
(Tzu-yin-chiang-huo-tang) 滋陰降火湯

Phragmites Stem Combination 832
(Wei-ching-tang) 葦莖湯

Pinellia and Agastache Combination 801
(Chung-cheng-tang) 中正湯

Pinellia and Areca Combination 804
(Hsia-pin-tang) 夏檳湯

Formula Index

Pinellia and Coptis Combination　　821
(Ping-kan-liu-chi-yin)　　　　　　　　　平肝流氣飲

Pinellia and Gardenia Combination　　598
(Li-ke-tang)　　　　　　　　　　　　　利膈湯

Pinellia and Gastrodia Combination　　614
(Pan-hsia-pai-chu-tien-ma-tang)　　　　半夏白朮天麻湯

Pinellia and Ginger Combination　　619
(Sheng-chiang-hsieh-hsin-tang)　　　　生薑瀉心湯

Pinellia and Jujube Combination　　831
(Tuan-li-tang)　　　　　　　　　　　　斷痢湯

Pinellia and Magnolia Combination　　613
(Pan-hsia-hou-pu-tang)　　　　　　　　半夏厚朴湯

Pinellia and Mume Combination　　789
(Chi-wei-ching-pi-tang)　　　　　　　　七味清脾湯

Pinellia and Sanguisorba Combination　　820
(Pan-hsia-ti-yu-tang)　　　　　　　　　半夏地榆湯

Pinellia and Trichosanthes Combination　　790
(Chia-wei-hsiao-hsien-hsiung-tang)　　加味小陷胸湯

Pinellia, Atractylodes, and Agastache Formula　　616
(Pu-huan-chin-cheng-chi-san)　　　　　不換金正氣散

Pinellia, Aurantium, and Polyporus Combination　　798
(Chiu-wei-pan-hsia-tang)　　　　　　　九味半夏湯

Pinellia, Bakeri, and Trichosanthes Combination　　811
(Kua-lu-hsieh-pai-pan-hsia-tang)　　　瓜呂薤白半夏湯

Pinellia Combination　　613
(Pan-hsia-hsieh-hsin-tang)　　　　　　半夏瀉心湯

Formula Index

Pinellia Formula   820
(Pan-hsia-san-liao)   半夏散料

Pinellia, Ginger, and Evodia Combination
(Chien-chin-pan-hsia-tang)   千金半夏湯

Pinellia, Ginseng, and Mel Combination   827
(Ta-pan-hsia-tang)   大半夏湯

Pinellia, Mume, and Zanthoxylum Combination   793
(Chiao-mei-hsieh-hsin-tang)   椒梅瀉心湯

Platycodon and Chih-shih Formula   611
(Pai-nung-san)   排膿散

Platycodon and Croton Formula   558
(Chieh-keng-pai-san)   桔梗白散

Platycodon and Fritillary Combination   562
(Ching-fei-tang)   清肺湯

Platycodon and Jujube Combination   612
(Pai-nung-tang)   排膿湯

Platycodon and Scute Combination   802
(Fei-yung-tang)   肺癰湯

Platycodon and Smilax Combination   793
(Chieh-keng-chieh-tu-tang)   桔梗解毒湯

Platycodon and Tang-kuei Four Combination   792
(Chia-wei-szu-wu-tang)   加味四物湯（回春）

Platycodon Combination   793
(Chieh-keng-tang) (for lung gangrene)   桔梗湯

Polyporus Combination   566
(Chu-ling-tang)   豬苓湯

Polyporus Combination with Tang-kuei Four Combination   799
(Chu-ling-tang-ho-szu-wu-tang)   豬苓湯合四物湯

Prunella Combination   803
(Hsia-ku-tsao-tang)   夏枯草湯

Pueraria and Ginger Combination   821
(Pen-tun-tang)   奔豚湯

Pueraria and Pinellia Combination   589
(Ko-ken-chia-pan-hsia-tang)   葛根加半夏湯

Pueraria Combination   589
(Ko-ken-tang)   葛根湯

Pueraria, Coptis, and Scute Combination   589
(Ko-ken-huang-lien-huang-chin-tang)   葛根黃連黃芩湯

Punica Combination   825
(Shih-liu-ken-tang)   石榴根湯

R

Rehmannia Eight Combination   820
(Pa-wei-ti-huang-tang)   八味地黃湯

Rehmannia Eight Formula   609
(Pa-wei-wan)   八味丸

Rehmannia and Sanguisorba Combination   797
(Ching-fei-tang) (for hemorrhoid bleeding)   清肺湯

Resin and Flava Wax Ointment   805
(Hsien-feng-kao)   先鋒膏

Rhinoceros and Rehmannia Combination Modified   790
(Chia-wei-hsi-chiao-ti-huang-tang)   加味犀角地黃湯

Rhubarb and Aconite Combination   628
(Ta-huang-fu-tzu-tang)   大黃附子湯

Formula Index

Rhubarb and Aquilaria Formula   813
(Kun-tan-wan)   滾痰丸

Rhubarb and Dragon Bone Combination   801
(Feng-yin-tang)   風引湯

Rhubarb and Leech Combination   633
(Ti-tang-tang)   抵當湯

Rhubarb and Licorice Formula   827
(Ta-kan-wan)   大甘丸

Rhubarb and Magnolia Combination   790
(Chia-wei-cheng-chi-tang)   加味承氣湯

Rhubarb and Mirabilitum Combination   633
(Tiao-wei-cheng-chi-tang)   調胃承氣湯

Rhubarb and Moutan Combination   628
(Ta-huang-mu-tan-pi-tang)   大黃牡丹皮湯

Rhubarb and Pueraria Combination   805
(Hsieh-wei-tang)   瀉胃湯

Rhubarb and Saltpeter Combination   827
(Ta-huang-hsiao-shih-tang)   大黃消石湯

Rhubarb and Trichosanthes Combination   806
(Hsien-hsiung-tang)   陷胸湯

Rhubarb, Ginger, and Croton Formula   820
(Pei-chi-tang)   備急丹

Rhubarb, Scute, and Coptis Formula   823
(San-huang-wan)   三黃丸

Rhubarb, Scute, Coptis, and Anemarrhena Combination   823
(San-huang-chih-mu-tang)   三黃知母湯

S

Saltpeter and Forsythia Formula   805
(Hsiao-tu-wan)   消毒丸

Saltpeter and Rhubarb Formula   805
(Hsiao-shih-ta-yuan)   消石大圓

Saussurea and Cardamon Combination   818
(Mu-hsiang-tiao-chi-yin)   木香調氣飲

Saussurea and Magnolia Combination   804
(Hsiang-pu-tang)   香朴湯

Saussurea and Mastic Formula   834
(Yen-ling-tang)   延齡湯

Schizandra and Ophiopogon Combination   640
(Wei-mai-i-chi-tang)   味麥益氣湯

Schizonepeta and Forsythia Combination   561, 796
(Ching-chieh-lien-chiao-tang)   荊芥連翹湯

Schizonepeta and Scute Combination   826
(Shou-lei-yin)   收淚飲

Scute and Coptis Formula   807
(Huang-chieh-wan)   黃解丸

Scute and Licorice Combination   580
(Huang-chin-tang)   黃芩湯

Scute and Mentha Combination   798
(Ching-wei-hsieh-huo-tang)   清胃瀉火湯

Scute, Pinellia, and Ginger Combination   579, 807
(Huang-chin-chia-pan-hsia-sheng-chiang-tang)   黃芩加半夏生薑湯

Scute Three Herb Combination   617
(San-wu-huang-chin-tang)   三物黃芩湯

Formula Index

Selinum Combination   824
(She-chuang-tzu-tang)   蛇床子湯

Siler and Forsythia Formula   798
(Chu-feng-chieh-tu-san)   驅風解毒散

Siler and Gardenia Combination   826
(Szu-shun-ching-liang-yin)   四順清涼飲

Siler and Plantago Formula   817
(Ming-yen-i-fang)   明眼一方

Siler and Platycodon Formula   568
(Fang-feng-tung-sheng-san)   防風通聖散

Siler Combination   565
(Ching-shang-fan-feng-tang)   清上防風湯

Silkworm and Glutinous Rice Formula   819
(Niang-ju-wan)   釀乳丸

Silkworm Molt Combination   816
(Ma-ming-tang)   馬明湯

Six Major Herb Combination   602
(Liu-chun-tzu-tang)   六君子湯

Sophora Combination   810
(Ku-sheng-tang)   苦參湯

Stephania and Astragalus Combination   567
(Fang-chi-huang-chi-tang)   防己黃耆湯

Stephania and Ginseng Combination   608
(Mu-fang-chi-tang)   木防己湯

Stephania and Ginseng Combination without Gypsum and incorporating Hoelen and Mirabilitum   607
(Mu-fang-chi-chu-shih-kao-chia-fu-ling-mang-hsiao-tang)
    木防己去石膏加茯苓芒硝湯

Stephania and Perilla Fruit Combination   *634*
(Tseng-sun-mu-fang-chi-tang)   增損木防己湯

Stephania and Smilax Combination   *826*
(Sou-feng-chieh-tu-tang)   搜風解毒湯

Succinum and Lygodium Formula   *806*
(Hu-po-san)   琥珀散

Sulfur and Rhubarb Formula   *830*
(Tu-hsien-san)   禿癬散

T

Tang-kuei and Arctium Formula   *576*
(Hsiao-feng-san)   清風散

Tang-kuei and Atractylodes Combination   *599*
(Lien-chu-yin)   連珠飲

Tang-kuei and Atractylodes Combination   *828*
(Tang-kuei-pai-chu-tang)   當歸白朮湯

Tang-kuei and Bulrush Combination   *826*
(Szu-wu-i-huang-tang)   四物一黃湯

Tang-kuei and Cimicifuga Combination   *564*
(Ching-je-pu-chi-tang)   清熱補氣湯

Tang-kuei and Cyperus Formula   *552*
(Nu-shen-san)   女神散

Tang-kuei and Eight Herb Formula   *609*
(Pa-wei-tai-hsia-fang)   八味帶下方

Tang-kuei and Evodia Combination   *640*
(Wen-ching-tang)   温經湯

Tang-kuei and Forsythia Combination   *828*
(Tang-kuei-lien-chiao-tang)   當歸連翹湯

Formula Index

Tang-kuei and Gardenia Combination   *641*
(Wen-ching-yin)   溫清飲

Tang-kuei and Gastrodia Formula   *825*
(Shen-ying-yang-shen-tan)   神應養神丹

Tang-kuei and Gelatin Combination   *566*
(Chiung-kuei-chiao-ai-tang)   芎歸膠艾湯

Tang-kuei and Ginseng Eight Combination   *608*
(Pa-chen-tang)   八珍湯

Tang-kuei and Jujube Combination   *630*
(Tang-kuei-szu-ni-tang)   當歸四逆湯

Tang-kuei and Kaolin Formula   *829*
(Ti-kang-san)   提肛散

Tang-kuei and Lindera Formula   *828*
(Tang-kuei-hsu-san)   當歸鬚散

Tang-kuei and Lycium Combination   *831*
(Tzu-yin-chih-pao-tang)   滋陰至寶湯

Tang-kuei and Magnolia Formula   *642*
(Wu-chi-san)   五積散

Tang-kuei and Paeonia Formula   *629*
(Tang-kuei-shao-yao-san)   當歸芍藥散

Tang-kuei and Saussurea Combination   *824*
(Shen-hsiao-tang)   神效湯

Tang-kuei and Six Yellow Combination   *828*
(Tang-kuei-liu-huang-tang)   當歸六黃湯

Tang-kuei and Tribulus Combination   *631*
(Tang-kuei-yin-tzu)   當歸飲子

Tang-kuei, Astragalus, and Paeonia Combination 811
(Kuei-chi-chien-chung-tang) 歸耆建中湯

Tang-kuei, Atractylodes, and Jujube Formula 824
(Shen-kung-nei-tuo-san) 神功內托散

Tang-kuei, Cinnamon, and Paeonia Combination 629
(Tang-kuei-chien-chung-tang) 當歸建中湯

Tang-kuei Combination 829
(Tang-kuei-tang) 當歸湯

Tang-kuei, Coptis, and Schizonepeta Combination 799
(Chu-lan-shui) 除爛燧

Tang-kuei, Evodia, and Ginger Combination 630
(Tang-kuei-szu-ni-chia-wu-chu-yu-sheng-chiang-tang)
當歸四逆加吳茱萸生薑湯

Tang-kuei Formula 828
(Tang-kuei-san-liao) 當歸散料

Tang-kuei Four Combination 625
(Szu-wu-tang) 四物湯

Tang-kuei Four Combination Modified 826
(Szu-wu-tang-chiao-chi-chia-chien) 四物湯脚氣加減

Tang-kuei, Fritillaria, and Sophora Formula 828
(Tang-kuei-pei-mu-ku-sheng-wan-liao) 當歸貝母苦參丸料

Tang-kuei, Paeonia, and Bupleurum Formula 819
(Pa-wei-hsiao-yao-san) 八味逍遙散

Tang-kuei, Paeonia, and Rehmannia Combination 829
(Tang-kuei-yang-hsieh-tang) 當歸養血湯

Tang-kuei, Persica, and Rhubarb Formula 793
(Chien-chin-chi-ming-san) 千金雞鳴散

Tang-kuei, Rehmannia, and Chin-chiu Combination   833
(Yang-hsieh-tang)   養血湯

Tang-kuei, Rehmannia, and Hoelen Combination   833
(Yang-hsieh-an-shen-tang)   養血安神湯

Tang-kuei, Rehmannia, and Persica Combination   831
(Tzu-hsieh-jun-chang-tang)   滋血潤腸湯

Tang-kuei, Siler, and Astragalus Combination   800
(Chu-yang-ho-hsieh-tang)   助陽和血湯

Terminalia Formula   802
(Ho-li-leh-wan)   訶梨勒丸

Tortoise Shell, Bupleurum, and Chih-shih Formula   793
(Chieh-lao-san)   解勞散

Tortoise Shell Formula   821
(Pieh-chia-chien-wan)   鱉甲煎丸

Trichosanthes and Chih-shih Combination   591
(Kua-lu-chih-shih-tang)   瓜呂枳實湯

Trichosanthes and Cinnamon Combination   811
(Kua-lu-kuei-chih-tang)   瓜呂桂枝湯

Trichosanthes and Dianthus Formula   810
(Kua-lu-chu-mai-wan)   瓜呂瞿麥丸

Trichosanthes and Oyster Shell Formula   811
(Kua-lu-mu-li-san)   瓜呂牡蠣散

Trichosanthes, Bakeri, and Vinegar Combination   810
(Kua-lu-hsieh-pai-pai-chu-tang)   瓜呂薤白白酒湯

Trichosanthes Seed Combination   811
(Kua-lu-tang)   瓜呂湯

Trichosanthes Seed Combination　794
(Chien-chin-kua-lu-tang) (Kua-lu-tang)　千金瓜呂湯（與瓜呂湯同）

Tu-huo Combination　831
(Tu-huo-tang)　獨活湯

Tu-huo and Pueraria Combination　831
(Tu-huo-ko-ken-tang)　獨活葛根湯

Tu-huo and Stephania Combination　797
(Ching-shih-tang)　清濕湯

Turtle Shell Combination　813
(Kuei-pan-tang)　龜板湯

V

Vitality Combination　556
(Chen-wu-tang)　眞武湯

Vitality Combination with Ginseng, Schizandra, and Ophiopogon Formula　788
(Chen-wu-tang-ho-sheng-mo-san)　眞武湯合生脈散

Vitex Formula　817
(Man-ching-tzu-san)　蔓荊子散

W

Wasp's Nest and Rehmannia Formula　830
(Tsuei-ju-fang)　催乳方

White Wax and Calomel Ointment　820
(Pai-yun-kao)　白雲膏

Wu-tou and Kaolin Formula　832
(Wu-tou-chih-shih-wan)　烏頭赤石丸

Wu-tou Combination　833
(Wu-tou-tang)　烏頭湯

Formula Index

Z

Zizyphus Combination 623
(Suan-tsao-jen-tang)

酸棗仁湯

FORMULA INDEX
CHINESE TO ENGLISH

A

Ah-chiao-fu-tzu-tang   阿膠附子湯
(Gelatin and Aconite Combination)   785

An-chung-san   安中散
(Cardamon and Fennel Formula)   551

C

Chai-hu-chia-lung-ku-mu-li-tang   柴胡加龍骨牡蠣湯
(Bupleurum and Dragon Bone Combination)   552

Chai-hu-chih-chieh-tang   柴胡枳桔湯
(Bupleurum, Chih-shih, and Platycodon Combination)   785

Chai-hu-ching-kan-tang   柴胡清肝湯
(Bupleurum and Rehmannia Combination)   553

Formula Index

Chai-hu-chiung-kuei-tang　　　　　　　　　　　　柴胡芎歸湯
(Bupleurum, Cnidium, and Tang-kuei Combination)　785

Chai-hu-chu-pan-hsia-chia-kua-lu-tang　　　　柴胡去半夏加瓜呂湯
(Bupleurum and Trichosanthes Root Combination)　786

Chai-hu-hou-pu-tang　　　　　　　　　　　　　　柴胡厚朴湯
(Magnolia and Bupleurum Combination)　786

Chai-hu-kuei-chih-kan-chiang-tang　　　　　　　柴胡桂枝乾薑湯
(Bupleurum, Cinnamon, and Ginger Combination)　554

Chai-hu-kuei-chih-tang　　　　　　　　　　　　　柴胡桂枝湯
(Bupleurum and Cinnamon Combination)　554

Chai-hu-pieh-chia-tang　　　　　　　　　　　　　柴胡鼈甲湯
(Bupleurum and Tortoise Shell Combination)　786

Chai-hu-shu-kan-san　　　　　　　　　　　　　　柴胡疏肝散
(Bupleurum and Gardenia Formula)　786

Chai-hu-shu-kan-tang　　　　　　　　　　　　　　柴胡疏肝湯
(Bupleurum and Cyperus Combination)　786

Chai-keng-pan-hsia-tang　　　　　　　　　　　　柴梗半夏湯
(Bupleurum, Platycodon, and Pinellia Combination)　786

Chai-ko-chieh-chi-tang　　　　　　　　　　　　　柴葛解肌湯
(Bupleurum and Pueraria Combination)　555

Chai-shao-liu-chun-tzu-tang　　　　　　　　　　柴芍六君子湯
(Bupleurum, Paeonia, and Six Major Herb Combination)　555

Chang-pin-tang　　　　　　　　　　　　　　　　　常檳湯
(Dichroa and Areca Seed Combination)　787

Chang-shan-tang　　　　　　　　　　　　　　　　常山湯
(Dichroa Combination)　787

Chang-yung-tang 腸癰湯
(Coix and Persica Combination)   787

Che-ku-tsai-tang 鷓鴣菜湯
(Digenea and Rhubarb Combination)   787

Chen-hsiang-chiang-chi-tang 沈香降氣湯
(Aquilaria and Cyperus Combination)   787

Chen-jen-yang-tsang-tang 眞人養臟湯
(Paeonia and Papaver Combination)   787

Chen-sha-tang 鍼砂湯
(Iron Powder Combination)   787

Chen-wu-tang 眞武湯
(Vitality Combination)   556

Chen-wu-tang-ho-sheng-mo-san 眞武湯合生脈散
(Vitality Combination with Ginseng, Schizandra, and Ophiopogon Formula)   788

Cheng-hsin-tang 正心湯
(Antelope Horn and Zizyphus Combination)   788

Cheng-yen-i-fang 蒸眼一方
(Alum and Licorice Formula)   788

Chi-fei-wan 起廢丸
(Lacca and Persica Formula)   788

Chi-hsien-san 七賢散
(Hoelen and Rehmannia Formula)   788

Chi-kan-wan 鷄肝丸
(Chicken Liver Formula)

Chi-ming-san-chia-fu-ling 鷄鳴散加茯苓
(Areca Seed and Chaenomeles Formula with Hoelen)   789

Chi-pi-tang
(Lotus and Citrus Combination)   656   啓 脾 湯

Chi-wei-che-ku-tsai-tang
(Cinnamon and Digenea Combination)   789   七味鷓鴣菜湯

Chi-wei-ching-pi-tang
(Pinellia and Mume Combination)   789   七味清脾湯

Chi-wei-pai-chu-san
(Ginseng, Pueraria, and Atractylodes Formula)   789   七味白朮散

Chia-chien-hsiao-chai-hu-tang
(Minor Bupleurum Combination Modified)   789   加減小柴胡湯

Chia-chien-hsieh-pai-san
(Morus and Lycium Formula Modified)   789   加減瀉白散

Chia-chien-liang-ke-san
(Forsythia and Paeonia Formula)   790   加減涼膈散

Chia-tzu-tang
(Ginger, Cinnamon. and Hoelen Combination)   790   甲 字 湯

Chia-wei-cheng-chi-tang
(Rhubarb and Magnolia Combination)   790   加味承氣湯

Chia-wei-chieh-tu-tang
(Coptis and Talc Combination)   790   加味解毒湯

Chia-wei-hsi-chiao-ti-huang-tang
(Rhinoceros and Rehmannia Combination Modified)   790   加味犀角地黃湯

Chia-wei-hsiao-hsien-hsiung-tang
(Pinellia and Trichosanthes Combination)   790   加味小陷胸湯

Chia-wei-hsiao-ke-tang
(Atractylodes and Licorice Combination)   791   加味消渴湯

Chia-wei-hsiao-yao-san 加味逍遙散
(Bupleurum and Paeonia Formula)   557

Chia-wei-liang-ke-san 加味涼膈散
(Forsythia and Gypsum Formula)   791

Chia-wei-ning-hsien-tang 加味寧癇湯
(Aquilaria and Hoelen Combination)   791

Chia-wei-pa-mo-san 加味八脈散
(Hoelen, Polyporus, and Alisma Formula)   791

Chia-wei-ping-wei-san 加味平胃散
(Magnolia and Ginger Formula Modified)   791

Chia-wei-szu-wu-tang 加味四物湯（正傳）
(Paeonia and Tang-kuei Four Combination)   791

Chia-wei-szu-wu-tang 加味四物湯（回春）
(Platycodon and Tang-kuei Four Combination)   792

Chia-wei-wen-tan-tang 加味溫膽湯
(Bamboo and Citrus Combination Modified)   792

Chiang-fan-wan 絳礬丸
(Melanterite and Citrus Formula)   792

Chiang-huo-yu-feng-tang 羌活愈風湯
(Ginger and Chianghuo Combination)   729

Chiang-shen-tang 強神湯
(Carthamus and Silkworm Combination)   792

Chiao-mei-hsieh-hsin-tang 椒梅瀉心湯
(Pinellia, Mume, and Zanthoxylum Combination)   793

Chiao-mei-tang 椒梅湯
(Mume and Zanthoxylum Combination)   793

Chieh-hsien-yu-yao-fang 疥癬浴藥方
(Paeonia and Lonicera Formula) 793

Chieh-keng-chieh-tu-tang 桔梗解毒湯
(Platycodon and Smilax Combination) 793

Chieh-keng-pai-san 桔梗白散
(Platycodon and Croton Formula) 558

Chieh-keng-tang (for lung gangrene) 桔 梗 湯
(Platycodon Combination) 793

Chieh-lao-san 解 勞 散
(Tortoise Shell, Bupleurum, and Chih-shih Formula) 793

Chien-chin-chi-ming-san 千金雞鳴散
(Tang-kuei, Persica, and Rhubarb Formula) 793

Chien-chin-kua-lu-tang (Kua-lu-tang) 千金瓜呂湯（與瓜呂湯同）
(Trichosanthes Seed Combination) 794

Chien-chin-nei-tu-san 千金內托散
(Astragalus and Platycodon Formula) 558

Chien-chin-pan-hsia-tang 千金半夏湯
(Pinellia, Ginger, and Evodia Combination)

Chih-chuan-i-fang 治喘一方
(Hoelen, Magnolia, and Apricot Formula) 794

Chih-hsiao-erh-ai-chih-ni-fang 治小兒愛吃泥方
(Gypsum, Citrus, and Quisqualis Formula) 794

Chih-hsiao-tou-tang 赤小豆湯（東洋）
(Phaseolus and Phytolacca Combination) 794

Chih-hsiao-tou-tang 赤小豆湯（濟生）
(Phaseolus and Alisma Combination) 794

Chih-kan-tsao-tang
(Baked Licorice Combination)   559   炙甘草湯

Chih-lei-pu-kan-tang
(Equisetum and Tribulus Combination)   794   止淚補肝湯

Chih-mu-fu-ling-tang
(Anemarrhena and Hoelen Combination)   795   知母茯苓湯

Chih-pan-wan
(Atractylodes and Citrus Formula)   795   治胖丸

Chih-shih-chih-tang
(Kaolin Combination)   559   赤石脂湯

Chih-shih-chih-tzu-shih-tang
(Chih-shih, Gardenia, and Soja Combination   795   枳實梔子豉湯

Chih-ta-pu-i-fang
(Cinnamon and Nuphar Formula)   治打撲一方

Chih-tou-chuang-i-fang
(Forsythia and Lonicera Formula)   560   治頭瘡一方

Chih-tzu-hou-pu-tang
(Gardenia and Magnolia Combination)   795   梔子厚朴湯

Chih-tzu-kan-chiang-tang
(Gardenia and Ginger Combination)   795   梔子乾薑湯

Chih-tzu-kan-lien-tang
(Gardenia, Licorice, and Coptis Combination)   795   梔子甘連湯

Chih-tzu-kan-tsao-shih-tang
(Gardenia, Licorice, and Soja Combination)   560   梔子甘草豉湯

Chih-tzu-sheng-chiang-shih-tang
(Gardenia, Ginger, and Soja Combination)   561   梔子生薑豉湯

Chih-tzu-shih-tang
(Gardenia and Soja Combination)   561   梔子豉湯

Chin-chiu-chiang-huo-tang
(Chin-chiu and Chiang-huo Combination)   796   秦艽羌活湯

Chin-chiu-fang-feng-tang
(Chin-chiu and Siler Combination)   796   秦艽防風湯

Chin-chiu-pieh-chia-tang
(Chin-chiu and Tortoise Shell Combination)   562   秦艽鱉甲湯

Chin-suo-shih
(Borax and Realgar Formula)   796   金鎖匙

Ching-chi-an-huei-tang
(Bupleurum and Digenea Combination)   796   清肌安蛔湯

Ching-chieh-lien-chiao-tang
(Schizonepeta and Forsythia Combination)   561, 796   荊芥連翹湯

Ching-chung-an-huei-tang
(Coptis and Mume Combination)   796   清中安蛔湯

Ching-fei-tang
(Platycodon and Fritillary Combination)   562   清肺湯

Ching-fei-tang (for hemorrhoid bleeding)
(Rehmannia and Sanguisorba Combination)   797   清肺湯

Ching-hsin-lien-tzu-yin
(Lotus Seed Combination)   563   清心蓮子飲

Ching-je-chieh-yu-tang
(Cyperus and Ginger Combination)   797   清熱解鬱湯

Ching-je-pu-chi-tang
(Tang-kuei and Cimicifuga Combination)   564   清熱補氣湯

Formula Index

Ching-je-pu-hsieh-tang 清熱補血湯
(Cnidium and Moutan Combination)　564

Ching-liang-yin 清涼飲
(Gardenia and Mentha Combination)　797

Ching-shang-fang-feng-tang 清上防風湯
(Siler Combination)　565

Ching-shang-yin 清上飲
(Bupleurum and Gardenia Combination)　797

Ching-shih-tang 清濕湯
(Tuhuo and Stephania Combination)　797

Ching-wei-hsieh-huo-tang 清胃瀉火湯
(Scute and Mentha Combination)　798

Chiu-ni-tang 救逆湯
(Cinnamon, Dichroa, Oyster Shell, and Dragon Bone Combination)　798

Chiu-wei-ching-pi-tang 九味清脾湯
(Hoelen and Citrus Combination)　798

Chiu-wei-pan-hsia-tang 九味半夏湯
(Pinellia, Aurantium, and Polyporus Combination)　798

Chiu-wei-ping-lang-tang 九味檳榔湯
(Areca Seed Nine Combination)

Chiung-huang-san 芎黃散
(Cnidium and Rhubarb Formula)　798

Chiung-kuei-chiao-ai-tang 芎歸膠艾湯
(Tang-kuei and Gelatin Combination)　566

Chiung-kuei-tang 芎歸湯
(Cnidium and Tang-kuei Combination)　798

883

Formula Index

Chu-feng-chieh-tu-san 驅風解毒散
(Siler and Forsythia Formula) 798

Chu-feng-chu-tung-tang 驅風觸痛湯
(Ophiopogon and Asarum Combination) 799

Chu-feng-pai-tu-san 祛風敗毒散
(Chih-shih and Tu-huo Formula) 799

Chu-lan-shui 除爛燧
(Tang-kuei, Coptis, and Schizonepeta Combination 799

Chu-ling-tang 豬苓湯
(Polyporus Combination) 566

Chu-ling-tang-ho-szu-wu-tang 豬苓湯合四物湯
(Polyporus Combination with Tang-kuei Four Combination) 799

Chu-pi-pan-hsia-tang 橘皮半夏湯
(Aurantium and Pinellia Combination) 799

Chu-pi-ta-huang-pu-hsiao-tang 橘皮大黃朴硝湯
(Aurantium, Rhubarb, and Mirabilitum Combination) 799

Chu-pi-ta-wan 竹皮大丸
(Gypsum and Bamboo Formula) 800

Chu-pi-tang 橘皮湯
(Aurantium Combination) 800

Chu-shih-pu-chi-tang 除濕補氣湯
(Bupleurum, Citrus, and Anemarrhena Combination) 800

Chu-yang-ho-hsieh-tang 助陽和血湯
(Tang-kuei, Siler, and Astragalus Combination) 800

Chu-yeh-shih-kao-tang 竹葉石膏湯
(Bamboo Leaves and Gypsum Combination) 567

Chuan-li-chung-tang 喘理中湯
(Cinnamon and Cardamon Combination)   *800*

Chang-yuan-tang 壯原湯
(Ginseng and Psoralea Combination)   *800*

Chui-feng-wan 追風丸
(Ho-shou-wu and Schizonepeta Formula)   *800*

Chung-cheng-tang 中正湯
(Pinellia and Agastache Combination)   *801*

Chung-huang-kao 中黃膏
(Phellodendron and Curcuma Ointment)   *801*

E

Erh-chen-tang 二陳湯
(Citrus and Pinellia Combination)   *551*

Erh-hsien-tang 二仙湯
(Paeonia and Scute Combination)   *801*

F

Fa-sheng-san 髮生散
(Adiantum and Viper Formula)   *801*

Fan-pi-chiao-kan-tan 反鼻交感丹料
(Hoelen and Viper Formula)   *801*

Fang-chi-huang-chi-tang 防已黃耆湯
(Stephania and Astragalus Combination)   *567*

Fang-feng-tung-sheng-san 防風通聖散
(Siler and Platycodon Formula)   *568*

Fei-kan-fang 肺疳方
(Akebia and Pinellia Formula)   *801*

Formula Index

Fei-yung-tang 肺癰湯
(Platycodon and Scute Combination) 802

Fen-hsiao-tang 分消湯
(Hoelen and Alisma Combination) 568

Feng-yin-tang 風引湯
(Rhubarb and Dragon Bone Combination) 801

Fu-ling-pu-hsin-tang 茯苓補心湯
(Hoelen Heart Tonic Combination) 802

Fu-ling-szu-ni-tang 茯苓四逆湯
(Hoelen, G. L. and Aconite Combination) 569

Fu-ling-tse-hsieh-tang 茯苓澤瀉湯
(Alisma, Hoelen, and Ginger Combination) 570

Fu-ling-yin 茯苓飲
(Hoelen Combination) 570

Fu-ling-yin-ho-pan-hsia-hou-pu-tang 茯苓飲合半夏厚朴湯
(Hoelen Combination with Pinellia and Magnolia Combination) 802

Fu-pi-sheng-mo-san-chia-pai-chi 扶脾生脈散加白及
(Ginseng and Bletilla Formula) 802

Fu-tzu-keng-mi-tang 附子粳米湯
(Aconite and Oryza Combination) 571

Fu-tzu-tang 附子湯
(Aconite Combination) 571

H

Ho-kou-san 和口散
(Bulrush and Cinnabar Formula) 802

Ho-li-leh-wan 訶梨勒丸
(Terminalia Formula) 802

Hou-pu-ma-huang-tang 厚朴麻黃湯
(Magnolia and Ma-huang Combination) 803

Hou-shih-hei-san 侯氏黑散
(Chrysanthemum and Siler Formula) 803

Hsi-kan-ming-mu-san 洗肝明目散
(Nandina and Gardenia Formula) 803

Hsi-kan-ming-mu-tang 洗肝明目湯
(Gardenia and Vitex Combination) 803

Hsia-ku-tsao-tang 夏枯草湯
(Prunella Combination) 803

Hsia-pin-tang 夏檳湯
(Pinellia and Areca Combination) 804

Hsiang-chiung-tang 香芎湯
(Cyperus and Cnidium Combination) 804

Hsiang-pu-tang 香朴湯
(Saussurea and Magnolia Combination) 804

Hsiang-sha-liu-chun-tzu-tang 香砂六君子湯
(Cyperus and Cardamon Combination) 572

Hsiang-sha-ping-wei-san 香砂平胃散
(Cyperus, Cardamon, and Atractylodes Formula) 804

Hsiang-su-san 香蘇散
(Cyperus and Perilla Formula) 572

Hsiao-chai-hu-chia-chieh-keng-shih-kao-tang
小柴胡加桔梗、石膏湯
(Bupleurum, Platycodon, and Gypsum Combination) 804

Formula Index

Hsiao-chai-hu-tang 小柴胡湯
(Minor Bupleurum Combination) 573

Hsiao-cheng-chi-tang 小承氣湯
(Minor Rhubarb Combination) 573

Hsiao-chien-chung-tang 小建中湯
(Minor Cinnamon and Paeonia Combination) 574

Hsiao-ching-lung-chia-shih-kao-tang 小青龍加石膏湯
(Minor Blue Dragon Combination incorporating Gypsum) 574

Hsiao-ching-lung-tang 小青龍湯
(Minor Blue Dragon Combination) 574

Hsiao-feng-san 消風散
(Tang-kuei and Arctium Formula) 576

Hsiao-hsien-hsiung-tang 小陷胸湯
(Minor Trichosanthes Combination) 575

Hsiao-kan-yin 消疳飲
(Cardamon and Shen-chu Combination) 576

Hsiao-pai-chung-yin 小百中飲
(Ginseng and Smilax Combination) 804

Hsiao-pan-hsia-chia-fu-ling-tang 小半夏加茯苓湯
(Minor Pinellia and Hoelen Combination) 577

Hsiao-pin-pen-tun-tang 小品奔豚湯
(Licorice and Pueraria Combination) 804

Hsiao-shih-ta-yuan 滑石大圓
(Saltpeter and Rhubarb Formula) 805

Hsiao-tu-wan 消毒丸
(Saltpeter and Forsythia Formula) 805

Hsieh-hsin-tao-chih-san 瀉心導赤散
(Ophiopogon and Hoelen Formula)   805

Hsieh-pi-tang 瀉 脾 湯
(Hoelen and Pinellia Combination)   805

Hsieh-tao-jen-ta-huang-tang 謝導人大黃湯
(Paeonia and Rhubarb Combination)   805

Hsieh-wei-tang 瀉 胃 湯
(Rhubarb and Pueraria Combination)   805

Hsien-feng-kao 先 鋒 膏
(Resin and Flava wax Ointment)   805

Hsien-hsiung-tang 陷 胸 湯
(Rhubarb and Trichosanthes Combination)   806

Hsin-i-ching-fei-tang 辛夷清肺湯
(Magnolia Flower and Gypsum Combination)   806

Hsing-ho-shao-yao-san 行和芍藥散
(Paeonia, Tang-kuei, and Coptis Formula)   806

Hsing-shih-pu-chi-yang-hsieh-tang 行濕補氣養血湯
(Ginseng and Lygodium Combination)   806

Hsu-ming-tang 續 命 湯
(Ma-huang and Ginseng Combination)   577

Hsuan-fu-hua-tai-che-shih-tang 旋覆花代赭石湯
(Inula and Hematite Combination)   578

Hu-po-san 琥 珀 散
(Succinum and Lygodium Formula)   806

Hua-shih-yang-pi-tang 化食養脾湯
(Cardamon and Six Major Herb Combination)   806

Hua-tu-wan 化 毒 丸
(Mastic and Realgar Formula)   807

Huan-hsien-tang 緩 痃 湯
(Bupleurum, Scute, and Licorice Combination)   807

Huang-chi-chien-chung-tang 黃耆建中湯
(Astragalus Combination)   578

Huang-chi-pieh-chia-tang 黃耆鱉甲湯
(Astragalus and Tortoise Shell Combination)   579

Huang-chi-tang 黃 耆 湯
(Astragalus and Ginger Combination)   807

Huang-chieh-san 黃 解 散
(Coptis and Scute Formula)   807

Huang-chieh-wan 黃 解 丸
(Scute and Coptis Formula)   807

Huang-chin-chia-pan-hsia-sheng-chiang-tang 黃芩加半夏生薑湯
(Scute, Pinellia, and Ginger Combination)   579, 807

Huang-chin-tang 黃 芩 湯
(Scute and Licorice Combination)   580

Huang-lien-ah-chiao-tang 黃連阿膠湯
(Coptis and Gelatin Combination)   580

Huang-lien-chieh-tu-tang 黃連解毒湯
(Coptis and Scute Combination)   581

Huang-lien-chu-pi-tang 黃連橘皮湯
(Coptis and Aurantium Combination)   808

Huang-lien-hsiao-tu-yin 黃連消毒飲
(Coptis and Stephania Combination)   808

Huang-lien-tang　　　　　　　　　　　　　黃　連　湯
(Coptis Combination)　581

Huang-tu-tang　　　　　　　　　　　　　　黃　土　湯
(Fu-lung-kan Combination)　582

Hui-shou-san　　　　　　　　　　　　　　　回　首　散
(Lindera and Chaenomeles Formula)　808

Huo-hsiang-cheng-chi-san　　　　　　　　藿香正氣散
(Agastache Formula)　582

Huo-hsieh-san-yu-tang　　　　　　　　　　活血散瘀湯
(Cnidium and Persica Combination)　808

I

I-chi-yang-jung-tang　　　　　　　　　　　益氣養榮湯
(Ginseng, Tang-kuei, and Cyperus Combination)　808

I-kan-fu-pi-san　　　　　　　　　　　　　　抑肝扶脾散
(Bupleurum and Atractylodes Formula)　809

I-kan-san-chia-chen-pi-pan-hsia　　　　　抑肝散加陳皮半夏
(Bupleurum, Pinellia, and Citrus Formula)　583

I-kan-san　　　　　　　　　　　　　　　　　抑　肝　散
(Bupleurum Formula)　583

I-tzu-tang　　　　　　　　　　　　　　　　　乙　字　湯
(Cimicifuga Combination)　584

I-yi-fu-tzu-pai-chiang-tang　　　　　　　　薏苡附子敗醬湯
(Coix, Aconite, and Thlaspi Combination)　584

I-yi-jen-san　　　　　　　　　　　　　　　　薏苡仁散
(Coix Formula)　809

I-yi-jen-tang　　　　　　　　　　　　　　　　薏苡仁湯
(Coix Combination)　585

Formula Index

J

Jen-sheng-hu-tao-tang 人參胡桃湯
(Ginseng and Walnut Combination)   *809*

Jen-sheng-san (Sheng-hui-jen-sheng-san) 人參散（聖惠人參散同）
(Ginseng and Ophiopogon Formula)   *809*

Jen-sheng-shun-chi-san 人參順氣散
(Ginseng, Cnidium, and Platycodon Formula)   *809*

Jen-sheng-tang 人　參　湯
(Ginseng and Ginger Combination)   *585*

Jen-sheng-yin-tzu 人參飲子
(Ginseng and Bamboo Leaves Combination)   *809*

Jun-chang-tang 潤　腸　湯
(Linum and Rhubarb Combination)   *586*

K

Kan-chiang-fu-tzu-tang 乾薑附子湯
(Ginger and Aconite Combination)   *810*

Kan-chiang-huang-chin-huang-lien-tang 乾薑黃芩黃連湯
(Ginger, Scute, and Coptis Combination)   *810*

Kan-lien-chih-tzu-tang 甘連梔子湯
(Licorice, Coptis, and Gardenia Combination)   *810*

Kan-mai-ta-tsao-tang 甘麥大棗湯
(Licorice and Jujube Combination)   *586*

Kan-tsao-fu-tzu-tang 甘草附子湯
(Licorice and Aconite Combination)   *587*

Kan-tsao-hsieh-hsin-tang 甘草瀉心湯
(Licorice and Pinellia Combination)   *587*

Kan-tsao-kan-chiang-tang 甘草乾薑湯
(Licorice and Ginger Combination) 588

Kan-tsao-ma-huang-tang 甘草麻黃湯
(Licorice and Ma-huang Combination) 810

Kan-tsao-tang 甘 草 湯
(Licorice Combination) 588

Ko-ken-chia-pan-hsia-tang 葛根加半夏湯
(Pueraria and Pinellia Combination) 589

Ko-ken-huang-lien-huang-chin-tang 葛根黃連黃芩湯
(Pueraria, Coptis, and Scute Combination) 589

Ko-ken-tang 葛 根 湯
(Pueraria Combination) 589

Kou-teng-san 鈎 藤 散
(Gambir Formula) 590

Ku-sheng-tang 苦 參 湯
(Sophora Combination) 810

Kua-lu-chih-shih-tang 瓜呂枳實湯
(Trichosanthes and Chih-shih Combination) 591

Kua-lu-chu-mai-wan 瓜呂瞿麥丸
(Trichosanthes and Dianthus Formula) 810

Kua-lu-hsieh-pai-pai-chu-tang 瓜呂薤白白酒湯
(Trichsanthes, Bakeri, and Vinegar Combination) 810

Kua-lu-hsieh-pai-pan-hsia-tang 瓜呂薤白半夏湯
(Pinellia, Bakeri, and Trichosanthes Combination) 811

Kua-lu-kuei-chih-tang 瓜呂桂枝湯
(Trichosanthes and Cinnamon Combination) 811

Kua-lu-mu-li-san 瓜呂牡蠣散
(Trichosanthes and Oyster Shell Formula)   811

Kua-lu-tang 瓜呂湯
(Trichosanthes Seed Combination)   811

Kua-tzu-jen-tang 瓜子仁湯
(Benincasa Combination)   811

Kuei-chi-chien-chung-tang 歸耆建中湯
(Tang-kuei, Astragalus and Paeonia Combination)   811

Kuei-chiang-tsao-tsao-huang-hsin-fu-tang 桂薑棗草黃辛附湯
(Cinnamon and Six Herbs Combination)   811

Kuei-chih-chia-fu-tzu-tang 桂枝加附子湯
(Cinnamon and Aconite Combination)   591

Kuei-chih-chia-huang-chi-tang 桂枝加黃耆湯
(Cinnamon and Astragalus Combination)   592

Kuei-chih-chia-ko-ken-tang 桂枝加葛根湯
(Cinnamon and Pueraria Combination)   592

Kuei-chih-chia-ling-chu-fu-ching-chieh-tang 桂枝加苓朮附荊芥湯
(Cinnamon, Aconite, and Schizonepeta Combination)   812

Kuei-chih-chia-ling-chu-fu-tang 桂枝加苓朮附湯
(Cinnamon and Atractylodes Combination)   593

Kuei-chih-chia-ling-chu-tang 桂枝加苓朮湯
(Cinnamon, Hoelen, and Atractylodes Combination)   812

Kuei-chih-chia-lung-ku-mu-li-tang 桂枝加龍骨牡蠣湯
(Cinnamon and Dragon Bone Combination)   593

Kuei-chih-chia-shao-yao-sheng-chiang-jen-sheng-tang
 桂枝加芍藥生薑人參湯
(Cinnamon and P. G. G. Combination)   812

Kuei-chih-chia-shao-yao-ta-huang-tang 桂枝加芍藥大黃湯
(Cinnamon, Paeonia, and Rhubarb Combination) 594

Kuei-chih-chia-shao-yao-tang 桂枝加芍藥湯
(Cinnamon and Paeonia Combination) 594

Kuei-chih-chu-shao-yao-chia-ma-huang-fu-tzu-hsi-hsin-tang
桂枝去芍藥加麻黃附子細辛湯
(Cinnamon, Ma-huang, Aconite, and Asarum Combination) 595

Kuei-chih-chu-shao-yao-chia-shu-chi-lung-ku-mu-li-chiu-ni-tang
桂枝去芍藥加蜀漆龍骨牡蠣救逆湯
(Cinnamon, Dichroa, Dragon Bone, and Oyster Shell Combination) 595

Kuei-chih-chu-shao-yao-tang 桂枝去芍藥湯
(Cinnamon minus Paeonia Combination) 812

Kuei-chih-erh-ma-huang-i-tang 桂枝二麻黃一湯
(Ma-huang and Double Cinnamon Combination) 812

Kuei-chih-erh-yueh-pei-i-tang 桂枝二越婢一湯
(Cinnamon, Ma-nuang, and Gypsum Combination) 813

Kuei-chih-fu-ling-wan 桂枝茯苓丸
(Cinnamon and Hoelen Formula) 596

Kuei-chih-jen-sheng-tang 桂枝人參湯
(Cinnamon and Ginseng Combination) 596

Kuei-chih-kan-tsao-lung-ku-mu-li-tang 桂枝甘草龍骨牡蠣湯
(Cinnamon, Licorice, Dragon Bone and Oyster Shell Combination) 813

Kuei-chih-kan-tsao-tang 桂枝甘草湯
(Cinnamon and Licorice Combination) 813

Kuei-chih-tang 桂 枝 湯
(Cinnamon Combination) 597

Kuei-chih-tao-jen-tang 桂枝桃仁湯
(Cinnamon, Persica, and Rehmannia Combination) 813

Kuei-pan-tang 龜板湯
(Turtle Shell Combination) 813

Kuei-pi-tang 歸脾湯
(Ginseng and Longan Combination) 597

Kuei-tzu-fu-ling-san 葵子茯苓散
(Abutilon and Hoelen Formula) 813

Kun-tan-wan 滾痰丸
(Rhubarb and Aquilaria Formula) 813

L

Li-hsiao-san 立效散
(Asarum and Cimicifuga Formula) 814

Li-ke-tang 利膈湯
(Pinellia and Gardenia Combination) 598

Li-tse-tung-chi-tang 麗澤通氣湯
(Angelica and Siler Combination) 814

Liang-chih-tang 良枳湯
(Galanga and Chih-shih Combination) 598

Lien-chiao-tang (for sudamina) 連翹湯
(Forsythia and Akebia Combination) 814

Lien-chiao-tang (for ophthalmology) 連翹湯
(Forsythia and Scute Combination) 814

Lien-chiao-tang (for erysipelas) 連翹湯
(Forsythia and Cimicifuga Combination) 814

Lien-chu-yin 連珠飲
(Tang-kuei and Atractylodes Combination) 599

Lien-li-tang 連理湯
(Ginseng, Ginger, and Coptis Combination) 814

Ling-chiang-chu-kan-tang 苓薑朮甘湯
(Ginger and Hoelen Combination) 599

Ling-kan-chiang-wei-hsin-hsia-jen-huang-tang 苓甘薑味辛夏仁黃湯
(Hoelen, Schizandra, and Rhubarb Combination) 600

Ling-kan-chiang-wei-hsin-hsia-jen-tang 苓甘薑味辛夏仁湯
(Hoelen and Schizandra Combination) 600

Ling-kuei-chu-kan-tang 苓桂朮甘湯
(Atractylodes and Hoelen Combination) 601

Ling-kuei-kan-tsao-tang 苓桂甘棗湯
(Hoelen, Licorice, and Jujube Combination) 601

Ling-kuei-wei-kan-tang 苓桂味甘湯
(Hoelen, Licorice, and Schizandra Combination) 602

Ling-yang-chiao-san 羚羊角散
(Antelope Horn Formula) 814

Ling-yang-chiao-tang 羚羊角湯
(Antelope Horn Combination) 815

Liu-chun-tzu-tang 六君子湯
(Six Major Herb Combination) 602

Liu-shen-wan 六神丸
(Bear Gall and Pearl Formula) 815

Liu-tu-chien 六度煎
(Paeonia and Tigers Shinebone Formula) 815

Liu-wei-hai-jen-tang 六味海人湯
(Digenea Six Combination) 815

Formula Index

Liu-wu-fu-tzu-tang 六物附子湯
(Aconite Six Combination) 815

Liu-wu-pai-tu-tang 六物敗毒湯
(Lonicera and Coix Combination) 815

Lu-fan-wan 綠礬丸
(Melanterite Formula) 816

Luan-fa-shuang 亂髮霜
(Human Hair Formula) 816

Lung-ku-tang 龍骨湯
(Dragon Bone Combination) 816

Lung-liu-wan 龍硫丸
(Dragon Bone and Sulfur Formula) 816

Lung-tan-hsieh-kan-tang 龍膽瀉肝湯
(Gentiana Combination) 603

M

Ma-hsing-i-kan-tang 麻杏薏甘湯
(Ma-huang and Coix Combination) 603

Ma-hsing-kan-shih-tang 麻杏甘石湯
(Ma-huang and Apricot Seed Combination) 604

Ma-huang-chia-chu-tang 麻黃加朮湯
(Ma-huang and Atractylodes Combination) 604

Ma-huang-hsi-hsin-fu-tzu-tang 麻黃細辛附子湯
(Ma-huang, Aconite, and Asarum Combination) 605

Ma-huang-tang 麻黃湯
(Ma-huang Combination) 605

Ma-huang-tso-ching-tang 麻黃左經湯
(Ma-huang and Chianghuo Combination) 816

Ma-ming-tang 馬明湯
(Silkworm Molt Combination)   816

Ma-tzu-jen-wan 麻子仁丸
(Linum and Apricot Seed Formula)   606

Mai-men-tung-tang 麥門冬湯
(Ophiopogon Combination)   606

Mai-men-tung-yin-tzu 麥門冬飲子
(Ophiopogon and Trichosanthes Combination)   607

Man-chien-tang 曼倩湯
(Aconite and Oyster Shell Combination)   816

Man-ching-tzu-san 曼荊子散
(Vitex Formula)   817

Miao-kung-san 妙功散
(Astragalus and Hoelen Formula)   817

Miao-kung-shih-i-wan 妙功十一丸
(Clove and Aquilaria Formula)   817

Ming-lang-yin 明朗飲
(Hoelen, Licorice, and Plantago Combination)   817

Ming-yen-i-fang 明眼一方
(Siler and Plantago Formula)   817

Mu-fang-chi-chu-shih-kao-chia-fu-ling-mang-hsiao-tang
木防己去石膏加茯苓芒硝湯
(Stephania and Ginseng Combination without Gypsum and incorporating Hoelen and Mirabilitum)   607

Mu-fang-chi-tang 木防己湯
(Stephania and Ginseng Combination)   608

Mu-hsiang-tiao-chi-yin 木香調氣飲
(Saussurea and Cardamon Combination)   818

Mu-li-san
(Oyster Shell Formula)   818   牡蠣散

Mu-li-tang
(Oyster Shell Combination)   818   牡蠣湯

Mu-li-tse-hsieh-san
(Oyster Shell and Alisma Formula)   818   牡蠣澤瀉散

Mu-tan-pi-san
(Moutan Formula)   818   牡丹皮散

N

Nei-shu-huang-lien-tang
(Coptis and Saussurea Combination)   818   內疏黃連湯

Nei-tuo-san
(Astragalus and Platycodon Formula)   819   內托散

Niang-ju-wan
(Silkworm and Glutinous Rice Formula)   819   釀乳丸

Niu-hsi-san
(Achyranthes Formula)   819   牛膝散

Niu-pang-tzu-tang
(Arctium Combination)   819   牛蒡子湯

Nu-shen-san
(Tang-kuei and Cyperus Formula)   552   女神散

P

Pa-chen-tang
(Tang-kuei and Ginseng Eight Combination)   608   八珍湯

Pa-wei-hsiao-yao-san
(Tang-kuei, Paeonia, and Bupleurum Formula)   819   八味逍遙散

Formula Index

Pa-wei-shan-chi-fang 八味疝氣方
(Cinnamon and Akebia Formula)   819

Pa-wei-shun-chi-san 八味順氣散
(Atractylodes and Lindera Formula)   820

Pa-wei-tai-hsai-fang 八味帶下方
(Tang-kuei and Eight Herb Formula)   609

Pa-wei-ti-huang-tang 八味地黃湯
(Rehmannia Eight Combination)   820

Pa-wei-wan 八味丸
(Rehmannia Eight Formula)   609

Pai-ho-ku-chin-tang 百合固金湯
(Lily Combination)   820

Pai-hu-chia-jen-sheng-tang 白虎加人參湯
(Ginseng and Gypsum Combination)   610

Pai-hu-chia-kuei-chih-tang 白虎加桂枝湯
(Gypsum and Cinnamon Combination)   611

Pai-hu-tang 白虎湯
(Gypsum Combination)   611

Pai-nung-san 排膿散
(Platycodon and Chih-shih Formula)   611

Pai-nung-tang 排膿湯
(Platycodon and Jujube Combination)   612

Pai-tou-weng-chia-kan-tsao-ah-chiao-tang 白頭翁加甘草阿膠湯
(Anemone, Licorice, and Gelatin Combination)   280

Pai-yun-kao 白雲膏
(White Wax and Calomel Ointment)   820

Formula Index

Pan-hsia-hou-pu-tang
(Pinellia and Magnolia Combination)　　*613*　　半夏厚朴湯

Pan-hsia-hsieh-hsin-tang
(Pinellia Combination)　　*613*　　半夏瀉心湯

Pan-hsia-pai-chu-tien-ma-tang
(Pinellia and Gastrodia Combination)　　*614*　　半夏白朮天麻湯

Pan-hsia-san-liao
(Pinellia Formula)　　*820*　　半夏散料

Pan-hsia-ti-yu-tang
(Pinellia and Sanguisorba Combination)　　*820*　　半夏地榆湯

Pei-chi-tang
(Rhubarb, Ginger, and Croton Formula)　　*820*　　備急丹

Pei-mu-tang
(Fritillaria Combination)　　*821*　　貝母湯

Pen-tun-tang
(Pueraria and Ginger Combination)　　*821*　　奔豚湯

Pieh-chia-chien-wan
(Tortoise Shell Formula)　　*821*　　鼈甲煎丸

Pien-chih-hsin-chi-yin
(Areca and Evodia Combination)　　*614*　　變製心氣飲

Ping-kan-liu-chi-yin
(Pinellia and Coptis Combination)　　*821*　　平肝流氣飲

Ping-wei-san
(Magnolia and Ginger Formula)　　*615*　　平胃散

Po-kuan-tang
(Persica and Morus Combination)　　*822*　　破棺湯

Po-yeh-tang
(Biota Leaves Combination)　　822　　　柏葉湯

Pu-chi-chien-chung-tang
(Magnolia and Alisma Combination)　　615　　　補氣健中湯

Pu-chung-chih-shih-tang
(Ginseng and Akebia Combination)　　822　　　補中治濕湯

Pu-chung-i-chi-tang
(Ginseng and Astragalus Combination)　　616　　　補中益氣湯

Pu-fei-tang
(Jujube and Ophiopogon Combination)　　822　　　補肺湯

Pu-huan-chin-cheng-chi-san
(Pinellia, Atractylodes, and Agastache Formula)　　616　　　不換金正氣散

Pu-kan-san
(Gypsum and Gastrodia Formula)　　822　　　補肝散

Pu-yang-huan-wu-tang
(Astragalus and Paeonia Combination)　　822　　　補陽還五湯

S

San-huang-chih-mu-tang
(Rhubarb, Scute, Coptis, and Anemarrhena Combination)　　823　　　三黃知母湯

San-huang-hsieh-hsin-tang
(Coptis and Rhubarb Combination)　　617　　　三黃瀉心湯

San-huang-wan
(Rhubarb, Scute, and Coptis Formula)　　823　　　三黃丸

San-pin-i-tiao-chiang
(Alum and Arsenic Formula)　　823　　　三品一條鎗

Formula Index

San-sheng-wan
(Limonite Three Formula)   823   三聖丸

San-sheng-yin
(Aconite and Arisaema Combination)   823   三生飲

San-wei-che-ku-tsai-tang
(Digenea and Rhubarb Combination)   823   三味鷓鴣菜湯

San-wu-huang-chin-tang
(Scute Three Herb Combination)   617   三物黃芩湯

Shan-hsiung-tang
(Digenea and Bulrush Combination)   823   芡凶湯

Shao-yao-kan-tsao-fu-tzu-tang
(Paeonia, Licorice, and Aconite Combination)   618   芍藥甘草附子湯

Shao-yao-kan-tsao-tang
(Paeonia and Licorice Combination)   618   芍藥甘草湯

Shao-yao-szu-wu-chieh-tu-tang
(Paeonia Four Combination)   824   芍藥四物解毒湯

She-chuang-tzu-tang
(Selinum Combination)   824   蛇床子湯

Shen-hsiao-tang
(Tang-kuei and Saussurea Combination)   824   神效湯

Shen-kung-nei-tuo-san
(Tang-kuei, Atractylodes, and Jujube Formula)   824   神功內托散

Shen-mi-tang
(Ma-huang and Magnolia Combination)   619   神秘湯

Shen-tan-tang
(Hoelen and Hao-pen Combination)   824   腎疸湯

Shen-ying-yang-shen-tan 神應養神湯
(Tang-kuei and Gastrodia Formula) 825

Shen-shui-kao 神水膏
(Mercury and Lard Ointment) 825

Sheng-chiang-hsieh-hsin-tang 生薑瀉心湯
(Pinellia and Ginger Combination) 619

Sheng-chin-tang 生津湯
(Ophiopogon and Rehmannia Combination) 825

Sheng-lien-tang 參連湯
(Chu-chieh Ginseng and Coptis Combination) 825

Sheng-ling-pai-chu-san 參苓白朮散
(Ginseng and Atractylodes Formula) 620

Sheng-shih-yin 勝勢飲
(Cyperus and Hoelen Combination) 825

Sheng-yang-san-huo-tang 升陽散火湯
(Bupleurum and Ginseng Combination) 825

Shih-chuan-ta-pu-tang 十全大補湯
(Ginseng and Tang-kuei Ten Combination) 620

Shih-liu-ken-tang 石榴根湯
(Punica Combination) 825

Shih-wei-pai-tu-tang 十味敗毒湯
(Bupleurum and Schizonepeta Combination) 621

Shou-lei-yin 收淚飲
(Schizonepeta and Scute Combination) 826

Shu-ching-huo-hsieh-tang 疏經活血湯
(Clematis and Stephania Combination) 622

Formula Index

Sou-feng-chieh-tu-tang
(Stephania and Smilax Combination)   826   搜風解毒湯

Su-tzu-chiang-chi-tang
(Perilla Fruit Combination)   622   蘇子降氣湯

Suan-tsao-jen-tang
(Zizyphus Combination)   623   酸棗仁湯

Szu-chun-tzu-tang
(Four Major Herb Combination)   623   四君子湯

Szu-ling-tang
(Hoelen and Polyporus Combination)   826   四苓湯

Szu-ni-chia-jen-sheng-tang
(G. L. and Aconite Combination with Ginseng)   624   四逆加人參湯

Szu-ni-san
(Bupleurum and Chih-shih Formula)   624   四逆散

Szu-ni-tang
(Aconite and G. L. Combination)   625   四逆湯

Szu-shun-ching-liang-yin
(Siler and Gardenia Combination)   826   四順清涼飲

Szu-shun-tang
(Fritillaria and Aster Combination)   826   四順湯

Szu-wu-i-huang-tang
(Tang-kuei and Bulrush Combination)   826   四物一黃湯

Szu-wu-tang
(Tang-kuei Four Combination)   625   四物湯

Szu-wu-tang-chiao-chi-chia-chien
(Tang-kuei Four Combination Modified)   826   四物湯脚氣加減

T

Ta-cheng-chi-tang　　　　　　　　　　　　　大承氣湯
(Major Rhubarb Combination)　　626

Ta-chien-chung-tang　　　　　　　　　　　　大建中湯
(Major Zanthoxylum Combination)　　626

Ta-ching-lung-tang　　　　　　　　　　　　　大青龍湯
(Major Blue Dragon Combination)　　627

Ta-fang-feng-tang　　　　　　　　　　　　　 大防風湯
(Major Siler Combination)　　627

Ta-huang-fu-tzu-tang　　　　　　　　　　　　大黃附子湯
(Rhubarb and Aconite Combination)　　628

Ta-huang-mu-tan-pi-tang　　　　　　　　　　 大黃牡丹皮湯
(Rhubarb and Moutan Combination)　　628

Ta-hsu-ming-tan　　　　　　　　　　大續命湯（續命湯）
(Ma-huang and Ginseng Combination)　　827

Ta-huang-hsiao-shih-tang　　　　　　　　　　大黃消石湯
(Rhubarb and Saltpeter Combination)　　827

Ta-kan-wan　　　　　　　　　　　　　　　　大　甘　丸
(Rhubarb and Licorice Formula)　　827

Ta-pai-chung-yin　　　　　　　　　　　　　　大百中飲
(Achyranthes and Smilax Combination)　　827

Ta-pan-hsia-tang　　　　　　　　　　　　　　大半夏湯
(Pinellia, Ginseng, and Mel Combination)　　827

Ta-san-chi-wu-san　　　　　　　　　　　　　 大三七五散
(Hoelen and Cornus Formula)　　827

Tang-chih-chung-i-fang　　　　　　　　　　　　　　　　　　唐痔中一方
(Areca Seed and Ginger Formula)　　827

Tang-kuei-chien-chung-tang　　　　　　　　　　　　　　　　當歸建中湯
(Tang-kuei, Cinnamon, and Paeonia Combination)　　629

Tang-kuei-hsu-san　　　　　　　　　　　　　　　　　　　　　當歸鬚散
(Tang-kuei and Lindera Formula)　　828

Tang-kuei-lien-chiao-tang　　　　　　　　　　　　　　　　　　當歸連翹湯
(Tang-kuei and Forsythia Combination)　　828

Tang-kuei-liu-huang-tang　　　　　　　　　　　　　　　　　　當歸六黃湯
(Tang-kuei and Six Yellow Combination)　　828

Tang-kuei-pai-chu-tang　　　　　　　　　　　　　　　　　　　當歸白朮湯
(Tang-kuei and Atractylodes Combination)　　828

Tang-kuei-pei-mu-ku-sheng-wan-liao　　　　　　　　　　當歸貝母苦參丸料
(Tang-kuei, Fritillaria, and Sophora Formula)　　828

Tang-kuei-san-liao　　　　　　　　　　　　　　　　　　　　　當歸散料
(Tang-kuei Formula)　　828

Tang-kuei-shao-yao-san　　　　　　　　　　　　　　　　　　當歸芍藥散
(Tang-kuei and Paeonia Formula)　　629

Tang-kuei-szu-ni-chia-wu-chu-yu-sheng-chiang-tang
　　　　　　　　　　　　　　　　　當歸四逆加吳茱萸生薑湯
(Tang-kuei, Evodia, and Ginger Combination)　　630

Tang-kuei-szu-ni-tang　　　　　　　　　　　　　　　　　　　當歸四逆湯
(Tang-kuei and Jujube Combination)　　630

Tang-kuei-tang　　　　　　　　　　　　　　　　　　　　　　　當　歸　湯
(Tang-kuei Combination)　　829

Tang-kuei-yang-hsieh-tang　　　　　　　　　　　　　　　　　當歸養血湯
(Tang-kuei, Paeonia, and Rehmannia Combination)　　829

Tang-kuei-yin-tzu 當歸飲子
(Tang-kuei and Tribulus Combination) *631*

Tao-chih-tung-ching-tang 導滯通經湯
(Atractylodes and Alisma Combination) *829*

Tao-ho-cheng-chi-tang 桃核承氣湯
(Persica and Rhubarb Combination) *631*

Tao-jen-tang 桃仁湯
(Persica Combination) *829*

Teng-lung-tang 騰龍湯
(Moutan and Persica Combination) *632*

Ti-kang-san 提肛散
(Tang-kuei and Kaolin Formula) *829*

Ti-tang-tang 抵當湯
(Rhubarb and Leech Combination) *633*

Tiao-jung-tang 調榮湯
(Ginseng, Tang-kuei, and Rehmannia Combination) *829*

Tiao-wei-cheng-chi-tang 調胃承氣湯
(Rhubarb and Mirabilitum Combination) *633*

Tien-hsiung-san 天雄散
(Aconite and Dragon Bone Formula) *830*

Ting-chi-yin 定悸飲
(Hoelen and Evodia Combination) *830*

Ting-fu-li-chung-tang 丁附理中湯
(Clove and Aconite Combination) *830*

Tsao-chia-wan 皂莢丸
(Gleditsia Formula) *830*

Tseng-sun-mu-fang-chi-tang
(Stephania and Perilla Fruit Combination)   634   增損木防己湯

Tsing-fu-tang
(Bupleurum and Pinellia Combination)   635   淨腑湯

Tsuei-ju-fang
(Wasp's Nest and Rehmannia Formula)   839   催乳方

Tso-tu-kao
(Asphalt Ointment)   830   左突膏

Tsou-ma-tang
(Croton and Apricot Seed Combination)   635   走馬湯

Tu-hsien-san
(Sulfur and Rhubarb Formula)   830   禿癬散

Tu-huo-ko-ken-tang
(Tu-huo and Pueraria Combination)   831   獨活葛根湯

Tu-huo-tang
(Tu-huo Combination)   831   獨活湯

Tu-sheng-tang
(Ginseng Combination)   831   獨參湯

Tuan-li-tang
(Pinellia and Jujube Combination)   831   斷痢湯

Tung-hsien-wan
(Fogopyrum and Rhubarb Formula)   831   通仙丸

Tung-mo-szu-ni-tang
(Licorice, Aconite, and Ginger Pulse Combination)   636   通脈四逆湯

Tou-li-hsiao-tu-yin
(Gleditsia Combination)   634   托裏消毒飲

Tzu-hsieh-jun-chang-tang 滋血潤腸湯
(Tang-kuei, Rehmannia, and Persica Combination) 831

Tzu-ken-mu-li-tang 紫根牡蠣湯
(Lithospermum and Oyster Shell Combination) 636

Tzu-yin-chiang-huo-tang 滋陰降火湯
(Phellodendron Combination) 637

Tzu-yin-chih-pao-tang 滋陰至寶湯
(Tang-kuei and Lycium Combination) 831

Tzu-yuan 紫圓
(Croton and Hematite Formula) 637

Tzu-yun-kao 紫雲膏
(Lithospermum Ointment) 638

W

Wei-ching-tang 葦莖湯
(Phragmites Stem Combination) 832

Wei-feng-tang 胃風湯
(Atractylodes and Setaria Combination) 639

Wei-ling-tang 胃苓湯
(Magnolia and Hoelen Combination) 639

Wei-mai-i-chi-tang 味麥益氣湯
(Schizandra and Ophiopogon Combination) 640

Wei-cheng-fang 痿證方
(Eucommia and Achyranthes Formula) 638

Wen-ching-tang 溫經湯
(Tang-kuei and Evodia Combination) 640

Formula Index

Wen-ching-yin 温清飲
(Tang-kuei and Gardenia Combination)   *641*

Wen-tan-tang 温膽湯（千金方）
(Bamboo and Chih-shih Combination)   *641*

Wu-chi-san 五積散
(Tang-kuei and Magnolia Formula)   *642*

Wu-chu-yu-tang 吳茱萸湯
(Evodia Combination)   *642*

Wu-hu-tang 五虎湯
(Gypsum and Apricot Seed Combination)   *832*

Wu-ling-san 五苓散
(Hoelen Five Herb Formula)   *643*

Wu-ling-tang 五苓湯
(Hoelen Five Herb Combination)   *832*

Wu-ling-tung-chi-san 烏苓通氣散
(Lindera and Hoelen Formula)   *832*

Wu-mei-wan 烏梅丸
(Mume Formula)   *643*

Wu-shen-tang 巫神湯
(Hoelen and Saussurea Combination)   *832*

Wu-tou-chih-shih-wan 烏頭赤石丸
(Wu-tou and Kaolin Formula)   *832*

Wu-tou-tang 烏頭湯
(Wu-tou Combination)   *833*

Wu-wu-chieh-tu-tang 五物解毒湯
(Cnidium and Lonicera Combination)   *833*

912

Y

Yang-fei-tang　養肺湯
(Fritillaria and Hoelen Combination)　833

Yang-hsieh-an-shen-tang　養血安神湯
(Tang-kuei, Rehmannia, and Hoelen Combination)　833

Yang-hsieh-tang　養血湯
(Tang-kuei, Rehmannia, and Chin-chiu Combination)　833

Yang-po-san　楊柏散
(Myrica and Phellodendron Formula)　833

Yeh-kan-ma-huang-tang　射干麻黃湯
(Belamcanda and Ma-huang Combination)　834

Yen-ling-tang　延齡湯
(Saussurea and Mastic Formula)　834

Yen-nien-pan-hsia-tang　延年半夏湯
(Evodia and Pinellia Combination)　644

Yin-chen-hao-tang　茵陳蒿湯
(Capillaris Combination)　644

Yin-chen-san　茵陳散
(Capillaris and Talc Formula)　834

Yin-chen-szu-ni-tang　茵陳四逆湯
(Capillaris and Aconite Combination)　834

Yin-chen-wu-ling-san　茵陳五苓散
(Capillaris and Hoelen Formula)　645

Yin-ching-tang　茵荊湯
(Capillaris and Schizonepeta Combination)　834

Formula Index

Ying-chung-san
(Cnidium and Rhubarb Formula)   834   應鐘散

Yu-tse-san
(Alum and Apricot Seed Formula)   834   羽澤散

Yueh-pi-chia-chu-tang
(Atractylodes Combination)   646   越婢加朮湯

Yueh-pi-chia-pan-hsia-tang
(Ma-huang, Gypsum, and Pinellia Combination)   645   越婢加半夏湯

Yueh-pi-tang
(Ma-huang and Gypsum Combination)   646   越婢湯

Other Publications of the Oriental Healing Arts Institute

SHANG HAN LUN

The *Shang han lun* as a medical classic ranks alongside the *I ching* and the works of Confucius and Lao-tzu. In conjunction with *The Yellow Emperor's Classic of Internal Medicine*, it serves as the wellspring of Chinese herbal medicine. Eighty percent of formulas used today come from the *Shang han lun*. This publication marks the first English edition of the classic. Hsu, Hong-yen, Ph.D., & Peacher, William, G., M. D., 1981. Hardback and paper. 261 Pages. Illustrated. $15.00 and 9.95

COMMONLY USED CHINESE HERB FORMULAS WITH ILLUSTRATIONS

An extensive compilation of the herbal formulas commonly prescribed by physicians who follow the Chinese herbal tradition. Twenty-four categories of formulas are presented according to their pharmaceutical action: emetics, purgatives, anthelmintics, *ch'i* formulas, sedatives, etc. Included in each formula's entry are its ingredients, indications, and discriminatory symptoms, plus an anatomical diagram showing the targets of treatment. Hsu, Hong-yen, Ph.D., & Hsu, Chau-shin, Ph.D., 1982. Hardback and paper. 671 Pages. Illustrated. $25.00 and 19.95

COMMON HEALTH COMPLAINTS

Sometimes minor physical problems hamper our full enjoyment of life. For such common complaints—headaches, stiff shoulders, acne, chilling, constipation, etc.—Chinese medicine over the centuries has devised herbal formulas which alleviate these annoyances and sometimes even eliminate them altogether. Many of these efficacious remedies are found in this book. Hsu, Hong-yen, Ph.D., 1982. Paper. 43 Pages. $3.00

CHINESE HERB MEDICINE & THERAPY

For the first time, this comprehensive introduction to Chinese medicine deals with the general conception of diagnosis in Chinese medicine, principles of treatment, and formulas for diseases and symptoms. Some 68 major prescriptions used by Chinese herbal physicians are discussed. This invaluable source book is a must for anyone interested in Chinese medicine. Hsu, Hong-yen, Ph.D., & Peacher, William G., M.D., 1976. Paper. 223 Pages. Illustrated. $10.00

HOW TO TREAT YOURSELF WITH CHINESE HERBS

This handbook explains in clear and concise language how the Chinese use herbs to achieve good health. The first section reviews 14 categories of chronic and acute illnesses and their therapies. The following sections include a discussion of 95 herbs and 128 formulas, their uses and healing properties. This is the most comprehensive and practical study of Chinese herbal formulas to appear in English. Hsu, Hong-yen, Ph.D., 1980. Paper. 296 Pages. Illustrated. $5.95

Available by mail from . . . .

ORIENTAL HEALING ARTS INSTITUTE
8820 S. SEPULVEDA BLVD., SUITE 218
LOS ANGELES, CALIFORNIA 90045

(Price includes postage and handling. California residents please add 6.5% sales tax.)